# Causes, Diagnosis and Management of Glaucoma

# Causes, Diagnosis and Management of Glaucoma

Edited by Collin Cruz

hayle
medical

New York

Hayle Medical,
750 Third Avenue, 9th Floor,
New York, NY 10017, USA

Visit us on the World Wide Web at:
www.haylemedical.com

ISBN: 978-1-63241-931-6

**Cataloging-in-Publication Data**

Causes, diagnosis and management of glaucoma / edited by Collin Cruz.
    p. cm.
Includes bibliographical references and index.
ISBN 978-1-63241-931-6
1. Glaucoma. 2. Glaucoma--Etiology. 3. Glaucoma--Diagnosis. 4. Glaucoma--Treatment.
5. Eye--Diseases. I. Cruz, Collin.
RE871 .C38 2020
617.741--dc23

# Table of Contents

**Permissions**

**List of Contributors**

**Index**

# Preface

This book has been an outcome of determined endeavour from a group of educationists in the field. The primary objective was to involve a broad spectrum of professionals from diverse cultural background involved in the field for developing new researches. The book not only targets students but also scholars pursuing higher research for further enhancement of the theoretical and practical applications of the subject.

Damage to the optic nerve causes gradual vision loss. This may occur due to a group of eye diseases called glaucoma. Open-angle glaucoma, closed-angle glaucoma and normal-tension glaucoma are some types of glaucoma. Testing for glaucoma comprises of an eye examination with measurements of the intraocular pressure, an anterior chamber angle examination, and optic nerve evaluation. Scanning laser polarimetry, optical coherence tomography and scanning laser ophthalmoscopy help in assessing the retinal nerve fiber. Vision loss due to glaucoma is permanent. If the disease is detected early, it may be possible to slow or even stop the progression of the disease with the aid of laser treatment, medication or surgery. These treatments seek to lower eye pressure. This book is a valuable compilation of topics, ranging from the basic to the most complex advancements in the diagnosis and management of glaucoma. From theories to research to practical applications, case studies related to all contemporary topics of relevance to this condition have been included herein. It will help new researchers by foregrounding their knowledge in glaucoma.

It was an honour to edit such a profound book and also a challenging task to compile and examine all the relevant data for accuracy and originality. I wish to acknowledge the efforts of the contributors for submitting such brilliant and diverse chapters in the field and for endlessly working for the completion of the book. Last, but not the least; I thank my family for being a constant source of support in all my research endeavours.

**Editor**

# *VAV2* and *VAV3* as Candidate Disease Genes for Spontaneous Glaucoma in Mice and Humans

**Keiko Fujikawa[1,3,6]\*, Takeshi Iwata[2], Kaoru Inoue[3], Masakazu Akahori[2], Hanako Kadotani[1], Masahiro Fukaya[4], Masahiko Watanabe[4], Qing Chang[5], Edward M. Barnett[5], Wojciech Swat[6]**

1 Department of Pathology and Immunology, Hokkaido University Graduate School of Medicine, Sapporo, Japan, 2 National Institute of Sensory Organs, National Hospital Organization Tokyo Medical Center, Tokyo, Japan, 3 Faculty of Health Science, Hokkaido University, Sapporo, Japan, 4 Department of Anatomy, Hokkaido University Graduate School of Medicine, Sapporo, Japan, 5 Department of Ophthalmology and Visual Sciences, Washington University School of Medicine, St. Louis, Missouri, United States of America, 6 Department of Pathology and Immunology, Washington University School of Medicine, St. Louis, Missouri, United States of America

## Abstract

*Background:* Glaucoma is a leading cause of blindness worldwide. Nonetheless, the mechanism of its pathogenesis has not been well-elucidated, particularly at the molecular level, because of insufficient availability of experimental genetic animal models.

*Methodology/Principal Findings:* Here we demonstrate that deficiency of Vav2 and Vav3, guanine nucleotides exchange factors for Rho guanosine triphosphatases, leads to an ocular phenotype similar to human glaucoma. Vav2/Vav3-deficient mice, and to a lesser degree Vav2-deficient mice, show early onset of iridocorneal angle changes and elevated intraocular pressure, with subsequent selective loss of retinal ganglion cells and optic nerve head cupping, which are the hallmarks of glaucoma. The expression of Vav2 and Vav3 tissues was demonstrated in the iridocorneal angle and retina in both mouse and human eyes. In addition, a genome-wide association study screening glaucoma susceptibility loci using single nucleotide polymorphisms analysis identified *VAV2* and *VAV3* as candidates for associated genes in Japanese open-angle glaucoma patients.

*Conclusions/Significance:* Vav2/Vav3-deficient mice should serve not only as a useful murine model of spontaneous glaucoma, but may also provide a valuable tool in understanding of the pathogenesis of glaucoma in humans, particularly the determinants of altered aqueous outflow and subsequent elevated intraocular pressure.

**Editor:** Patrick Callaerts, Katholieke Universiteit Leuven, Belgium

**Funding:** The work described in this report was funded in parts by a grant from the Ministry of Education, Culture, Sports, Science and Technology in Japan. The funders had no role in study design, data collection and analysis, decision to publish, or preparation of the manuscript.

**Competing Interests:** The authors have declared that no competing interests exist.

\* E-mail: fujikawa@med.hokudai.ac.jp

## Introduction

The critical importance of elevated intraocular pressure (IOP) in the pathogenesis of glaucomatous optic neuropathy is widely recognized [1,2]. While compromise of aqueous humor outflow is the key determinant of elevation in IOP [3,4], the molecular mechanisms underlying changes in the outflow pathway that lead to elevated IOP remain to be elucidated. For this reason, mouse genetic knockout models of spontaneous glaucoma are highly sought after.

The Vav proteins are the best-characterized family of guanine nucleotide exchange factors (GEFs) that activates Rho guanosine triphosphatases (GTPases) in a phosphorylation-dependent manner [5]. Rho GTPases control cell behavior via regulating the specific filamentous actin structures involved in migration, adhesion, and morphogenesis, by acting as binary switches cycling between an inactive (GDP-bound) and active (GTP-bound) state [6]. The three mammalian Vav proteins, Vav1, Vav2, and Vav3, share a Dbl homology domain for their enzymatic activity as GEFs and contain a common structural array characteristic of proteins involved in signal transduction. Regardless of the structural similarity, Vav proteins differ in their tissue distribution. Vav1 is expressed specifically in lymphoid lineage cells, whereas Vav2 and Vav3 are more widely expressed [5,7]. Genetic approaches using knockout mice have provided valuable information on the function of Vav proteins *in vivo*. Vav proteins are crucial for the development and function of hematopoietic lineage cells such as lymphocytes, neutrophils, natural killer cells, and osteoclasts [8–16]. Individual Vav proteins exhibit both redundant and specialized functions. Despite the wide distribution of Vav2 and Vav3 proteins in mouse tissues, little is known about their specific function in non-hematopoietic cells.

While trying to better elucidate the functions of Vav2 and Vav3 in non-hematopoietic cells, we discovered that Vav2/Vav3-deficient mice have a significant ocular phenotype. Specifically, we show that Vav2/Vav3-deficient mice have elevated IOP, which eventually manifests as buphthalmos. Loss of Vav2 and Vav3 expression is associated with changes in the iridocorneal angle, with eventual chronic angle closure. The elevation of IOP in Vav2/Vav3-deficient mice is accompanied by an optic neuropathy characterized by selective loss of retinal ganglion cells (RGCs) and optic nerve head (ONH) excavation and is therefore consistent with glaucoma. In addition, both *VAV2* and *VAV3* are shown to be susceptibility loci by single nucleotide polymorphisms (SNPs) study of Japanese primary open-angle glaucoma patients.

## Results

### Vav2/Vav3-Deficient Mice Develop Buphthalmos

Eyes of Vav2/Vav3-deficient ($Vav2^{-/-}$ $Vav3^{-/-}$) mice were noted to develop buphthalmos starting between 6 and 12 weeks of age (Figure 1). This enlargement was typically seen unilaterally at first, with frequent bilateral involvement over the next 1–2 months, and continued enlargement until the mice were 6-months

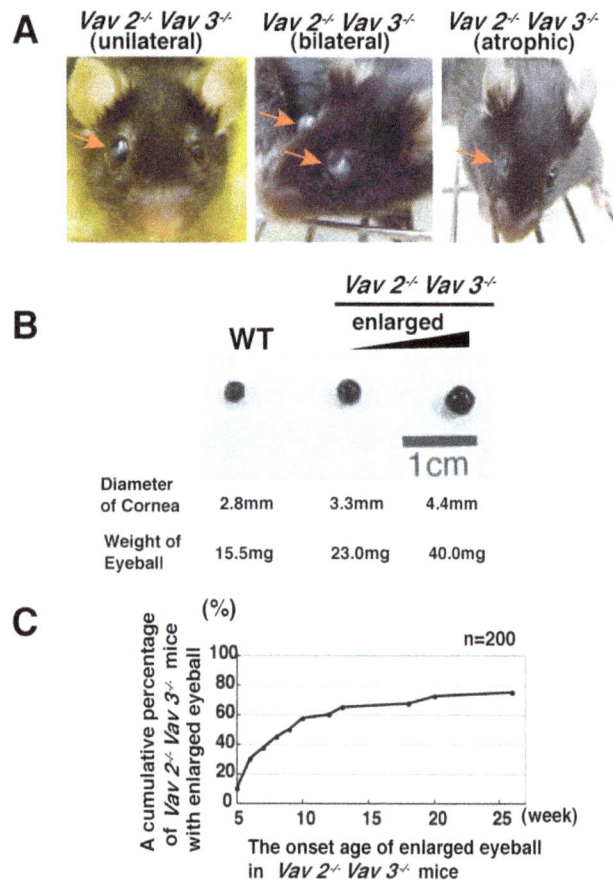

**Figure 1. Vav2/Vav3-deficient mice develop buphthalmos.** Eyes of Vav2/Vav3-deficient ($Vav2^{-/-}$ $Vav3^{-/-}$) mice develop buphthalmos between 6 and 12 weeks of age. **A**. Left photo: Representative photo of unilateral enlarged eye in 10-week-old $Vav2^{-/-}$ $Vav3^{-/-}$ mice. Centre photo: Representative photo of bilateral enlarged eyes in 16-week-old $Vav2^{-/-}$ $Vav3^{-/-}$ mice. Right photo: Representative photo of enlarged eye becoming atrophic in 8-week-old $Vav2^{-/-}$ $Vav3^{-/-}$ mice. **B**. Comparison of eye sizes. Left panel: Representative eye of 10-week-old wild-type (WT) mice as a control (n = 20). Cornea diameter is 2.9±0.1 mm. Weight is 15.8±1.1 mg. Centre panel: Representative first-recognized enlarged eye of $Vav2^{-/-}$ $Vav3^{-/-}$ mice (9- to 10-week-old, n = 20). The cornea diameter is 3.3±0.1 mm. Weight is 23.7±4.4 mg. P<0.001. Right panel: Representative moderately enlarged eye of 12-week-old $Vav2^{-/-}$ $Vav3^{-/-}$ mice (n = 20). The cornea diameter is 4.2±0.4 mm. Weight is 38.0±4.0 mg. **C**. Age of onset of enlarged eyes up to 25 weeks of age in $Vav2^{-/-}$ $Vav3^{-/-}$ mice (n = 200). The vertical axis is a cumulative percentage of $Vav2^{-/-}$ $Vav3^{-/-}$ mice with enlargement of the eyes.

old. Eventually, some of the eyes, became atrophic and phthisical in appearance (Figure 1A). In order to confirm our initial observations, we measured the corneal diameters and weights of $Vav2^{-/-}$ $Vav3^{-/-}$ mice eyes and compared them with age-matched wild-type mice eyes (Figure 1B). The examination clearly showed our observations were relevant. We observed 200 $Vav2^{-/-}$ $Vav3^{-/-}$ mice at 6 months of age and almost 75% of them showed the enlarged eyes (Figure 1C). In addition, histological study indicated that there were no abnormal findings in the tissues both around the enlarged eyes such as inflammation, tumor, or hyperplasia, and in the thyroid of the $Vav2^{-/-}$ $Vav3^{-/-}$ mice (data not shown).

### Elevation of Intraocular Pressure of Vav-Deficient Mice

As we observed the development of buphthalmos, we assessed for elevated IOP in $Vav2^{-/-}$ $Vav3^{-/-}$, Vav2-deficient ($Vav2^{-/-}$), and Vav3-deficient ($Vav3^{-/-}$) mice. IOP was measured using a rodent tonometer (Tonolab) starting at 4 weeks post-natal and were compared with age-matched wild-type C57BL/6 mice. Reliable measurement of IOP before 4 weeks of age was not possible. At 6 weeks of age, $Vav2^{-/-}$ $Vav3^{-/-}$ mice first showed increased IOP (18.2±3.1 vs. 14.0±2.4 mmHg, p<0.05), with further increases out to 10 weeks of age (22.5±7.4 vs. 14.6±4.2 mmHg, p<0.01) (Figure 2A). IOP measurements in $Vav2^{-/-}$ $Vav3^{-/-}$ mice ranged from 11–40 mmHg between 7 weeks and 16 weeks of age. There was a statistically significant difference in IOP between the $Vav2^{-/-}$ $Vav3^{-/-}$ and wild-type mice at all time points demonstrated. The phenotype of littermate wild type mice was identical to that of the "inbred" C57BL/6 strain (Figure S1).

In $Vav2^{-/-}$ mice, elevated IOP was first detected at 7 weeks of age. The IOP for $Vav2^{-/-}$ mice was found to be increased at 8 weeks of age compared to wild-type mice (15.5±3.7 vs. 14.0±4.2 mmHg, p<0.05)(Figure 2B). The IOP of $Vav2^{-/-}$ mice showed further increases at 10 weeks of age (18.1±3.7 vs. 14.6±4.2 mmHg, p<0.01) and remained significantly higher at 12 weeks. In contrast, the IOP of $Vav3^{-/-}$ mice did not differ significantly from wild-type mice between 8 and 12 weeks (Figure 2C). The phenotype of littermate wild type mice was identical to that of inbred strain "C57BL/6". We also demonstrated that the phenotype of Vav2 and Vav3 heterozygous littermate mice ($Vav2^{+/-}$, and $Vav3^{+/-}$) were same as that of wild type (Figure S1).

### Retinal Ganglion Cell Loss and Optic Nerve Head Changes in Vav2/Vav3-Deficient Mice

We next examined whether Vav2/Vav3-deficient ($Vav2^{-/-}$ $Vav3^{-/-}$) mice showed changes in the retinal ganglion cell (RGC) layer and optic nerve head (ONH). At 3 weeks of age, $Vav2^{-/-}$ $Vav3^{-/-}$ mice did not show any histological difference in the ONH or the number of RGCs compared to that of age-matched wild-type mice (Figure 3A). At 10 weeks of age, following several weeks of IOP elevation, early signs of ONH cupping and cell body loss in the RGC layer were apparent in $Vav2^{-/-}$ $Vav3^{-/-}$ mice (Figure 3B). At 15 and 30 weeks of age, $Vav2^{-/-}$ $Vav3^{-/-}$ mice showed further evidence of ONH cupping and RGC loss in the context of an otherwise normal retinal architecture. These findings are consistent with a selective loss of RGCs with corresponding changes in the ONH, which are the hallmarks of glaucoma.

### Iridocorneal Angle Histopathology in Vav-Deficient Mice

As histopathological examination of globes from mice with buphthalmos frequently demonstrated angle closure, we compared

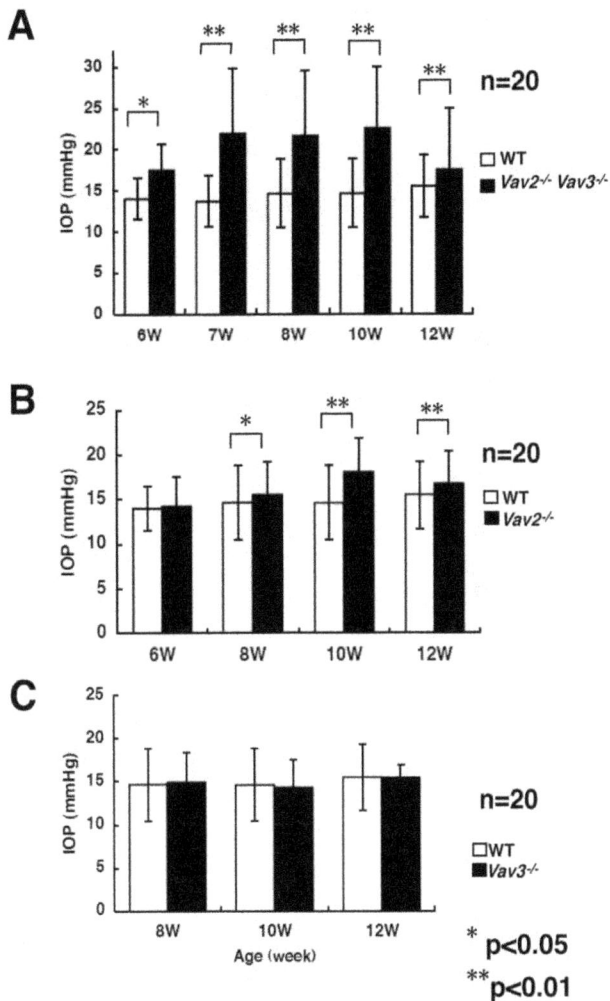

**Figure 2. Elevated intraocular pressure of $Vav2^{-/-} Vav3^{-/-}$ and $Vav2^{-/-}$ mice.** The intraocular pressure (IOP) of Vav2/Vav3-deficient ($Vav2^{-/-} Vav3^{-/-}$), Vav2-deficient ($Vav2^{-/-}$), and Vav3-deficient ($Vav3^{-/-}$) mice were measured between 10–12 AM. At the indicated ages, twenty mice were examined, respectively. For the IOP measurement of each Vav-deficient mouse, IOP of an age-matched wild-type (WT) mouse was also measured under the same conditions. We confirmed that these results were reproducible with four independent examinations. **A.** IOPs of $Vav2^{-/-} Vav3^{-/-}$ mice were dramatically elevated at 6 weeks of age. **B.** $Vav2^{-/-}$ mice also showed elevated IOP from around 8 weeks of age. **C.** $Vav3^{-/-}$ mice have normal range of IOP at any age. Error bars represent S.D. *P<0.05, **P<0.01 versus WT mice.

the iridocorneal angle histology of 20 Vav2/Vav3-deficient ($Vav2^{-/-} Vav3^{-/-}$) mice with wild-type mice at both 7 and 12 weeks of age. Angles were classified as either being completely open, displaying evidence of partial occlusion of the trabecular meshwork (TM) as manifest by peripheral anterior synechiae (PAS), or being completely closed (total occlusion of the trabecular meshwork)(Figure 4A). Over half of the Vav2/Vav3-deficient mice already showed evidence of angle closure by 7 weeks of age, increasing to nearly 80% in 12-week-old mice (Figure 4B).

We also examined the correlation between elevated IOP and angle changes in 7-week-old $Vav2^{-/-} Vav3^{-/-}$ mice respectively (n = 20) (Figure S2). The mean and standard deviation of IOP in 7-week-old wild-type mice (n = 18) were $13.7 \pm 3.12$ mmHg respectively. The 95th percentile of those IOPs using a normal

curve was 18.8 mmHg. So that IOP over 18.8 mmHg was regarded as elevated IOP. $Vav2^{-/-} Vav3^{-/-}$ mice with elevated IOP showed evidence of angle closure by histological analysis, while $Vav2^{-/-} Vav3^{-/-}$ mice with non-elevated IOP displayed either open angles or evidence of early angle closure (PAS) and angle closure.

In addition, to characterize the progression of angle changes, two additional time points were added to this analysis of the iridocorneal angle $-18$ days and 4 weeks of age (n = 20 each). While at 18 days of age nearly half of the eyes demonstrated open angles, a large percentage already showed evidence of PAS (Figure 4B). By 4 weeks of age, $Vav2^{-/-} Vav3^{-/-}$ mice showed increasing frequencies of both PAS and angle closure. Taken as a whole, the data showed a gradual progression from open angles to PAS formation to closed angle from 18 days to 12 weeks.

The iridocorneal angles of Vav2-deficient ($Vav2^{-/-}$) and Vav3-deficient ($Vav3^{-/-}$) mice were examined histologically and graded in a similar manner. The iridocorneal angles of $Vav2^{-/-}$ mice also demonstrated evidence of progressive angle closure, but to a lesser extent as compared with $Vav2^{-/-} Vav3^{-/-}$ mice (Figure 4B). $Vav3^{-/-}$ mice had normal appearing open angles without evidence of PAS formation or angle closure (Figure 4B).

In order to better investigate the status of iridocorneal angles in $Vav2^{-/-} Vav3^{-/-}$ mice, we stained for myocilin as a marker for TM cells, as myocilin is strongly expressed in TM cells [17]. We examined 7-week-old $Vav2^{-/-} Vav3^{-/-}$ mice with non-elevated IOP who had either open angles or who displayed evidence of angle closure. As shown in Figure S3, myocilin was not detected in the iridocorneal angle of $Vav2^{-/-} Vav3^{-/-}$ mice with angle closure, but was seen in mice with open angles similar to those of wild-type mice.

## Effects of Ocular Hypotensives in Vav2/Vav3 -Deficient Mice

We next tested the efficacy of ocular hypotensives used for human glaucoma in $Vav2^{-/-} Vav3^{-/-}$ mice with elevated IOP (Figure S4). The elevated IOP of 7-week-old $Vav2^{-/-} Vav3^{-/-}$ mice was dramatically reduced by ocular hypotensives used in humans, such as latanoprost, a prostaglandin analogue (Figure S4A). We also tested the IOP-lowering effect in $Vav2^{-/} Vav3^{-/}$ mice by two other ocular hypotensives, dorzolamide and timolol, whose mechanisms of action differ from that of latanoprost [18–20], being aqueous suppressants (Figure S4B). Furthermore, we tested Y-27632, a Rho-associated protein kinase inhibitor, that has been reported to cause a reduction in IOP presumably by altering cellular behavior of TM cells [21–23]. Y-27632 showed no effect of lowering IOPs against $Vav2^{-/-} Vav3^{-/-}$ mice, while it lowered the IOP significantly in age-matched wild-type mice (Figure S4C).

## Expression of Vav2 and Vav3 in Mouse and Human Eyes

In order to understand the pathogenesis of the Vav2/Vav3-deficient eye phenotype, we examined the mRNA and protein expression patterns of Vav2 and Vav3 in the eye (Figure 5). Quantitative real-time PCR revealed that Vav2 and Vav3 mRNA are expressed in TM, cornea, retina, lens, iris, and ciliary body in the mouse eye (Figure 5A). Vav3 mRNA was more abundantly expressed than that of Vav2 in the TM and the retina. Gene expression levels of both Vav2 and Vav3 in the eye were comparable to levels found in immune cells where Vavs play a critical role [5,7–16]. Next, the Vav2 and Vav3 mRNA localization in mouse eye was examined by in situ hybridization (ISH) analysis (Figure 5B). Both Vav2 and Vav3 oligo probes (antisense), we used here, have been examined the specificities before and proved to have its specificity. As negative controls for

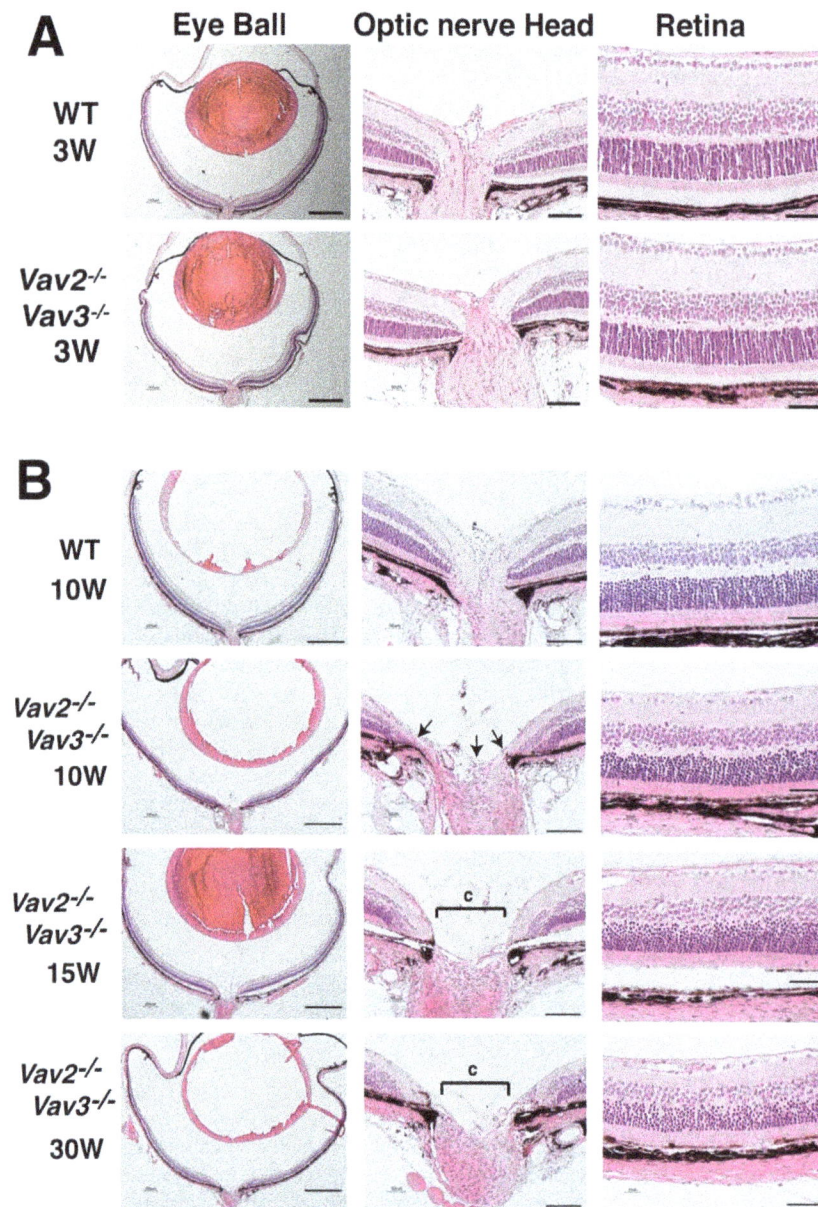

**Figure 3. Optic nerve head degeneration and decrease in RGCs observed in $Vav2^{-/-} Vav3^{-/-}$ mice with elevated IOP.** Light-microscopic histological examination is conducted to evaluate retinal neuropathy in Vav2/Vav3-deficient ($Vav2^{-/-} Vav3^{-/-}$) mice. **A**. At the age of 3 weeks, $Vav2^{-/-} Vav3^{-/-}$ mice exhibited impairment of angle status, but no abnormal findings of Optic nerve head degeneration (ONH) or retinal ganglion cells (RGCs) in the retinas. Scale bars, from left to right side: 500 μm, 100 μm, and 50 μm. **B**. After elevation of IOP, compared to control wild-type (WT) mice in the upper panel, ONH in 10-, 15-, and 30-week-old $Vav2^{-/-} Vav3^{-/-}$ mice present so-called capping (shown in c) and thin retinal neural layers (indicated by arrows in the photos). In those retinas, RGCs are decreased. Scale bars, from left to right side: 500 μm, 100 μm, and 50 μm. Sections are representative from 6–12 samples.

these experiments, we used sense probes of Vav2 and Vav3, respectively, which showed no detectable signal (Figure S5). Both genes expression were widely distributed in the ocular tissues including the iridocorneal angle, retina, cornea, and sclera. The co- localization of Vav2 and Vav3 mRNA expression in iridocorneal angle, such as TM, was confirmed by ISH. Also, we assessed Vav2 and Vav3 protein expression by immunoblotting in both mouse and human eyes (Figure 5C). In mouse eyes, expression of both Vav2 and Vav3 was demonstrated in several ocular tissues including the iridocorneal angle, retina, cornea, and sclera. Both Vav2 and Vav3 proteins were also expressed in

human retina and iridocorneal angle. The migrated bands were absent in the liver extracts of the $Vav2^{-/-} Vav3^{-/-}$ mice. Results of densitometric ratio (Vav3/Vav2) from normalized protein loading in each lane revealed that Vav3 was more abundantly expressed than Vav2 in the iridocorneal angle tissues of both mouse and human eyes and also in the retina.

## Single Nucleotide Polymorphisms in Japanese Primary Open-Angle Glaucoma Patients

We observed Vav2 and Vav3 proteins expression in the tissues of human iridocorneal angle and retina. In order to investigate the

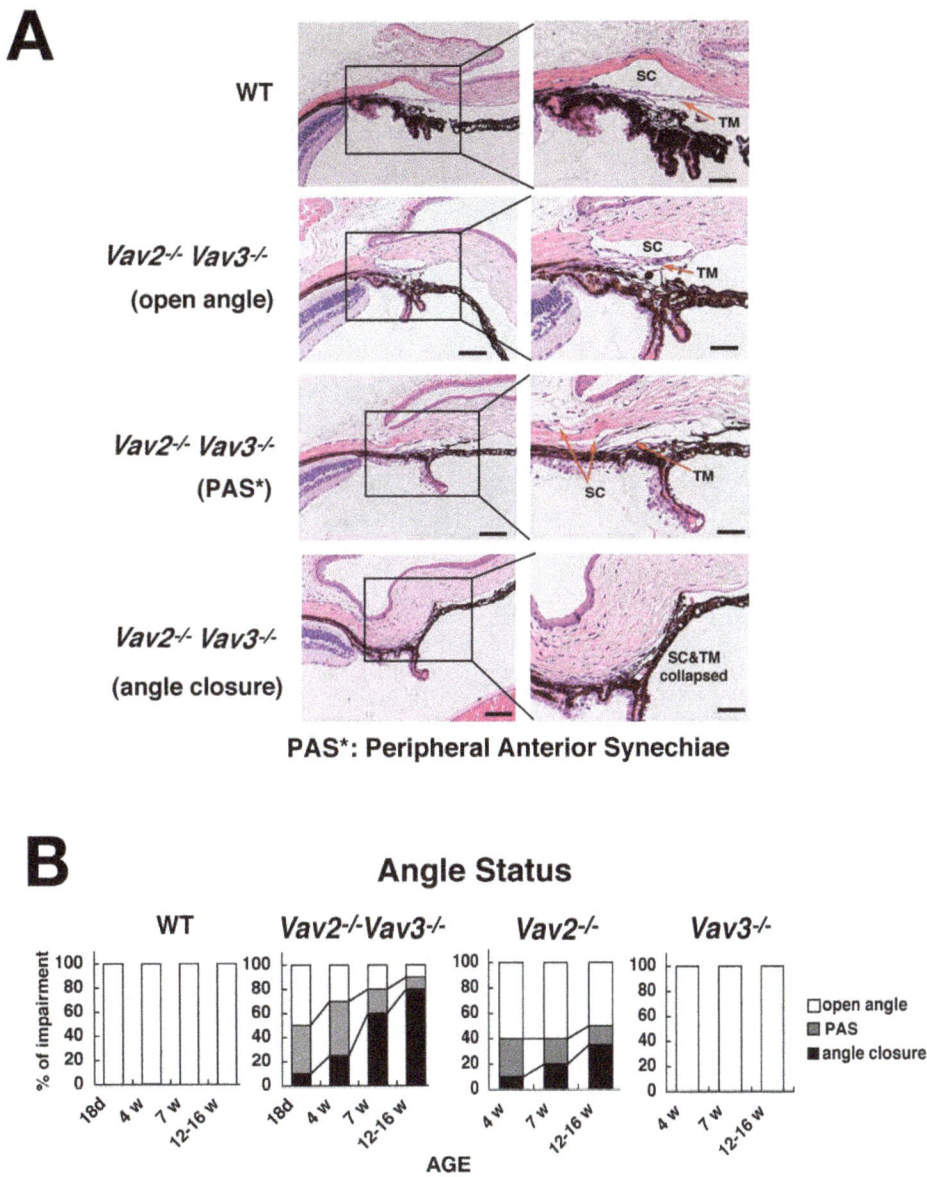

**Figure 4. Characterization of progressive iridocorneal angle closures in $Vav2^{-/-}Vav3^{-/-}$ and $Vav2^{-/-}$ mice.** The aqueous humor outflow facility, trabecular meshwork (TM) and Schlemm's canal (SC) (iridocornial angle) in Vav2/Vav3-deficient ($Vav2^{-/-}Vav3^{-/-}$) mice are evaluated in histological manner. Vav2-deficient ($Vav2^{-/-}$) mice also have the same changes, but of lower severity. **A.** Representative photos of normal TM and SC histology of 12-week-old wild-type (WT) mice as a control. Representative photos of normal open angle, peripheral anterior synechiae (PAS) in 12-week-old $Vav2^{-/-}Vav3^{-/-}$ mice, and angle closure status in 12-week-old $Vav2^{-/-}Vav3^{-/-}$ mice. Sections used here are all representative from 20 samples. Scale bars: left photos, 200 μm; right photos, 100 μm. **B.** Changes of angle status appear at the early ages. We classify angle status of $Vav2^{-/-}$ $Vav3^{-/-}$, $Vav2^{-/-}$, and $Vav3^{-/-}$ mice into open angle, PAS, and angle closure by histological evaluation. We find the changes of angle status at the early ages, such as in 18-day-old $Vav2^{-/-}Vav3^{-/-}$ mice (n = 20) and in 4-week-old of $Vav2^{-/-}Vav3^{-/-}$ mice (n = 20). We took four ($Vav2^{-/-}Vav3^{-/-}$) and three ($Vav2^{-/-}$, $Vav3^{-/-}$) different age groups, with 20 mice examined, respectively.

relevant association of *VAV2* and *VAV3* in human glaucoma patients, we carried out a genome-wide association study using the Affymetrix GeneChip Human Mapping 500 K Array Set. We examined Japanese primary open–angle glaucoma (POAG) cases and age-matched non-glaucoma controls. Both *VAV2* and *VAV3* loci in Japanese POAG patients showed SNPs against the non-glaucoma controls for dbSNPs rs2156323 and rs2801219, respectively. We reported the most extreme (Table 1). Both were intronic SNPs, SNP rs2156323 lying in intron3 of *VAV2* and SNP rs2801219 lying in intron1 of *VAV3*. *VAV2* SNP rs2156323 in particular indicated significant association with Japanese POAG,

including a 5.65 heterozygote odds ratio (95% confidence interval (CI): 1.99–16.0), 4.34 heterozygote relative risk (95% CI: 1.72–10.44) and $4.38 \times 10^{-4}$ genotypic *P* value with respect to risk allele A.

Judging from alleric *P*-values distribution for detecting *VAV2* ranking and genotypic *P*- values distribution for *VAV3* ranking, we observed that *VAV2* and *VAV3* showed high scores ($-\log_{10}(P)$) among approximately 380,000 SNPs analyzed in this study (Figure 6). On the contrary, *VAV1* showed no association with the POAG. These data strongly suggest that *VAV2* and *VAV3* genes are susceptibility loci in Japanese POAG.

**Table 1.** Vav2, Vav3, Vav1 association study for POAG using the Affymetrix GeneChip.

| Gene | VAV2 | VAV3 | VAV1 |
|---|---|---|---|
| SNP ID | rs2156323 | rs2801219 | rs2617815 |
| Chromosome Location | 9q34.1 | 1p13.3 | 19p13.2 |
| Position | 133750375 | 108214454 | 6746147 |
| Genotypic $P$ value | $4.38 \times 10^{-4}$ | $5.42 \times 10^{-4}$ | $4.41 \times 10^{-2}$ |
| Allele | AG | AC | AG |
| Risk allele | A | C | G |
| Minor allele | A | C | G |
| Heterozygote odds ratio (95%CI) | 5.65 (1.99–16.0) | 2.03 (1.01–4.09) | 1.04 (0.52–2.08) |
| Heterozygote relative risk (95%CI) | 4.34 (1.72–10.44) | 1.31 (1.00–1.75) | 1.01 (0.82–1.23) |
| Homozygote odds ratio | Not Available | Not Available | Not Available |
| Exon Intron | VAV2 Intron3 | VAV3 Intron1 | VAV1 Intron1 |
| SNP type | iSNP*1 | iSNP | iSNP |

*1: intronic S.

## Discussion

To our knowledge, this is the first report of a spontaneous glaucoma phenotype in Vav2 $(Vav2^{-/-})$ or Vav2/Vav3-deficient $(Vav2^{-/-} Vav3^{-/-})$ mice. Vav2/Vav3-deficiency is associated with progressive iridocorneal angle changes and elevation of IOP in mice. Subsequent selective loss of RGCs and progressive ONH cupping are associated with this elevated IOP, as has previously been demonstrated in other rodent models of glaucoma [24]. The finding that Vav2-deficiency alone results in a glaucoma phenotype suggests that the absence of Vav2 plays a critical role in the development of this phenotype. Despite our finding that Vav3-deficiency did not result in either iridocorneal angle changes or elevated IOP, the more severe glaucomatous phenotype demonstrated in $Vav2^{-/-} Vav3^{-/-}$ mice as compared with $Vav2^{-/-}$ mice is consistent with an additive effect.

A number of induced glaucoma models have been established in rats and mice [24]. Each model has advantages and disadvantages, related to factors such as the ease of inducing elevated IOP, the magnitude, duration and variability of elevated IOP, and secondary effects on the eye. Due to the ease of genetic manipulation, mouse models are becoming increasingly popular over those in rats. Despite the lack of a lamina cribosa as found in human eyes, the mouse is a good genetic model to study the pathogenesis of human glaucoma as aqueous physiology and anterior segment anatomy are similar to that found in humans [25].

Other spontaneous models of glaucoma have been described in mice, most notably in DBA/2J mice. The pigmentary glaucoma phenotype demonstrated in the DBA/2J mice has been extensively studied at genetic, clinical, morphological and pathological levels [26–29]. A limitation of this model is that the elevated IOP phenotype is not primary but secondary due to the systemic pigment dispersion syndrome with the associated mutations in the *Gpnmb* and *Tyrp1* loci [26–30]. In these mice, recessive mutations in these 2 genes are associated with iris degeneration characterized by iris stromal atrophy and pigment dispersion with subsequent reduced outflow facility secondary to pigment and cell debris. Therefore, it is difficult to tie-in the identified mutations to the pathogenesis of any primary form of human glaucoma.

The Vav2/Vav3-deficient mouse has several characteristics which make it particularly useful as an animal glaucoma model.

The elevated IOP occurs spontaneously in these genetically manipulated mice and does not require the ocular manipulation necessary in induced models. The frequency of the ocular phenotype is high and onset occurs at a relatively young age. In addition, ocular hypotensives commonly used to treat human glaucoma show efficacy in lowering IOP in this model. The most significant advantage of this mouse glaucoma model is that the deleted genes, Vav2 and Vav3, are well-focused targets that have been studied over 20 years providing a useful starting point for further investigation of the potential molecular mechanisms underlying this phenotype.

Several aspects of this model of spontaneous glaucoma will require further study and clarification, although we speculated from our histological results and the correlation between elevated IOP and angle status changes that anatomic angle closure is the possible mechanism for elevated IOP in this model. While progressive angle closure may be the etiology prior to elevated IOP in mice lacking Vav2 and Vav3 function, it may alternatively be a subsequent change related to other alterations in angle structures which might also affect aqueous humor outflow. In addition, since the expression of Vav2 and Vav3 was detected in ocular tissues other than those comprising the iridocorneal angle, it will be necessary in future studies to consider how their deficiency in these tissues might have potentially contributed to the spontaneous glaucoma phenotype in any way.

While so far there are several reports of glaucoma associated candidate genes based on the single nucleotide polymorphisms (SNPs) study in the Japanese population [31–36], our data first suggest that *VAV2* and *VAV3* are susceptibility loci in Japanese primary open–angle glaucoma (POAG) cases. In addition, so far we could not find the report of non-Japanese glaucoma association case study that demonstrated *VAV2* and/or *VAV3* as candidate gene loci for glaucoma [37–43]. They demonstrated glaucoma associated candidate genes study with SNPs analysis focusing on the other specific target genes, although we are interested in the *VAV2* and/or *VAV3* glaucoma association study using the different populations. This work would be important investigation to be done.

Although our current findings do not address the molecular mechanisms underlying glaucoma phenotypes, it is interesting to consider possible mechanisms based on what is currently known about Vav protein function. The TM has been regarded as a key determinant of IOP and has been implicated as the major site of

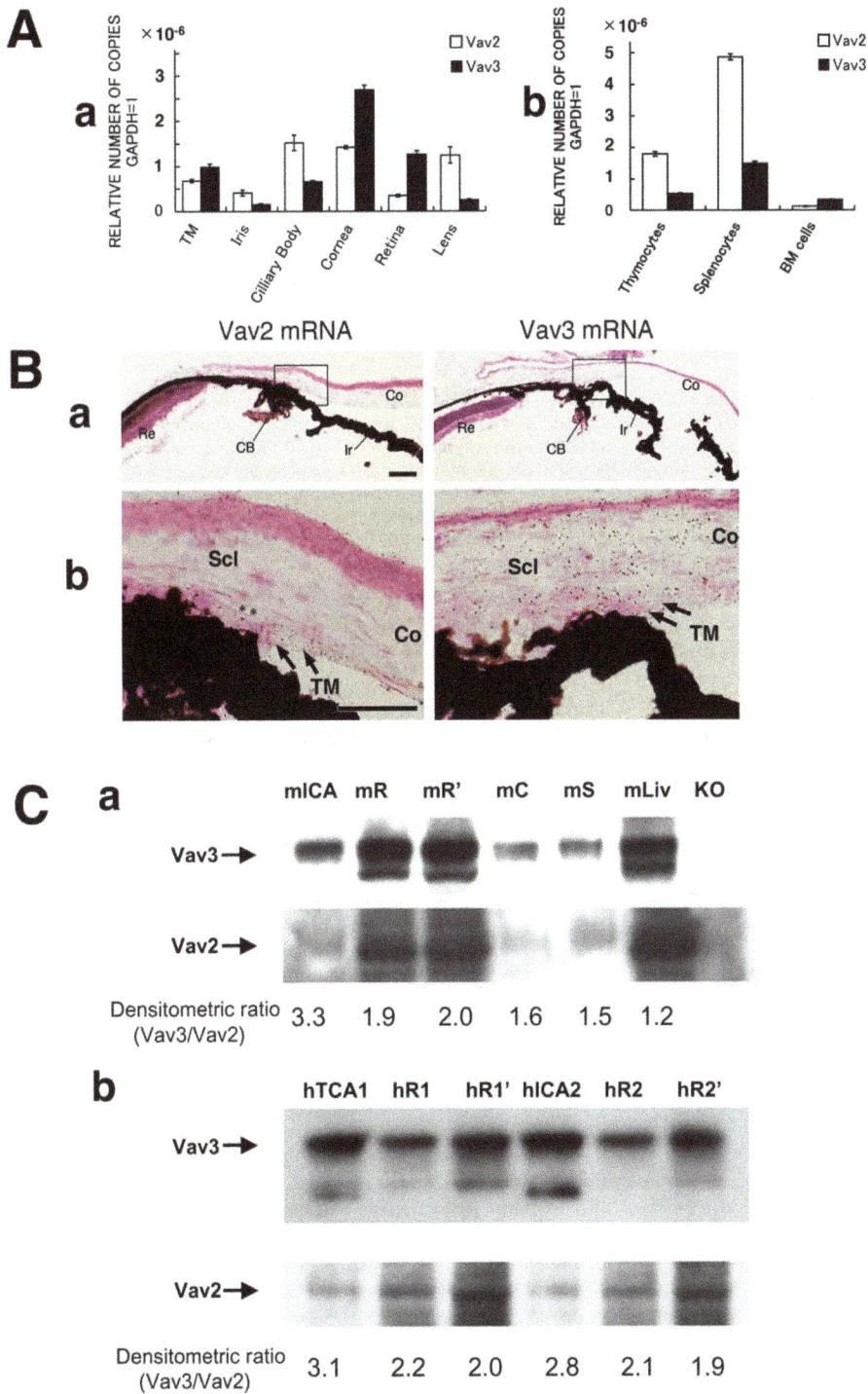

**Figure 5. Vav2 and Vav3 expression in mouse and human eyes. A**. Quantitative real time PCR analysis is performed for Vav2 and Vav3 mRNA expression study. The vertical axis is the copy number of Vav2 or Vav3 mRNA when that of mGAPDH is taken as 1. The assay method is absolute quantification (standard curve). **a.** Both Vav2 and Vav3 mRNA are expressed in all tissues of the murine eyes including the trabecular meshwork (TM), cornea, sclera, and retina. **b.** Vav2 and Vav3 mRNA expression level of murine immune cells. The levels of Vav2 and Vav3 expression in eye tissues are the same as those of the immune cells where Vav2 and Vav3 play the critical role. **B. a.** In situ hybridization analysis of emulsion-dipped sections display the distribution of Vav2 and Vav3 mRNA in the anterior chamber. The localization of Vav2 and Vav3 mRNA in trabecular meshwork(TM), ciliary body (CB), cornia(CO), iris(Ir), sclera (Scl) and retina(Re) by in situ hybridization. **b.** Vav2 and Vav3 mRNA expression are both detected in iridocorneal angle, such as TM (indicated by arrows in the photos). Scale bars, 50 μm. **C.** Expression of Vav2 and Vav3 proteins in mouse (**a**) and human (**b**) eyes. Vav2 and Vav3 proteins were detected in mouse or human ocular extracts (from two independent postmortem eye globe samples; at death age of 58 (1) and 87 (2)) by western blotting. Densitometric ratios (Vav3/Vav2) were shown under the blotting panels. mICA: mouse iridocorneal angle tissues, mR: mouse retina, mR': 3-fold increased loading mouse retina, mC: mouse cornea, mS: mouse sclera, mLiv: normal mouse liver(positive control), KO: Vav2/Vav3-deficient mouse as a negative control, hICA: human iridocorneal angle tissue,hR1: human retina 1, hR1': human retina1' (3-fold loading).

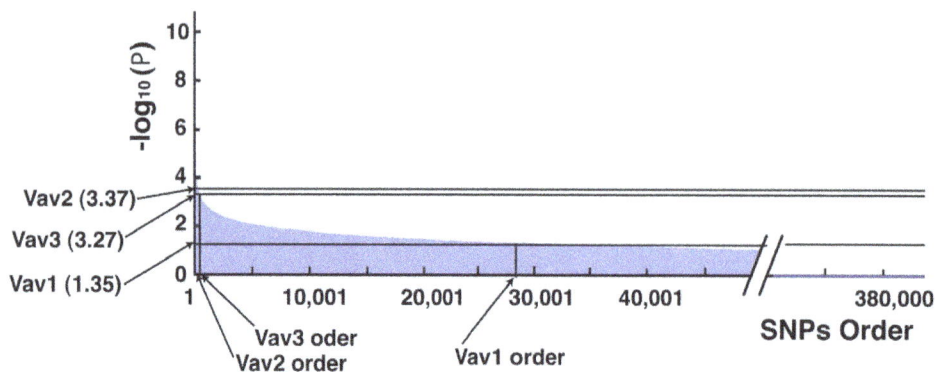

**Figure 6.** *VAV2* **and** *VAV3* **genome-wide SNPs high ranking of** *P*-value **scores.** Genome-wide ranking orders of *P*-value indicate that *VAV2* and *VAV3* are strongly susceptible genes with Japanese POAG cases. Clinically diagnosed Japanese POAG 100 cases and non-glaucoma age-matched 100 controls are examined for this study. The analysed SNPs number is about 380,000 by the Affymetrix GeneChip 500 K Mapping Array Set. The SNPs data under the 85% call rate, under 0.001 Hardy-Weinberg equilibrium (HWE), and under 5% minor allele frequencies are excluded. Allelic frequency $\chi2$ test and genotypic frequency $\chi2$ test are calculated respectively. The vertical axis is $-\log10$ (*P*) and the horizontal axis is SNPs order which showed high scores from left to right. The Upper graph is alleric *P*-values distribution of *VAV2* analysis and the lower graph is genotypic *P*-values for *VAV3* and *VAV1* study. *VAV2* is located at high position in rank and *VAV3* also located at high position in rank. *VAV1* shows no association for POAG cases here.

increased resistance to aqueous outflow which occurs in human glaucoma [44,45]. Recent findings indicate that signals emanating from integrins, key regulators of the actin cytoskeleton in trabecular meshwork cells, may be involved in control of outflow facility and Rho GTPases would be important downstream effectors of integrin-mediated actin cytoskeletal dynamics [4,46–48]. Considering the Vavs function as GEF, dysregulation of Rho is one possible mechanism by which pathology in the iridocorneal angle might result and is one that deserves further study.

In summary, we had demonstrated that Vav2/Vav3-deicient mice develop a spontaneous glaucoma phenotype. In addition, our data first suggest that *VAV2* and *VAV3* are susceptibility loci in Japanese primary open-angle glaucoma (POAG) cases. We believe that Vav2/Vav3-deficient mice will serve not only as a useful murine model of spontaneous glaucoma, but may also provide a valuable tool in understanding of the pathogenesis of glaucoma in humans, particularly the determinants of altered aqueous outflow and elevated IOP.

## Materials and Methods

### Mice

$Vav3^{-/-}$, $Vav2^{-/-}$ and $Vav2^{-/-} Vav3^{-/-}$ mice were described previously [15]. Mice were backcrossed at least 9 times with C57BL/6 mice (Clea Japan, Tokyo, Japan) to have the C57BL/6 background. All mice used in these experiments were bred and maintained in the SPF Facility of Hokkaido University Graduate School of Medicine in a 12-hour light-dark cycle. All mice experiments were approved by the Animal Ethics Committee of Hokkaido University Graduate School of Medicine and were conducted in accordance with the ARVO Statement for the Use of Animals in Ophthalmic and Vision Research.

### Tissue Preparation and Histology

Eyes were quickly enucleated from each age group of knock-out mice and C57BL/6 wild-type control mice after deep anesthesia with pentobarbital sodium solution, then immediately fixed with solution of 2.5% glutaraldehyde (TAAB, EM Grade) in 10% formalin neutral buffer-methanol solution deodorized for anterior chamber study, or fixed with Davidson' solution for retinal analysis for 12 hours. Following this, the eyes were embedded in paraffin and dissected sagittally using a microtome into 5 µm sections.

After deparaffinization and rehydration, the sections were stained with hematoxylin and eosin (Sigma).

### Immunohistochemistry

The eyes were sectioned at 5 µm thickness along the vertical meridian through the optic nerve head. After deparaffinization and rehydration, the tissue sections were incubated with blocking solution containing 1% BSA in PBS for 1 hour. This was followed by 1 hour incubation with rabbit polyclonal antibody to myocilin at 1:200 in blocking solution as first antibody for 1 hour at room temperature. Anti-rabbit IgG conjugated with Alexa 488 (Molecular Probes, Eugene, OR) at 1:400 in PBS containing 0.1% Tween 20 was used as secondary antibody for 1 hour at room temperature. The stained tissues were examined using confocal fluorescence laser microscope (Radius 2000, Bio-Rad, Hercules, CA). For negative control of the immunohistochemical staining, the sections were incubated with blocking solution without primary antibody (data not shown).

### Real Time PCR

Each tissue was freshly taken from SPF level C57BL/6 mice and immediately used for generating RNA by TRIzol reagent (Invitrogen). Templates for real time PCR were made by Cloned AMV Reverse Transcriptase (Invitrogen). Probes of mVav2 and mVav3 were TaqMan probes (Vav2: Mm00437287_m1, Vav3: Mm00445082_m1) purchased from Applied Biosystems (Foster city, CA). The standard curves were constructed by mVav2, mVav3 inserted plasmids, normalized by mGAPDH (Product Code: 4352339E, Applied Biosystems). All the PCR studies were performed by Applied Biosystems 7500 Real Time PCR System following the manufacturer's recommended procedures. The assay method was absolute quantification (standard curve).

### In Situ Hybridization

The detailed procedure was described as previously [49]. Briefly, to detect mRNAs for Vav2 and Vav3, specific antisense oligonucleotide probes were synthesizedas follows:(2275–2319;45mers)5′-AGCTG-GAGACCGGCTTGAGGCC CTGCTGGTGGTTCGCTCCCG-AGA-3′ for Vav2 mRNA (GenBank accession No. NM_009500) and (2346–2302;45mers)5′–GTTGCCTGTTCTATTACCCCTCTG T CCAGCTGGCTGTTCTGGCTC-3′ for Vav3 mRNA (accession No. NM_020505). Oligonucleotide probes were labeled with [33P] dATP using terminal deoxyribonucleotidyl transferase (Invitrogen, Carlsbad, CA). Under deep pentobarbital anesthesia, the eyeballs were freshly obtained from Adult C57BL/6J mice. Fresh frozen sections (20 μm thickness) were cut with a cryostat (CM1900, Leica, Nussloch,Germany) and mounted on glass slides precoated with 3-aminopropyltriethoxysilane. Sections were exposed to Nuclear Track emulsion (NTB-2, Kodak) for 5 weeks. Emulsion-dipped sections were stained with methyl green pyronine solution. The specificity of the hybridizing signals was verified by the disappearance of signals when hybridization was carried out with sense probes.

## Western Blotting

Mouse Ocular Tissue Dissection: 8-week male C57BL/6J mice (Jackson Laboratory, ME) were used for ocular tissue samples. The animals were euthanized by carbon dioxide inhalation in an induction chamber. The globes were promptly enucleated after euthanization and washed in ice-cold PBS. Ocular tissues were microscopically dissected. Dissection of Postmortem Human Eye Globes: Human eyes without previous eye diseases including glaucoma were acquired from a local eye bank (Heartland Lions Eye Banks; Columbia, MO) within 6 hours post-mortem. Dissected mouse and postmortem human ocular tissues were lysed in a tissue extraction buffer (BioChain, CA). The concentration of protein supernatants was determined by a protein assay kit (Bio-Rad, CA). Rabbit polyclonal anti-mouse Vav2 (1:1000) (Santa Cruz Biotechnology, CA), monoclonal anti-human Vav2 (1:2000) (Cell Signaling Technology, MA), polyclonal anti-mouse and anti-human Vav3 (1:3000 for each) (Millipore, CA) antibodies were used for detection.

## Intraocular Pressure (IOP) Measurement

IOP was measured using the TonoLab rebound tonometer for rodents (Tiolat i-care, Finland) according to the manufacturer's recommended procedures. All IOP measurements were performed between 10 AM and noon in conscious condition. Mice were gently restrained first by hand and placed on a soft towel bed on the desk and usually appeared calm and comfortable. These data were confirmed to be reproducible by three additional different independent studies (n = 20).

## Evaluation of Eye Drop Medications for High Intra-Ocular Pressure of Vav2Vav3-Deficient Mice

$Vav2^{-/-} Vav3^{-/-}$ mice were housed in SPF barrier facility in standard lighting conditions (12-hour light-dark cycle). The 7–9 week after birth mice were used for the experiment. Four independent experiments were carried out to confirm the results reproducible.

## Preparation and Application of Ophthalmic Solution

Latanoprost was purchased from Cayman Chemical Co. (Ann Arbor, MI) and dissolved in its vehicle solution (0.02% benzalkonium chloride, 0.5% monosodium phosphate monohydrate, 0.6% disodium hydrogen phosphate dihydrate and 0.4% sodium chloride). With a micropipette, 3 μl of PG analogue (latanoprost; prostaglandin F2α) solution or vehicle was randomly applied to the eyes of $Vav2^{-/-} Vav3^{-/-}$ mice. Before administration, IOP was measured with the tonometer from 10–12 AM and then the PG analogue 0.005% 3 μl or vehicle solution was applied in a masked manner. Evaluation of IOP-lowering effect was performed by measuring the IOP with the tonometer at 3 hours after drug instillation also in a masked manner. Furthermore, two different mechanistic medications, 3 μl of timolol maleate (0.5%, Merck, Whitehouse Station, NJ) or 3 μl of dorzolamide hydrochloride

(1%, Trusopt; Merck), was also tested, respectively, after measuring the IOP under the same conditions as those of the Latanoprost application. Evaluation of IOP-lowering effects was performed by measuring the IOP with tonometer at 2 hours after drug instillation under blinded test protocols. Y-27632 was purchased from Carbiochem (La Jolla, CA) and dissolved in its vehicle solution (phosphate buffered saline). Y-27632 (1 mM) or vehicle solution was administered to the central cornea as a 3 μl drop by pipetting in a masked manner. Evaluation of IOP-lowering effect was performed by measuring the IOP with the tonometer at 1 hour after drug instillation.

## Statistical Analysis of IOPs

Data are reported as means ± S.D. Two-tailed Student's t-test was used to compare between two groups of results. Differences between any two groups were regarded as significant when $P < 0.01$ (**) or $P < 0.05$ (*).

## Disease Associated Genome-Wide Analysis

One hundred clinically-diagnosed cases (male 46; female 54) with primary open-angle glaucoma over 30 years of age (mean age, 71.60 years; SD, 9.33 years) and non-glaucoma age-matched controls (mean age, 66.71 years; SD, 12.00 years) in a Japanese population were examined for this study. Informed consent was obtained from all participants, and the procedures used conformed to the tenets of the Declaration of Helsinki. Genomic DNAs were isolated from the peripheral blood of the POAG cases and age-matched controls for genotyping analysis. Genotyping was performed using the Affymetrix GeneChip Human Mapping 500 K Array Set (Affymetrix Services Laboratory, California). We omitted the SNP data under an 85% call rate, under 0.001 Hardy-Weinberg equilibrium (HWE), and under 5% minor allele frequency. Data analysis was performed using the LaboServer System (World Fusion, Tokyo Japan). An allelic frequency $\chi^2$ test and genotypic frequency $\chi^2$ test were calculated, respectively with respect to risk allele. The Odds ratio was calculated in three manners such as per allele odds ratio, heterozygote odds ratio, and homozygote odds ratio. Relative risk was also calculated, the same as for the odds ratio. The most significant SNPs were chosen in this report to evaluate the association of *VAV2*, *VAV3*, and *VAV1* in the cases.

## Supporting Information

**Figure S1** The comparison of intraocular pressures in age matched wild-type inbred C57BL/6 mice, wild-type littermate controls, and Vav2 and Vav3 heterozygous mice ($Vav2^{+/-}$, and $Vav3^{+/-}$). Intraocular pressures (IOPs) were measured using the TonoLab rebound tonometer for rodents from 6-week to 12-week, as described in the Methods. The phenotype of littermate wild-type mice was identical to that of the "inbred" C57BL/6 strain. The phenotype of Vav2 and Vav3 heterozygous mice were similar to that of wild-type. n = 20.
Found at: doi:10.1371/journal.pone.0009050.s001 (0.45 MB TIF)

**Figure S2** The correlation between elevated IOP and angle changes in Vav2/Vav3-deficient mice. The IOP was measured in 7-week-old Vav2/Vav3-deficient ($Vav2^{-/-}Vav3^{-/-}$) mice (n = 20), followed by examination of the angle status by histology. While $Vav2^{-/-}Vav3^{-/-}$ mice with elevated IOP displayed histological evidence of angle closure, mice without elevated IOP showed either normal open angles or evidence of angle changes, angle closure or peripheral anterior synechiae. The mean and standard deviation of IOP in wild-type mice at 7-week-old (n = 18) were 13.7±3.12 mmHg, respectively. The 95th percentile of those

IOPs using a normal curve was 18.8 mmHg. IOP over 18.8 mmHg was regarded here as elevated IOP.
Found at: doi:10.1371/journal.pone.0009050.s002 (0.57 MB TIF)

**Figure S3** Anti-myocilin staining of trabecular meshwork in Vav2/Vav3-deficient mice. Immunohistochemical staining of trabecular meshwork with anti-myocilin antibody in representative iridocorneal angle sections of age-matched wild-type and Vav2/Vav3-deficient (Vav2$^{-/-}$Vav3$^{-/-}$) 7-week-old mice with normal IOP, with either evidence of angle closure, or normal open angles similar to wild type mice. Myocilin (green-labeled), which is strongly expressed in TM cells, was regarded as a marker for TM cells. In Vav2$^{-/-}$Vav3$^{-/-}$ mice with angle closure, myocilin was not detected in the iridocorneal angle (indicated by arrows). Conversely, it was detected in sections from mice with normal open angles, similar to those in wild type mice. Blue fluorescence is DAPI counter staining. Scale bars, 20 um.
Found at: doi:10.1371/journal.pone.0009050.s003 (2.19 MB TIF)

**Figure S4** Effects of ocular hypotensives in Vav2/Vav3-deficient mice. A. Ocular hypotensives used for human glaucoma, latanoprost, a prostaglandin analogue was tested in 7-week-old Vav2/Vav3-deficient (Vav2$^{-/-}$Vav3$^{-/-}$) mice with elevated IOP (n = 20). The IOP was measured 3 hours before and after topical application of 3 μl of 0.01% latanoprost in a masked manner. Vehicle was used as a control. Latanoprost lowered the IOP significantly in Vav2$^{-/-}$Vav3$^{-/-}$ mice (26.3±5.0 mmHg versus 15.8±5.1 mmHg; n = 20), while the IOP was not altered by the vehicle alone. The latanoprost-induced reduction of IOP in Vav2$^{-/-}$Vav3$^{-/-}$ mice was statistically significant (**P<0.01, n = 20). The data shown are representative of three independent experiments performed. Error bars represent S.D. **P<0.01 versus vehicle-treated Vav2$^{-/-}$Vav3$^{-/-}$ mice. B. Using three different drugs for lowering IOP, we compared the effects by percentages of elevated IOP reduction. These data are representative from three independent experiments, respectively (n = 20).

Error bars represent S.D. **P<0.01 versus vehicle-treated Vav2$^{-/-}$Vav3$^{-/-}$ mice. C. Rho-associated protein kinase Inhibitor, Y-27632 was tested for lowering IOP on Vav2$^{-/-}$Vav3$^{-/-}$ mice (n = 20). Y27632 administration has no effect against Vav2$^{-/-}$Vav3$^{-/-}$ mice (before, 19.69±4.98 mmHg; after, 18.83±5.60 mmHg; n = 20), while Y-27632 lowered the IOP significantly in age-matched wild-type mice (13.58±2.27 mmHg versus 12.31±1.94 mmHg; n = 20. p<0.05) and the IOP was not altered by the vehicle solution (13.25±1.71 mmHg versus 13.18±3.17 mmHg; n = 20). These data are representative from four independent experiments, respectively. Error bars represent S.D. *P<0.05 versus vehicle-treated WT mice.
Found at: doi:10.1371/journal.pone.0009050.s004 (0.41 MB TIF)

**Figure S5** Sense probe staining for in situ hybridization experiments in ocular tissues. In situ hybridization with Vav2 and Vav3 sense probes were carried out as negative controls for the experiments. C57BL/6 mouse ocular tissue sections including the iridocorneal angle, sclera and cornea were used. With sense probes, there was no detectable signal around mouse iridocorneal angle tissues. TM; trabecular meshwork. Scl; sclera.
Found at: doi:10.1371/journal.pone.0009050.s005 (4.14 MB TIF)

## Acknowledgments

The authors thank Professor Duco Hamasaki (Bascom Palmer Eye Institute, University of Miami School of Medicine, Florida) and Morton Smith, M.D. (Washington University Department of Ophthalmology & Visual Sciences) for helpful suggestions and discussion; and Mr. Tsutomu Osanai and Ms. Takae Oyama for technical help.

## Author Contributions

Conceived and designed the experiments: KF TI KI. Performed the experiments: KF TI MA HK MF QC. Analyzed the data: KF TI KI MA MF MW EMB WAS. Contributed reagents/materials/analysis tools: KF TI KI MW WAS. Wrote the paper: KF KI EMB WAS.

## References

1. Kass MA, Heuer DK, Higginbotham EJ, Johnson CA, Keltner JL, et al. (2002) The ocular hypertension treatment study: a randomized trial determines that topical ocular hypotensive medication delays or prevents the onset of primary open-angle glaucoma. Arch Ophthalmol 120: 701–713.
2. AGIS investigators (2002) The advanced glaucoma intervention study (AGIS): 7. The relationship between control of intraocular pressure and visual field deterioration. Am J Ophthalmol 130: 429–440.
3. Gabelt BT, Kaufman PL (2005) Changes in aqueous humor dynamics with age and glaucoma. Prog Retin Eye Res 24: 612–637.
4. Tan JC, Peters DM, Kaufman PL (2006) Recent developments in understanding the pathophysiology of elevated intraocular pressure. Curr Opin Ophthalmol 17: 168–174.
5. Bustelo XR (2001) Vav protein, adaptors and cell signaling. Oncogene 20: 6372–6381.
6. Schmidt A, Hall A (2002) Guanine nucleotide exchange factors for Rho GTPases: turning on the switch. Genes Dev 16: 1587–1609.
7. Turner M, Billadeau DD (2002) VAV proteins as signal integrators for multi-subunit immune-recognition receptors. Nat Rev Immunol 2: 476–486.
8. Swat W, Fujikawa K (2005) The Vav family: at the crossroads of signaling pathways. Immunol Res 32: 259–265.
9. Riteau B, Barber DF, Long EO (2003) Vav1 phosphorylation is induced by β2 integrin engagement on natural killer cells upstream of actin cytoskeleton and lipid raft reorganization. J Exp Med 198: 469–474.
10. Gakidis MAM, Cullere X, Olson T, Wilsbacher JL, Zhang B, et al. (2004) Vav GEFs are required for β2 integrin-dependent functions of neutrophils. J Cell Biol 166: 273–282.
11. Holsinger LJ, Graef IA, Swat W, Chi T, Bautista DM, et al. (1998) Defects in actin-cap formation in Vav-deficient mice implicate an actin requirement for lymphocyte signal transduction. Curr Biol 8: 563–572.
12. Cella M, Fujikawa K, Tassi I, Kim S, Latinis K, et al. (2004) Differential requirements for Vav proteins in DAP10- and ITAM-mediated NK cell cytotoxicity. J Exp Med 200: 817–823.
13. Doody GM, Bell SE, Vigorito E, Clayton E, McAdam S, et al. (2001) Signal transduction through Vav-2 participates in humoral immune responses and B cell maturation. Nat Immunol 2: 542–547.
14. Faccio R, Teitelbaum SL, Fujikawa K, Chappel J, Zallone A, et al. (2005) Vav3 regulates osteoclast function and bone mass. Nat Med 11: 284–290.
15. Fujikawa K, Miletic AV, Alt FW, Faccio R, Brown T, et al. (2003) Vav1/2/3-null mice define an essential role for Vav family proteins in lymphocyte development and activation but a differential requirement in MAPK signaling in T and B cells. J Exp Med 198: 1595–1608.
16. Tybulewicz VLJ, Ardouin L, Prisco A, Reynolds LF (2003) Vav1: a key signal transducer downstream of the TCR. Immunol Rev 192: 42–52.
17. Karali A, Russell P, Stefani FH, Tamm ER (2000) Localization of myocilin/trabecular meshwork-inducible glucocorticoid response protein in the human eye. Invest Ophthalmol Vis Sci 41: 729–740.
18. Weinreb RN, Toris CB, Gabelt BT, Lindsey JD, Kaufman PL (2002) Effects of prostaglandins on the aqueous humor outflow pathways. Surv Ophthalmol 47 (suppl. 1): S53–S64.
19. Neufeld AH (1979) Experimental studies on the mechanism of action of timolol. Surv Ophthalmol 23: 363–370.
20. Pfeiffer N (1997) Dorzolamide: Development and clinical application of a topical carbonic anhydrase inhibitor. Surv Ophthalmol 42: 137–151.
21. Tanihara H, Inatani M, Honjo M, Tokushige H, Azuma J, et al. (2008) Intraocular pressure-lowering effects and safety of topical administration of a selective ROCK inhibitor, SNJ-1656, in healthy volunteers. Arch Ophthalmol 126: 309–315.
22. Rao PV, Peterson YK, Inoue T, Casey PJ (2008) Effects of pharmacologic inhibition of protein geranylgeranyltransferase type I on aqueous humor outflow through the trabecular meshwork. Invest Ophthalmol Vis Sci 49: 2464–2471.
23. Honjo M, Tanihara H, Inatani M, Kido N, Sawamura T, et al. (2001) Effects of Rho-associated protein kinase inhibitor, Y-27632, on intraocular pressure and outflow facility. Invest Ophthalmol Vis Sci 42: 137–144.
24. Pang IH, Clark AF (2007) Rodent models for glaucoma retinopathy and optic neuropathy. J Glaucoma 16: 483–505.
25. Aihara M, Lindsey JD, Weinreb RN (2003) Aqueous humor dynamics in mice. Invest Ophthalmol Vis Sci 44: 5168–5173.
26. Chang B, Smith RS, Hawes NL, Anderson MG, Zabaleta A, et al. (1999) Interacting loci cause severe iris atrophy and glaucoma in DBA/2J mice. Nat Genet 21: 405–409.

27. John SW, Smith RS, Savinova OV, Hawes NL, Chang B, et al. (1998) Essential iris atrophy, pigment dispersion, and glaucoma in DBA/2J mice. Invest Ophthalmol Vis Sci 39: 951–962.

28. Goldblum D, Kipfer-Kauer A, Sarra GM, Wolf S, Frueh BE (2007) Distribution of amyloid precursor protein and amyloid-beta immunoreactivity in DBA/2J glaucomatous mouse retinas. Invest Ophthalmol Vis Sci 48: 5085–5090.

29. Schlamp CL, Li Y, Dietz JA, Janssen KT, Nickells RW (2006) Progressive ganglion cells loss and optic nerve degeneration in DBA/2J mice is variable and asymmetric. BMC Neurosci 7: 66.

30. Anderson MG, Smith RS, Hawes NL, Zabaleta A, Chang B, et al. (2002) Mutations in genes encoding melanosomal proteins cuase pigmentary glaucoma in DBA/2J mice. Nat Genet 1: 81–85.

31. Nakano M, Ikeda Y, Taniguchi T, Yagi T, Fuwa M, et al. (2009) Three susceptible loci associated with primary open-angle glaucoma identified by genome-wide association study in a Japanese population. Proc Natl Acad Sci U S A 106(31): 12838–12842.

32. Tanito M, Minami M, Akahori M, Kaidzu S, Takai Y, et al. (2008) LOXL1 variants in elderly Japanese patients with exfoliation syndrome/glaucoma, primary open-angle glaucoma, normal tension glaucoma, and cataract. Mol Vis 14: 1898–1905.

33. Shibuya E, Meguro A, Ota M, Kashiwagi K, Mabuchi F, et al. (2008) Association of Toll-like receptor 4 gene polymorphisms with normal tension glaucoma. Invest Ophthalmol Vis Sci 49: 4453–4457.

34. Funayama T, Mashima Y, Ohtake Y, Ishikawa K, Fuse N, et al. (2006) SNPs and interaction analyses of noelin 2, myocilin, and optineurin genes in Japanese patients with open-angle glaucoma. Invest Ophthalmol Vis Sci 47: 5368–5375.

35. Inagaki Y, Mashima Y, Fuse N, Funayama T, Ohtake Y, et al. (2006) Polymorphism of b-adrenergic receptors and susceptibility to open-angle glaucoma. Mol Vis 12: 673–680.

36. Ishikawa K, Funayama T, Ohtake Y, Kimura I, Ideta H, et al. (2005) Association between glaucoma and gene polymorphism of endothelin type A receptor. Mol Vis 11: 431–437.

37. Jiao X, Yang Z, Yang X, Chen Y, Tong Z, et al. (2009) Common variants on chromosome 2 and risk of primary open-angle glaucoma in the Afro-Caribbean population of Barbados. Proc Natl Acad Sci U S A 106(40): 17105–17110.

38. Wolf C, Gramer E, Müller-Myhsok B, Pasutto F, Reinthal E, et al. (2009) Evaluation of nine candidate genes in patients with normal tension glaucoma: a case control study. BMC Med Genet 10: 91.

39. Narooie-Nejad M, Paylakhi SH, Shojaee S, Fazlali Z, Rezaei Kanavi M, et al. (2009) Loss of function mutations in the gene encoding latent transforming growth factor beta binding protein 2, LTBP2, cause primary congenital glaucoma. Hum Mol Genet 18(20): 3969–3977.

40. Sud A, Del Bono EA, Haines JL, Wiggs JL (2008) Fine mapping of the GLC1K juvenile primary open-angle glaucoma locus and exclusion of candidate genes. Mol Vis 4: 1319–1326.

41. Liu Y, Schmidt S, Qin X, Gibson J, Hutchins K, et al. (2008) Lack of association between LOXL1 variants and primary open-angle glaucoma in three different populations. Invest Ophthalmol Vis Sci 49(8): 3465–3468.

42. Thorleifsson G, Magnusson KP, Sulem P, Walters GB, Gudbjartsson DF, et al. (2007) Common sequence variants in the LOXL1 gene confer susceptibility to exfoliation glaucoma. Science 317(5843): 1397–1400.

43. Kumar A, Basavaraj MG, Gupta SK, Qamar I, Ali AM, et al. (2007) Role of CYP1B1, MYOC, OPTN, and OPTC genes in adult-onset primary open-angle glaucoma: predominance of CYP1B1 mutations in Indian patients. Mol Vis 13: 667–676.

44. Bill A, Svedberg B (1972) Scanning electron microscopic studies of the trabecular meshwork and the canal of Schlemm: an attempt to localize the main resistance to outflow of aqueous humor in man. Acta Ophthalmol 50: 295–320.

45. Wiedelholt M, Bielka S, Schweig F, Lütjen-Drecoll E, Lepple-Wienhues A (1995) Regulation of outflow rate and resistance in the perfused anterior segment of the bovine eye. Exp Eye Res 61: 223–234.

46. Filla MS, Woods A, Kaufman PL, Peters DM (2006) Beta1 and beta3 integrins cooperate to induce syndecan-4-containing cross-linked actin networks in human trabecular meshwork cells. Invest Ophthalmol Vis Sci 47(5): 1956–1967.

47. Peterson JA, Sheibani N, David G, Garcia-Pardo A, Peters DM (2005) Heparin II domain of fibronectin uses alpha4beta1 integrin to control focal adhesion and stress fiber formation, independent of syndecan-4. J Biol Chem 25 280(8): 6915–6922.

48. Diskin S, Cao Z, Leffler H, Panjwani N (2009) The role of integrin glycosylation in galectin-8-mediated trabecular meshwork cell adhesion and spreading. Glycobiology 19(1): 29–37.

49. Fukaya M, Hayashi Y, Watanabe M (2005) NR2 to NR3B subnit switchover of NMDA receptors in early postnatal motoneurons. Eur J Neurosci 21: 1432–1436.

# 2

# Association of *Glutathione S transferases* Polymorphisms with Glaucoma

**Yibo Yu¹, Yu Weng², Jing Guo³, Guangdi Chen³\*, Ke Yao¹\***

**1** Eye Center of the 2^nd Affiliated Hospital, Zhejiang University School of Medicine, Hangzhou, China, **2** Department of Clinical Laboratory, Sir Run Run Shaw Hospital, Zhejiang University School of Medicine, Hangzhou, China, **3** Department of Public Health, Zhejiang University School of Medicine, Hangzhou, China

## Abstract

**Background:** *Glutathione S transferase* (*GST*) polymorphisms have been considered risk factors for the development of glaucoma, including primary open angle glaucoma (POAG) and other types of glaucoma. However, the results remain controversial. In this study, we have conducted a meta-analysis to assess the association between polymorphisms of *GSTM1*, *GSTT1* and *GSTP1* and glaucoma risk.

**Methods:** Published literature from PubMed and other databases were retrieved. All studies evaluating the association between *GSTM1*, *GSTT1* and *GSTP1* polymorphisms and glaucoma risk were included. Pooled odds ratio (OR) and 95% confidence interval (CI) were calculated using random- or fixed-effects model.

**Results:** Twelve studies on *GSTM1* (1109 cases and 844 controls), ten studies on *GSTT1* (709 cases and 664 controls) and four studies on *GSTP1* (543 cases and 511 controls) were included. By pooling all the studies, either *GSTM1* or *GSTT1* null polymorphism was not associated with a POAG risk, and this negative association maintained in Caucasian. The *GSTP1* Ile 105 Val polymorphism was significantly correlated with increased POAG risk among Caucasian in a recessive model (Val/Val *vs.* Ile/Ile+Ile/Val: OR, 1.62, 95%CI: 1.00–2.61). Interestingly, increased glaucoma risk was associated with the combined *GSTM1* and *GSTT1* null genotypes (OR, 2.20; 95% CI, 1.47–3.31), and with the combined *GSTM1* null and *GSTP1* Val genotypes (OR, 1.86; 95% CI, 1.15–3.01).

**Conclusions:** This meta-analysis suggests that combinations of *GST* polymorphisms are associated with glaucoma risk. Given the limited sample size, the associations between single *GST* polymorphism and glaucoma risk await further investigation.

**Editor:** Yingfeng Zheng, Zhongshan Ophthalmic Center, China

**Funding:** This work was supported by the Zhejiang Key Innovation Team Project of China (No. 2009R50039), the Zhejiang Key Laboratory Fund of China (No. 2011E10006), the National Natural Science Foundation of China (No. 30900273), the Qianjiang Talents Program of Zhejiang Province (2012R10023) and the Fundamental Research Funds for the Central Universities (No. 2011QNA7018, 2012QNA7019). Dr. Guangdi Chen was supported by Technology Foundation for Excellent Overseas Chinese Scholar, Zhejiang Province Human Resources and Social Security Bureau. The funders had no role in study design, data collection and analysis, decision to publish, or preparation of the manuscript.

**Competing Interests:** The authors have declared that no competing interests exist.

\* E-mail: chenguangdi@gmail.com (GC); xlren@zju.edu.cn (KY)

## Introduction

Glaucoma is a heterogeneous group of diseases characterized by the death of the retinal ganglion cells and progressive degeneration of the optic nerve. It is, the second most frequent cause of irreversible blindness in the world and affects primarily the older population, estimated to affect about 80 million people worldwide by 2020 [1]. However, the etiology of glaucoma remains obscure. Risk factors for glaucoma include aging, elevated intraocular pressure, variable susceptibility of the optic nerve, vascular factors (ischemia), diabetes, myopia, cigarette smoking and positive family history [2]. Glaucoma can be inherited as a Mendelian autosomal-dominant or autosomal-recessive trait, or as a complex multifactorial trait [3]. Genetic approaches have defined the causative genes (e.g., *MYOC*, *OPTN* and *WDR36*) for juvenile-onset and late-onset primary open angle glaucoma (POAG) [4]. In addition to these genes, over 20 gene variants were found to be associated with glaucoma [5]. Recently, large-scale genome-wide association studies have been conducted to map the genes for glaucoma [6,7,8].

Growing evidence supports the involvement of oxidative stress as a common component of glaucomatous neurodegeneration in different subcellular compartments of retinal ganglion cells (RGCs), by acting as a second messenger and/or modulating protein function by redox modifications of downstream effectors through enzymatic oxidation of specific substrates [9]. There are many defensive mechanisms against this oxidative damage, including catalase, superoxide dismutase, glutathione peroxidase, and glutathione S transferase (GST) in the eye for protection. Among them, GST is a multigene family with different enzymes that play an important role in the anti-oxidation, detoxification and elimination of xenobiotics, including carcinogens, oxidants, toxins, and drugs [10]. Human GST enzymes mainly include members of eight classes, assigned on the basis of sequence similarity: Alpha (GSTA), Mu (GSTM), Pi (GSTP), Theta

(GSTT), Kappa (GSTK), Zeta (GSTZ), Omega (GSTO), and Sigma (GSTS) [11].

Previous studies of allelic variants in these classes have identified two major polymorphisms of the *GSTT1* and *GSTM1* genes caused by a deletion in each gene, and a single-nucleotide polymorphism (SNP) of *GSTP1* resulting in the coding sequence change Ile 105 Val [11]. The deletion of *GSTT1* or *GSTM1*, or *GSTP1* Ile 105 Val polymorphism results in an absence of their enzyme activity [12,13,14], and these polymorphisms of *GST* have been associated with altered risk of a variety of pathologies including cancer [15], cardiovascular disease [16], respiratory disease [17], and ophthalmologic problems such as cataract [18,19]. The relationship between *GST* polymorphisms and risk of glaucoma has been studied for more than 10 years. Several studies have found *GST* polymorphisms to be protective or risk factors in POAG [20,21,22,23,24,25,26] or other types of glaucoma [27], but other studies show no association between *GST* polymorphisms and risk of glaucoma [28,29]. These studies revealed an inconsistent conclusion, probably due to the relatively small size of subjects, since individual studies are usually underpowered in detecting the effect of low penetrance genes; therefore, in this study we conducted a meta-analysis to investigate the associations between *GSTM1*, *GSTT1*, and *GSTP1* polymorphisms and the risk for glaucoma.

## Materials and Methods

### Identification and Eligibility of Relevant Studies

To identify all articles that examined the association of *GST* polymorphism with glaucoma, we conducted a literature search in the PubMed databases up to August 2012 using the following MeSH terms and keywords: "glutathione S transferase", "polymorphism" and "glaucoma". Additional studies were identified by a manual search from other sources (e.g., Web of Knowledge), references of original studies or review articles on this topic. Eligible studies included in this meta-analysis had to meet the following criteria: (a) evaluation of the association between *GSTM1* or *GSTT1* null genotypes, or *GSTP1* Ile 105 Val polymorphism and glaucoma, (b) an unrelated case-control study, if studies had partly overlapped subjects, only the one with a larger sample size was selected, (c) available genotype frequency, (d) sufficient published data for estimating an odds ratio (OR) with 95% confidence interval (CI), and (e) papers published in English from 2000.

### Data Extraction

Two investigators independently assessed the articles for inclusion/exclusion and extracted data, and reached a consensus on all of the items. For each study, the following information was extracted: name of the first author; publication year; ethnicity (country); sample size (numbers of cases and controls); gene polymorphisms investigated; types of glaucoma; sources of samples; genotyping methods.

### Statistical Analysis

The association between *GSTM1*, *GSTT1* or *GSTP1* polymorphism and glaucoma was estimated by calculating pooled odd ratios (ORs) and 95% CIs. The significance of the pooled OR was determined by Z test ($P<0.05$ was considered statistically significant). The risk of *GSTM1* or *GSTT1* null genotype on glaucoma was evaluated by comparing with their reference wild type homozygote. For the *GSTP1* polymorphism, we first estimated the risks of the Ile/Val and Val/Val genotypes on glaucoma, compared with the reference Ile/Ile homozygote, and then evaluated the risks of (Ile/Val+Val/Val *vs.* Ile/Ile) and (Val/Val *vs.* Ile/Ile+Ile/Val) on glaucoma, assuming dominant and recessive effects of the variant Val/Val allele, respectively. The $I^2$-based Q statistic test was performed to evaluate variations due to heterogeneity rather than chance. A random-effects (DerSimonian-Laird method) or fixed-effects (Mantel-Haenszel method) model was used to calculate pooled effect estimates in the presence ($P\leq0.10$) or absence ($P>0.10$) of heterogeneity. Publication bias was detected by Egger's test [30] and Begg's [31] test for the overall pooled analysis of *GSTM1* and *GSTT1* null genotypes, and recessive model of *GSTP1*. Additionally, Begg's funnel plot was drawn. Asymmetry of the funnel plot means a potential publication bias. Stratified analyses were also performed by types of glaucoma and ethnicities of study populations. For the one-way sensitivity analysis, one single study was excluded each time, and the new pooled results could reflect the influence of that deleted study to the overall summary OR. All analyses were done with Stata software (version 11.0; Stata Corp LP, College Station, TX), using two-sided *P* values.

## Results

### Characteristics of Studies

Thirteen abstracts were retrieved through the search "glutathione S transferase", "polymorphism" and "glaucoma", and ten studies meeting the inclusion criteria were identified as eligible [20,22,23,24,26,27,28,29,32,33]. Out of the thirteen, one was commentary [34], and one was *in vitro* study to evaluate the sensitivity to oxidative stress of anterior chamber tissues [35]. One article was excluded due to the study on the relationship between GST polymorphisms and risk of age-related macular degeneration [36]. We also included two eligible studies with manual searching [21,25]. As a result, a total of twelve studies met the inclusion criteria and were identified as eligible articles (Figure 1).

Twelve studies were included in the meta-analysis of *GSTM1* genotype (1908 cases, 1457 controls), ten studies for *GSTT1* genotype (1414 cases, 1177 controls) and four studies for *GSTP1* polymorphism (543 cases, 511 controls). For the ethnicities, eleven studies of Caucasians and one study of Asians were included on the *GSTM1* genotype. As to *GSTT1*, night studies of Caucasians and one study of Asians were included. The four studies on *GSTP1* were all based on the Caucasians. For the glaucoma type, this meta-analysis included ten, eight, and three studies on the relationship between *GSTM1*, *GSTT1*, and *GSTP1* polymorphism and risk of POAG (the most common form of glaucoma), respectively. In addition, we included four and three studies on the association between the *GSTM1* and *GSTT1* polymorphism and risk of other types of glaucoma (including exfoliative glaucoma and primary closed angle glaucoma), respectively. In addition to the study by Juronen et al. [20], in which the *GSTM1* and *GSTT1* phenotypes were determined with monoclonal antibody based enzyme-linked immunosorbent assay (ELISA), the genotyping for *GSTM1*, *GSTT1* or GSTP1 was performed using polymerase chain reaction (PCR) in all other studies. The detailed characteristics of each study included in the meta-analysis are presented in Table 1, and the *GST* polymorphism genotype distributions from each study are presented in Table S1 and S2.

### Quantitative Synthesis

Table 2 shows the results of the meta-analysis on the association between *GSTM1* or *GSTT1* null polymorphism and risk of glaucoma. By pooling all the studies, either *GSTM1* or *GSTT1* null polymorphism was not associated with a glaucoma risk, and this negative association maintained in Caucasian (Table 2, and

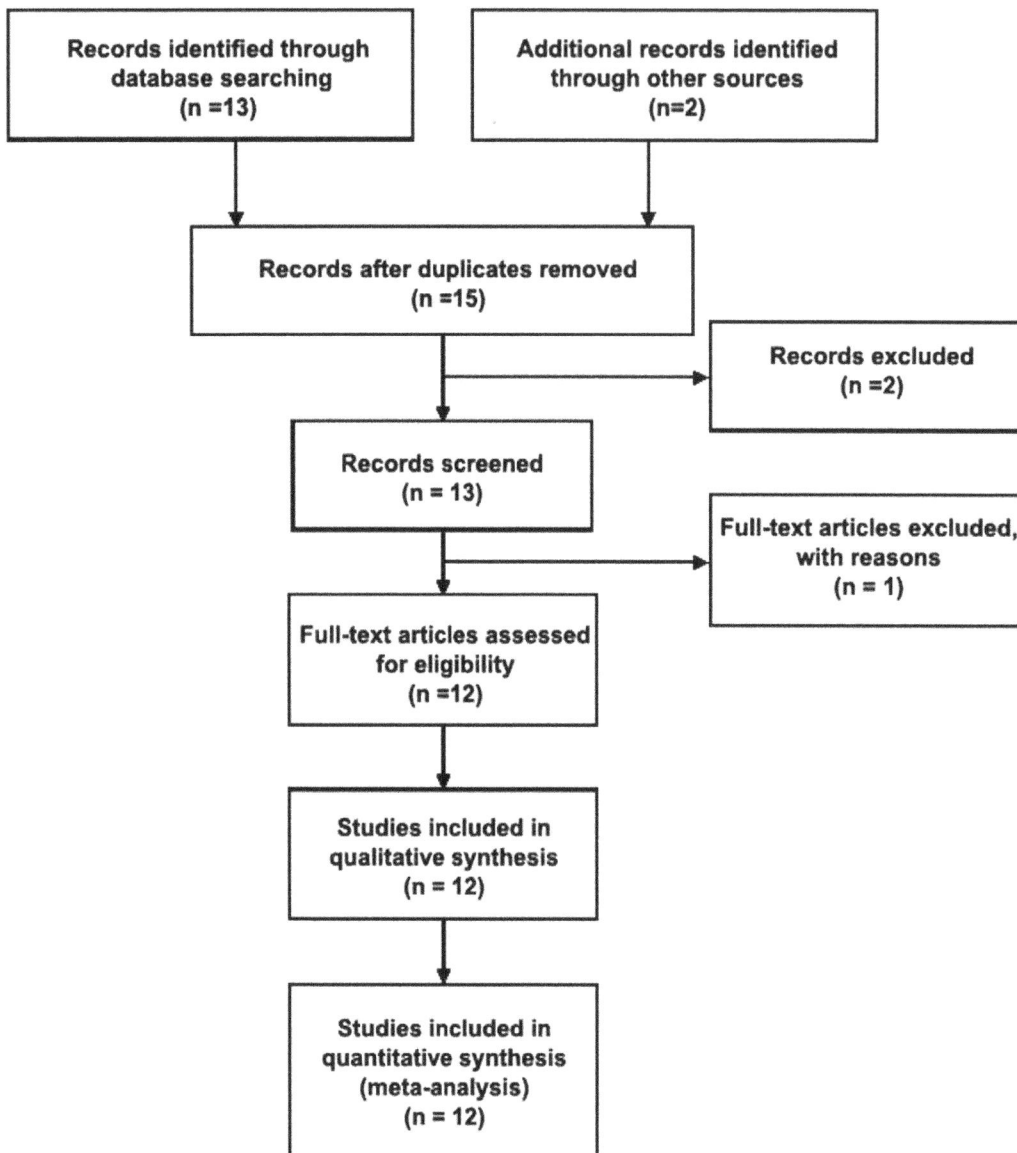

**Figure 1. Flow diagram of studies identification.**

Figure S1 and S2). When stratified by glaucoma types, no association was found between *GSTM1* or *GSTT1* null polymorphism and risk of POAG, or other types of glaucoma, in all populations or in Caucasians.

We also examined the association between *GSTP1* Ile 105 Val polymorphism and glaucoma risk, and the overall result showed that *GSTP1* polymorphism was not correlated with glaucoma risk in all four models by pooling all four studies (Table 3 and Figure S3). In subgroup analysis, we found that *GSTP1* Ile 105 Val polymorphism was significantly correlated with increased POAG risk in a recessive model (Val/Val *vs.* Ile/Ile+ Ile/Val: OR, 1.62; 95%CI, 1.00–2.61; *P* = 0.049) but not in other three models. Interestingly, these three studies were all based on Caucasian populations, thus, *GSTP1* Ile 105 Val polymorphism in recessive model was associated with increased POAG risk in Caucasians (Table 3).

To investigate if the profiles of *GST* genotypes were associated with the risk of glaucoma, we first examined the association

between combinations of *GSTM1* and *GSTT1* null genotypes and the risk of glaucoma, in which the reference group consisted of individuals with both putative low-risk genotypes, i.e., the presence of *GSTM1* and *GSTT1* genotypes [22]. Table 4 displays the risk of glaucoma associated with combinations of *GST* null genotypes as well as the trend in risk associated with each putative high-risk null genotype. The data showed a significant association between increased glaucoma risk and the combined *GSTM1* and *GSTT1* null genotypes in all population (OR, 2.20; 95% CI, 1.47–3.31; *P*<0.001). When stratified by the types of glaucoma, combination of *GSTM1* and *GSTT1* null genotypes was associated with increased risk of POAG (OR, 1.90; 95% CI, 1.15–3.13; *P* = 0.013) but not other types of glaucoma (OR, 3.04; 95% CI, 0.95–9.72; *P* = 0.061). We also examined if the risk of glaucoma was associated with combinations of *GSTP1* and *GSTM1*, or *GSTT1* genotypes, in which the homozygous Ile/Ile genotype for *GSTP1* was used as reference and the individuals heterozygous and homozygous for the Ile 105 Val allele was combined [22]. The

**Table 1.** Characteristics of literatures included in the meta-analysis.

| Author/Year [Reference] | Origin | Ethnicity | Case/control | GST family | Glaucoma Type* | Samples | Genotype |
|---|---|---|---|---|---|---|---|
| Juronen 2000 [20] | Estonia | Caucasian | 250/202 | GSTM1/GSTT1/GSTP1 | POAG | Blood | ELISA |
| Izzotti 2003 [21] | Italy | Caucasian | 45/46 | GSTM1/GSTT1 | POAG | Trabecular meshwork | PCR |
| Jansson 2003 [33] | Sweden | Caucasian | 388/200 | GSTM1 | POAG/Others | Blood | PCR |
| Yilmaz 2005 [28] | Turkey | Caucasian | 53/65 | GSTM1/GSTT1/GSTP1 | Others | Blood | PCR |
| Yildirim 2005 [22] | Turkey | Caucasian | 153/159 | GSTM1/GSTT1/GSTP1 | POAG | Blood | PCR |
| Unal 2007 [23] | Turkey | Caucasian | 144/121 | GSTM1/GSTT1 | POAG | Blood | PCR |
| Abu-Amero 2008 [24] | Saudi Arabia | Caucasian | 107/120 | GSTM1/GSTT1 | POAG/Others | Blood | PCR |
| Rasool 2010 [25] | Egypt | Caucasian | 32/16 | GSTM1/GSTT1 | POAG | Trabeculectomy specimens | PCR |
| Fan 2010 [29] | China | Asian | 405/201 | GSTM1/GSTT1 | POAG | Blood | PCR |
| Khan 2010 [27] | Pakistan | Caucasian | 165/162 | GSTM1/GSTT1 | Others | Blood | PCR |
| Izzotti 2010 [32] | Italy | Caucasian | 100/100 | GSTM1 | POAG | Trabecular meshwork | PCR |
| Rocha 2011 [26] | Brazil | Caucasian | 87/85 | GSTM1/GSTT1/GSTP1 | POAG | Blood | PCR |

*Others: including exfoliative and primary closed angle glaucoma.
Abbreviations: POAG, primary closed angle glaucoma; PCR, Polymerase chain reaction; ELISA, enzyme-linked immunosorbent assay.

**Table 2.** Subgroup Analysis of the Association between GSTM1 and GSTT1 Polymorphisms and the Risk for Glaucoma.

| Groups | n[†] | Statistical Method | OR (95% CI) | P |
|---|---|---|---|---|
| **All Glaucoma** | | | | |
| GSTM1 null | | | | |
| Pooled | 12 | Random | 1.25 (0.82- 1.90) | 0.290 |
| Caucasian | 11 | Random | 1.25 (0.77- 2.04) | 0.361 |
| Asian | 1 | | | |
| GSTT1 null | | | | |
| Pooled | 10 | Random | 1.37 (0.82- 2.28) | 0.229 |
| Caucasian | 9 | Random | 1.49 (0.83- 2.67) | 0.183 |
| Asian | 1 | 1 | | |
| **POAG** | | | | |
| GSTM1 null | | | | |
| Pooled | 10 | Random | 1.23 (0.74- 2.03) | 0.426 |
| Caucasian | 9 | Random | 1.24 (0.68- 2.27) | 0.474 |
| Asian | 1 | | | |
| GSTT1 null | | | | |
| Pooled | 8 | Random | 1.42 (0.80- 2.52) | 0.237 |
| Caucasian | 7 | Random | 1.61 (0.80- 3.24) | 0.182 |
| Asian | 1 | | | |
| **Others*** | | | | |
| GSTM1 null | | | | |
| Pooled | 4 | Random | 1.64 (0.82–3.28) | 0.164 |
| GSTT1 null | | | | |
| Pooled | 3 | Random | 2.13 (0.59–7.72) | 0.248 |

*Others: including exfoliative and primary closed angle glaucoma.
[†]n: number of studies.
Abbreviations: POAG, primary closed angle glaucoma.

results showed that that increased glaucoma risk was associated with the combined GSTM1 null and GSTP1 Val genotypes (OR, 1.86; 95% CI, 1.15–3.01; $P=0.012$), but the combined GSTT1 null and GSTP1 Val genotypes played a protective role in glaucoma risk which, which remained of borderline statistical significance (OR, 0.60; 95% CI, 0.36–1.00; $P=0.051$).

## Potential Publication Bias and Sensitivity Analysis

Publication bias was firstly detected by Begg's test for the overall pooled analysis of GSTM1 and GSTT1 null genotypes, and the recessive model of GSTP1 polymorphism. The Begg's test showed that the P value for GSTM1, GSTT1 and GSTP1 polymorphism was 1.00, 0.371 and 1.00 respectively, and the corresponding funnel plots showed symmetric distribution (Figure 2). The Egger's test also showed that All the P values were more than 0.05 (Data not shown). Thus, no evident publication bias was found in present study. Sensitivity analysis was conducted by deleting each study in turn from the pooled analysis to examine the influence of the removed data set to the overall ORs. As shown in Figure S4, S5, S6, exclusion of each study did not influence the result in specific genotype comparison for GST polymorphism, suggesting that the results of synthetic analysis were robust.

## Discussion

In the present study, we systemically reviewed all available published studies and performed a meta-analysis to examine the association between the GST polymorphisms and susceptibility to glaucoma. Our meta-analysis showed that single GSTM1 or GSTT1 null polymorphism was not associated with glaucoma risk, and GSTP1 Ile 105 Val polymorphism in recessive model was positively correlated with increased glaucoma risk. The combination of GSTM1 null and GSTT1 null, or GSTM1 null and GSTP1 genotype was associated with increased risk of glaucoma. Although different types of glaucoma have their own clinical characteristics and pathogenesis, our meta-analysis indicates that GST polymorphisms may contribute to increased risk of glaucoma.

**Table 3.** Meta-analysis of the *GSTP1* Ile105Val polymorphism on glaucoma risk.

| Groups | n[†] | Ile/Val vs. Ile/Ile | | Val/Val vs. Ile/Ile | | Ile/Val +Val/Val vs. Ile/Ile (dominant) | | Val/Val vs. Ile/Ile +Ile/Val (recessive) | |
|---|---|---|---|---|---|---|---|---|---|
| | | OR (95% CI) | P | OR (95% CI) | P | OR (95% CI) | P | OR (95% CI) | P |
| All glaucoma | | | | | | | | | |
| Pooled | 4 | 0.95(0.73–1.24) | 0.700 | 1.17(0.51–2.68) | 0.706[‡] | 1.00(0.78–1.29) | 0.987 | 1.18(0.50–2.80) | 0.708[‡] |
| Glaucoma type | | | | | | | | | |
| POAG | 3 | 0.92(0.70–1.23) | 0.587 | 1.55(0.94–2.55) | 0.087 | 1.03(0.79–1.34) | 0.836 | 1.62(1.00–2.61) | 0.049 |
| Others[*] | 1 | | | | | | | | |

*Others: including exfoliative glaucoma.
[†]Number of studies.
[‡]A random-effects model was used to calculate pooled effect estimates.
Abbreviations: POAG, primary closed angle glaucoma.

Previously, the study by Juronen et al. suggests that the *GSTM1* positive phenotype may be a genetic risk factor for development of POAG [20]. However, the following studies show that the *GSTM1*

**Table 4.** Subgroup Analysis of the Association between *GSTM1*, *GSTT1* and *GSTP1* Polymorphisms and the Risk for Glaucoma.

| Groups[*] | n[†] | Statistical Method | OR (95% CI) | P |
|---|---|---|---|---|
| ***GSTM1 GSTT1*** | | | | |
| Pooled | | | | |
| *GSTM1* null | 7 | Random | 1.42 (0.66- 3.04) | 0.373 |
| *GSTT1* null | 7 | Random | 1.79 (0.76- 4.21) | 0.180 |
| *GSTM1* null+*GSTT1* null | 7 | Fixed | 2.20 (1.47- 3.31) | <0.001 |
| POAG | | | | |
| *GSTM1* null | 5 | Random | 1.32 (0.43- 4.08) | 0.633 |
| *GSTT1* null | 5 | Random | 1.99 (0.64- 6.19) | 0.236 |
| *GSTM1* null+*GSTT1* null | 5 | Fixed | 1.90 (1.15- 3.13) | 0.013 |
| Others[*] | | | | |
| *GSTM1* null | 3 | Random | 2.72 (1.05- 7.00) | 0.039 |
| *GSTT1* null | 3 | Random | 2.40 (0.61- 9.53) | 0.212 |
| *GSTM1* null+*GSTT1* null | 3 | Random | 3.04 (0.95- 9.72) | 0.061 |
| ***GSTM1 GSTP1*** | | | | |
| Pooled | | | | |
| *GSTM1* null | 3 | Fixed | 1.16 (0.74- 1.83) | 0.523 |
| *GSTP1* Val allele | 3 | Fixed | 0.69 (0.44- 1.07) | 0.099 |
| *GSTM1* null+*GSTP1* Val allele | 3 | Fixed | 1.86 (1.15- 3.00) | 0.011 |
| ***GSTT1 GSTP1*** | | | | |
| Pooled | | | | |
| *GSTT1* null | 3 | Fixed | 1.07 (0.62- 1.83) | 0.818 |
| *GSTP1* Val allele | 3 | Fixed | 1.17 (0.81- 1.69) | 0.395 |
| *GSTT1* null+*GSTP1* Val allele | 3 | Fixed | 0.60 (0.36- 1.00) | 0.051 |

*Others: including exfoliative, pseudoexfoliative and primary closed angle glaucoma.
[†]n: number of studies.
Abbreviations: POAG, primary closed angle glaucoma.

null genotype is a risk factor for development of POAG [22,26], while another study showed otherwise [33]. By pooled 10 studies, we did not find an association between *GSTM1* polymorphism and POAG, suggesting that previous controversial data may be due to small size of population. As to *GSTP1*, previous studies did not identify differences between POAG patients and control individuals in the frequencies of *GSTP1* Ile 105 Val genotypes [20,22,26,28]; however, by pooled these studies, we found that *GSTP1* polymorphism was significantly correlated with increased POAG risk in Caucasian in a recessive model. It should be noted that the statistical significance of the association between the *GSTP1* polymorphism and POAG risk was at borderline level. The *GSTP1* 105-Val allele homozygote was correlated with increased POAG risk but the difference did not reach statistical significance (OR, 1.55; 95% CI, 0.94–2.55). Since the studies included were very limited, it is necessary to validate the association between *GSTP1* Ile 105 Val polymorphism and glaucoma risk in future studies.

To the best of our knowledge, this is the first meta-analysis assessing the association between single *GST* polymorphism, or combination of *GST* polymorphisms and glaucoma. Previously, Yildirin et al. reported an increasing glaucoma risk with higher numbers of the combined of *GSTM1* null and *GSTP1* 105-Val allele genotypes but this association was not significant [22]. Our meta-analysis results showed that the association between combined of *GSTM1* and *GSTT1* null genotypes, or *GSTM1* null and *GSTP1* Val genotypes, and the risk for glaucoma is statistically significant in Caucasians. The study by Yildirin et al. also found a trend of increasing glaucoma risk with higher numbers of the combined *GSTM1* null, *GSTT1* null and *GSTP1* 105-Val allele genotypes (OR, 2.3; 95% CI: 0.75–7.08) [22]. Due to the limited studies, we did not perform meta-analysis for association between the combined *GSTM1* null, *GSTT1* null and *GSTP1* 105-Val allele genotypes and glaucoma risk. The current available data support the multifactorial nature of glaucoma, and both genetic and environmental factors are involved in pathogenesis of glaucoma. However, most studies did not provide *GST* polymorphisms when stratified by environmental factors (e. g., smoking). The relationship between polymorphic *GST* with other genetic and environmental glaucoma risk factors may be highly complicated, and extensive research is required to ascertain how exactly the *GST* genotype affects the individual susceptibility to glaucoma.

Meta-analysis has advantages compared to individual studies, however, some potential limitations in our study should be considered. First, this meta-analysis was limited by the small

## Begg's funnel plot with pseudo 95% confidence limits

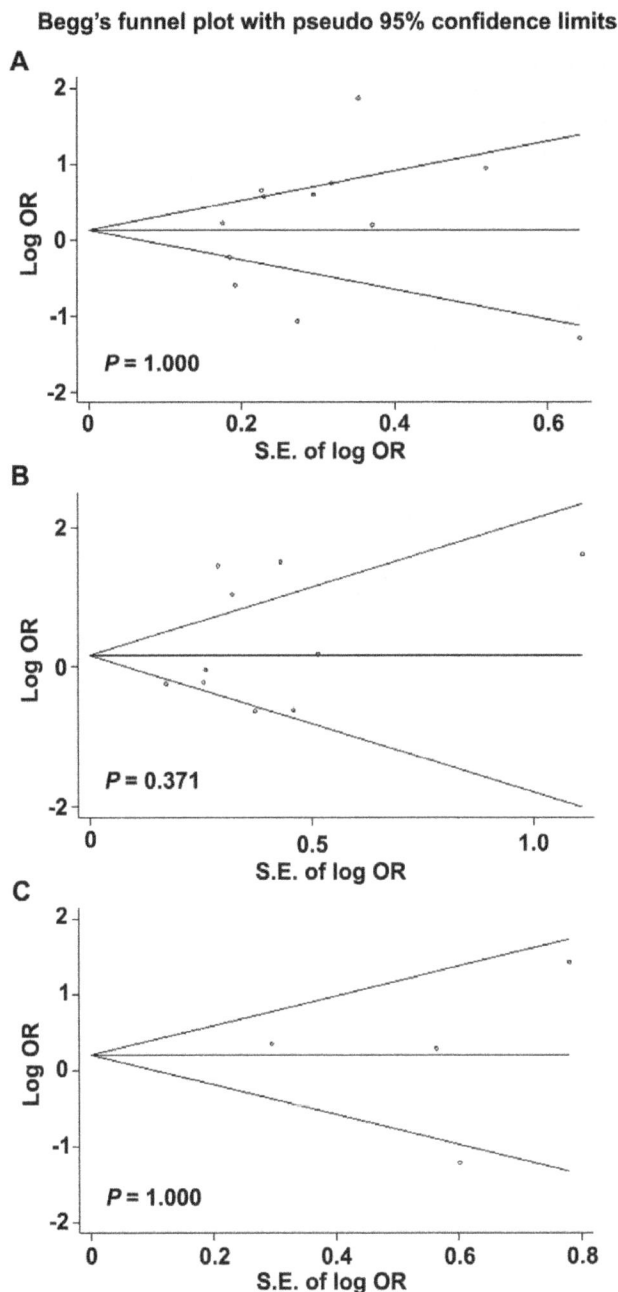

**Figure 2. Funnel plots showed symmetric distribution.** Log OR is plotted against the standard error of log OR for studies on *GSTM1* null (A), *GSTT1* null (B) and *GSTP1* Ile 105 Val (recessive model) (C) polymorphism. The dots represent specific studies for the indicated association.

sample size, especially in subgroup analysis aforementioned (e.g., studies on *GSTP1* polymorphism), which needs further investigations. Second, basic methodological differences among the studies might have affected the results. In addition to three studies [20,22,28], the controls recruited in other studies were hospital-based [21,23,24,25,26,27,29,32,33]. Most of studies used PCR methods for genotyping, but the study by Juronen et al. [20] used enzyme-linked immunosorbent assay. Although excluding this study did not affect the result of *GSTM1* and *GSTT1* genotypes, the association between *GSTP1* polymorphism and POAG risk in

Caucasian was not significant due to the limited studies (n = 2) (Data not shown). Third, the studies differed in their procedure for sampling. Three studies used trabeculectomy specimens [25,32,33] while other studies used blood. We found no association between each single *GST* polymorphism and glaucoma risk in each subgroup analysis when the samples were stratified as trabeculectomy specimens or blood, and excluding one study using trabeculectomy specimens as samples did not affect the results on the associations between the combinations of *GST* polymorphisms and glaucoma risk (Data not shown). Fourth, most of the studies included in this meta-analysis did not categorize the POAG patients as high- and normal-tension glaucoma. So, we did not analyze the association between *GST* polymorphism and risk of high- or normal-tension glaucoma, and future studies should address this point. Last, the Caucasian group might have been genetically heterogeneous, with differences in terms of lifestyle and environment (e.g., European *vs.* Arabian). These factors may explain the heterogeneity in meta-analysis for Caucasian populations.

In summary, the present meta-analysis suggested that combination of *GSTM1* and *GSTT1* null genotypes, and *GSTM1* null and *GSTP1* 105-Val allele genotypes are associated with increased risk for glaucoma in Caucasian populations. The association between single *GST* polymorphism and glaucoma is either negative or evidence limited. More epidemiologic studies are suggested to further ascertain the relationship between *GST* polymorphisms and genetic predisposition to glaucoma.

## Supporting Information

**Figure S1 Forest plots of the association between *GSTM1* null polymorphism and glaucoma risk.**

**Figure S2 Forest plots of the association between *GSTT1* null polymorphism and glaucoma risk.**

**Figure S3 Forest plots of the association between *GSTP1* Ile 105 Val polymorphism and glaucoma risk.**

**Figure S4 Sensitivity analysis for *GSTM1* null polymorphism.**

**Figure S5 Sensitivity analysis for *GSTT1* null polymorphism.**

**Figure S6 Sensitivity analysis for *GSTP1* Ile 105 Val polymorphism.**

**Table S1 *GSTM1 and GSTT1* polymorphism genotype distribution of each study included in the meta-analysis.**

**Table S2 *GSTP1* Ile 105 Val polymorphism genotype distribution of each study included in the meta-analysis.**

## Author Contributions

Conceived and designed the experiments: YY KY GC. Performed the experiments: YY YW JG. Analyzed the data: YY JG GC. Contributed reagents/materials/analysis tools: KY GC. Wrote the paper: YY YW KY GC.

# References

1.  Quigley HA, Broman AT (2006) The number of people with glaucoma worldwide in 2010 and 2020. Br J Ophthalmol 90: 262–267.
2.  Worley A, Grimmer-Somers K (2011) Risk factors for glaucoma: what do they really mean? Aust J Prim Health 17: 233–239.
3.  Wiggs JL (2007) Genetic etiologies of glaucoma. Arch Ophthalmol 125: 30–37.
4.  Fan BJ, Wang DY, Lam DS, Pang CP (2006) Gene mapping for primary open angle glaucoma. Clin Biochem 39: 249–258.
5.  Allingham RR, Liu Y, Rhee DJ (2009) The genetics of primary open-angle glaucoma: a review. Exp Eye Res 88: 837–844.
6.  van Koolwijk LM, Ramdas WD, Ikram MK, Jansonius NM, Pasutto F, et al. (2012) Common genetic determinants of intraocular pressure and primary open-angle glaucoma. PLoS Genet 8: e1002611.
7.  Vithana EN, Khor CC, Qiao C, Nongpiur ME, George R, et al. (2012) Genome-wide association analyses identify three new susceptibility loci for primary angle closure glaucoma. Nat Genet 44: 1142–1146.
8.  Wiggs JL, Yaspan BL, Hauser MA, Kang JH, Allingham RR, et al. (2012) Common variants at 9p21 and 8q22 are associated with increased susceptibility to optic nerve degeneration in glaucoma. PLoS Genet 8: e1002654.
9.  Tezel G (2006) Oxidative stress in glaucomatous neurodegeneration: mechanisms and consequences. Prog Retin Eye Res 25: 490–513.
10. Eaton DL, Bammler TK (1999) Concise review of the glutathione S-transferases and their significance to toxicology. Toxicol Sci 49: 156–164.
11. Josephy PD (2010) Genetic variations in human glutathione transferase enzymes: significance for pharmacology and toxicology. Hum Genomics Proteomics 2010: 876940.
12. Johansson AS, Stenberg G, Widersten M, Mannervik B (1998) Structure-activity relationships and thermal stability of human glutathione transferase P1–1 governed by the H-site residue 105. J Mol Biol 278: 687–698.
13. Hayes JD, Strange RC (2000) Glutathione S-transferase polymorphisms and their biological consequences. Pharmacology 61: 154–166.
14. Ginsberg G, Smolenski S, Hattis D, Guyton KZ, Johns DO, et al. (2009) Genetic Polymorphism in Glutathione Transferases (GST): Population distribution of GSTM1, T1, and P1 conjugating activity. J Toxicol Environ Health B Crit Rev 12: 389–439.
15. Ye Z, Song H (2005) Glutathione s-transferase polymorphisms (GSTM1, GSTP1 and GSTT1) and the risk of acute leukaemia: a systematic review and meta-analysis. Eur J Cancer 41: 980–989.
16. Ramprasath T, Senthil Murugan P, Prabakaran AD, Gomathi P, Rathinavel A, et al. (2011) Potential risk modifications of GSTT1, GSTM1 and GSTP1 (glutathione-S-transferases) variants and their association to CAD in patients with type-2 diabetes. Biochem Biophys Res Commun 407: 49–53.
17. Minelli C, Granell R, Newson R, Rose-Zerilli MJ, Torrent M, et al. (2010) Glutathione-S-transferase genes and asthma phenotypes: a Human Genome Epidemiology (HuGE) systematic review and meta-analysis including unpublished data. Int J Epidemiol 39: 539–562.
18. Juronen E, Tasa G, Veromann S, Parts L, Tiidla A, et al. (2000) Polymorphic glutathione S-transferases as genetic risk factors for senile cortical cataract in Estonians. Invest Ophthalmol Vis Sci 41: 2262–2267.
19. Sun L, Xi B, Yu L, Gao XC, Shi DJ, et al. (2010) Association of glutathione S-transferases polymorphisms (GSTM1 and GSTT1) with senile cataract: a meta-analysis. Invest Ophthalmol Vis Sci 51: 6381–6386.
20. Juronen E, Tasa G, Veromann S, Parts L, Tiidla A, et al. (2000) Polymorphic glutathione S-transferase M1 is a risk factor of primary open-angle glaucoma among Estonians. Exp Eye Res 71: 447–452.
21. Izzotti A, Sacca SC, Cartiglia C, De Flora S (2003) Oxidative deoxyribonucleic acid damage in the eyes of glaucoma patients. Am J Med 114: 638–646.
22. Yildirim O, Ates NA, Tamer L, Oz O, Yilmaz A, et al. (2005) May glutathione S-transferase M1 positive genotype afford protection against primary open-angle glaucoma? Graefes Arch Clin Exp Ophthalmol 243: 327–333.
23. Unal M, Guven M, Devranoglu K, Ozaydin A, Batar B, et al. (2007) Glutathione S transferase M1 and T1 genetic polymorphisms are related to the risk of primary open-angle glaucoma: a study in a Turkish population. Br J Ophthalmol 91: 527–530.
24. Abu-Amero KK, Morales J, Mohamed GH, Osman MN, Bosley TM (2008) Glutathione S-transferase M1 and T1 polymorphisms in Arab glaucoma patients. Mol Vis 14: 425–430.
25. Rasool HA, Nowier SR, Gheith M, Saif AS, Ismail S (2010) The Risk of Primary Open Angle Glaucoma and Glutathione S Transferase M1 and T1 Polymorphism among Egyptians. J Am Sci 6: 375–381.
26. Rocha AV, Talbot T, Magalhaes da Silva T, Almeida MC, Menezes CA, et al. (2011) Is the GSTM1 null polymorphism a risk factor in primary open angle glaucoma? Mol Vis 17: 1679–1686.
27. Khan MI, Micheal S, Akhtar F, Ahmed W, Ijaz B, et al. (2010) The association of glutathione S-transferase GSTT1 and GSTM1 gene polymorphism with pseudoexfoliative glaucoma in a Pakistani population. Mol Vis 16: 2146–2152.
28. Yilmaz A, Tamer L, Ates NA, Yildirim O, Yildirim H, et al. (2005) Is GST gene polymorphism a risk factor in developing exfoliation syndrome? Curr Eye Res 30: 575–581.
29. Fan BJ, Liu K, Wang DY, Tham CC, Tam PO, et al. (2010) Association of polymorphisms of tumor necrosis factor and tumor protein p53 with primary open-angle glaucoma. Invest Ophthalmol Vis Sci 51: 4110–4116.
30. Hayashino Y, Noguchi Y, Fukui T (2005) Systematic evaluation and comparison of statistical tests for publication bias. J Epidemiol 15: 235–243.
31. Begg CB, Mazumdar M (1994) Operating characteristics of a rank correlation test for publication bias. Biometrics 50: 1088–1101.
32. Izzotti A, Sacca SC, Longobardi M, Cartiglia C (2010) Mitochondrial damage in the trabecular meshwork of patients with glaucoma. Arch Ophthalmol 128: 724–730.
33. Jansson M, Rada A, Tomic L, Larsson LI, Wadelius C (2003) Analysis of the Glutathione S-transferase M1 gene using pyrosequencing and multiplex PCR– no evidence of association to glaucoma. Exp Eye Res 77: 239–243.
34. Izzotti A, Sacca SC (2004) Glutathione S-transferase M1 and its implications in glaucoma pathogenesis: a controversial matter. Exp Eye Res 79: 141–142.
35. Izzotti A, Sacca SC, Longobardi M, Cartiglia C (2009) Sensitivity of ocular anterior chamber tissues to oxidative damage and its relevance to the pathogenesis of glaucoma. Invest Ophthalmol Vis Sci 50: 5251–5258.
36. Othman H, Gholampour AR, Saadat I, Farvardin-Jahromoi M, Saadat M (2012) Age-related macular degeneration and genetic polymorphisms of glutathione S-transferases M1 (GSTM1) and T1 (GSTT1). Mol Biol Rep 39: 3299–3303.

# 3

# CXCR3 Antagonism of SDF-1(5-67) Restores Trabecular Function and Prevents Retinal Neurodegeneration in a Rat Model of Ocular Hypertension

Alexandre Denoyer[1,2,3,4]*, David Godefroy[1,2,3], Isabelle Célérier[5], Julie Frugier[1,2,3], Julie Degardin[1,2,3], Jeffrey K. Harrison[6], Francoise Brignole-Baudouin[1,2,3,7], Serge Picaud[1,2,3], Francoise Baleux[8], José A. Sahel[1,2,3,4], William Rostène[1,2,3⑨], Christophe Baudouin[1,2,3,4⑨]

1 UPMC University Paris 6, Institut de la Vision, UMRS968, Paris, France, 2 INSERM, U968, Paris, France, 3 CNRS, U7210, Paris, France, 4 Quinze-Vingts National Ophthalmology Hospital, Paris, France, 5 Team 1, Centre de Recherche des Cordeliers, INSERM, U872, Paris, France, 6 Department of Pharmacology & Therapeutics, College of Medicine, University of Florida, Gainesville, Florida, United States of America, 7 Department of Toxicology, Faculty of Biological and Pharmacological Sciences, University René Descartes Paris 05, Paris, France, 8 Unité de chimie des biomolécules, Institut Pasteur, CNRS 2128, Paris, France

## Abstract

Glaucoma, the most common cause of irreversible blindness, is a neuropathy commonly initiated by pathological ocular hypertension due to unknown mechanisms of trabecular meshwork degeneration. Current antiglaucoma therapy does not target the causal trabecular pathology, which may explain why treatment failure is often observed. Here we show that the chemokine CXCL12, its truncated form SDF-1(5-67), and the receptors CXCR4 and CXCR3 are expressed in human glaucomatous trabecular tissue and a human trabecular cell line. SDF-1(5-67) is produced under the control of matrix metallo-proteinases, TNF-$\alpha$, and TGF-$\beta$2, factors known to be involved in glaucoma. CXCL12 protects in vitro trabecular cells from apoptotic death via CXCR4 whereas SDF-1(5-67) induces apoptosis through CXCR3 and caspase activation. Ocular administration of SDF-1(5-67) in the rat increases intraocular pressure. In contrast, administration of a selective CXCR3 antagonist in a rat model of ocular hypertension decreases intraocular pressure, prevents retinal neurodegeneration, and preserves visual function. The protective effect of CXCR3 antagonism is related to restoration of the trabecular function. These data demonstrate that proteolytic cleavage of CXCL12 is involved in trabecular pathophysiology, and that local administration of a selective CXCR3 antagonist may be a beneficial therapeutic strategy for treating ocular hypertension and subsequent retinal degeneration.

**Editor:** Demetrios Vavvas, Massachusetts Eye & Ear Infirmary, Harvard Medical School, United States of America

**Funding:** This work was supported by INSERM grants for AD, DG, JD, WR and CB, by a UPMC grant for IC and JF, and by an NIH grant for JKH (AI058256). The funders had no role in study design, data collection and analysis, decision to publish, or preparation of the manuscript.

**Competing Interests:** The authors have declared that no competing interests exist.

* E-mail: alexandre.denoyer@gmail.com

⑨ These authors contributed equally to this work.

## Introduction

Primary open-angle glaucoma affects about 70 million people and is predicted to account for over 11 million cases of blindness by 2020 [1,2]. Its prevalence continues to increase as the population ages. Glaucoma is a retinal neuropathy characterized by retinal ganglion cell death. Pathological elevation of intraocular pressure (IOP), namely ocular hypertension (OHT), is the most critical risk factor for both the development and the progression of the disease [3]. OHT is often diagnosed several years before detecting the neuropathy. It is attributed to a decrease in trabecular meshwork (TM) outflow facility to aqueous humor (AH) caused by tissue degeneration whose primary mechanisms are still unclear. Classical antiglaucoma treatments reduce the abnormally elevated IOP but do not target directly the initial TM pathology. In clinical practice, progressive therapeutic inefficiency in controlling both the elevation of IOP and neuropathy often occurs [4]. The lack of specific therapies for the TM pathology, which is still developing in well-treated patients, could be

responsible for progressive treatment inefficiency coupled with neuropathy worsening and sometimes blindness.

TM degeneration has largely been demonstrated as the main cause of aqueous outflow resistance leading to OHT in primary open-angle glaucoma (5). The main glaucoma-related trabecular modifications resemble age-related TM degeneration and involve accumulation of trabecular extracellular matrix together with a decrease in TM cellularity as previously described by our group and others [6–9]. Trabecular cell (TC) loss that occurs in glaucoma is known to develop through apoptotic phenomena and was found as a characteristic of primary open-angle glaucoma [10], but its causal mechanisms are still unknown.

Stromal cell-derived factor-1 (SDF-1), termed CXCL12, belongs to the CXC subfamily of chemokines. CXCL12 is known to bind mainly to a G-protein coupled receptor, CXCR4. Recently, CXCR7 has been identified as an additional receptor for CXCL12 [11–13]. Interestingly, CXCL12 is not only involved in the immune system, but also in axonal development and neurotransmission [14,15], migration, proliferation, and survival of cancer cells [16], and extracellular matrix adhesion of haematopoietic cells in bone marrow or damaged tissues [17,18]. In the eye, CXCL12 and CXCR4 have been hypothesized to play a role in neovascularization and in ocular inflammation since they were detected in the retina [19,20], the cornea [21], and the AH [22]. Matrix metalloproteinase (MMP) proteolysis is one of the regulating factors for chemokine activity [23,24]. Proteolytic processing of CXCL12 yields a wide variety of amino-terminal truncated proteins that lose their ability to bind to CXCR4 [25] as this chemokine–receptor interaction requires the CXCL12 N-terminal residues [26]. One of the cleaved forms of CXCL12, SDF-1(5-67), has been reported to induce neuronal apoptosis during HIV brain infection [27]. Recently, SDF-1(5-67) has been shown to bind specifically to another chemokine receptor, CXCR3, where it induces direct neuronal apoptosis [28].

In the present study, highly selective non-peptide antagonists of CXCR3 and CXCR4 were studied for their effects on OHT and related retinal neurodegeneration. We show that ocular administration of a CXCR3 antagonist lowers IOP, prevents retinal ganglion cell degeneration, and protects visual function in an animal model of OHT. The chemokine and both receptors were detected in human glaucomatous trabecular tissue and a trabecular cell line. SDF-1(5-67) was found to be produced by trabecular cells under the control of MMPs and cytokines known to be involved in glaucoma. We demonstrate that SDF-1(5-67) induces TC apoptosis through CXCR3, and that blocking CXCR3 restores the filtrating function of the TM and protects the retina against OHT-related degeneration. Collectively, the results suggest that pathological enhancement of a SDF-1(5-67)/CXCR3 interaction is involved in trabecular degeneration and this chemokine/chemokine receptor axis may represent a new therapeutic target to prevent the deleterious effect of OHT on the visual function.

## Methods

### Reagents

Recombinant human CXCL12 (7.8 kDa), TNF-α (17.5 kDa), TGF-β2 (12.8 kDa), CXCL10 (8.7 kDa) and TIMP-1 (20.6 kDa) were obtained from R&D Systems (Minneapolis, MN, USA). CXCL11 (8.3 kDa) was obtained from Preprotech (Rocky Hill, NJ, USA). Exogenous CXCL12 and truncated SDF-1(5-67) (7.4 kDa) were synthesized by F. Baleux. NBI-74330, a non-peptide antagonist of CXCR3 [29,30], and AMD-3100, a non-peptide antagonist of CXCR4 [31], were synthesized by Orga-Link (Gif-sur-Yvette, France). Batimastat was a gift from E. Gabison and S. Menashi (CNRS UMR 7149, University of Paris 12, Créteil, France). Cell antigens (Ag) were detected in TCs using the following antibodies (Ab): mouse IgG1 anti-human CXCL12 mAb (1:200, clone 79018, R&D Systems), mouse IgG2B anti-human CXCR4 mAb (1:200, clone 44716, R&D Systems), mouse IgG1 anti-human CXCR3 mAb (1:200, clone 49801, R&D Systems), anti-caspase 3 (clone 92-605, BD Biosciences), secondary antibodies Alexa Fluor488 goat anti-mouse IgG (1:500, Molecular Probes, Montluçon, France), and FITC-conjugated goat anti-mouse Fab (1:500, DakoCytomation, Glostrup, Denmark). Rat TM were assessed for inflammatory cell infiltration using primary rabbit anti-CD45 pAb (1:100, ab10558. Abcam, Cambridge, MA, USA) and mouse anti-rat CD11b mAb (1:200, ab8879, Abcam). Anti-SDF-1(5-67) (1:100) was a generous gift from C. Overall (University of British Columbia, Vancouver, Canada), and anti-CXCR7 (1:200) was given by M. Thelen (Institute for Research in Biomedicine, Bellinzona, Switzerland).

Isotype-matched antibodies from R&D Systems were used as negative controls.

### Human Trabecular Meshwork Specimens

Human TMs were obtained from 15 patients undergoing surgery for primary open-angle glaucoma. All patients included in the study were diagnosed for glaucoma at least 1 year before and presented no other ocular pathology or systemic disease. The TM was selectively removed during non-penetrating deep sclerectomy. Experiments were conducted in the Clinical Investigation Centre for Ocular Surface Pathology (Centre Hospitalier National d'Ophtalmologie des Quinze-Vingts, Paris, France) in accordance with the Declaration of Helsinki, Scotland amendment, 2000. National ethics committee approval was obtained (INSERM-DHOS CIC, 503) and all patients signed the informed consent form before surgery.

### Human Glaucomatous Trabecular Cell Line

For *in vitro* experiments, the human glaucomatous TC line HTM3 was used, which has been previously characterized [32]. HTM3 cells were routinely cultured in standard humidified 5% $CO_2$ atmosphere in serum-free Dulbecco's Modified Eagle Medium (DMEM. GIBCO, Invitrogen, Carlsbad, CA, USA) supplemented with 4 mM L-glutamine, 10% fetal bovine serum, and 50 µg/mL gentamicin. For passages, monolayers were rinsed with PBS, dislodged by trypsinization (0.25% trypsin, 0.02% EDTA), then cultured from an initial concentration of 60,000 cells/mL. For immunofluorescence, TCs were grown on 22-mm glass cover-slips, then dried and fixed in 4% paraformaldehyde for 15 min. All cells were used at passage 10 to 20.

### Animal Model

Male 8-week-old Long-Evans rats weighing 300–350 g were used. Animals were kept in pathogen-free conditions with food and water available *ad libitum* and housed in a 12-h light/12-h dark cycle. Ocular integrity was checked using the slit lamp biomicroscope. The surgical model of OHT was induced in the right eye of each rat by cauterization of three episcleral veins after conjunctival dissection under general anesthesia (intraperitoneal injection of ketamine 75 mg/kg and xylazine 10 mg/kg) as reported elsewhere [33]. The left eyes underwent conjunctival dissection only as controls. After the surgery, the animals were maintained for a 21-day period and monitored for IOP three times a week using a handheld tonometer (TonoLab, Medtronics, Jacksonville, FL, USA) without sedation. Animals presenting low or instable IOP were then excluded, and the experiments were carried out at least one month after the surgery. Institutional review board approved the animal ethics for this study. All experiments were conducted in accordance with the Association for Research in Vision and Ophthalmology for the Use of Animals in Ophthalmic research.

### Real-time PCR

mRNA levels in human tissues and TC line were assessed using RT 7300 (Applied Biosystems) and assays-on-demand primers for human CXCL12 (ID Hs00171022m1), human CXCR4 (ID Hs00607978s1), and human CXCR3 (ID Hs00171041m1). Total mRNA was isolated from cultured TCs using the NucleoSpin RNA II extraction kit (Macherey-Nagel, Düren, Germany), and was then reverse-transcribed (TaqMan Reverse Transcription Reagents, Applied Biosystems). mRNA in human TM tissue was extracted using the NucleoSpin RNA XS kit (Macherey-Nagel), then conditioned and determined following the same above-described procedure. Relative quantitation of target genes was calculated according to the comparative Ct method, *i.e.* normalized to an endogenous control S18 gene and relative to a calibrator after calculating the efficiency coefficient. The results are presented as the inverse of the normalized Ct value (InvCt) or as the relative fold change compared to unstimulated control. A negative control was routinely used omitting mRNA from the RT reaction mixture.

## Immunohistofluorescence

Protein expression of CXCR3, CXCR4, and CXCL12 was detected in tissues and in the HTM3 cell line by indirect immunofluorescence using a laser confocal microscope (E800, PCM2000, Nikon, Champigny-sur-Marne, France). Nonspecific Ab binding was blocked with normal goat serum or with fetal bovine serum in PBS/0.1% Triton for 60 min, washed three times, then incubated overnight at 4°C with primary Ab. After three more washes, cells were counterstained with secondary fluorescent Ab for 2 h at room temperature. Specimens were finally washed three times in PBS, incubated in propidium iodide for 3 min (Sigma-Aldrich, France) or in DAPI for 1 min, and mounted in gel mounting medium. Isotype-matched mAbs were used as controls for each sample and each primary Ab.

## Flow Cytometry

Total and cell membrane surface expression of proteins was analyzed on a FC 500 flow cytometer (Beckman Coulter, Miami, FL, USA). TCs (120,000 per well) were plated in six-well plates (Costar, Cambridge, MA, USA) and grown to 80% confluence. The cells were cultured in complete medium for 24 h and subsequently incubated with serum-free DMEM, supplemented CXCL12, or SDF-1(5-67) for 12 h. Cells were carefully detached, suspended in PBS containing 1% BSA, blocked with normal rabbit serum, and stained with primary Ab for 1 h on ice, washed three times with cold 1% BSA PSB, followed by counterstaining with the corresponding fluorescein isothiocyanate-conjugated secondary antibody (DakoCytomation) for 30 min. Cells were preincubated and immunostained adding or not 0.5 mg/mL saponin in order to determine total or surface expression respectively. Isotype-matched antibodies were used as negative controls. For each specimen, at least 1,000 cells per antibody were analyzed. The results are reported as mean fluorescence intensity (MFI) normalized to isotypic control.

## ELISA

The amount of CXCL12 released into TC supernatants was measured by an in-house ELISA kit (ref. DY350, R&D Systems). Cells were cultured and stimulated as described above, and supernatants were isolated after centrifugation. 96-well microtitre plates were coated overnight with mouse anti-CXCL12 capture mAb then nonspecific binding was blocked for 2 h with 1% BSA in PBS. Duplicate samples (100 μL) of cell supernatants or serial dilutions of standards of human recombinant CXCL12 were incubated for 2 h, washed, then incubated with goat anti-CXCL12 mAb for 2 h, followed by 20-min incubation with HRP-conjugated streptavidin. Reaction product was detected using color reagent (ref. DY999, R&D Systems). Optical density was read (450–570 nm, SpectraFluor, TECAN, Switzerland) and averaged from ten measurements per well. The limit of sensitivity for this assay was 15 pg/mL.

## Western Blot Analysis

Protein extracts were prepared from TCs (120,000 cells per well) grown to 80% confluence in six-well plates. The cells were maintained with medium for 24 h, then incubated subsequently for 24 h with supplemented DMEM only or with specific inhibitors, detached and homogenized in cell lysis buffer. Equal amounts of proteins were separated on 4%–12% Tris-Glycine gel (Novex, Invitrogen), transferred to nitrocellulose, and probed overnight with anti-SDF-1(5-67) neoepitope polyclonal antibody (1:100, 30-min preincubated with CXCL12 to improve the antibody specificity) following carefully the same procedure as previously described [28]. Primary Ab binding was revealed using HRP-conjugated goat anti-rabbit IgG (1:3000, Vector, AbCys, Paris, France) for 1 hour and developed with ECL Plus detection reagents (GE healthcare, Orsay, France). β-actin (Abcam) was used as internal control. Signal intensity of anti-SDF-1(5-67) binding was quantitated using ImageJ software and normalized to β-actin detection. Recombinant CXCL12 and SDF-1(5-67) were used in Western Blots in order to control the antibody for specificity against SDF-1(5-67) neoepitope only.

## TUNEL Labeling

A terminal deoxynucleotidyl transferase-mediated dUTP nick-end labeling (TUNEL) assay (Roche Diagnostics, Meylan, France) was performed to detect apoptosis in rat eye cryosections following the manufacturer's instructions. Controls were done in each eye using a 10-min pretreatment with DNAse or omitting the transferase solution as positive or negative control, respectively. Specimens were mounted in aqueous mounting medium with DAPI to be further analyzed using light epifluorescence microscopy. TUNEL-labeled TCs were observed and counted in five 0.01 mm$^2$ fields per sample in order to compare apoptotic TC density between groups. TUNEL-labeled retinal ganglion cells were counted in five fields per sample and normalized to the observed retinal inner layer length.

## Cell Viability Assays

The effects of CXCL12 and SDF-1(5-67) on the cell proliferation and apoptosis were analyzed in a previously used cellular model of toxicity [34]: 80% confluent TCs were incubated in PBS with 0.01% benzalkonium chloride for 15 min in order to induce approximately 50% apoptosis. Cells were washed with PBS, incubated in free medium (control) or with CXCL12, SDF-1(5-67), and inhibitors during a 24-h recovery period. Microplate cytofluorometry was performed on Saphire Microplate reader (Tecan Instruments, Lyon, France) in 96-well microtitre plates: neutral red staining (Fluka, Ronkonkoma, NY, USA) was used to evaluate membrane integrity that closely correlates with cell viability [35]; apoptosis was quantified with the nuclear dye Hoechst33258 (Hoechst, Germany) combined with propidium iodide in order to exclude necrosis [36]. Apoptosis was calculated as the ratio of apoptotic cells on the total cell viability, and expressed as relative fold changes compared to control.

## Animal Experiments

For evaluation of the effect of non-peptide antagonists on IOP, forty animals presenting stable OHT were included and randomly divided into four equal groups: in both eyes, ten rats received one subconjunctival injection of the CXCR4 antagonist AMD3100 (1 μM, 100 μL), ten received a single injection of the CXCR3 antagonist NBI-74330 (1 μM, 100 μL), ten received one injection of NBI-74330 followed by a second one 4 days after, and ten rats received the vehicle only. IOP was monitored every two days by an independent person *i.e.* who was blind to the treatment. At the end of the experiments, animals were euthanized and the eyes were immediately removed, fixed in 4% paraformaldehyde, embedded in an optimal cutting-temperature compound (OCT, Tissue-Tek, Miles Inc, Bayer Diagnostic, Püteaux, France) and cut into 15-μm cryosections. For the NBI-74330 dose-response study, twenty animals presenting stable OHT were randomly divided into four equal groups to receive either NBI-74330 injections (100 μL) at three different concentrations (0.01 μM, 0.1 μM, and 1 μM) or the vehicle only. IOPs were averaged from days 6, 8, and 10.

For the evaluation of AH outflow, twenty animals presenting stable OHT were randomly divided into two equal groups to receive either NBI-74330 injections (1 μM, 100 μL) or the vehicle only. AH outflow was assessed at day 8 using *in vivo* fluorophotometry [37,38]. Briefly, 1 μL fluorescein was injected using a 33G needle into the anterior chamber under general anesthesia. One hour after, AH decrease in anterior chamber fluorescence has been recorded *in vivo* for 30 minutes using Micron III fluorescent imaging device (Phoenix research laboratories, San Ramon, CA) and ImageJ software (NIH). Mean fluorescence intensities were normalized to the initial intensity and drawn in semi-log graphs as a function of time in order to calculate the AH outflow depending on the curve slope. To label the hydrodynamic patterns of trabecular outflow passage, ocular perfusion of fluorescent microsphere was performed as reported elsewhere [39,40]. Ocular anterior chamber was exchanged with red-fluorescent microspheres in BSS (0.1 μm, 0.02%v/v, Invitrogen) using a double 30G needle infusion, and followed by a 30-minute perfusion at the IOP measured before death. Anterior chamber contents were washed with BSS and eyes were immediately removed and fixed in 4% paraformaldehyde for 15 minutes. Anterior segments were quadrisected and flat-mounted on coverglass after exposing the TM by gently moving the iris tissue. TM was observed under laser confocal microscope using a 20× objective lens regardless of the presence of microsphere accumulation. An index of the trabecular filtration, namely trabecular percent effective filtration length (PEFL), was calculated as the length ratio of the zones wherein tracer accumulated to the total length of the inner wall in at least 8 images per eye [39].

For the *in vivo* evaluation of retinal atrophy and visual function, twenty animals with stable OHT were injected in one eye with either NBI-74330 (1 μM, 100 μL) or vehicle (100 μM) following the same protocol as described above. IOP was monitored once a week. Retinal nerve fiber density was assessed *in vivo* 2 months after the treatment using confocal scanning laser ophthalmoscopy (HRA, Heidelberg Engineering, Heidelberg, Germany). The eyes were dilated with 0.5% tropicamide and 0.5% phenylephrine hydrochloride eye drops (Santen, Osaka, Japan). Each rat was gently held manually to keep the eye in position for imaging the retina. Dynamic retinal images were recorded in the center of the fundus and in the four mildperipheral areas. The density of retinal nerve fiber was calculated in each image and averaged using Metamorph software (Molecular Device, Sunnyval, CA, USA). Visual function was evaluated using an optokinetic apparatus consisting of interchangeable circular drums with black and white stripes rotating around a stationary holder in which the rat sits, as previously described [41]. Rats were tested at spatial frequencies of 0.125, 0.25, and 0.5 cycles/degree (2 turns/minute) under photopic conditions. Each rat was tested for one minute for each eye and each frequency during one session. Digital recordings of the head movements were analyzed and the amount of time the rat spent head tracking was calculated separately for each eye in a masked manner.

To study the effect of the chemokine on IOP, intraocular injections with CXCL12 or SDF-1(5-67) (100 ng/mL [13 nM], 5 μL) or vehicle only were performed in ten normal rats. The IOP was measured every 12 hours using Tonolab tonometer during five days.

## Statistical Analysis

All data in text and in bar graphs are reported as means ± SEM and represent at least three independent experiments. Analysis was performed using NCSS software (NCSS, Kaysville, UT, USA). Data were tested for distribution in order to perform the adequate parametric (Student's t-test or one-way ANOVA followed by Tukey's post hoc test) or nonparametric test (Mann-Whitney or Kruskal-Wallis tests) for the comparisons. A value of $P<0.05$ was considered to be significant.

## Results

### Human Glaucomatous Trabecular Tissue and A Trabecular Cell Line Express CXCL12, SDF-1(5-67), CXCR3 and CXCR4

We first checked whether human glaucomatous trabecular tissue and cells were able to express the chemokine and chemokine receptors. CXCL12, CXCR3, and CXCR4 were detected by immunofluorescence and flow cytometry in unstimulated cells (**Fig. 1A–E**). mRNAs for CXCL12, CXCR3 and CXCR4 were also detected in both human tissue and trabecular cell line (**Fig. 1F**). Finally, TCs were able to release CXCL12 as determined by ELISA of cell supernatants (22.8±5.28 pg/ml [2.9±0.7 pM] from 100,000 cells/mL grown during 48 h). Western blot analysis of unstimulated HTM3 cells, using a polyclonal anti-SDF-1(5-67) neoepitope-specific antibody, identified SDF-1(5-67) (**Fig. 2A,B**). Incubation (24-h) with MMP inhibitors batimastat (100 nM) or TIMP-1 (0.5 nM) significantly reduced the amount of SDF-1(5-67), confirming that it originated from MMP activity produced by TCs. 24-h incubation of TCs with either TNF-α (50 ng/mL [2.9 nM]) or TGF-β2 (10 ng/mL [0.8 nM]), both known to be involved in glaucoma, increased the production of SDF-1(5-67) (**Fig. 2A,B**).

### CXCL12 Protects TCs from Apoptotic Stress Whereas SDF-1(5-67) Induces Apoptosis

In a TC model of toxic-induced apoptosis [34], addition of CXCL12 (10 ng/mL [1.3 nM]) decreased apoptosis, whereas SDF-1(5-67) (10 ng/mL [1.3 nM]) potentiated apoptosis (**Fig. 3A**). Both the protective effect of CXCL12 and the deleterious effect of SDF-1(5-67) were concentration-dependent, with a maximal effect of either chemokine observed at 10 ng/mL (**Fig. 3B**).

### SDF-1(5-67) Induces Apoptosis via CXCR3 and Caspase-3 Activation

In order to test that CXCL12 and its cleaved form were acting *via* two different receptors, the effect of CXCL12/SDF-1(5-67) on receptor cell membrane expression was assessed using flow cytometry. We observed that exogenous CXCL12 (10 ng/mL [1.3 nM], 6 h) downregulated cell surface expression of CXCR4 but not CXCR3. In contrast, stimulation with SDF-1(5-67) reduced the membrane expression of CXCR3 but not CXCR4 (**Fig. S1**). TC expression of CXCR7, an additional CXCL12 receptor, was not affected by either CXCL12 or by SDF-1(5-67), (1±0.2, 1.2±0.1, and 0.95±0.05 for normalized mean fluorescence intensity in unstimulated, CXCL12- and SDF-1(5-67)-stimulated cells, respectively). Blockade of CXCR4 with AMD3100 (1 μM) inhibited the protective effect of CXCL12 and induced apoptosis, mimicking the apoptotic effect of SDF-1(5-67) (**Fig. 3C**). I-TAC/CXCL11, a ligand for CXCR3 and

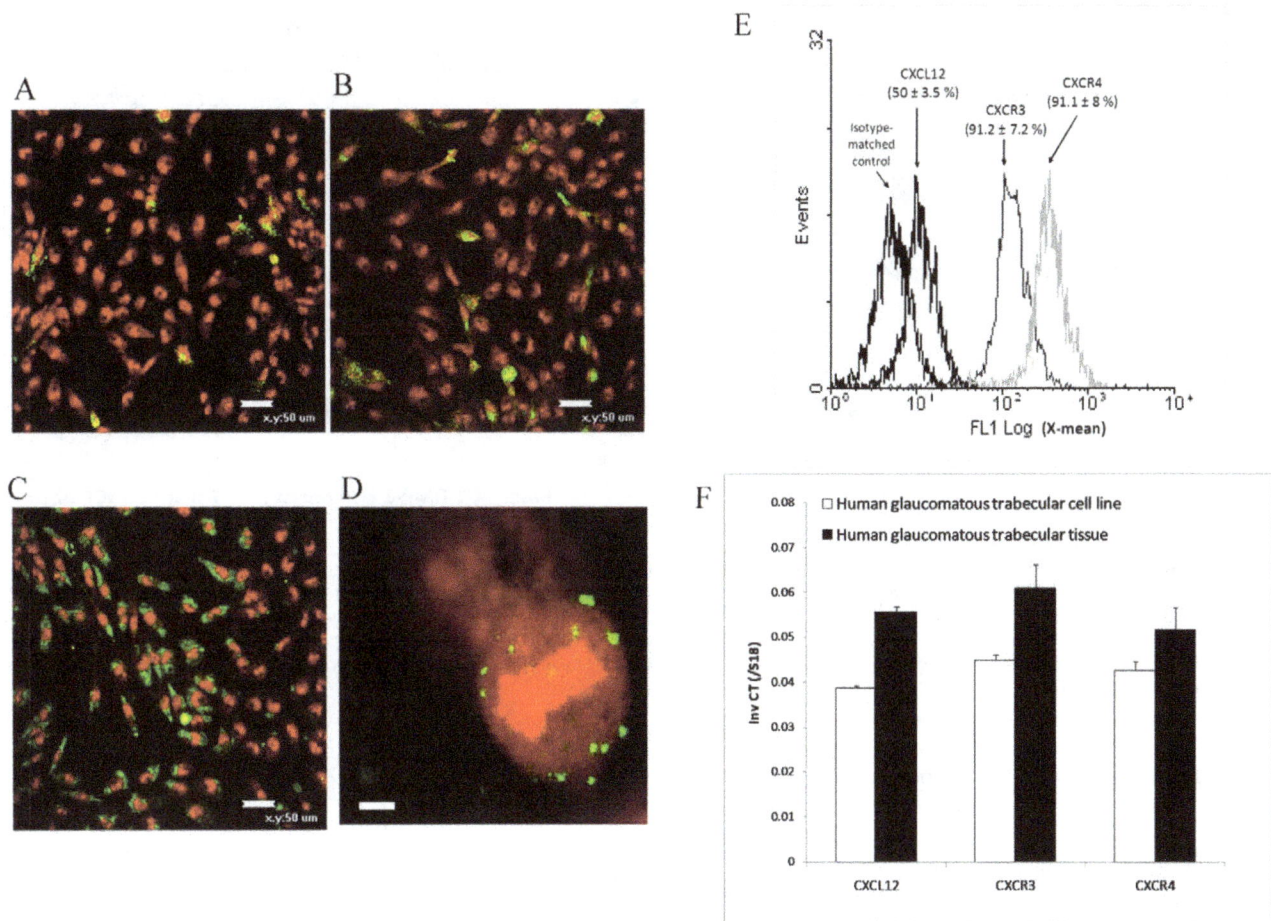

**Figure 1. CXCL12, CXCR3, and CXCR4 expression by human glaucomatous trabecular tissue and a trabecular cell line.** *(A–C)* The chemokine CXCL12 *(A)* and receptors CXCR3 *(B)* and CXCR4 *(C)* are detected in unstimulated human glaucomatous trabecular cells HTM3 by indirect immunofluorescence (secondary antibody in green, propidium iodide in red, scale bar: 50 µm, magnification ×200). *(D)* Chemokine receptor CXCR4 appears as distinct spots located at the cell membrane surface (scale bar: 5 µm, mag. ×800). Representative images of three independent experiments are depicted. *(D)* Cell expression of CXCL12 and receptors is also detected and quantified by immunoflowcytometry. Representative results obtained over 6 independent experiments, mean ± SEM of positive cells. *(E)* Chemokine and receptor mRNAs are detected in human glaucomatous trabecular tissues (n = 15) and in the HTM3 trabecular cell line. Data in the bar graph are presented as means ± SEM.

CXCR7, had no effect on TC apoptosis (1.04±0.12, 1.11±0.10, and 1.03±0.14 fold over control for a 24-h incubation with CXCL11 at 1 ng/mL, 10 ng/mL, and 100 ng/mL respectively) confirming that the protective effect of CXCL12 was mediated by CXCR4. In contrast, selective blockade of CXCR3 with NBI-74330 (1 µM) inhibited the apoptotic effect of SDF-1(5-67) (10 ng/mL) (**Fig. 3C**). Moreover, 24-h incubation with CXCL10 (10 ng/mL [1.1 nM]), another ligand for CXCR3, induced cell apoptosis that was prevented by NBI-74330. SDF-1(5-67) increased active caspase-3 and this effect was also inhibited by the CXCR3 antagonist (**Fig. 3D**).

## In vivo Treatment with a CXCR3 Antagonist Reduces Ocular Hypertension in a Rat Model of Ocular Hypertension

In order to extent our *in vitro* data, we tested *in vivo* whether CXCR3 and/or CXCR4 were implicated in the regulation of IOP by using highly selective non-peptide antagonists of both chemokine receptors in a rat model of OHT and related retinal

degeneration, which was induced by episcleral vein cauterization [29]. AMD-3100 [31] (1 µM, 100 µL) or NBI-74330 [29,30] (1 µM, 100 µL), selective antagonists for CXCR4 and CXCR3 respectively, were administrated in the subconjunctival space of rat eyes. A single administration of NBI-74330 induced a decrease in IOP 4 days after the treatment, reaching the normal IOP values observed in normotensive control eyes (**Fig. 4A**). This decrease in IOP was transient since IOP returned to elevated values of untreated eyes after 6 days. When a second administration was given at the time of maximal decrease, IOP remained low during a period of 6 weeks (**Fig. 4B**). NBI-74330 reduced IOP in a dose-dependent manner (**Fig. 4C**). In contrast, subconjunctival administration of a CXCR4 selective antagonist did not influence IOP in eyes with OHT (**Fig. S2**). In control eyes, the antagonists had no effect. In parallel, CXCL12 and SDF-1(5-67) were tested in normal rat eyes for their ability to modify IOP. CXCL12 ocular injections had no significant effect on IOP, whereas two injections of SDF-1(5-67) significantly increased IOP that remained elevated for 3 days (**Fig. S3**).

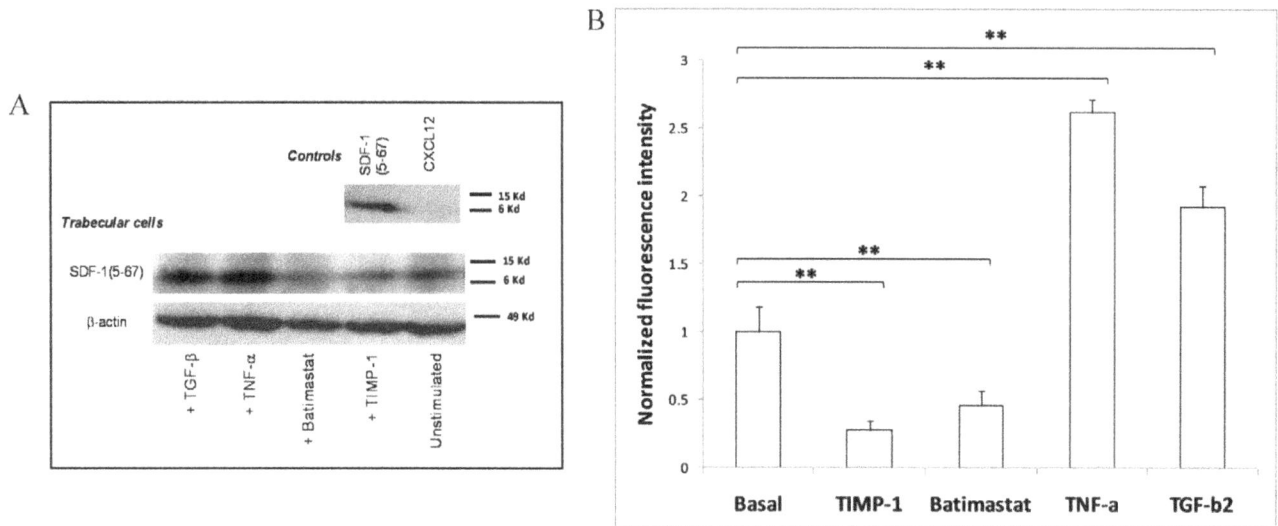

**Figure 2. Human glaucomatous trabecular cells produce SDF-1(5-67).** *(A,B)* SDF-1(5-67), a truncated form of CXCL12, is detected in the human glaucomatous trabecular cell line HTM3 using a specific anti-SDF-1(5-67) neoepitope antibody. MMP inhibitors batimastat (100 nM) and TIMP-1 (0.5 nM) induce a decrease in SDF-1(5-67) production, whereas TNF-α (50 ng/mL [2.9 nM]) and TGF-β2 (10 ng/mL [0.8 nM]) enhance the production of SDF-1(5-67). ** $P < 0.01$. Exogenous SDF-1(5-67) and CXCL12 were used as positive and negative controls respectively for the antibody specificity as presented in the upper membrane (controls) of a representative western blot *(A)* taken from three independent experiments. Data in bar graphs are presented as means ± SEM.

## CXCR3 Antagonist Improves Trabecular Function and Reduces Trabecular Cell Apoptosis

Investigations were conducted in the anterior segment of the eye in order to study mechanisms involved in the NBI-74330-related decrease in IOP. In our animal model, we observed a decrease in AH outflow together with a decrease in the TM filtrating surface in hypertensive eyes compared to normotensive controls, one month after the surgical procedure (**Fig. 5A,B,C,D**). AH outflow impairment was significantly counteracted by treatment with NBI-74330 (**Fig. 5A**). Furthermore, trabecular filtrating surface was also significantly improved by the selective CXCR3 antagonist (**Fig. 5B,C,D**). TC apoptosis was significantly detected in hypertensive eyes as compared to normotensive controls (**Fig. 5E,F,G**). In hypertensive eyes, apoptosis was significantly decreased by NBI-74330 as compared to untreated eyes. There was no inflammatory cell infiltration in the TM whatever the group as revealed by a lack of either anti-CD45 or anti-CD11b reactive cells. These data together suggested that blocking CXCR3 may lower OHT by restoring the trabecular filtrating function and protecting directly TCs from apoptosis.

## CXCR3 Antagonist Prevents Retinal Neuropathy and Protects Visual Function

In parallel, OHT-related retinal degeneration and related visual degradation were studied. In our animal model, retinal nerve fiber density was significantly decreased in eyes with OHT compared to controls three months after the surgery as assessed *in vivo* by confocal scanning laser ophthalmoscopy (**Fig. 6A**). Eyes treated with selective CXCR3 antagonist presented higher nerve fiber density than untreated hypertensive eyes (**Fig. 6A**). Similarly, the visual function was better in NBI-74330-treated eyes than in untreated controls as assessed by optokinetic measurements (**Fig. 6B**). *Ex vivo*, NBI-74330-related reduction in IOP was associated with a decrease in retinal ganglion cell apoptosis as assessed by TUNEL-labeling (**Fig. 6C**).

## Discussion

Several recent data have demonstrated that chemokines are not only involved in inflammatory/immune processes but also in the regulation of tissue microenvironment as well as in degenerative disorders [42]. In this study, we addressed the involvement of a balance between the full length chemokine CXCL12 and its truncated form SDF-1(5-67) in the regulation of IOP by modulating the TM filtrating function *via* the chemokine receptors CXCR4 and CXCR3. We describe the successful use *in vivo* of a non-peptide selective antagonist of CXCR3 to decrease elevated IOP and protect the retina in an animal model of OHT, establishing this chemokine receptor as a new therapeutic target to prevent the trabecular degeneration and its deleterious effects on the visual function.

We report that CXCL12, CXCR3, and CXCR4 are expressed in human trabecular tissue of glaucomatous patients as well as in a human glaucomatous TC line. In the eye, CXCL12 mRNA has been previously detected in TCs using gene microarrays [43]; CXCR4 has been investigated in the retina and in the cornea [19–21] but not in the TM; no data are available on the expression of CXCR3. TCs play a crucial role in IOP regulation because of their phagocytic activity and their ability to produce extracellular matrix components and MMPs [44,45]. It has been recently demonstrated that MMP cleavage of CXCL12 yields a toxic truncated form, SDF-1(5-67), causing direct apoptosis *via* CXCR3 [27,28]. MMPs have been reported to be significantly involved in mechanisms associated with TM degeneration in primary open-angle glaucoma [46]. Here we observed a basal production of SDF-1(5-67) by TCs, which originated from MMP activity on full length CXCL12. Interestingly, TNF-α and TGF-β2, cytokines known to be overexpressed in glaucoma [47,48], increased the production of SDF-1(5-67). *In vitro*, we described a constitutive autocrine function of CXCL12/CXCR4 in TCs, as previously described in the brain [49], which protected TCs against apoptosis. Indeed, a direct protective role of full length CXCL12 has been reported in meningioma [50] and in a primary neuronal cell line [51] without any involvement of inflammatory cells. Recently, another chemokine receptor,

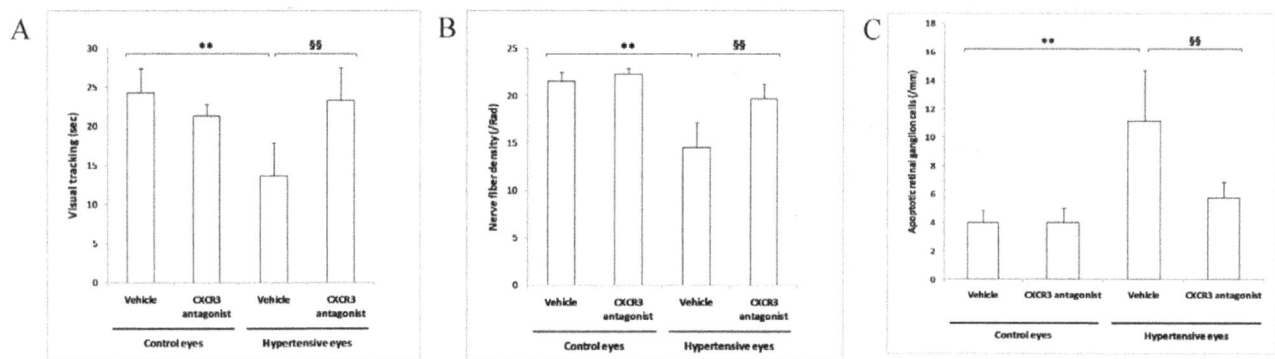

**Figure 6. CXCR3 antagonism-induced lowering of intraocular pressure prevents retinal neurodegeneration and protects visual function in a rat model of ocular hypertension.** *(A,B)* Ocular hypertension during 3 months is associated with a degradation in the visual function *(A)* as assessed by the duration of visual tracking during a 1-min optokinetic testing (spatial frequency, 0.5 cycle/degree), and with a decrease in retinal nerve fiber density *(B)* as measured *in vivo* by scanning light ophthalmoscopy. Ophthalmic treatment with CXCR3 antagonist significantly protects the visual function and prevents retinal nerve fiber loss (n = 10 each). *(C)* Ocular hypertension during one month is associated with an increase in retinal ganglion cell apoptosis (reported as the number of TUNEL-labeled cells normalized to the observed retinal layer length), which is reversed 15 days after the treatment with CXCR3 antagonist (n = 10 each). ** $P<0.01$ vs. normotensive eyes, §§ $P<0.01$ vs. untreated hypertensive eyes. Data in graphs are presented as means ± SEM.

dysfunction occurring after the initial vein obstruction. At the cellular level, we observed an increase in TC apoptosis similarly to what is observed in glaucoma in humans [10]. Ophthalmic treatment with NBI-74330 reduced IOP and related retinal degeneration by restoring the trabecular filtrating function and protecting TCs from apoptosis Even if the trabecular pathology in primary glaucoma is currently considered as a degenerative process, the relationship between glaucoma and inflammation has to be pointed out. It is noted that no inflammatory cell infiltration was found in rat TMs. Accordingly, our team previously found very few inflammatory cells in the TM of glaucomatous patients as assessed *ex vivo* by confocal microscopy [9]. Together these findings suggest that CXCL12 acts in autocrine/paracrine manner in the TM, and that glaucomatous trabecular degeneration is likely to develop without involving immune cells, further confirming that NBI-74330 acts directly on trabecular cells. Moreover, we reported *in vivo* that subconjunctival injections of SDF-1(5-67) in healthy rat eyes induced OHT. The transient effect of SDF-1(5-67) on IOP elevation may suggest that other factors can be implicated. Though our study focused on CXCL12, we cannot exclude that other chemokines could also play a role in the TM regulation, such as CXCL8, CCL2 and CXCL6 that were recently detected in cultured TCs, but whose effects are still unknown [62].

Here we originally suggest that the chemokine CXCL12 plays a crucial role in the initial pathogenesis of trabecular degeneration: (i) CXCL12 acts physiologically as a protective chemokine in an autocrine CXCL12/CXCR4 signaling mechanism; (ii) cytokine- and MMP-related pathological overexpression and processing of CXCL12 into SDF-1(5-67) decrease CXCL12-related CXCR4 activation and induce morphological changes and apoptosis *via* CXCR3, leading to TM dysfunction, OHT, and retinal degeneration; and (iii) CXCR3 blockade *in vivo* by ophthalmic treatment with a selective antagonist can restore trabecular function, prevent the retinal neuropathy and protect the visual function in an animal model of OHT. Current antiglaucoma treatment to decrease OHT is still non-curative because it does not treat the TM degeneration responsible for OHT that leads to retinal neurodegeneration and visual impairments. Here we propose that SDF-1(5-67)/CXCR3 interaction may be targeted in order to treat the causal trabecular pathology.

## Supporting Information

**Figure S1  CXCL12 and its truncated form SDF-1(5-67) bind to two different chemokine receptors.** Human glaucomatous trabecular cell line HTM3 was assessed for membrane expression of CXCR3 and CXCR4 using immuno-flowcytometry. 3-h stimulation with exogenous CXCL12 (10 ng/mL [1.3 nM]) decreases membrane expression of CXCR4 but not CXCR3, whereas 3-h stimulation with SDF-1(5-67) (10 ng/mL [1.3 nM]) decreases the membrane expression of CXCR3 but not CXCR4; ** $P<0.01$. Data are presented as means ± SEM.

**Figure S2  Lack of effect of a CXCR4 antagonist on intraocular pressure in a rat model of ocular hypertension.** Ophthalmic administration of a CXCR4 antagonist (AMD-3100, 1 µM, 100 µL) in the subconjunctival space does not modify intraocular pressure in control and surgically-induced hypertensive rat eyes (n = 10 in each group). Data are presented as means ± SEM.

**Figure S3  SDF-1(5-67) increases intraocular pressure.** Two intraocular injections (black arrows) of exogenous SDF-1(5-67) (100 ng/mL [13 nM], 5 µL) in the anterior chamber of healthy rat eyes induce a transient ocular hypertension (n = 10 each); ** $P<0.01$ vs. vehicle-injected eyes. Data are presented as means ± SEM.

## Acknowledgments

The authors thank Christopher Overall and Amanda Starr (University of British Columbia, Vancouver, Canada) for providing the anti-SDF-1(5-67) antibody, and Marcus Thelen (Institute for Research in Biomedicine, Bellinzona, Switzerland) for the anti-CXCR7 antibody. We also thank Nathalie Rouach (INSERM U840, Collège de France, Paris, France) for her helpful advice.

## Author Contributions

Conceived and designed the experiments: AD FB-B WR CB. Performed

## References

1. Quigley HA, Broman AT (2006) The number of people with glaucoma worldwide in 2010 and 2020. Br. J. Ophthalmol. 90, 262–267.
2. Cedrone C, Mancino R, Cerulli A, Cesareo M, Nucci C (2008) Epidemiology of primary glaucoma: prevalence, incidence, and blinding effects. Prog. Brain. Res. 173, 3–14.
3. Sommer A (1989) Intraocular pressure and glaucoma. Am. J. Ophthalmol. 107, 186–188.
4. Kass MA, Heuer DK, Higginbotham EJ, Johnson CA, Keltner JL, et al. (2002) The Ocular Hypertension Treatment Study: a randomized trial determines that topical ocular hypotensive medication delays or prevents the onset of primary open-angle glaucoma. Arch. Ophthalmol. 120, 701–713.
5. Tektas OY, Lütjen-Drecoll E (2009) Structural changes of the trabecular meshwork in different kinds of glaucoma. Exp. Eye Res. 88, 769–775.
6. Alvarado J, Murphy C, Juster R (1984) Trabecular meshwork cellularity in primary open-angle glaucoma and non-glaucomatous normals. Ophthalmology 91, 564–579.
7. Rohen JW, Lutjen-Drecoll E, Flugel C, Meyer M, Grierson I (1993) Ultrastructure of the trabecular meshwork in untreated cases of primary open-angle glaucoma. Exp. Eye Res. 56, 683–692.
8. Grierson I, Howes RC (1987) Age-related depletion of the cell population in the human trabecular meshwork. Eye 1, 204–210.
9. Hamard P, Valtot F, Sourdille P, Bourles-Dagonet F, Baudouin C (2002) Confocal microscopic examination of trabecular meshwork removed during ab externo trabeculectomy. Br. J. Ophthalmol. 86, 1046–1052.
10. Baleriola J, Garcia-Feijoo J, Martinez-de-la-Casa JM, Fernandez-Cruz A, de la Rosa EJ, et al. (2008) Apoptosis in the trabecular meshwork of glaucomatous patients. Mol. Vis. 14, 1513–1516.
11. Balabanian K, Lagane B, Infantino S, Chow KY, Harriague J, et al. (2005) The chemokine SDF-1/CXCL12 binds to and signals through the orphan receptor RDC1 in T lymphocytes. J. Biol. Chem. 280, 35760–35766.
12. Burns JM, Summers BC, Wang Y, Melikian A, Berahovich R, et al. (2006) A novel chemokine receptor for SDF-1 and I-TAC involved in cell survival, cell adhesion, and tumor development. J. Exp. Med. 203, 2201–2213.
13. Thelen M, Thelen S (2008) CXCR7, CXCR4 and CXCL12: an eccentric trio? J. Neuroimmunol. 198, 9–13.
14. Li M, Ransohoff RM (2008) Multiple roles of chemokine CXCL12 in the central nervous system: a migration from immunology to neurobiology. Prog. Neurobiol. 84, 116–131.
15. Rostene W, Kitabgi P, Parsadaniantz SM (2007) Chemokines: a new class of neuromodulator? Nat. Rev. Neurosci. 8, 895–903.
16. Muller A, Homey B, Soto H, Ge N, Catron D, et al. (2001) Involvement of chemokine receptors in breast cancer metastasis. Nature 410, 50–56.
17. Lapidot T, Dar A, Kollet O (2005) How do stem cells find their way home? Blood 106, 1901–1910.
18. Son BR, Marquez-Curtis LA, Kucia M, Wysoczynski M, Turner AR, et al. (2006) Migration of bone marrow and cord blood mesenchymal stem cells in vitro is regulated by stromal-derived factor-1-CXCR4 and hepatocyte growth factor-c-met axes and involves matrix metalloproteinases. Stem Cells 24, 1254–1264.
19. Crane IJ, Wallace CA, McKillop-Smith S, Forrester JV (2000) CXCR4 receptor expression on human retinal pigment epithelial cells from the blood-retina barrier leads to chemokine secretion and migration in response to stromal cell-derived factor 1 alpha. J. Immunol. 165, 4372–4378.
20. Bhutto IA, McLeod DS, Merges C, Hasegawa T, Lutty GA (2006) Localisation of SDF-1 and its receptor CXCR4 in retina and choroid of aged human eyes and in eyes with age related macular degeneration. Br. J. Ophthalmol. 90, 906–910.
21. Bourcier T, Berbar T, Paquet S, Rondeau N, Thomas F, et al. (2003) Characterization and functionality of CXCR4 chemokine receptor and SDF-1 in human corneal fibroblasts. Mol. Vis. 9, 96–102.
22. Curnow SJ, Wloka K, Faint JM, Amft N, Cheung CM, et al. (2004) Topical glucocorticoid therapy directly induces up-regulation of functional CXCR4 on primed T lymphocytes in the aqueous humor of patients with uveitis. J. Immunol. 172, 7154–7161.
23. McQuibban GA, Gong JH, Tam EM, McCulloh CA, Clark-Lewis I, et al. (2000) Inflammation dampened by gelatinase A cleavage of monocyte chemoattractant protein-3. Science 289, 1202–1206.
24. Zhang H, Trivedi A, Lee JU, Lohela M, Lee SM, et al. (2011) Matrix metalloproteinase-9 and stromal cell-derived factor-1 act synergistically to support migration of blood-borne monocytes into the injured spinal cord. J. Neurosci. 9, 143–149.
25. McQuibban GA, Butler GS, Gong JH, Bendall L, Power C, et al. (2001) Matrix metalloproteinase activity inactivates the CXC chemokine stromal cell-derived factor-1. J. Biol. Chem. 276, 43503–43508.
26. Valenzuela-Fernandez A, Planchenault T, Baleux F, Staropoli I, Le-Barillec K, et al. (2002) Leukocyte elastase negatively regulates Stromal cell-derived factor-1 (SDF-1)/CXCR4 binding and functions by amino-terminal processing of SDF-1 and CXCR4. J. Biol. Chem. 277, 15677–15689.

the experiments: AD DG IC JF JD WR. Analyzed the data: AD JKH FB-B SP FB JS WR CB. Contributed reagents/materials/analysis tools: DG IC JKH FB. Wrote the paper: AD WR.

27. Zhang K, McQuibban GA, Silva C, Butler GS, Johnston JB, et al. (2003) HIV-induced metalloproteinase processing of the chemokine stromal cell derived factor-1 causes neurodegeneration. Nat. Neurosci. 6, 1064–1071.
28. Vergote D, Butler GS, Ooms M, Cox JH, Silva C, et al. (2006) Proteolytic processing of SDF-1alpha reveals a change in receptor specificity mediating HIV-associated neurodegeneration. Proc. Natl. Acad. Sci. U.S.A. 103, 19182–19187.
29. Medina J (2004) Discovery and Development of a CXCR3 antagonist T487 as therapy for Th1-mediated immune disorders. 29th National Medicinal Chemistry Symposium.
30. Heise CE, Pahuja A, Hudson SC, Mistry MS, Putnam AL, et al. (2005) Pharmacological characterization of CXC chemokine receptor 3 ligands and a small molecule antagonist. J. Pharmacol. Exp. Ther. 313, 1263–1271.
31. Donzella GA, Schols D, Lin SW, Esté JA, Nagashima KA, et al. (1988) AMD3100, a small molecule inhibitor of HIV-1 entry via the CXCR4 co-receptor. Nat. Med. 4, 72–77.
32. Pang IH, Shade DL, Clark AF, Steely HT, DeSantis L (1994) Preliminary characterization of a transformed cell strain derived from human trabecular meshwork. Curr. Eye Res. 13, 51–63.
33. Garcia-Valenzuela E, Shareef S, Walsh J, Sharma SC (1995) Programmed cell death of retinal ganglion cells during experimental glaucoma. Exp. Eye. Res. 61, 33–44.
34. Hamard P, Blondin C, Debbash C, Warnet JM, Baudouin C, et al. (2003) In vitro effects of preserved and unpreserved antiglaucoma drugs on apoptotic marker expression by human trabecular cells. Graefes Arch. Clin. Exp. Ophthalmol. 241, 1037–1043.
35. Borenfreund E, Puerner JA (1985) Toxicity determined in vitro by morphological alterations and neutral red absorption. Toxicol. Lett. 24, 119–124.
36. Debbasch C, Brignole F, Pisella PJ, Warnet JM, Rat P, et al. (2001) Quaternary ammoniums and other preservatives' contribution in oxidative stress and apoptosis on Chang conjunctival cells. Invest. Ophthalmol. Vis. Sci. 42, 642–652.
37. Jones RF, Maurice DM (1966) New methods of measuring the rate of aqueous flow in man with fluorescein. Exp. Eye. Res. 5, 208–220.
38. Yablonski ME, Zimmerman TJ, Waltman SR, Becker B (1978) A fluorophotometric study of the effect of topical timolol on aqueous humor dynamics. Exp. Eye. Res. 25, 135–142.
39. Lu Z, Overby DR, Scott PA, Freddo TF, Gong H (2008) The mechanism of increasing outflow facility by rho-kinase inhibition with Y-27632 in bovine eyes. Exp. Eye. Res. 86, 271–281.
40. Zhang Y, Toris CB, Liu Y, Ye W, Gong H (2009) Morphological and hydrodynamic correlates in monkey eyes with laser induced glaucoma. Exp. Eye. Res. 89, 748–756.
41. Thomas BB, Seiler MJ, Sadda SR, Coffey PJ, Aramant RB (2004) Optokinetic test to evaluate visual acuity of each eye independently. J. Neurosci. Methods 138, 7–13.
42. Rostène W, Dansereau MM, Godefroy D, Van Steenwinckel J, Reaux-Le Goazio A, et al. (2011) Neurochemokines: a ménage a trois providing new insights on the functions of chemokines in the central nervous system. J. Neurochem. 118, 680–694.
43. Zhao X, Ramsey KE, Stephan DA, Russell P (2004) Gene and protein expression changes in human trabecular meshwork cells treated with transforming growth factor-beta. Invest. Ophthalmol. Vis. Sci. 45, 4023–4034.
44. Sherwood ME, Richardson TM, Epstein DL (1988) Phagocytosis by trabecular meshwork cells: Sequence of events in cats and monkeys. Exp. Eye Res. 46, 881–895.
45. Hernandez MR, Weinstein BI, Schwartz J, Ritch R, Gordon GG (1987) Human trabecular meshwork cells in culture: Morphology and extracellular matrix components. Invest. Ophthalmol. Vis. Sci. 28, 1655–1660.
46. Acott TS, Kelley MJ (2008) Extracellular matrix in the trabecular meshwork. Exp. Eye Res. 86, 543–561.
47. Tripathi RC, Li J, Chan WF, Tripathi BJ (1994) Aqueous humor in glaucomatous eyes contains an increased level of TGF-beta 2. Exp. Eye. Res. 59, 723–727.
48. Sawada H, Fukuchi T, Tanaka T, Abe H (2010) Tumor necrosis factor-alpha concentrations in the aqueous humor of patients with glaucoma. Invest. Ophthalmol. Vis. Sci. 51: 903–906.
49. Pujol F, Kitabgi P, Boudin H (2005) The chemokine SDF-1 differentially regulates axonal elongation and branching in hippocampal neurons. J. Cell. Sci. 118, 1071–1080.
50. Barbieri F, Bajetto A, Stumm R, Pattarozzi A, Porcile C, et al. (2006) CXC receptor and chemokine expression in human meningioma: SDF1/CXCR4 signaling activates ERK1/2 and stimulates meningioma cell proliferation. Ann. N.Y. Acad. Sci. 1090, 332–343.
51. Khan MZ, Brandimarti R, Shimizu S, Nicolai J, Crowe E, et al. (2008) The chemokine CXCL12 promotes survival of postmitotic neurons by regulating Rb protein. Cell Death Differ. 15, 1663–1672.

52. Lasagni L, Francalanci M, Annunzuato F, Lazzeri E, Giannini S, et al. (2003) An alternatively spliced variant of CXCR3 mediates the inhibition of endothelial cell growth induced by IP-10, Mig, and I-TAC, and acts as functional receptor for platelet factor 4. J. Exp. Med. 197, 1537–1549.

53. Zhu Y, Vergote D, Pardo C, Noorbakhsh F, McArthur JC, et al. (2009) CXCR3 activation by lentivirus infection suppresses neuronal autophagy: neuroprotective effects of antiretroviral therapy. FASEB J. 23, 2928–2941.

54. Jopling LA, Watt GF, Fisher S, Birch H, Coggon S, et al. (2007) Analysis of the pharmacokinetic/pharmacodynamic relationship of a small molecule CXCR3 antagonist, NBI-74330, using a murine CXCR3 internalization assay. Br. J. Pharmacol. 152, 1260–1271.

55. Verzijl D, Storelli S, Scholten DJ, Bosch L, Reinhart TA, et al. (2008) Noncompetitive antagonism and inverse agonism as mechanism of action of nonpeptidergic antagonists at primate and rodent CXCR3 chemokine receptors. J. Pharmacol. Exp. Ther. 325, 544–555.

56. van Wanrooij EJ, de Jager SC, van Es T, de Vos P, Birch HL, et al. (2008) CXCR3 antagonist NBI-74330 attenuates atherosclerotic plaque formation in LDL receptor-deficient mice. Arterioscler. Thromb. Vasc. Biol. 28, 251–257.

57. Liu C, Luo D, Reynolds BA, Meher G, Katritzky AR, et al. (2011) Chemokine receptor CXCR3 promotes growth of glioma. Carcinogenesis 32, 129–137.

58. Danias J, Shen F, Kavalarakis M, Chen B, Goldblum D, et al. (2006) Characterization of retinal damage in the episcleral vein cauterization rat glaucoma model. Exp. Eye. Res. 82, 219–228.

59. Yu S, Tanabe T, Yoshimura N (2006) A rat model of glaucoma induced by episcleral vein ligation. Exp. Eye. Res. 83, 758–770.

60. Morrison JC, CepurnaYing Guo WO, Johnson EC (2011) Pathophysiology of human glaucomatous optic nerve damage : insights from rodent models of glaucoma. Exp. Eye Res. 93, 156–64.

61. Nissirios N, Chanis R, Johnson E, Morrison J, Cepurna WO, et al. (2008) Comparison of anterior segment structures in two rat glaucoma models: an ultrasound biomicroscopic study. Invest. Ophthalmol. Vis. Sci. 49, 2478–2482.

62. Shifera AS, Trivedi S, Chau P, Bonnemaison LH, Iguchi R, et al. (2010) Constitutive secretion of chemokines by cultured human trabecular meshwork cells. Exp. Eye Res. 91, 42–47.

# 4

# Molecular Basis for Involvement of CYP1B1 in MYOC Upregulation and its Potential Implication in Glaucoma Pathogenesis

**Suddhasil Mookherjee**¤a, **Moulinath Acharya**¤b, **Deblina Banerjee, Ashima Bhattacharjee**¤c, **Kunal Ray***

Molecular & Human Genetics Division, CSIR-Indian Institute of Chemical Biology, Kolkata, India

## Abstract

*CYP1B1* has been implicated in primary congenital glaucoma with autosomal recessive mode of inheritance. Mutations in *CYP1B1* have also been reported in primary open angle glaucoma (POAG) cases and suggested to act as a modifier of the disease along with *Myocilin* (*MYOC*). Earlier reports suggest that over-expression of myocilin leads to POAG pathogenesis. Taken together, we propose a functional interaction between CYP1B1 and myocilin where 17β estradiol acts as a mediator. Therefore, we hypothesize that 17β estradiol can induce *MYOC* expression through the putative estrogen responsive elements (EREs) located in its promoter and CYP1B1 could manipulate *MYOC* expression by metabolizing 17β estradiol to 4-hydroxy estradiol, thus preventing it from binding to *MYOC* promoter. Hence any mutation in *CYP1B1* that reduces its 17β estradiol metabolizing activity might lead to *MYOC* upregulation, which in turn might play a role in glaucoma pathogenesis. It was observed that 17β estradiol is present in Human Trabecular Meshwork cells (HTM) and Retinal Pigment Epithelial cells (RPE) by immunoflouresence and ELISA. Also, the expression of enzymes related to estrogen biosynthesis pathway was observed in both cell lines by RT-PCR. Subsequent evaluation of the EREs in the *MYOC* promoter by luciferase assay, with dose and time dependent treatment of 17β estradiol, showed that the EREs are indeed active. This observation was further validated by direct binding of estrogen receptors (ER) on EREs in *MYOC* promoter and subsequent upregulation in *MYOC* level in HTM cells on 17β estradiol treatment. Interestingly, *CYP1B1* mutants with less than 10% enzymatic activity were found to increase the level of endogenous myocilin in HTM cells. Thus the experimental observations are consistent with our proposed hypothesis that mutant CYP1B1, lacking the 17β estradiol metabolizing activity, can cause MYOC upregulation, which might have a potential implication in glaucoma pathogenesis.

**Editor:** Robert Lafrenie, Sudbury Regional Hospital, Canada

**Funding:** This work was supported by Council of Scientific and Industrial Research, India [Grant number SIP-007 and MLP-0016.]. The funders had no role in study design, data collection and analysis, decision to publish, or preparation of the manuscript.

**Competing Interests:** The authors have declared that no competing interests exist.

* E-mail: kunalray@gmail.com

¤a Current address: National Eye Institute, National Institute of Health, Bethesda, Maryland, United States of America
¤b Current address: National Institute of Biomedical Genomics, Kalyani, India
¤c Current address: Department of Physiology, Johns Hopkins University, Baltimore, Maryland, United States of America

## Introduction

Glaucoma is a multifactorial optic disc neuropathy in which there is characteristic acquired loss of retinal ganglion cells and atrophy of the optic nerve [1]. It is the second largest blinding disorder after cataract [2]. According to the latest estimates, worldwide 5.7 million people are visually impaired and about 3.1 million people are blind due to glaucoma [2].

Among the various glaucoma subtypes, primary open angle glaucoma (POAG) occurs most frequently. Transmission of the disease occurs mostly in monogenic form in juvenile onset POAG (JOAG) and complex form in adults. The complex nature of the POAG has been reviewed recently [3]. It has been reported that 72% of POAG cases have an inherited component [4]. Thirty three chromosomal loci have so far been implicated in POAG, of which four genes, *Myocilin* (*MYOC*) on *GLC1A* (1q32) [5], *Optineurin* (*OPTN*) [6] on *GLC1E* (10p25), *WDR36* on *GLC1G* (5q22.3) [7] and *NTF4* on *GLC1O* (19q13.3) [8,9] have been characterized. In most cases, however, in spite of clear familial clustering, POAG

does not follow a Mendelian pattern of inheritance. All studies carried out on the role of *MYOC* in POAG including the largest study done on 1703 patients [10] reported similar frequency (2–4%) of mutations in *MYOC*.

In 1997, *CYP1B1* was first identified as a causal gene for primary congenital glaucoma (PCG) [11]. Later, it was reported as a modifier locus for POAG that together with *MYOC* mutation expedite the disease progression from adult onset to a juvenile form in a digenic mode of inheritance [12]. Screening *CYP1B1* in 236 unrelated French Caucasian POAG patients unraveled mutations in 4.6% (n = 11) of the patients with no mutation in *MYOC* [13]. We observed that on rare occasion even *CYP1B1* alone could be responsible for JOAG [14].

CYP1B1 is a multifactorial enzyme involved in fatty acid, retinoic acid and 17β estradiol metabolism. Multiple studies have demonstrated that mutations in *CYP1B1* results in the loss of one or more of its enzymatic activity, stability and relative abundance [15–19] but no studies have been done yet to determine the mechanism operating in digenic scenarios in POAG cases involving both *CYP1B1* and *MYOC* mutations. We here propose a mechanism based on our experimental data that could potentially explain monogenic as well as digenic association of *CYP1B1* along with *MYOC* in POAG. We hypothesize that CYP1B1 can manipulate myocilin expression by metabolizing 17β estradiol to 4-hydroxy estradiol in Human Trabecular Meshwork (HTM) cells preventing it from binding the Estrogen Receptors (ER) present in cells and thus limiting the activation of the putative EREs present in the *MYOC* promoter region. Mutant CYP1B1, lacking 17β estradiol metabolizing activity, may lead to accumulation of higher level of 17β estradiol in cells, thus leading to prolonged activation of the EREs in the *MYOC* promoter region via ERs and upregulate myocilin expression by transcriptional activation. We attempted to prove this hypothesis by providing supporting evidence for the following biological events: (1) 17β estradiol is present in HTM cells and is synthesized in the trabecular meshwork itself; (2) the EREs in the *MYOC* promoter region are active; (3) 17β estradiol via EREs can cause transcriptional activation of *MYOC* by nuclear localization of ERα and direct binding of ERα-17β estradiol complex to the EREs; and (4) specific CYP1B1 mutants, lacking 17β estradiol metabolizing activity, can upregulate endogenous myocilin in HTM cells.

## Results

### 17β Estradiol is Present in HTM and RPE Cells

To probe the presence of 17β estradiol in ocular cells, HTM and RPE cells were grown approximately for 36 hours in culture media and treated with 17β estradiol antibody followed by FITC conjugated anti-mouse secondary antibody. Immunofluoresence assay showed scattered expression of 17β estradiol in the cytosol of HTM (Figure 1A) and RPE (Figure 1B) that was absent in the negative control (cells treated only with FITC conjugated anti-mouse secondary antibody). To eliminate the possibility of experimental artifact due to non-specific binding, same experiment was performed with HEK293 (Human Embryonic Kidney) cells that revealed the presence of 17β estradiol at a very low level in these cells (Figure 1C).

Under normal condition, these cells were grown in a media containing FBS. Thus these cells might have contaminating amount of the hormone carried by FBS used in cell culture. In order to eliminate such a possibility, HTM and RPE cells were grown for several passages in media supplemented with charcoal treated FBS to remove 17β-estradiol. Both cell types as well as the culture media were treated with di-ethyl ether to extract 17β-estradiol. The concentration of the extracted estradiol was determined from the standard curve and was found to be 70,000 pg/ml and 150,000 pg/ml in HTM and RPE cell lines respectively and the media was found to contain ≤200 pg/ml 17β estradiol (Figure 1D). These observations strongly suggested the presence of 17β estradiol in HTM and RPE cells.

### Presence of Estrogen Biosynthesis Pathway Enzymes in HTM and RPE Cells

To gather additional support in favor of intracellular synthesis of 17β estradiol in HTM and RPE, we examined for the presence of the enzymes involved in the biosynthetic pathway of estradiol from cholesterol in these cell lines. In both HTM and RPE cells, expression of *P450SCC, CYP17, 3β-HSD, 17β-HSD* and *Aromatase* (Figure 2A) were found by RT-PCR (Figure 2B) using gene specific primer pairs that encompass an intron to distinguish the amplified products from genomic sequences. The PCR products were

further sequenced to confirm the identity of the target region (data not shown).

### EREs in the *MYOC* Promoter are Functionally Active

To provide evidence for 17β estradiol mediated upregulation of *MYOC*, it was important to examine the responsiveness of EREs in the *MYOC* promoter in the presence of estradiol. To examine this possibility, deletion constructs (M700, M900, M1449 & M3194 in Figure 3A) of *MYOC* promoter region containing ERE & AP1 sites were generated and cloned in a promoter-less pGL3 basic vector containing luciferase as the reporter gene. To test the functionality of the EREs and AP1 cis-elements, the deletion clones were transfected into human RPE cells, followed by a dose (250 nM and 1000 nM) and time (0–16 hrs) dependent treatment of 17β estradiol, 40 hours post transfection. Based on experiments shown in Figure 3B, two different time points (4 hrs and 8 hrs) were selected for further downstream analysis to determine the ratio of induced and uninduced cells with different dosages of 17β estradiol (Figure 3C). The largest construct (M3194) containing all 3 EREs was observed to induce maximum luciferase activity proportional to dose and duration of estradiol treatment. However, other clones either lacking (M700 & M900) or containing half-ERE (M1449) were unresponsive to 17β estradiol treatment (Figure 3B & 3C).

### Inhibition of *MYOC* Promoter Activity by 17β-estradiol Competitor

To further confirm that the putative EREs in the *MYOC* promoter are active, we treated the cells with Estrogen Receptor (ER) competitor 4-hydroxy tamoxifen (4-OHT). RPE cells were transfected with the largest *MYOC* promoter construct containing all the EREs (M3194) followed by treatment with increasing concentration of 4-OHT. It was found that with increasing concentration of 4-OHT, the basal promoter activity reduced. This observation provided further support that the putative EREs of the *MYOC* promoter are functionally active (Figure 3D).

### 17β Estradiol Elevates the Level of Endogenous Myocilin in Human TM Cells

To further validate the functionality of the putative EREs in *MYOC* promoter, HTM cells were treated with 1000nM of 17β estradiol for 24 hrs. A subsequent increase in the level of endogenous myocilin was observed post treatment (Figure 3E). Thus, this further substantiates the activity of the EREs on *MYOC* promoter and that the increased concentration of 17β estradiol can upregulate *MYOC* in HTM cells.

### 17β Estradiol is Responsible for Nuclear Localization of ERα in HTM and RPE Cells

To examine the presence of ERα in HTM and RPE cells and its nuclear translocation on steroid treatment, the cells were treated with 17β estradiol with similar dosage(250 nM and 1000 nM) in a time dependent manner (4 hrs and 8 hrs). Then the cells were treated with human specific ERα antibody raised in rabbit followed by treatment with Alexa Fluor® 488 conjugated anti-rabbit secondary antibody. Confocal images of the HTM and RPE cells revealed that nuclear localization of ERα was maximum after 8hours at both 250 nM and 1000 nM concentrations of 17β estradiol (Figure 4 and 5).

### ERα Binds to Putative EREs in *MYOC* Promoter

Since increased concentration of 17β estradiol in HTM cells can upregulate endogenous myocilin and also cause nuclear localiza-

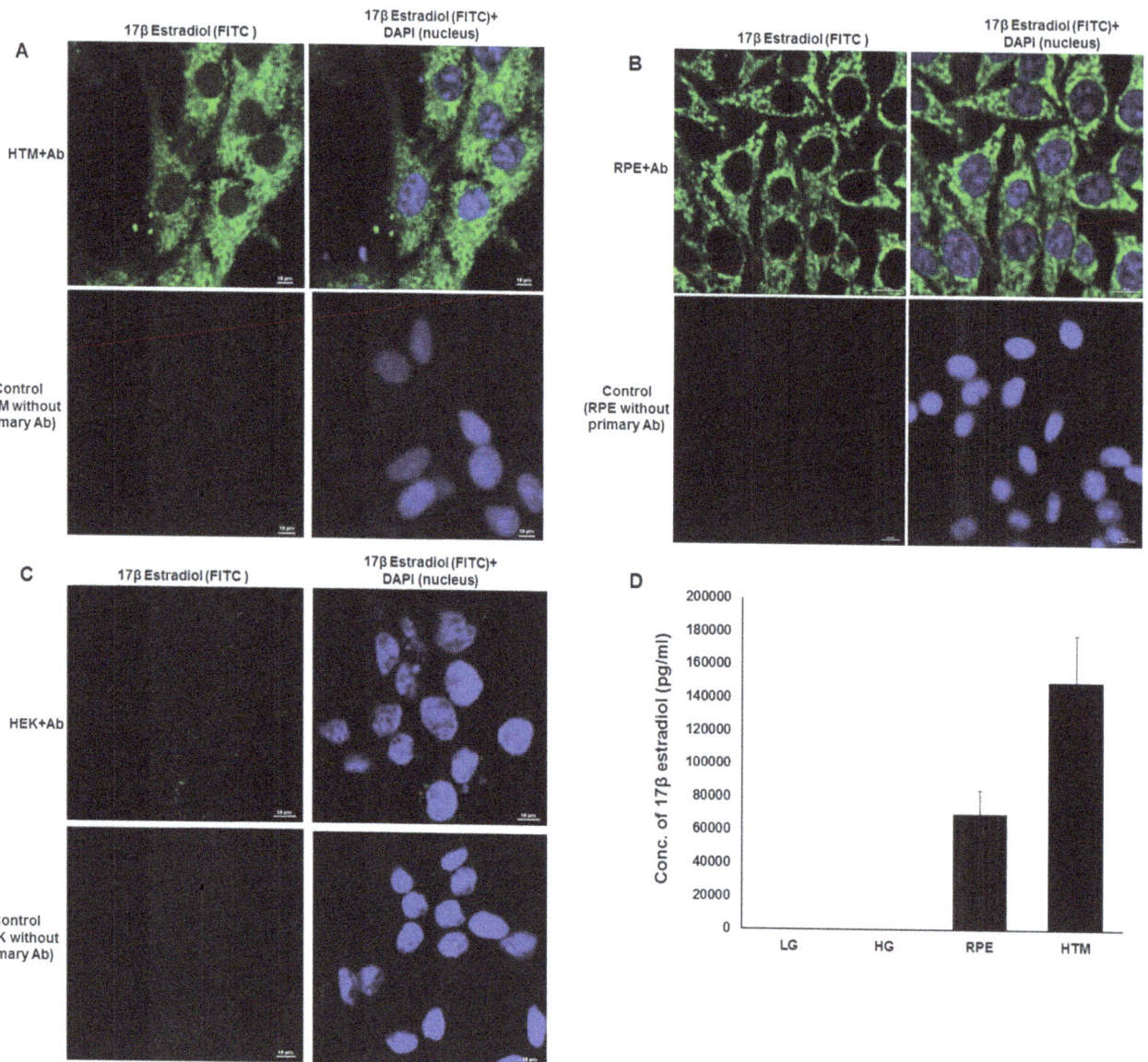

**Figure 1. Presence of 17β estradiol in ocular cells.** Confocal images are shown for HTM (*Panel A*), RPE (*Panel B*) and HEK 293 (*Panel C*) cells using anti-17β estradiol antibody and counterstained with FITC labeled secondary antibody. DAPI was used to stain the nucleus. In each panel control cells were treated only with FITC labeled secondary antibody, but not primary antibody, to assess the background noise. The scale of magnification is shown in each panel. The level of 17β estradiol in HTM and RPE cell lines were estimated by ELISA (*Panel D*). Similar estimation in low glucose (LG) and high glucose (HG) media containing 10% charcoal treated FBS did not show presence of 17β estradiol. The experiments were done in triplicate.

tion of ERα, we intended to test the direct binding of ERs to the *MYOC* promoter element by chromatin immunoprecipitation (ChIP) assay. In HTM cells, treated with 1000 nM of 17β-estradiol for 48 hrs, ChIP was done using anti-ERα antibody and the precipitated DNA was PCR amplified with primers specific to a 308 bp region of the *MYOC* promoter (Figure 6). Positive amplification of the specific region on *MYOC* promoter was observed in HTM cells treated with 17β-estradiol indicating that ERα specifically binds to the EREs in the *MYOC* promoter and transactivates it. In order to further evaluate the specificity of the ChIP assay, a second PCR amplification was done with the same DNA sample immumoprecipitated with ERα antibody using primers specific to the *Tyrosinase (TYR)* promoter which is devoid of any putative ERE; absence of any PCR product strongly

suggests the specific binding of the ERα to the EREs in the *MYOC* promoter (Figure 6).

## CYP1B1 Mutant Proteins Show Reduced Enzymatic Activity

The enzymatic activity of normal and mutant CYP1B1 was analyzed to explore whether the mutant CYP1B1 clones (E229K, R368H and R532T) lack 17β estradiol metabolizing activity, leading to accumulation of higher level of the steroid in cells. Among the mutants, E229K has been reported as a hypomorphic *CYP1B1* variant [16]. The R523T variant has been reported as a cause of JOAG in an East Indian family [14] and R368H is a predominant mutation in *CYP1B1* in Indian PCG as well as POAG patients [20], [21]. The level of activity of transfected CYP1B1 was measured using P450-Glo assay kit with appropriate

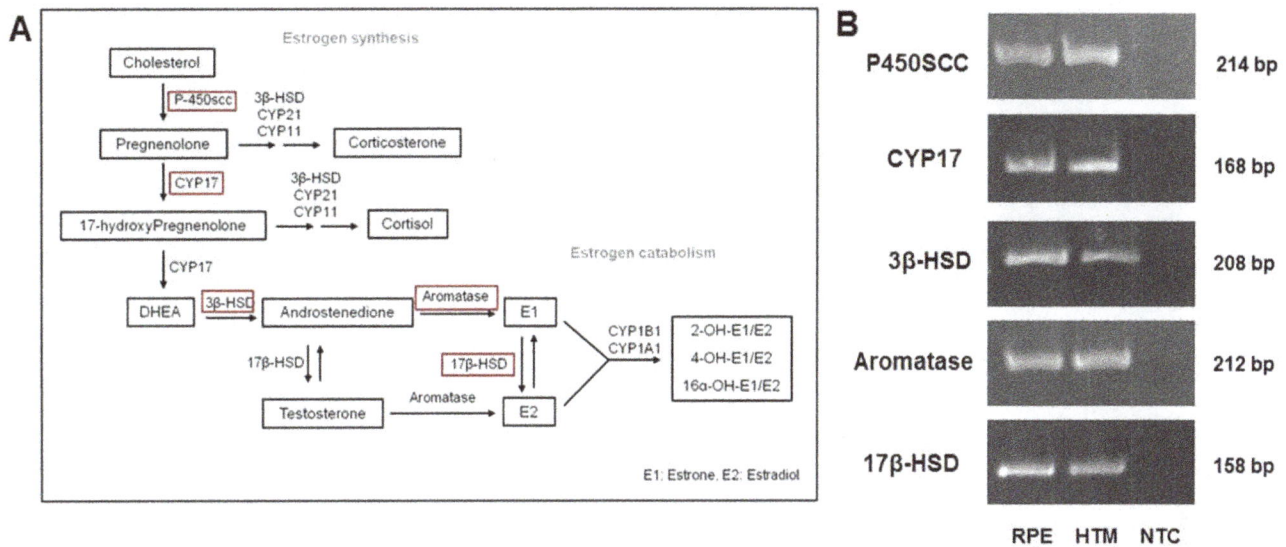

**Figure 2. Expression of 17β estradiol synthesizing enzymes in HTM and RPE cells. A:** 17β estradiol synthesis pathway. The key enzymes are highlighted by red squares. **B:** Semi-quantitative RT-PCR showing the presence of key 17β estradiol synthesizing enzymes in HTM and RPE cells. Three independent experiments were done for each enzyme in both cell lines. The identity of each product was confirmed by sequencing (data not shown). NTC: No cDNA template control.

controls in each step which includes (i) equal seeding density, (ii) normalization of endogenous CYP1B1, activity, and (iii) transfection efficiency. For each mutant or wild type CYP1B1 enzyme activity was normalized with the transfection efficiency as determined by the mRNA level by real-time PCR (Figure 7B). All three mutants showed <10% 17β metabolizing activity as compared to the wild type CYP1B1 (Figure 7A).

## Elevation of Endogenous Myocilin Level in Mutant CYP1B1 Background

To delineate the effect of CYP1B1 mutants on the expression of myocilin, the level of endogenous myocilin in HTM cell line was analyzed in cells transfected with mutant CYP1B1 constructs. The cells were harvested 36 hrs after transfection with normal and mutant CYP1B1 constructs (E229K, R523T and R368H). Myocilin expression in the background of R368H and R523T mutants was found to be significantly higher leading to 180% (p value: 0.023) and 165% (p value: 0.014) expression of MYOC, respectively, compared to normal CYP1B1. The E229K mutant of CYP1B1, though over expressed myocilin by 144% as compared to wild type CYP1B1, the expression was not found to be statistically significant (p value: 0.086) (Figure 8). Thus, in cells expressing mutant CYP1B1 consistent overexpression of MYOC was observed.

## Discussion

To date multiple genetic evidences of involvement of *CYP1B1* in POAG have been reported [12–14,22,23]. From these reports, it appears that *CYP1B1* has a larger role to play in glaucoma pathogenesis, which includes causation of PCG, acting as a modifier for POAG and on rare occasions, being the primary cause of JOAG. In addition, digenic inheritance in POAG suggested genetic correlation between *MYOC* and *CYP1B1* that requires to be understood at the functional level. In our present study, we deciphered that CYP1B1 plays a role in transcriptional activation of *MYOC*, by regulating the level of 17β estradiol, the substrate of *CYP1B1*.

It was observed that 17β estradiol is present in ocular cells (HTM and RPE), which was further supported by the expression of the enzymes required to synthesize estrogen from cholesterol in these cells. Previous studies have demonstrated presence of estradiol synthesizing enzymes in human ocular surface and adnexal tissues (lacrimal and meibomian glands, corneal and conjunctival epithelium, ciliary epithelium etc.) [24,25]. Expression of sex steroid hormone receptors were also found in multiple ocular tissues (cornea, conjunctiva, ciliary body, retina, RPE etc.) in different animals [26]. These observations together point that potential local sex steroid biosynthetic and effector mechanisms are available in the eye.

To support our hypothesis, we established that the EREs in the *MYOC* promoter [27] could induce its transcription in the presence of 17β estradiol. Also by the introduction of 17β estradiol competitor it was found that the basal promoter activity of the *MYOC* promoter is inhibited, which further proves that the EREs of the *MYOC* promoter are active. In addition, a twofold higher expression of endogenous myocilin was observed in HTM cell line upon treatment with 17β estradiol. This was further supported by observed nuclear localization of estrogen receptor-alpha on 17β estradiol induction. This transactivation was eventually brought about by binding of estrogen receptor and 17β estradiol complex on the ERE elements of the *MYOC* promoter, as evidenced from our ChIP experiment results.

It is well known that CYP1B1 plays an important role in steroid metabolism (4-hydroxylation of 17β estradiol). Induction of *MYOC* by dexamethasone, which is a corticosteroid by nature [28] and association of early menopause with POAG [29], point towards the fact that regulation of 17β estradiol by CYP1B1 is likely to have a role in POAG. In fact, we detected the over-expression of endogenous myocilin in HTM cell line in the presence of mutated CYP1B1. The three *CYP1B1* mutants (E229K, R368H and R523T), earlier detected in East Indian POAG patients [14], were selected for the present study and were found to have <10% of relative enzymatic activity compared to the wild type. Among these three mutations, R368H is one of the predominant mutations in India in both PCG and POAG and R523T is a novel

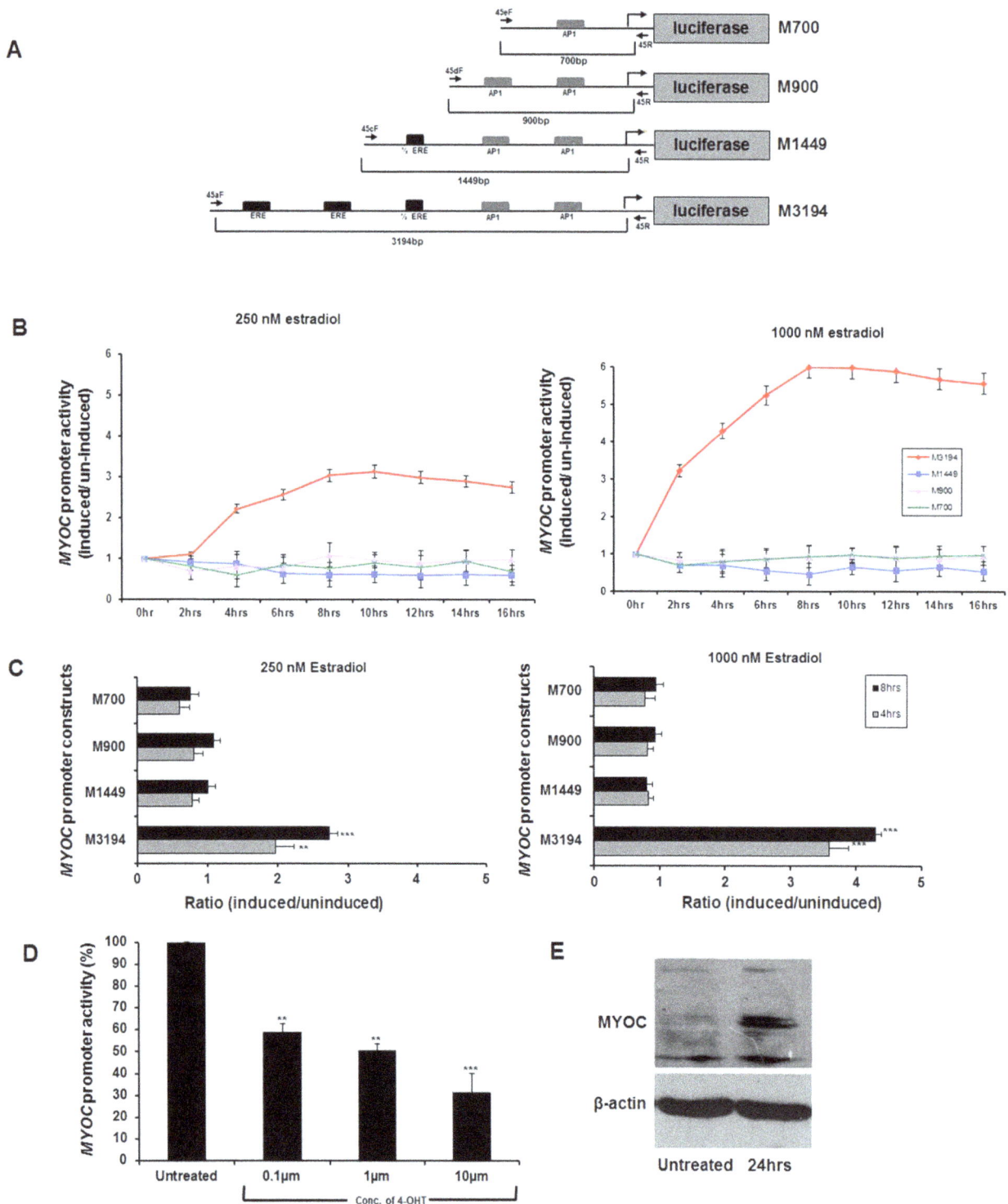

**Figure 3. Functional evaluation of putative EREs in *MYOC* promoter. *A*:** Serial constructs of *MYOC*-promoter region containing ERE and AP1 sites cloned in promoter less PGL3 basic vector. Black solid arrows indicate the forward and reverse primers used to amplify the inserts for subcloning. Also, the alphanumeric nomenclature of the constructs corresponds to the first initial of *myocilin* (M) followed by the size of the insert in base pairs. *B*: Luciferase activity in extracts from RPE cells transfected with the clones containing *MYOC* constructs and treated with 17β estradiol (250 nM or 1000 nM). *C*: Ratio of luciferase activity in cell extracts between induced and uninduced RPE cells for all 4 serial constructs upon dose (250 nM and 1000 nM) and time (4 hrs & 8 hrs) dependent treatment of 17β estradiol. The time points were taken based on the previous experiment in *Panel B*. *D*: The M3194 construct was transfected in RPE cells and subjected to increasing amount of 4-hydroxy tamoxifen (4-OHT; 17β estradiol competitor) treatment followed by luciferase assay. A gradual decrease in *MYOC* promoter activity was observed with increasing amount of 4-OHT. *E*: Significant upregulation of endogenous myocilin with 17β estradiol treatment in HTM cell. (**p-value<0.001, ***p-value<0.0001). Three independent replicates were performed for all the experiments described here.

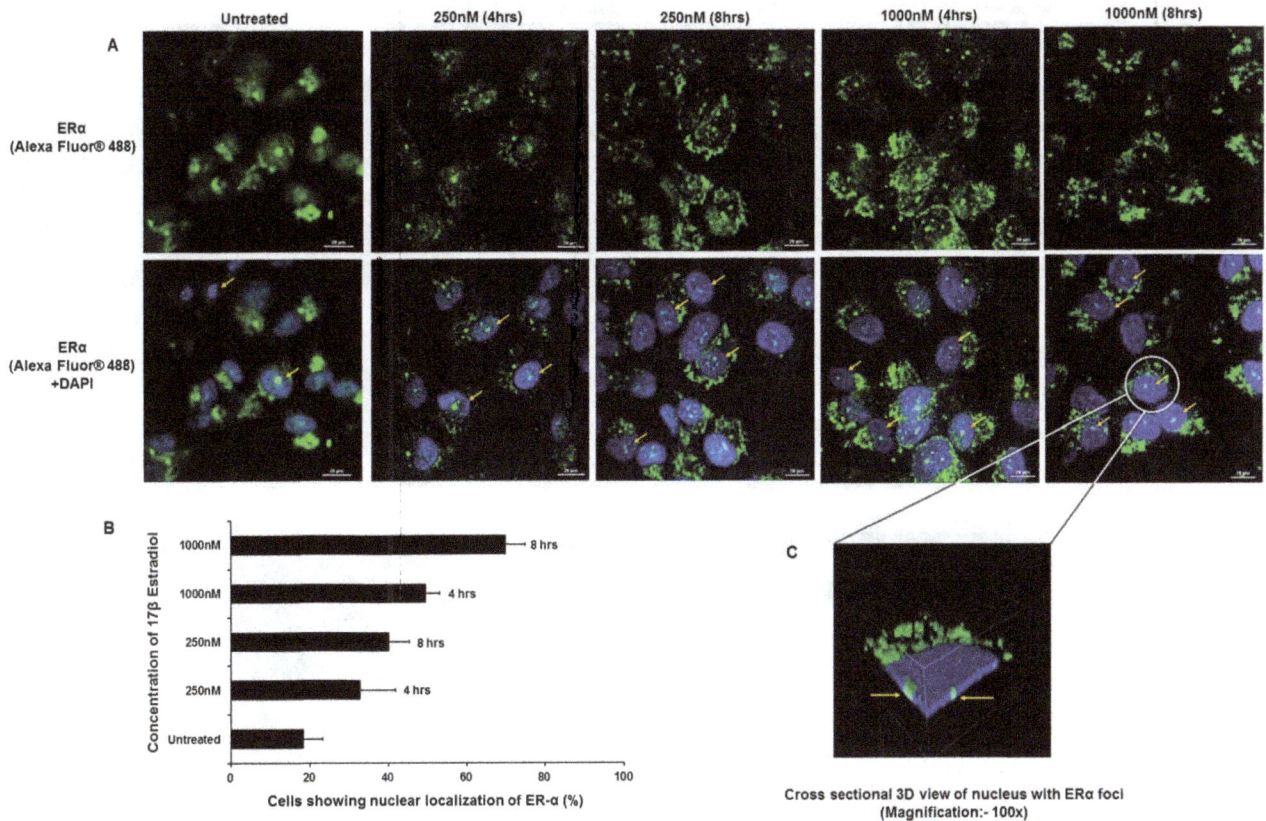

**Figure 4. Nuclear localization of ERα on 17β estradiol treatment in HTM cells.** *A:* Confocal images of HTM cells upon dose (250 mM & 1000 mM) and time (4 hr and 8 hr) dependent treatment with 17β estradiol. Cells were stained with human specific ERα-antibody followed by Alexa Fluor® 488 labeled anti-rabbit secondary antibody (*Upper panel*). For all conditions, corresponding superimposed image with DAPI are given (*Lower panel*). Arrows point to the cells where nuclear localization of ERα was observed. *B:* Histogram showing the percentage of HTM cells with ERα localized in the nucleus upon treatment with 17β estradiol in a dose and time dependent manner. Each experiment was done in triplicate. *C:* Cross sectional 3D view of nuclear localization of ERα in HTM cell is shown [Scale bar: 20 μm].

mutation found to cause JOAG in autosomal recessive mode of inheritance. Interestingly, for both the mutations significant increase in myocilin expression was found. Although E229K did not elicit significant overexpression of myocilin, it is possible that, similar to other multifactorial diseases, additional underlying factor(s) might precipitate the disease. E229K has been previously characterized as a hypomorphic allele [16]. Nevertheless, the activity for the variant (E229K) has been reported to be 26–40% [15,16] while we observed it to be <10%. The difference in *in-vitro* assessment of the enzyme activity may be due to the usage of different cells (RPE, HEK-293 or yeast cells), assay method and method for normalization (protein vs mRNA). In addition, relatively lower stability of E229K [16] could further complicate the precise assessment of the enzyme activity. Also, it is predicted to act as a risk factor for both PCG and POAG [14,20,21]. However, this variant has not yet been found in homozygous state in PCG patients [16]. Even when found in compound heterozygous state with another mutation, E229K was not found to be fully penetrant [23,30]. Interestingly, we found that this variant does not significantly overexpress myocilin.

*CYP1B1* mutation has also been found in sporadic POAG patients and on rare occasions, can cause JOAG in autosomal recessive mode of inheritance [14]. *MYOC* mutation when present along with *CYP1B1* mutation is reported to expedite the disease condition [31]. Also, mutated myocilin has been reported to form protein aggregates in the cell, in cytoplasm as well as in

endoplasmic reticulum which ultimately results in cell death [32]. Therefore, over expression of mutated myocilin as a result of mutant CYP1B1 would be expected to hasten up the cell death. Over expression of wild type myocilin is also believed to be involved in glaucoma pathogenesis. It is believed that in case of steroid induced glaucoma, over expression myocilin is one of the triggering factors for glaucoma causation; however, the notion is still controversial [33]. Over expression of myocilin has been shown to compromise the adhesive property of the cultured HTM cells through activation of cAMP/PKA and inhibition of Rho kinase [34]. Human myocilin over expression in the eyes of *Drosophila melanogaster* results in distortion of ommatidia (the 'eye' of Drosophila) which is accompanied by fluid discharge [35] and also activates the UPR (Unfolded protein response) [36]. On the contrary, BAC mediated myocilin overexpression in mouse does not produce any glaucoma phenotype [37]. This is not rare that mutations in homologues genes in mouse do not produce similar phenotype observed in human, which also varies depending on the mouse strain used in the specific study. Intravitreal administration of adenoviral vector with Y437H myocilin mutation in four different mouse strain (A/J, BALB/cJ, C57BL/6J, and C3H/HeJ) elevated the IOP level in three (BALB/cJ, C57BL/6J, and A/J) and considerable damage to the optic nerve was found in only one strain (A/J) [38].

*CYP1B1* represents the first example where mutation in a member of the cytochrome P450 superfamily results in a primary

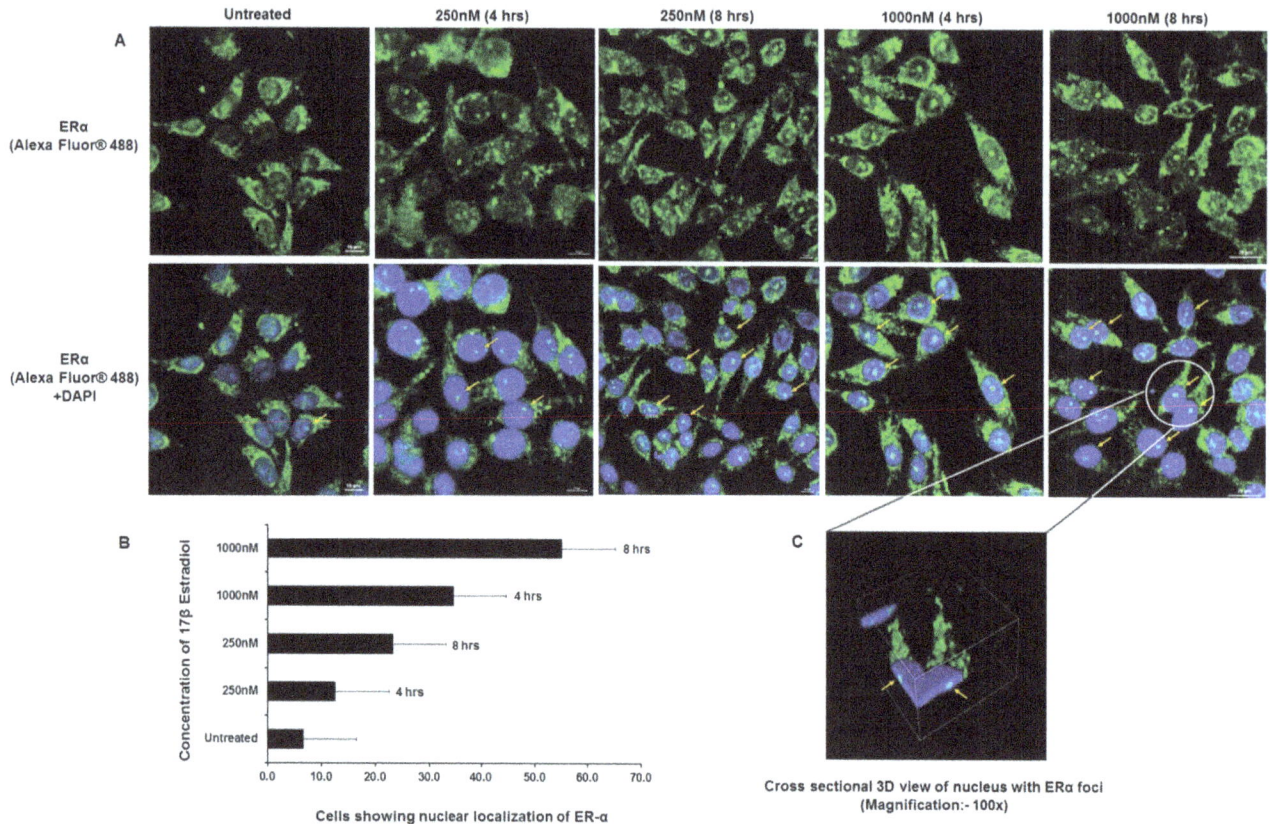

**Figure 5. Nuclear localization of ERα upon 17β estradiol treatment in human RPE cells. A:** Confocal images of human RPE cells upon dose (250 mM & 1000 mM) and time (4 hr and 8 hr) dependent treatment with 17β estradiol. Cells were stained with human specific ERα-antibody followed by Alexa Fluor® 488 labeled anti-rabbit secondary antibody (*Upper panel*). For all conditions, corresponding superimposed image with DAPI are given (*Lower panel*). Arrows point to the cells where nuclear localization of ERα was observed. **B:** Histogram showing the percentage of RPE cells with ERα localized in the nucleus upon treatment with 17β estradiol in a dose and time dependent manner. Each experiment was done in triplicate. **C:** Cross sectional 3D view of nuclear localization of ERα in RPE cell is shown [Scale bar: 10 μm].

developmental defect in terms of PCG [11]. It has also been found to be associated with head and neck squamous cell carcinoma and breast cancer [39,40]. It has been speculated earlier that CYP1B1 participates in the metabolism of an as-yet-unknown biologically active molecule that is a participant in eye development [11]. Vincent *et al* (2001) [12] suggested that *MYOC* and *CYP1B1* possibly interact through a common pathway and proposed that myocilin function could potentially be influenced by mutation in

CYP1B1. Also, polymorphisms in *CYP1B1* are known to be associated with its functional differences in estrogen hydroxylation activity [41]. Here we tried to elucidate a possible underlying mechanism where regulation of 17β estradiol by CYP1B1 plays a key role in the cascade of events that may lead to glaucoma (Figure 9). However, further *in-vivo* studies on animal models are necessary to provide additional supporting evidence for CYP1B1

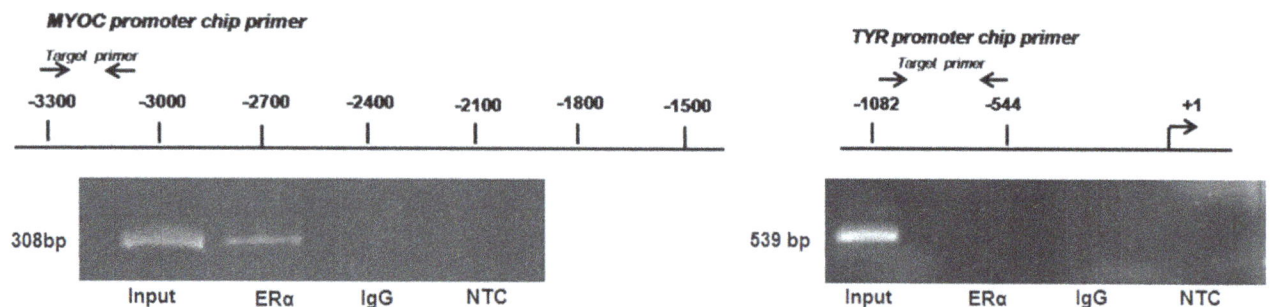

**Figure 6. Direct binding of ER-α- 17β estradiol complex to EREs in *MYOC* promoter.** ChIP (Chromatin-immunoprecipitation) assay results showing the presence of specific 308 bp band for *myocilin* promoter in the sample immunoprecipitated with the anti-estrogen receptor antibody. No specific band was observed for *Tyrosinase* gene promoter devoid of any EREs. In both the cases no amplification was observed on immunoprecipitation with immunoglobulin (IgG). Three independent replicates were performed for this experiment. NTC: No Template Control.

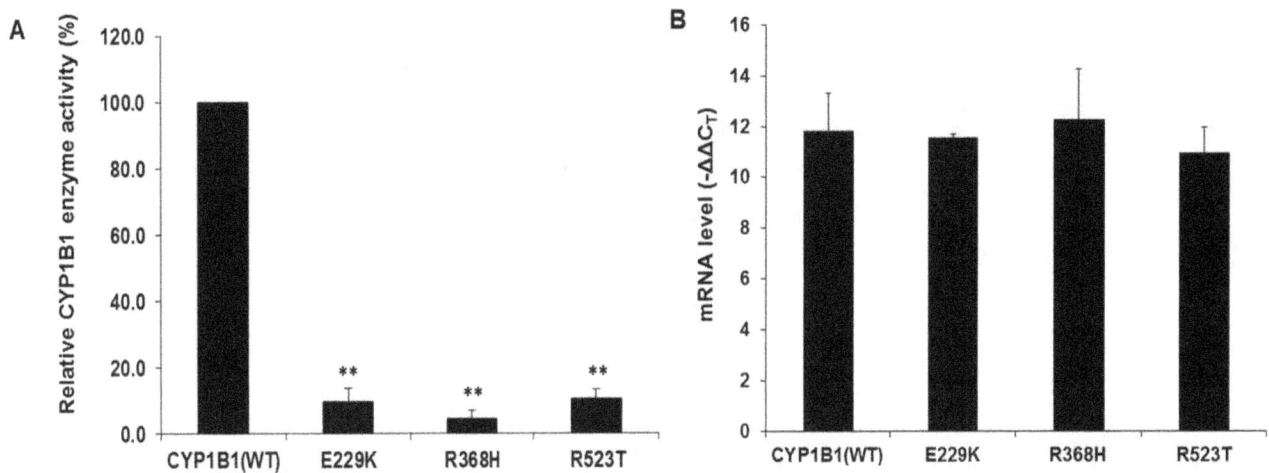

**Figure 7. CYP1B1 mutants have lower 17β estradiol metabolizing activity compared to wild type protein.** *A:* The enzyme activity of the mutant proteins was expressed as percentage of the activity retained as compared to the native (wild type) enzyme. Mutant constructs of CYP1B1 (i.e. E229K, R368H and R523T) showed <10% of 17β estradiol metabolizing activity (**p-value<0.001). *B:* Histogram showing the expression level of the transfected wild type and mutant constructs of *CYP1B1* in RPE cells as detected by RT-PCR. Three independent replicates were performed for this experiment.

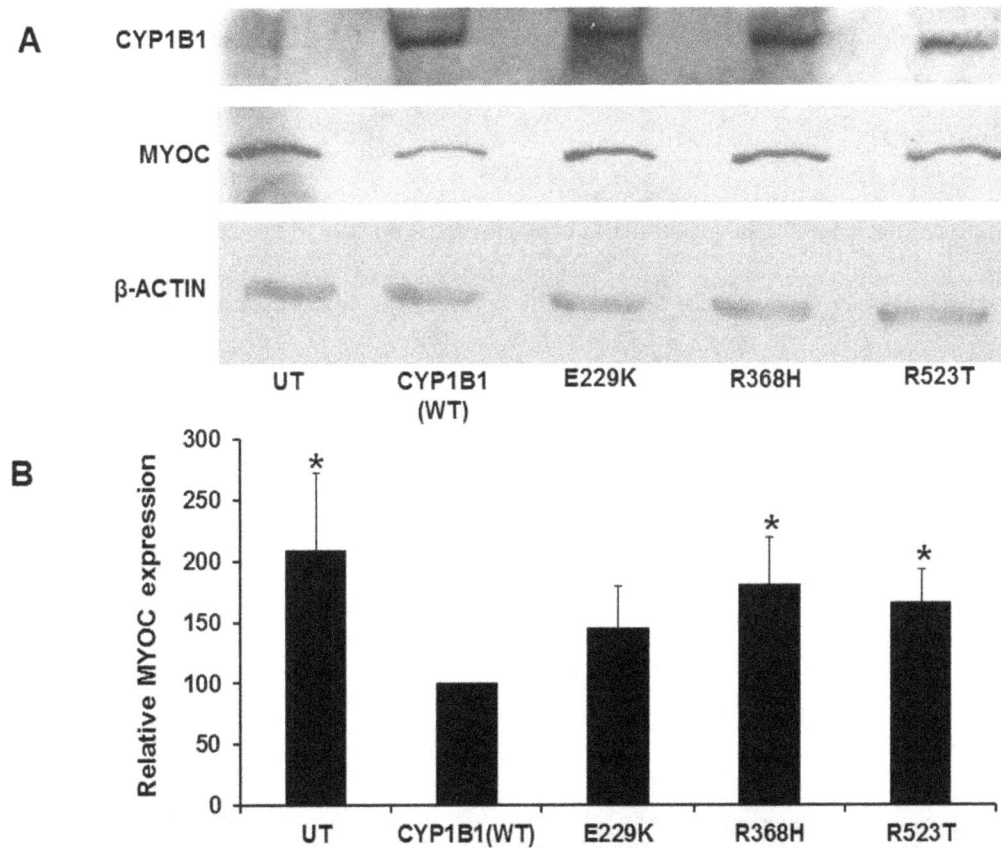

**Figure 8. CYP1B1 mutants cause upregulation of MYOC in HTM cells.** *A: Increased MYOC expression with mutant CYP1B1.* Western blot analysis of mutant CYP1B1 and myocilin showed increased expression of MYOC in the presence of mutant CYP1B1 clones with reduced (<10%) 17β estradiol metabolizing activity. *B: Quantitative analysis of MYOC expression.* The histogram shows levels of expression of endogenous MYOC in HTM cells transfected with wild type and mutant CYP1B1 clones. All the three mutants of CYP1B1 (i.e. E229K, R368H and R523T) considerably over-expressed MYOC compared to the normal CYP1B1. The R368H and R523T showed statistically significant over expression of myocilin with a p-value of 0.023 and 0.014, respectively. However, the effect of E229K mutant was not found to be statistically significant. This experiment was repeated three times [*p-value- <0.05].

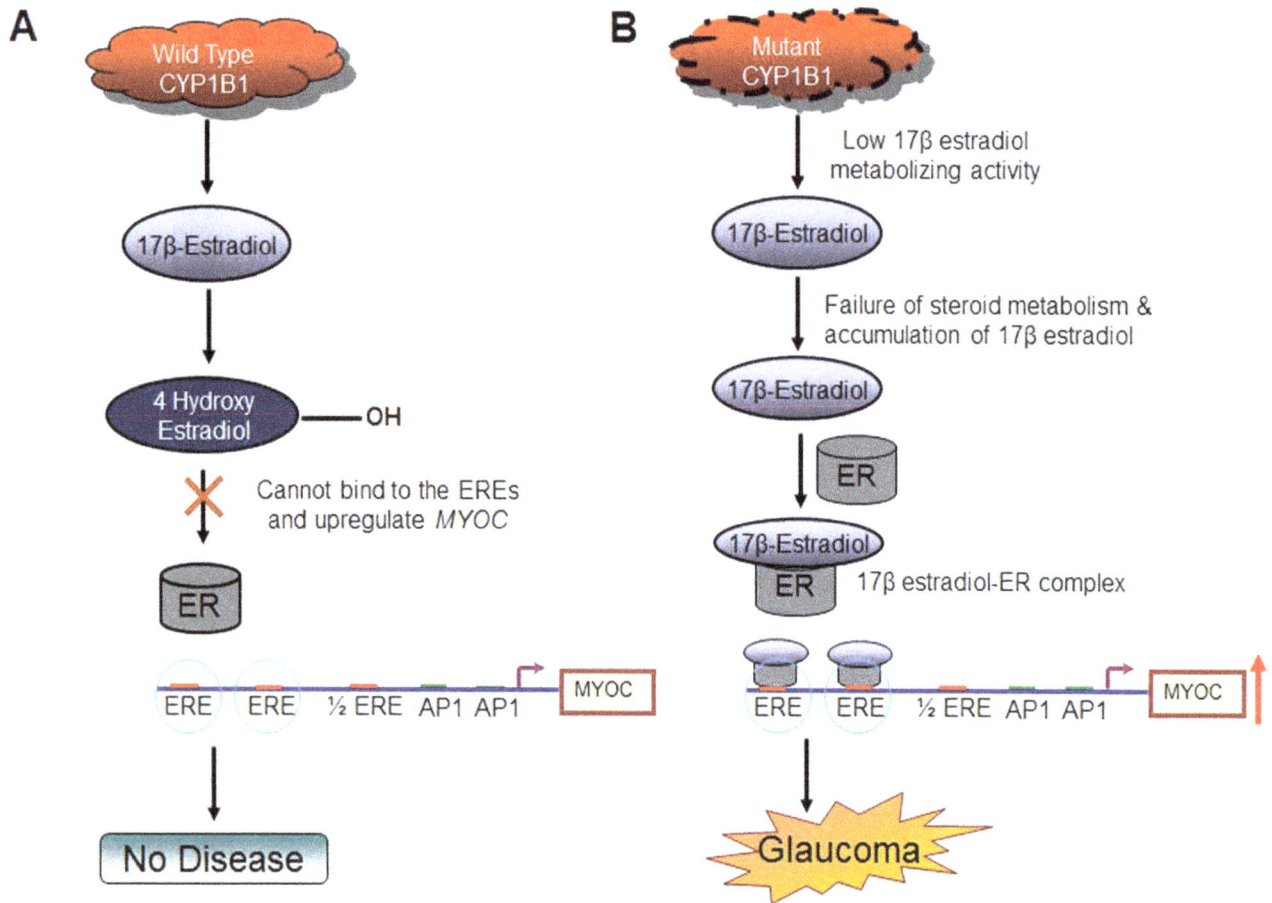

**Figure 9. Schematic diagram showing potential influence of CYP1B1 mutants on MYOC expression.** In *Panel A* fully functional wild-type CYP1B1 metabolizes 17β-Estradiol; thus limiting the steroid to form the hormone-receptor complex (17β-Estradiol-ER) whereas in *Panel B* restricted CYP1B1 enzymatic activity results in higher levels of the steroid available for formation of 17β-Estradiol-ER complex which in turn leads to *MYOC* upregulation through estrogen response elements (EREs) in *MYOC* promoter. The latter condition might have a potential implication in glaucoma pathogenesis.

mediated MYOC upregulation as a molecular basis for glaucoma pathogenesis.

## Methods

### Mammalian Cell Culture

The human retinal pigment epithelium cell line RPE8319 (kind gift from Dr. Frans Cremers, Univ. Medical Center, Nijmegen, The Netherlands), HEK293, and Human Trabecular Meshwork (HTM) cell line (originally developed by Polansky *et al* and kindly gifted by Dr. Michael Walter, University of Alberta, Edmonton, Canada) were maintained in DMEM (Dulbecco's modified Eagle Medium, GIBCO BRL) at pH 7.4 supplemented with 10% fetal bovine serum (GIBCO BRL) containing penicillin/streptomycin/gentamycin in the presence of 5% $CO_2$ at 37°C. While RPE and HEK293 cell lines were maintained with high glucose concentration (4 g/L), HTM cell line was maintained in media containing lower glucose concentration (1 g/L).The identity of the HTM cell line was verified by upregulation of endogenous myocilin by dexamethasone treatment (Figure S1). Transient transfections of human RPE and HTM cell lines were performed with the Lipofectamine 2000 system according to the manufacturer's instructions (Invitrogen Inc., USA).

## Immunocytochemistry

For the immunofluorescence assay, HTM and RPE cells (approximately $3 \times 10^5$ cells) were cultured on coverslips in a 35 mm culture dish for 14 hrs. The cells were rinsed twice with cold PBS and fixed with cold acetone:methanol (1:1) fixing solution for 5 mins at $-20°C$. After fixing, the cells were washed with PBS 3 to 4 times. Only in case of ER-α, cells were permealized using 0.1% Triton-X (Sigma-Aldrich, USA) at room temperature for 3 mins. The cells were then incubated in 5% BSA (Bangalore Genei, India) in PBS for 1hour at room temperature. This was followed by overnight incubation with either human ER-α specific primary antibody (1:100 dilution) raised in rabbit (Sigma Biologicals, Germany) or human 17β estradiol specific primary antibody (1:50 dilution) raised in mouse (Geneway, USA) at 4°C. On the following day, the excess primary antibody was washed off with PBS thrice and the cells were incubated with Alexa Fluor® 488 anti rabbit (1:200 dilutions) (Invitrogen, USA) or FITC conjugated anti mouse secondary antibody (1:200 dilutions) (Bangalore Genei, India) for 2hours at room temperature. The cells were again washed with PBS thrice and the cover slips were mounted on glass slides with Prolong Gold Antifade reagent with DAPI (Invitrogen, USA). The confocal imaging was done using A1R confocal microscope (Nikon, Japan).

To quantify ERα nuclear localization 3 to 4 fields were randomly chosen and percentage of cells showing ERα foci in the nucleus was determined for each field (for both RPE and HTM cells). The experiment was done in triplicate. In each case nuclear localization of the ER-α was confirmed by 3D imaging of the cells.

## Detection of 17β Estradiol in HTM, RPE and Culture Media by ELISA

Assessment of 17β estradiol in cells and cell culture media was done using estradiol bioassay kit (Stressgene, USA) with a modified protocol. The HTM and RPE cells were grown to confluency in a 6 cm culture dish in a media containing charcoal treated FBS for several passages. The confluent HTM and RPE cells were treated with 500 μl of NP40 lysis buffer and the lysate was collected in a tube. Estradiol was extracted from cell lysate with diethyl-ether. Estradiol was also extracted from the "virgin" culture media (not used in cell culture procedure) with charcoal treated FBS to estimate the level of estradiol in the media. After extraction the ether was evaporated under nitrogen and the extracted estradiol was re-suspended in assay buffer provided with the kit.

The kit is provided with a 96 well ELISA plate pre-coated with goat anti rabbit secondary antibody. The external antigen i.e 17β estradiol has to compete with an ALP (alkaline phosphatase) conjugated 17β estradiol competitor provided with the kit for binding with estradiol specific primary antibody raised in rabbit. So, as the amount of the external antigen increases the ALP signal is decreased. The amount of external antigen was calculated from the standard graph prepared with known amount of 17β estradiol. This experiment was repeated three times.

## Construction of MYOC-promoter Clones in PGL3 Basic Vector

Serial fragments containing AP1 and EREs in the promoter region of MYOC were amplified from genomic DNA using the respective oligonucleotide pairs (Table S1). All the oligonucleotides used for this purpose contained XhoI and HindIII restriction site at their 5'- and 3' ends respectively. The fragments were then cloned either directly or via TA vector (pCR2.1, Invitrogen, USA) mediated cloning into PGL3 basic vector (Promega, USA) after digestion with XhoI and HindIII (New England Biolabs, USA) using T4 DNA ligase (Invitrogen, USA). Recombinant plasmids were isolated using QIAGEN plasmid midi kit (Qiagen, Germany) from transformed E.coli cells in ampicillin mediated selection condition. These constructs were first checked on 0.8–1.0% agarose gel after digestion with above mentioned enzymes and then sequenced using respective amplification primers (Table S1) on one end and PGL3 specific primer PGLR (5'-CTTTATGTTTTTGGCGTCTTCCA-3') from the other end.

## Assay for Luciferase Activity Following Treatment with 17β Estradiol and 4-hydroxy-tamoxifen (4-OHT)

Human RPE cells were (approximately $1 \times 10^6$ cells/per well) seeded on 6-well plate and left overnight (~14 hrs). Cells were transiently transfected with empty pGL3 vector as control and MYOC promoter constructs. For consistency each transfection was carried out with 2 μg of either MYOC promoter constructs or pGL3 control vector from a single plasmid preparation. After 36 hours of transfection RPE cells were subjected to dose and time dependent treatment of 17β estradiol followed by luciferase assay. The luciferase activity was normalized with protein concentration and the ratio between estradiol treated and untreated cells were taken. This experiment was repeated three times and statistical significance was calculated using student's t-test.

For examining the inhibition of myocilin promoter activity by estrogen receptor competitor, human RPE cells (approximately $1 \times 10^6$ cells/per well) were seeded on 6-well plate and cultured overnight (~14 hrs). The cells were then treated with 0.1 μM, 1 μM and 10 μM of 4-OHT (Sigma, USA) for 8 hrs, post 36 hrs of transfection with M3194 (2μg/per well); the largest construct containing all the EREs followed by luciferase assay. For consistency replicate experiments were carried out with plasmids from single preparation. Here also the luciferase activity was normalized with protein concentration and the fold differences between 4-OHT treated and untreated cells were taken. For each dose luciferase activity was measured for three independent experiments and statistical significance was calculated using student's t-test.

The luciferase activity was determined as light units using the Luciferase Assay Kit (Promega, Madison, USA). For the assay, the cells were washed with phosphate buffered saline and lysed in the luciferase cell culture lysis buffer provided with the Luciferase Assay Kit. Twenty five micro-liter of cell lysate was then added to 25 μl of luciferase assay substrate (Luciferase Assay Kit) and the luminescence was measured as light units in a Monolight 2010 luminometer (Analytical Luminescence, San Diego, CA). The protein concentration in each lysate was determined with a protein assay kit (Bio-Rad, USA) and used to normalize the luciferase activity.

## Chromatin Immunoprecipitation (ChIP) Assay

For ChIP assay HTM cells were treated with 17β estradiol for 48 hrs. Then the cells were processed for ChIP reaction with IMGENEX quick ChIP kit (IMGENEX, USA) according to the manufacturer's protocol using estrogen receptor specific antibody (Sigma, USA) or IgG (negative control) (primer lists are available in Table S2).

## Site Directed Mutagenesis

A CYP1B1 cDNA construct in the pcDNA3 mammalian expression vector (kindly gifted by Dr. Thomas. H. Friedberg University of Dundee, UK) was used to generate mutant CYP1B1 clones: c.1057 G>A (E229K), c.1475 G>A (R368H) and c.1940 G>C (R523T). Site-directed mutagenesis and subsequent transformation of the mutant clones were performed using the QuikChange XL Site-Directed Mutagenesis Kit (Stratagene, La Jolla, CA, USA) according to the manufacturer's protocol with specific primers (Table S3). Plasmid isolation was done for all the three variants c.1057 G>A (E229K), c.1475 G>A (R368H) and c.1940 G>C (R523T) cloned in the pcDNA3 vector, using a QIAGEN plasmid mini kit (Qiagen, Germany) according to the manufacturer's protocol. The targeted changes in the recombinant clones generated were confirmed by sequencing.

## Determination of Wild Type and Mutant CYP1B1 Enzyme Activity

RPE cells (approximately $3 \times 10^5$ cells per well) were grown on 12 well culture plates. After 24 hrs, cells were transfected with 2 μg wild type and mutant CYP1B1 (pE229K, pR368H and pR523T). Forty hours post transfection CYP1B1 activity was measured using the CYP450-GLO™ Assay kit (catalog number V8762; Promega, Madison, WI) with a modified protocol. The media was changed and the luciferin-CEE substrate (0.1 mM final concentration) was added to each well with 500 μl of media. After 3 ½hrs incubation most of the luciferin-CEE was converted to luciferin and secreted out in the media. The medium was collected from each well and processed according to the manufacturer's protocol. The final amount of luciferin was determined using luminometer.

For each observation total media (500 µl) was taken out and 3 aliquots of 50µl of media for each mutant as well as the wild type construct were used for final reading from luminometer. The relative luminescence unit (RLU) obtained was normalized with respective mRNA levels of the wild type and mutant CYP1B1, as determined by Real-Time PCR, to nullify the difference in transfection efficiency. The enzyme activity of the mutant proteins were expressed as percentage of activity retained as compared to wild type protein. For each mutant three independent observations were made and statistical significance was calculated using Student's t-test.

### Preparation of cDNA from RNA (RT) and PCR

To determine the RNA levels of 17β estradiol synthesizing enzymes and the wild type and mutant CYP1B1, cells were collected from respective wells after determination of the luciferase activity from the media. Total RNA was extracted from each by using TriZol$^{TM}$ (Invitrogen, USA) as per the manufacturer's protocol. Preparation of cDNA was done using SUPERSCRIPT$^{TM}$ First – Strand Synthesis System (Invitrogen, USA) for RT-PCR at 42°C for 50 min following the manufacturer's instructions.

For PCR about 2 µl of cDNA was amplified in a 30 µl reaction volume containing 10 mM Tris-HCl, pH 8.3; 50 mM KCl, 2.5 mM or 2.0 mM MgCl$_2$ as required, 0.26mM of each dNTPs and 25 pmol of each primer and 0.5U Taq DNA polymerase (GIBCO-BRL, Gaithersburg, MD). To determine the expression of the enzymes required for estrogen synthesis from cholesterol, cDNAs of HTM and RPE cells were amplified with primer pairs (Table S4) from coding sequence but encompassing an intron such that amplified cDNA product could be distinguished from the gDNA by the known difference in sizes of the amplicons.

### Quantitative Real Time-PCR for Normal and Mutant CYP1B1

The mRNA expression of normal and mutant (c.1057 G>A, c.1475 G>A and c.1940 G>C) variants of *CYP1B1* was determined by Real-Time PCR in the 7500 Real Time PCR System (Applied Biosystems, Foster City, CA) using SYBR Green Jumpstart Taq Ready Mix (Sigma, St.Louis, MO). The following primers were used: CYP1B1 F 5'-GGAGAACGTACCGGC-CACTATC-3' and R 5'-CTTGGGTTTAATGGTTAGACC-3' and human β-actin F 5'-TGACGGGGGTCACCCA-CACTGTGCCCATCTA- 3' and R 5'-CTAGAAG-CATTGCGGTGGACGATGGAGGG- 3'. The threshold cycle C$_T$ of duplicate samples was determined using 7500 System SDS software (Applied Biosystems, Foster City, CA). The levels of both normal and mutant *CYP1B1* were normalized to β-actin levels by calculating the ΔC$_T$ value, which is the C$_T$ (threshold cycle) of the housekeeping gene (β-actin) subtracted from the C$_T$ of the target gene (*CYP1B1*). As CYP1B1 mRNA is expressed in RPE cells, we further normalized the data by calculating the ΔΔC$_T$ value which is a subtraction of ΔC$_T$ value of untransfected cells from each ΔC$_T$ value of both cells transfected with normal and mutant *CYP1B1*. All calculations were done according to the published paper in 2001 by Giulietti et al [42].

### Protein Electrophoresis and Western Blotting

Human trabecular meshwork (HTM) cells were grown on 6 well culture plates. After 24 hrs, cells were transfected with 4 µg of wild type and mutant CYP1B1 constructs. After transfection, the cells were treated with monensin sodium salt (3.2 µg/ml of media) for 36 hrs. Thirty six hrs post transfection cells were lysed using NP-

40 lysis buffer (150 mM Tris-Cl, 50 mM EDTA, pH. 8.0, 1%NP40) supplemented with protease inhibitor cocktail (1ul/ 106 cell; Sigma, St.Louis, MO) and was sonicated in a water bath for 5 mins. Total protein was estimated using Bradford assay, which is necessary for equal loading of the lysates. Fifty microgram of each protein sample were resolved in 10% SDS-polyacrylamide (MiniPROTEAN III; BioRad, Herucles, CA) and transferred onto a PVDF membrane (Hybond-P; GE Healthcare, Bedford, UK) by electroblotting using the ECL semi-dry transfer unit (Amersham Biociences, USA). Membranes were then blocked in 5% BSA in TBS for 3 hrs at room temperature and incubated with respective primary antibody [anti-CYP1B1 polyclonal antibody (1:1000) (Abcam, UK), anti-MYOC polyclonal antibody (1:250) (Santa-Cruz, USA) and Anti-β actin (1:2000) antibody (Sigma-Aldrich, USA)] overnight at 4°C. *B*eta- actin was used as the loading control. The membranes were washed thrice with TBST [25 mM Tris-HCl (pH 7.5), 150 mM NaCl, 0.05% tween-20] at 10 mins interval followed by incubation with appropriate secondary antibody conjugated with HRP [Anti-rabbit (1:60,000) and anti-mouse (1:2000)] (Bangalore Genei, India) for 2 hrs at room temperature. The secondary antibody was washed thrice with TBST followed by two washes with TBS. The ECL-western blotting detection kit (Pierce, USA) was used for chemiluminiscent detection. Densitometry for protein band quantitation was performed on scanned films using Image J software on triplicated independent experiments. The results were compared using Student's t-test.

## Supporting Information

**Figure S1 Upregulation of myocilin upon dexamethasone treatment.** A considerable overexpression of myocilin in HTM cell line is observed upon treatment with 100 mM dexamethasone for 5 days

**Table S1 Primer sequences and PCR conditions for serial amplification of promoter regions in *MYOC*.**

**Table S2 Primers used for ChIP assay.**

**Table S3 Primers for site directed mutagenesis of CYP1B1 constructs.**

**Table S4 Primers used for RT-PCR to amplify genes in estrogen synthesis pathway.**

## Acknowledgments

The authors are grateful to Dr. Frans Cremers, University Medical Center, Nijmegen, The Netherlands for providing the human RPE cells, Dr. Michael Walter, University of Alberta, Edmonton, Canada for the HTM cell line, Dr. Thomas.H.Friedberg University of Dundee, UK for the CYP1B1-pcDNA3 mammalian expression vector. We are thankful to Dr. Anupam Banerjee for helping us with the confocal imaging. We thank CSIR, India for providing pre-doctoral fellowships to SM, MA, DB and AB.

## Author Contributions

Conceived and designed the experiments: SM MA DB AB KR. Performed the experiments: SM MA DB AB. Analyzed the data: SM MA DB. Contributed reagents/materials/analysis tools: KR. Wrote the paper: SM MA DB AB KR.

# References

1. Libby RT, Gould DB, Anderson MG, John SW (2005) Complex genetics of glaucoma susceptibility. Annu Rev Genomics Hum Genet 6: 15–44.
2. Pascolini D, Mariotti SP (2012) Global estimates of visual impairment: 2010. Br J Ophthalmol 96: 614–618.
3. Ray K, Mookherjee S (2009) Molecular complexity of primary open angle glaucoma: current concepts. J Genet 88: 451–467.
4. Gong G, Kosoko-Lasaki S, Haynatzki G, Lynch HT, Lynch JA, et al. (2007) Inherited, familial and sporadic primary open-angle glaucoma. J Natl Med Assoc 99: 559–563.
5. Stone EM, Fingert JH, Alward WL, Nguyen TD, Polansky JR, et al. (1997) Identification of a gene that causes primary open angle glaucoma. Science 275: 668–670.
6. Rezaie T, Child A, Hitchings R, Brice G, Miller L, et al. (2002) Adult-onset primary open-angle glaucoma caused by mutations in optineurin. Science 295: 1077–1079.
7. Monemi S, Spaeth G, DaSilva A, Popinchalk S, Ilitchev E, et al. (2005) Identification of a novel adult-onset primary open-angle glaucoma (POAG) gene on 5q22.1. Hum Mol Genet 14: 725–733.
8. Pasutto F, Matsumoto T, Mardin CY, Sticht H, Brandstatter JH, et al. (2009) Heterozygous NTF4 mutations impairing neurotrophin-4 signaling in patients with primary open-angle glaucoma. Am J Hum Genet 85: 447–456.
9. Vithana EN, Nongpiur ME, Venkataraman D, Chan SH, Mavinahalli J, et al. (2010) Identification of a novel mutation in the NTF4 gene that causes primary open-angle glaucoma in a Chinese population. Mol Vis 16: 1640–1645.
10. Fingert JH, Heon E, Liebmann JM, Yamamoto T, Craig JE, et al. (1999) Analysis of myocilin mutations in 1703 glaucoma patients from five different populations. Hum Mol Genet 8: 899–905.
11. Stoilov I, Akarsu AN, Sarfarazi M (1997) Identification of three different truncating mutations in cytochrome P4501B1 (CYP1B1) as the principal cause of primary congenital glaucoma (Buphthalmos) in families linked to the GLC3A locus on chromosome 2p21. Hum Mol Genet 6: 641–647.
12. Vincent AL, Billingsley G, Buys Y, Levin AV, Priston M, et al. (2002) Digenic inheritance of early-onset glaucoma: CYP1B1, a potential modifier gene. Am J Hum Genet 70: 448–460.
13. Melki R, Colomb E, Lefort N, Brezin AP, Garchon HJ (2004) CYP1B1 mutations in French patients with early-onset primary open-angle glaucoma. J Med Genet 41: 647–651.
14. Acharya M, Mookherjee S, Bhattacharjee A, Bandyopadhyay AK, Daulat Thakur SK, et al. (2006) Primary role of CYP1B1 in Indian juvenile-onset POAG patients. Mol Vis 12: 399–404.
15. Campos-Mollo E, Lopez-Garrido MP, Blanco-Marchite C, Garcia-Feijoo J, Peralta J, et al. (2009) CYP1B1 mutations in Spanish patients with primary congenital glaucoma: phenotypic and functional variability. Mol Vis 15: 417–431.
16. Chavarria-Soley G, Sticht H, Aklillu E, Ingelman-Sundberg M, Pasutto F, et al. (2008) Mutations in CYP1B1 cause primary congenital glaucoma by reduction of either activity or abundance of the enzyme. Hum Mutat 29: 1147–1153.
17. Choudhary D, Jansson I, Sarfarazi M, Schenkman JB (2008) Characterization of the biochemical and structural phenotypes of four CYP1B1 mutations observed in individuals with primary congenital glaucoma. Pharmacogenet Genomics 18: 665–676.
18. Lopez-Garrido MP, Blanco-Marchite C, Sanchez-Sanchez F, Lopez-Sanchez E, Chaques-Alepuz V, et al. (2010) Functional analysis of CYP1B1 mutations and association of heterozygous hypomorphic alleles with primary open-angle glaucoma. Clin Genet 77: 70–78.
19. Pasutto F, Chavarria-Soley G, Mardin CY, Michels-Rautenstrauss K, Ingelman-Sundberg M, et al. (2010) Heterozygous loss-of-function variants in CYP1B1 predispose to primary open-angle glaucoma. Invest Ophthalmol Vis Sci 51: 249–254.
20. Reddy AB, Kaur K, Mandal AK, Panicker SG, Thomas R, et al. (2004) Mutation spectrum of the CYP1B1 gene in Indian primary congenital glaucoma patients. Mol Vis 10: 696–702.
21. Kumar A, Basavaraj MG, Gupta SK, Qamar I, Ali AM, et al. (2007) Role of CYP1B1, MYOC, OPTN, and OPTC genes in adult-onset primary open-angle glaucoma: predominance of CYP1B1 mutations in Indian patients. Mol Vis 13: 667–676.
22. Chakrabarti S, Kaur K, Komatireddy S, Acharya M, Devi KR, et al. (2005) Gln48His is the prevalent myocilin mutation in primary open angle and primary congenital glaucoma phenotypes in India. Mol Vis 11: 111–113.
23. Lopez-Garrido MP, Sanchez-Sanchez F, Lopez-Martinez F, Aroca-Aguilar JD, Blanco-Marchite C, et al. (2006) Heterozygous CYP1B1 gene mutations in Spanish patients with primary open-angle glaucoma. Mol Vis 12: 748–755.
24. Coca-Prados M, Ghosh S, Wang Y, Escribano J, Herrala A, et al. (2003) Sex steroid hormone metabolism takes place in human ocular cells. J Steroid Biochem Mol Biol 86: 207–216.
25. Schirra F, Suzuki T, Dickinson DP, Townsend DJ, Gipson IK, et al. (2006) Identification of steroidogenic enzyme mRNAs in the human lacrimal gland, meibomian gland, cornea, and conjunctiva. Cornea 25: 438–442.
26. Wickham LA, Gao J, Toda I, Rocha EM, Ono M, et al. (2000) Identification of androgen, estrogen and progesterone receptor mRNAs in the eye. Acta Ophthalmol Scand 78: 146–153.
27. Nguyen TD, Chen P, Huang WD, Chen H, Johnson D, et al. (1998) Gene structure and properties of TIGR, an olfactomedin-related glycoprotein cloned from glucocorticoid-induced trabecular meshwork cells. J Biol Chem 273: 6341–6350.
28. Polansky JR, Fauss DJ, Chen P, Chen H, Lutjen-Drecoll E, et al. (1997) Cellular pharmacology and molecular biology of the trabecular meshwork inducible glucocorticoid response gene product. Ophthalmologica 211: 126–139.
29. Hulsman CA, Westendorp IC, Ramrattan RS, Wolfs RC, Witteman JC, et al. (2001) Is open-angle glaucoma associated with early menopause? The Rotterdam Study. Am J Epidemiol 154: 138–144.
30. Firasat S, Riazuddin SA, Khan SN, Riazuddin S (2008) Novel CYP1B1 mutations in consanguineous Pakistani families with primary congenital glaucoma. Mol Vis 14: 2002–2009.
31. Vincent AL, Billingsley G, Buys Y, Levin AV, Priston M, et al. (2002) Digenic inheritance of early-onset glaucoma: CYP1B1, a potential modifier gene. Am J Hum Genet 70: 448–460.
32. Liu Y, Vollrath D (2004) Reversal of mutant myocilin non-secretion and cell killing: implications for glaucoma. Hum Mol Genet 13: 1193–1204.
33. Clark AF, Wordinger RJ (2009) The role of steroids in outflow resistance. Exp Eye Res 88: 752–759.
34. Shen X, Koga T, Park BC, SundarRaj N, Yue BY (2008) Rho GTPase and cAMP/protein kinase A signaling mediates myocilin-induced alterations in cultured human trabecular meshwork cells. J Biol Chem 283: 603–612.
35. Borras T, Morozova TV, Heinsohn SL, Lyman RF, Mackay TF, et al. (2003) Transcription profiling in Drosophila eyes that overexpress the human glaucoma-associated trabecular meshwork-inducible glucocorticoid response protein/myocilin (TIGR/MYOC). Genetics 163: 637–645.
36. Carbone MA, Ayroles JF, Yamamoto A, Morozova TV, West SA, et al. (2009) Overexpression of myocilin in the Drosophila eye activates the unfolded protein response: implications for glaucoma. PLoS ONE 4: e4216.
37. Gould DB, Miceli-Libby L, Savinova OV, Torrado M, Tomarev SI, et al. (2004) Genetically increasing Myoc expression supports a necessary pathologic role of abnormal proteins in glaucoma. Mol Cell Biol 24: 9019–9025.
38. McDowell CM, Luan T, Zhang Z, Putliwala T, Wordinger RJ, et al. (2012) Mutant human myocilin induces strain specific differences in ocular hypertension and optic nerve damage in mice. Exp Eye Res.
39. Clemons M, Goss P (2001) Estrogen and the risk of breast cancer. N Engl J Med 344: 276–285.
40. Ko Y, Abel J, Harth V, Brode P, Antony C, et al. (2001) Association of CYP1B1 codon 432 mutant allele in head and neck squamous cell cancer is reflected by somatic mutations of p53 in tumor tissue. Cancer Res 61: 4398–4404.
41. Hanna IH, Dawling S, Roodi N, Guengerich FP, Parl FF (2000) Cytochrome P450 1B1 (CYP1B1) pharmacogenetics: association of polymorphisms with functional differences in estrogen hydroxylation activity. Cancer Res 60: 3440–3444.
42. Giulietti A, Overbergh L, Valckx D, Decallonne B, Bouillon R, et al. (2001) An overview of real-time quantitative PCR: applications to quantify cytokine gene expression. Methods 25: 386–401.

# 5

# Crystallins are Regulated Biomarkers for Monitoring Topical Therapy of Glaucomatous Optic Neuropathy

**Verena Prokosch[1], Maurice Schallenberg[1], Solon Thanos[1,2]\***

**1** Institute of Experimental Ophthalmology, School of Medicine, University of Münster, Albert-Schweitzer-Campus 1, Münster, Germany, **2** Interdisciplinary Center for Clinical Research, Albert-Schweitzer-Campus 1, Münster, Germany

## Abstract

Optic nerve atrophy caused by abnormal intraocular pressure (IOP) remains the most common cause of irreversible loss of vision worldwide. The aim of this study was to determine whether topically applied IOP-lowering eye drugs affect retinal ganglion cells (RGCs) and retinal metabolism in a rat model of optic neuropathy. IOP was elevated through cauterization of episcleral veins, and then lowered either by the daily topical application of timolol, timolol/travoprost, timolol/dorzolamide, or timolol/brimonidine, or surgically with sectorial iridectomy. RGCs were retrogradely labeled 4 days prior to enucleation, and counted. Two-dimensional polyacrylamide gel electrophoresis (2D-PAGE), matrix-assisted laser desorption ionization mass spectrometry, Western blotting, and immunohistochemistry allowed the identification of IOP-dependent proteomic changes. Genomic changes were scrutinized using microarrays and qRT-PCR. The significant increase in IOP induced by episcleral vein cauterization that persisted until 8 weeks of follow-up in control animals ($p < 0.05$) was effectively lowered by the eye drops ($p < 0.05$). As anticipated, the number of RGCs decreased significantly following 8 weeks of elevated IOP ($p < 0.05$), while treatment with combination compounds markedly improved RGC survival ($p < 0.05$). 2D-PAGE and Western blot analyses revealed an IOP-dependent expression of crystallin cry-$\beta$b2. Microarray and qRT-PCR analyses verified the results at the mRNA level. IHC demonstrated that crystallins were expressed mainly in the ganglion cell layer. The data suggest that IOP and either topically applied antiglaucomatous drugs influence crystallin expression within the retina. Neuronal crystallins are thus suitable biomarkers for monitoring the progression of neuropathy and evaluating any neuroprotective effects.

**Editor:** Andreas Ohlmann, University of Regensburg, Germany

**Funding:** The work was supported by the Deutsche Forschungsgemeinschaft (DFG, grant Th386 18-1 to S.T.), the IZKF (grant Tha3/002/09 to S.T.), and the Medical Faculty of the University of Münster. The funders have no role in study design, data collection and analysis, decision to publish, or preparation of the manuscript.

**Competing Interests:** The authors have declared that no competing interests exist.

\* E-mail: solon@uni-muenster.de

## Introduction

Elevated intraocular pressure (IOP) is a major risk factor in glaucomatous optic neuropathy [1] for review and the mainstay of glaucoma treatment continues to be lowering of the IOP by pharmacological or surgical methods [2]. However, retinal ganglion cell (RGC) loss and damage to the optic nerve may continue despite significant reductions in IOP [3–11].

It has been assumed that inflammatory and metabolic processes are involved in glaucomatous neuron death. Crystallins, which belong to the family of small heat shock proteins (HSPs) and comprise three major families ($\alpha$, $\beta$, and $\gamma$ crystallins), have been found within RGCs [12,13]. Both neuroregenerative [13] and neurodegenerative [14] properties have been attributed to retinal crystallins. Specific regulation of crystallins has been observed in the context of neurodegenerative diseases such as glaucoma [12,15]. Furthermore, human glaucoma patients exhibit increased titers of antibodies against small HSPs [14,16–17]. Crystallins may act as critical modulators in glaucoma and thus be integral to the process of glaucomatous neurodegeneration [14].

The retina and the optic nerve provide an easily accessible and relevant model with which to study central nervous system injury and postinjury repair. Experimental, genetic, and hereditary mutant animal models of glaucoma provide suitable tools with which to study the complex process of neuronal degeneration in glaucoma [18–20]. We hypothesized that IOP elevation causes alterations in gene and protein expressions within retinal cells. Based on this hypothesis, different drugs may alter the expressions of such molecules, which can be analyzed by two-dimensional gel electrophoresis (2DE) and matrix-assisted laser desorption ionization (MALDI) mass spectrometry (MS) in order to identify disease- or treatment-associated proteins. In addition, proteomic–genomic correlations may help to identify novel pharmacological targets [21,22].

Several families of drugs that aim at limiting the risk for retinal and optic nerve neuropathy are in clinical use, and all of them are designed to normalize IOP. In addition to surgical procedures, $\alpha$-2a [23] and $\beta$-adrenergic [24] receptor agonists, prostaglandin F2$\alpha$ analogues [25], and carbonic anhydrase inhibitors [26] are the most important classes of drugs used in this context [27]. Some of these drugs are suspected to act neuroprotectively by altering retinal protein metabolism and activating signaling cascades in favor of RGC survival.

The purpose of the present study was to identify metabolic retinal changes at the genomic and proteomic levels using 2DE, MALDI-MS, microarray analysis, quantitative real-time polymerase chain reaction (qRT-PCR), Western blotting (WB), and immunohistochemistry (IHC).

## Methods

### Animals and drugs

Ethical statement and animals: All experiments were conducted in accordance with the Association for Research in Vision and Ophthalmology (ARVO) Statement on the Use of Animals in Ophthalmic and Vision Research. Sprague-Dawley rats were housed in a standard animal room under a 12-h light/dark cycle with food and water provided *ad libitum*. The ethics committee (Bezirksregierung Münster, i.e. regional government of Münster) specially approved this study (Permission Nr.: 84-02.04.2011.A132). Animals were housed in a standard animal facility with food and water *ad libitum* and a 12 hrs light-dark cycle. Surgical procedures were performed unilaterally, on the left eye of rats weighing 180–250 g, under general anesthesia induced by a mixture of 2 mg/kg body weight ketamine and 2 mg/kg body weight xylazine (Ceva-Sanofi, Düsseldorf, Germany), administered intraperitoneally. After each surgical intervention, gentamicin eye ointment (Gentamytrex, Dr. Mann Pharma, Berlin, Germany) was applied topically. The animals' health and behavior were monitored postoperatively at regular intervals. The experimental follow-up after cauterization lasted 8 weeks. Each experimental group comprised 9 animals, except for the normotensive and hypertensive groups, which each comprised 18 animals.

### Induction of glaucoma and intraocular-pressure measurement

IOP was elevated through thermic cauterization of three episcleral veins as follows. The limbus-draining veins travel close to the sclera from the limbus backwards and anastomose at the equator of the eye, and were exposed by incision of the conjunctiva where they form four to five major venous trunks almost equidistant around the circumference of the globe. Ophthalmic cautery was applied to three of these large veins per eye, resulting in blockage of more than 50% of the venous outflow (Fig. 1A) [4]. Care was taken not to damage the sclera during this procedure. IOP measurements were made before and immediately after cauterization, and then every week between 9.00 a.m. and 12.00 a.m. under light anesthesia with isoflurane (Isofluran DeltaSelect, Actavis, Langenfeld, Germany) and topically applied 0.5% proparacaine (URSA-Pharm, Saarbrücken, Germany). Ten tonometer readings were taken directly from the instrument display for each eye measurement, recorded, and averaged. "Off" (or outlier) readings and instrument-generated averages were ignored. An uncauterized group ($n = 18$) served as the normotensive control. The IOP appeared to have increased 10 days after cauterization, and it remained elevated for the entire duration of the experiment. Animals in which the IOP returned to normal levels were excluded from the study. None of the animals exhibited an enlarged globe or edematous cornea. Four weeks after the IOP elevation, the hypotensive treatment was begun either surgically by iridectomy or by daily application of topical IOP-lowering eye drops for the subsequent 4 weeks of follow-up. One group of animals ($n = 18$) remained untreated, with a persistent elevated IOP; this group served as the corresponding hypertensive control.

### Application of eye drops

Eye drops containing either only 0.5% timolol (Ti, $n = 9$; 0.5% TimOphtal; Winzer Pharma, Berlin, Germany), or combinations of 0.5% T and dorzolamide (Ti/D, $n = 7$; Cosopt, Chibret, München, Germany), 0.5% T and travoprost (Ti/Tr, $n = 7$;

Duotrav, Alcon, Hünenberg, Switzerland), or 0.5% T and brimonidine (TiB, $n = 9$; Combigan, Allergan, Irvine, CA, USA) were applied topically to the left eye daily between 8.00 a.m. and 10.00 a.m. over a 4-week period. Each drop was kept in situ for at least 30 s by manually holding the eye open.

### Retrograde labeling and quantification of retinal ganglion cells

Four days prior to enucleation of the eye, three rats from each experimental group were anesthetized and their RGCs retrogradely labeled from the superior colliculus (SC) using the fluorescent dye hydroxystilbamidine methanesulfonate (5% FluoroGold (5-FG)] in phosphate-buffered saline (PBS; Invitrogen, Eugene, OR, USA). This results in the exclusive labeling of RGCs in a uniform manner across the entire retina, thus enabling their quantification on retinal flat-mounts [28]. Briefly, after surgical exposure, a few solid crystals of 5-FG were inserted into the superficial layers of the contralateral right SC. The cortical cavity was filled with Gelfoam (Pharmacia and Upjohn, Kalamazoo, MI, USA) and the skin wound was sutured. The animals were subsequently allowed to survive for 4 days to allow the dye to be taken up by the axon terminals of the RGCs in the SC and transported retrogradely to the RGC somata in the retina.

Animals were killed under a carbon dioxide atmosphere, and their retinas isolated, flat-mounted, and fixed in 4% paraformaldehyde overnight at 4°C. RGCs were visualized with the aid of a fluorescence microscope (Axiophot, Carl Zeiss, Oberkochen, Germany) using a 360-nm excitation filter and a 460-nm bandpass emission filter. Images of five areas at five different eccentricities (uniform central to peripheral distribution) were obtained in each retinal quadrant at a final magnification of ×200. The optic disc served as the point of reference. RGCs were counted in a 150-$\mu m^2$ area in each image. The number of RGCs per square millimeter was determined and averaged for each group.

### Two-dimensional gel electrophoresis and matrix-assisted laser desorption ionization mass spectrometry

2DE and MALDI-MS were performed on retinal samples from normotensive and hypertensive retinas modified with and without hypotensive treatment. 2DE was conducted using a method initially described by O'Farrell [29]. Retinal explants were harvested and boiled in 10% sodium dodecylsulfate (SDS; Sigma, Taufkirchen, Germany) and homogenized in 2DE lysis buffer (7 M urea and 2 M thiourea; Merck, Darmstadt, Germany), 4% 3-[(3-cholamidopropyl)-dimethylammonio]-1-propane sulfonate (USB, Cleveland, OH, USA), 40 mM Tris base (Carl Roth, Karlsruhe, Germany), 1 mM phenylmethylsulfonyl fluoride (Sigma), and 10 mM dithiothreitol (DTT; Roche, Mannheim, Germany). The final SDS concentration was 0.25%. Soluble protein (200 µg according to the Bradford test) together with 2% immobilized pH-gradient (IPG) buffer (pH 3–10; Amersham Biosciences Europe, Freiburg, Germany) and 20 mM DTT were loaded onto Immobiline DryStrips (pH 3–10, 18 cm; Amersham Biosciences Europe) and rehydrated overnight. The rehydrated strips were focused on a Multiphor II system (Amersham Biosciences Europe) at approximately 80 kVh. Focused IPG strips were incubated twice for 15 min in equilibration solution [50 mM Tris HCl (pH 8.8), 6 M urea, 30% glycerol, 2% w/v SDS, and a trace of bromophenol blue (Merck)], with 1% β-mercaptoethanol and 2.5% iodoacetacetamide added to the first and second equilibration steps, respectively. For the second dimension, the equilibrated IPG strips were fixed with 0.5% w/v melted agarose

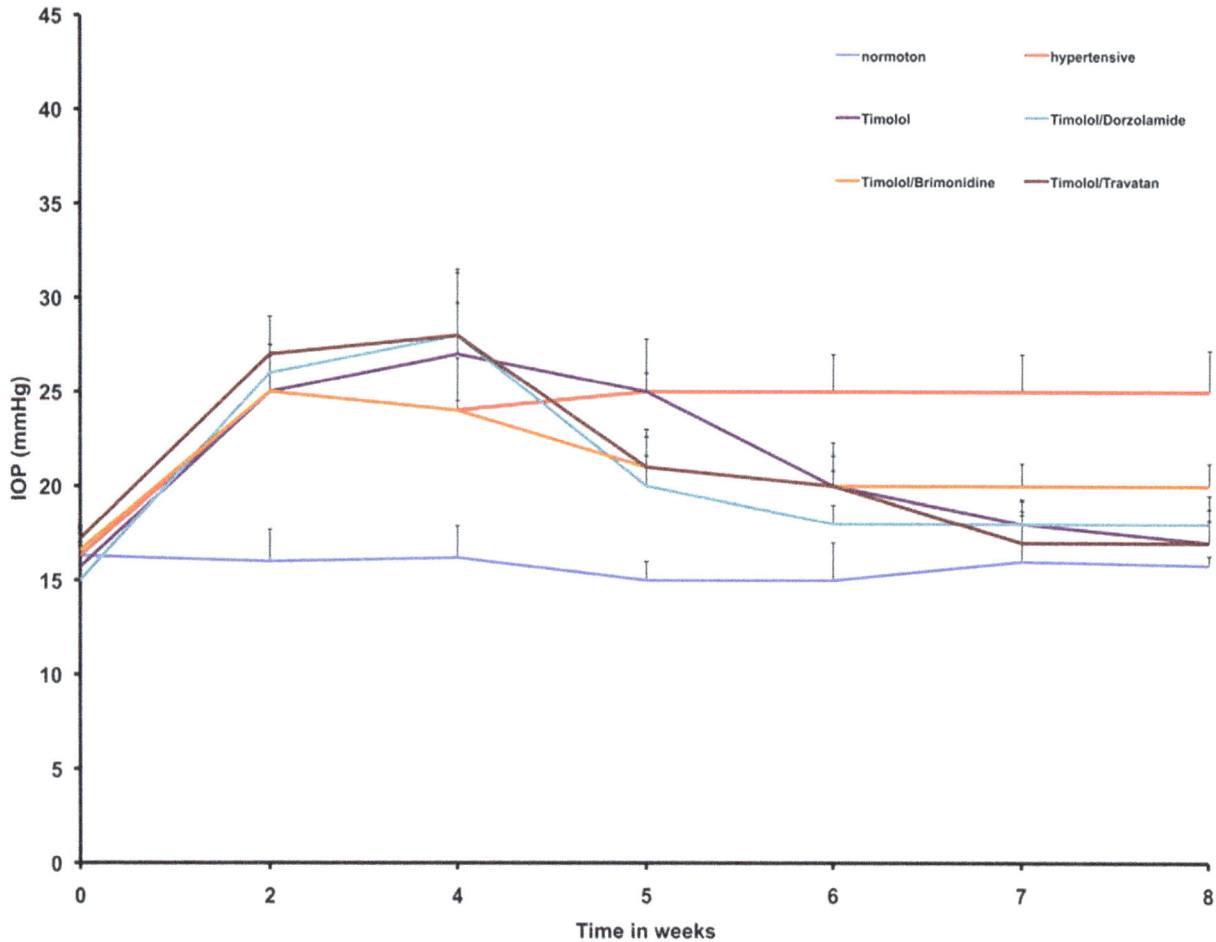

**Figure 1. IOP readings in an experimental model of ocular hypertension.** A significant increase in IOP (*$p<0.05$) was observed in eyes after cauterization of three episcleral veins in all groups relative to the normal control group (blue line) after 2 weeks. After the initiation of a medical hypotensive treatment, marked by a black arrow, the IOP was reduced significantly (**$p<0.05$) in all groups, whereas it remained elevated throughout the experimental period in the control group without hypotensive treatment (red line).

(Merck) on homogeneous 12.5% SDS gels (Rotiphorese Gel 30, Carl Roth). Proteins were separated by vertical SDS–polyacrylamide gel electrophoresis (SDS-PAGE; BioRad, München, Germany) according to Laemmli [30]. Protein spots were initially labeled with colloidal Coomassie Blue 250 (Merck). Spots were manually excised, tryptically digested in the gel, extracted, purified using Zigtips (microbed C18, Millipore, Bedford, MA, USA), and then subjected to MS. Peptide maps were generated using TOF-Spec-2E (Micromass, Manchester, UK), and selected retinal peptides were sequenced using nano-high-performance liquid chromatography MS/MS (Ultimate, LC Packings, Amsterdam, The Netherlands; Esquire 3000, Bruker Daltonics, Bremen, Germany). Three gel replicates were compared. National Center for Biotechnology Information and SWISS-PROT databases were searched using Mascot software (Matrix Science, London, UK). Additional image analyses were performed on gels stained with silver nitrate.

## Western blotting

The eyes of normotensive rats with elevated IOP and those subsequently treated with Ti or Ti/D, Ti/B, or Ti/Tr were enucleated, the retina was isolated, embedded in Tissue-Tek

(Sakura-Finetek, Torrance, CA, USA), and frozen in liquid nitrogen. The probes were homogenized in SDS sample buffer (62.5 mM Tris HCl, 2% w/v SDS, 10% glycerol, 50 mM DTT, and 0.01% w/v bromophenol blue). After sonicating and heating the sample, the protein concentration was determined using Bradford reagents. Fifty micrograms of protein from each sample was fractionated on 8%, 10%, or 12% SDS-PAGE (depending on the examined protein) with a protein marker (BioRad, San Diego, CA, USA). After electrophoresis, proteins were transferred to a nitrocellulose membrane. The blots were incubated in blocking solution (5% fat-free dry milk and 0.1% Tween-20 in PBS) for 1 h, followed by incubation overnight at 4°C with polyclonal antigoat βb2 crystallin (cryβb2; Santa Cruz Biotechnology, Santa Cruz, CA, USA) used at a dilution of 1:700. The polyclonal antigoat βb3 crystallin (cryβb3; Santa Cruz Biotechnology), the polyclonal antisheep βH crystallin (cryβH; Biogenesis, New Fields UK), the polyclonal antisheep βL crystallin (cryβL; Biogenesis), and µ crystallin (cryµ; Sigma-Aldrich, München, Germany) antibodies were used at dilutions of 1:700, 1:1000, 1:600, and 1:1000, respectively. Polyclonal antigoat HSP-90 (Santa Cruz Biotechnology), polyclonal antirabbit HSP-70 (Cell Signaling, Boston, MA, USA), polyclonal antirabbit HSP-25 (Upstate Biotechnology, Lake

Placid, NY, USA), and polyclonal antirabbit γ crystallin (cryγ; Santa Cruz Biotechnology) antibodies were used at dilutions of 1:1000, 1:1000, 1:10,000, and 1:200, respectively. The applied control antibodies, anticalnexin (Sigma-Aldrich), antiactin (Sigma-Aldrich), and anti-GAPDH (Sigma-Aldrich), were used at a dilution of 1:10,000. The membrane was then incubated with the secondary antibody conjugated with horseradish peroxidase in blocking solution for 1 h at room temperature. Antibody detection was performed with enhanced chemiluminescence (Amersham Biosciences, Rockville, MD, USA). The relative densities of the protein spots were analyzed using Alpha Ease (Alpha Ease FC software 4.0, Alpha Innotech, Biozym Scientific, Vienna, Austria). The protein density of a fixed area was determined for each spot after subtracting the specific background density of the same area. The spot density was correlated and normalized to the relative density of the particular application control. The normotensive spot density was defined as the reference mark, and the relative relationships were determined and processed.

## Immunohistochemistry

Frozen 10-μm-thick sections of isolated retina samples obtained from normotensive eyes and hypertensive eyes after IOP elevation were fixed in cold acetone for 10 min. They were washed three times for 5 min each in PBS and blocked with 10% fetal calf serum (FCS) for 30 min. The sections were then incubated overnight at 4°C with a primary antibody, polyclonal anti-rabbit β crystallin (gift from the Department of Biochemistry, Hyderabad, India), which was diluted at 1:400 in 10% FCS. After rinsing the slides three times each in PBS for 5 min, the sections were incubated with the secondary anti-rabbit Cy2 antibody (Dianova, Hamburg, Germany) diluted at 1:200 in 10% FCS for 30 min at room temperature, and then washed three times for 5 min each in PBS. Finally, the slides were coverslipped with Mowiol (Höchst, Frankfurt, Germany). The nuclei of retinal cells were stained by adding 4′,6-diamino-2-phenylindole dihydrochloride hydrate (Sigma-Aldrich) to the Mowiol embedding medium. Slides were examined with the aid of a fluorescence microscope (Axiophot, Carl Zeiss) with the appropriate filters. Negative controls comprised sections processed without addition of the primary antibodies. Control and experimental sections were stained simultaneously to avoid variations in immunohistochemical staining.

## Microarrays

Retinal samples obtained from normotensive ($n = 3$) and hypertensive ($n = 3$) rats 4 weeks after IOP elevation were used for the microarray analysis. Animals were killed in a carbon dioxide chamber, and their eyes were immediately enucleated and placed on ice. The retina was removed quickly and collected in RLT buffer, a component of the RNeasy kit (Qiagen, Hilden, Germany). A minimum of 10 μg of total RNA/retina was isolated using the RNeasy kit using the procedure described in the manufacturer's instructions. Total RNA was then shipped on dry ice to MWG Biotech (Ebersberg, Germany), where an aliquot of the RNA was subjected to quality analysis using the 2100 Bioanalyzer system. The RNA was then amplified with T7 polymerase following reverse transcription into cDNA, during which fluorescence-labeled nucleotides (Cy3/Cy5) were incorporated. The labeled probes were hybridized to 10 k chips (MWG Biotech). Three separate hybridizations per group were carried out with cDNA derived from three separate animals. The 10-k chip consists of 9715 rat genes (5535 Rat 5 k genes) spotted onto one array with an additional 4180 annotated open reading frames

from an in-house MWG Biotech expressed sequence tag sequencing project.

To design microarrays with optimal hybridization conditions, existing databases are filtered for redundant sequences and the oligonucleotides are designed with the Oligos-4-Array (developed by MWG Biotech). This requires that nontarget genes be less than 75% similar over a 50-base target region. In fact, if the 50-base target region is marginally similar (50–75%), it must not include a stretch of complementary sequence of >15 contiguous bases. The oligonucleotide design thus guarantees the exclusion of both dimer and secondary structure formation. Cross-hybridization is minimized by exhaustive BLAST and global Smith-Waterman searches. The microarrays were scanned at a resolution of 10 μm at three photomultiplier gain settings in order to optimize the dynamic range. The resulting three images were integrated into one intensity value for each spot using the software packages ImaGene and GeneSight (MWG Biotech), and MAVI (MWG Biotech).

The fluorescent signals were corrected and normalized for the difference between Cy3 and Cy5. Samples from each of the three cohybridizations were compared independently of each other. The signal values of probe sets that were reliably detected in most of the experiments in each group were used in two-sample, two-tailed $t$-tests between the "experimental" and "control" groups (nonglaucomatous vs. glaucomatous retina). Probe sets were selected from candidate genes using a $t$-test based on $p < 0.05$, and the ratio of means (relative change) between the two groups was calculated with "control" as the denominator. The final relative changes quoted here are the average values of three independent experiments. The cut-off values for up- and down-regulation were set at >3.0-fold and <0.3-fold, respectively. The biological function of differentially expressed genes with a change of >3.0-fold or <0.3-fold were modeled according to their biological process using the Protein ANalysis THrough Evolutionary Relationships (PANTHER) classification system (Applied Biosystems, San Diego, CA, USA). The PANTHER classification system allows high-throughput analysis of proteins (and their genes), which can be classified according to families and subfamilies, molecular functions, biological processes, and pathways.

## Quantitative real-time polymerase chain reaction

The real-time PCR was implemented in an ABI PRISM 7900 sequence detector (Applied Biosystems) in 384-well plates. For the qRT-PCR, total RNA was isolated from the retinas of a second set of animals, because there was insufficient RNA from the microarray experiments for both experiments. Five rats with IOP elevation and five animals with a normal IOP were used for qRT-PCR experiments. One microgram of total RNA was first reverse transcribed using the Omniscript Reverse Transcriptase (5 mM dNTPs, 10×RT buffer, 10 units/μl RNase inhibitor, and 10 μM Oligo-dT primer; MWG Biotech) in a total volume of 20 μl for 1 h at 37°C. The enzyme was inactivated by heating at 95°C for 5 min. The cDNA was diluted twofold, and a 1-μl aliquot was used for each 20-μl PCR using the TaqMan Universal PCR Master Mix and Assays-on-Demand (Applied Biosystems). Assays-on-Demand gene expression products consisted of a 20× mix of unlabeled PCR primers and a TaqMan MGB probe (labeled with FAM-TAMRA dye), and they were used to quantify the expression of seven genes: αA crystallin (cryαA), αB crystallin (cryαB), βB1 crystallin (cryβb1), cryβb2, cryβb3, and βA4 crystallin (cryβb4), with the 18S RNA (Assay Hs99999901_s1) gene serving as an endogenous control. The assays are designed for the detection and quantitation of specific rat genetic sequences in RNA samples converted to cDNA. The reaction components

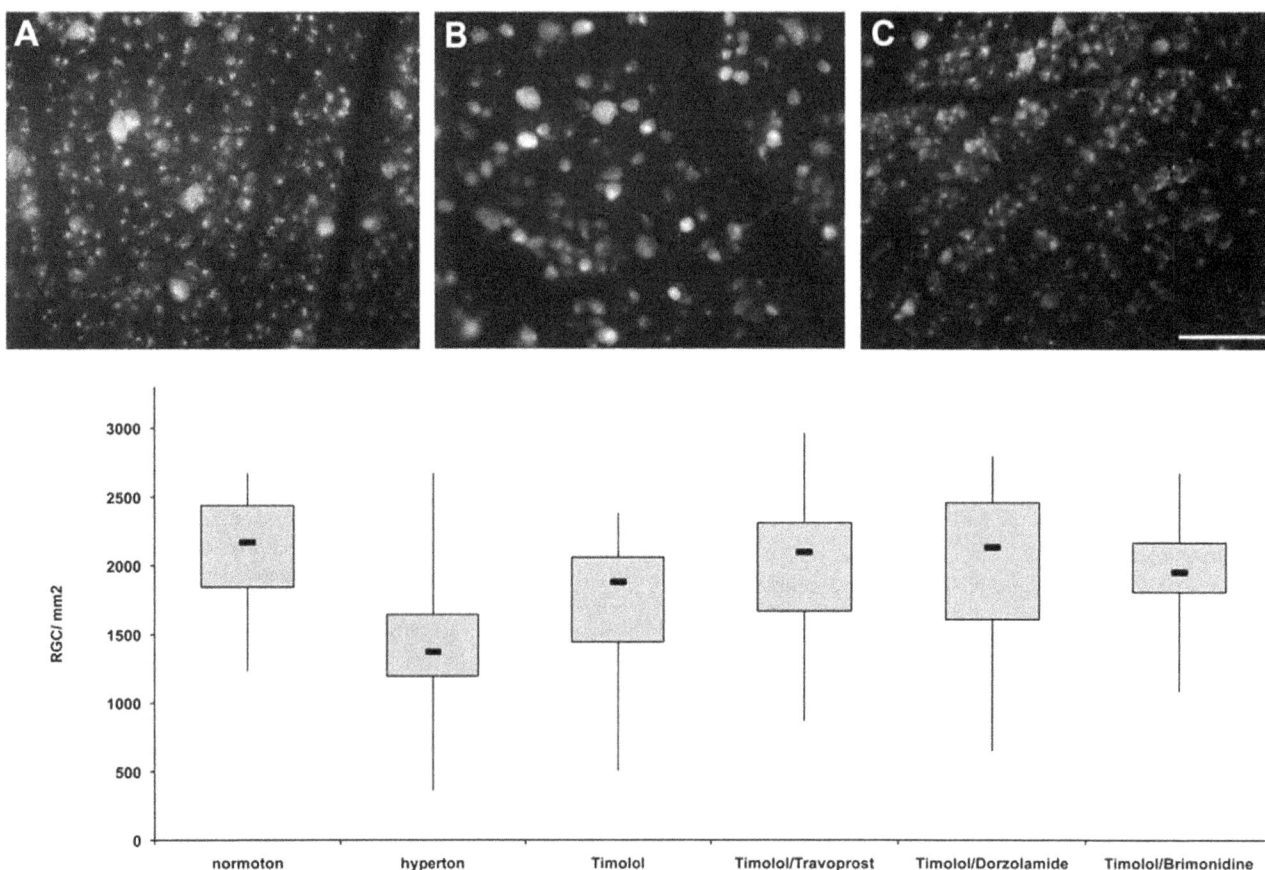

**Figure 2. Densities of retinal ganglion cells (RGCs) labeled with 5% FluoroGold 8 weeks after the induction of elevated IOP.** A RGCs in a normotensive, sham-treated retina. **B** RGCs in an untreated retina with elevated IOP without hypotensive treatment. **C** RGCs in a retina with elevated IOP treated with 0.5% timolol (Ti) and travoprost (Ti/Tr) for 4 weeks [the results were the same for those treated with 0.5% Ti and dorzolamide (Ti/D), and 0.5% Ti and brimonidine (Ti/B)]. **D** Boxplots illustrating the total RGC survival within the different experimental groups. IOP elevation significantly decreased the number of RGCs (*$p<0.05$) compared with the normotensive, sham-treated group, while 4 weeks of treatment with hypotensive eye drops (i.e., with Ti/Tr, Ti/D, or Ti/B), which began 4 weeks after IOP elevation, significantly improved RGC survival (**$p<0.05$) relative to the untreated hypertensive group. Treatment with Ti (0.5%) alone did not substantially improve RGC survival.

consisted of 10 µl of TaqMan Universal PCR Master Mix, AmpErase uracil-*N*-glycosylase (UNG; 2×), 1 µl of Assay-on-Demand (20×), and 1 µl of cDNA in a 20-µl reaction. The PCR conditions for all genes were as follows: UNG activation, 50°C for 2 min; preheating, 95°C for 10 min; then 40 cycles of denaturation (95°C for 15 s) and annealing/elongation (60°C for 1 min). Each sample was run in duplicate.

The data were analyzed using SDS 2.2 software (Applied Biosystems). 18S RNA served as the endogenous control against which to normalize the amount of cDNA added to each reaction (ΔCt), and the mean ΔCt of control samples was used as the calibrator to calculate ΔΔCt. The comparative Ct method was employed, whereby the relative quantity of the respective target gene mRNA—normalized to the endogenous control and relative to the calibrator—is expressed as the relative change: 2–ΔΔCt.

### Statistical analysis

All data regarding IOP recordings, RGC densities of retinal whole-mounts, and relative protein densities in WBs are presented as mean±SD values. Data were analyzed statistically using the two-independent-samples test (SPPS, Statistica version 7) for Gaussian distributions, with the remaining quantitative data analyzed using two-way analysis of variance (Statistica version 7)

with post-hoc analyses using the Tukey HSD test to identify possible differences among the experimental groups. If the distribution was not Gaussian, the Kruskal-Wallis *H* test was used.

### Results

#### Pharmacological effects on intraocular pressure

The baseline IOP in the normotensive sham-treated group was 15.8±1.5 mmHg. By 10–12 days after episcleral vein cauterization, the IOP had increased significantly by 1.6-fold to 24.8±1.7 mmHg ($p<0.001$). These values are consistent with those obtained by other groups, and are nearly identical to those recorded in humans, rabbits, and anesthetized monkeys [31]. The recordings were sustained for the entire duration of the experimental period if animals remained untreated. If treated hypotensively, IOP was reduced effectively as follows ($p<0.05$):

1. Ti lowered IOP to 20.00±1.65 mmHg ($p<0.05$).
2. Ti/B reduced IOP to 20.5±1.4 mmHg ($p<0.03$).
3. Ti/D and Ti/Tr produced more distinctive reductions in IOP (18.50±1.35 and 18.75±1.80 mmHg, respectively; $p<0.001$).

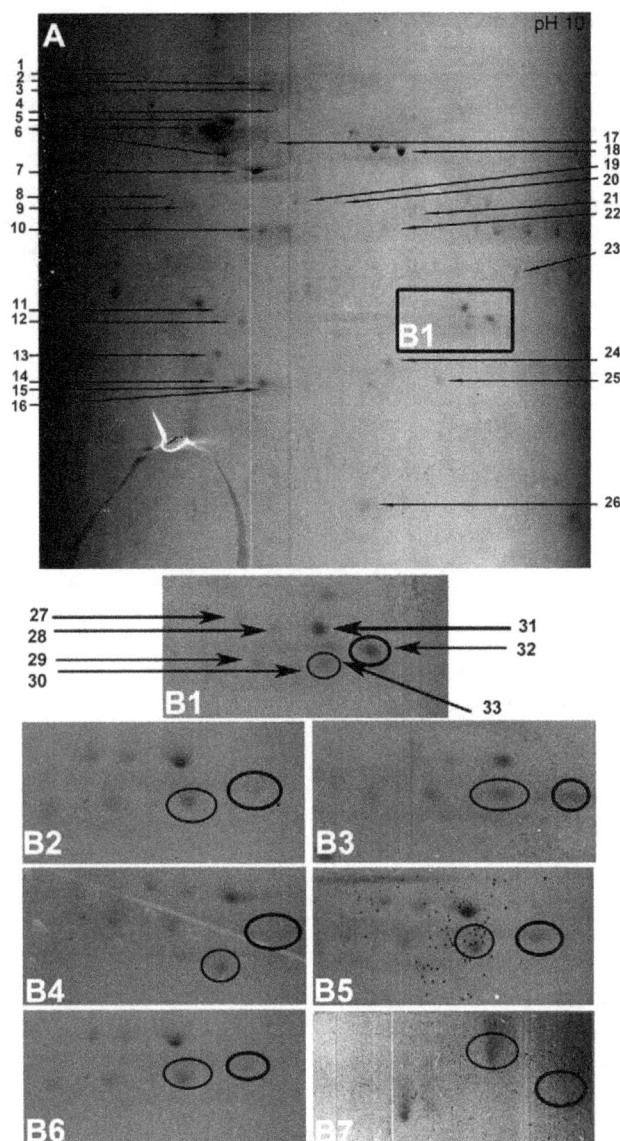

**Figure 3. Two-dimensional gelelectrophoresis of retinal proteins.** A Peptide mapping of a retina obtained from a Sprague-Dawley rat with untreated, sustained elevated IOP 8 weeks after IOP induction. Hypertensive retinal samples showed a marked increase in βb2-crystallin (cryβb2) expression (area marked by a black box in **A**, shown at higher magnification in **B1** compared to a normotensive sham-treated retina, **B2**). The 4 weeks of IOP-lowering treatment with topical treatment with Ti (**B3,B4**), Ti/T (**B5**), Ti/D (**B6**), and Ti/B (**B7**) decreased cryβb2 expression to baseline levels. The proteins identified, which are marked by an arrow in **A** and **B1**, are listed in Table 1 according to the number given.

These recorded readings remained constant over the 4 weeks of antihypertensive treatment. IOP recordings are illustrated in detail in Fig. 1.

## Quantification of retinal ganglion cells

The density of RGCs in retinal whole-mounts of normotensive animals ($n = 3$) was $2112 \pm 369$ RGCs/mm$^2$. IOP elevation ($n = 3$) significantly reduced the RGC density to $1488 \pm 532$ RGCs/mm$^2$ ($p < 0.001$) at 8 weeks after cauterization. These data are in agreement with previous RGC quantifications in glaucoma using

5-FG. Topical treatment with the combination compounds Ti/Tr, Ti/D, and Ti/B strongly enhanced RGC survival, preserving $2020 \pm 548$ RGCs/mm$^2$ ($p < 0.001$; $n = 3$), $2031 \pm 734$ RGCs/mm$^2$ ($p < 0.004$; $n = 3$), and $1956 \pm 340$ RGCs/mm$^2$ ($p < 0.001$; $n = 3$), respectively. The RGC densities in the experimental groups are illustrated in Fig. 2.

## Retinal protein profiling

Several protein spots were reproducibly detected with 2DE (those for the hypertensive group are shown in Fig. 3A). Landmark protein spots that appeared with consistent staining intensities in all experimental groups were first mapped and identified (listed in Table 1). In addition, a conspicuous group of proteins appeared in the middle range of molecular masses (20–30 kDa) at slightly basic pH values (Fig. 3A). This area (within the rectangular frame in Fig. 3A, labeled 3B1) also contained several enzymes (marked by a black arrow in Fig. 3B1 and listed in Table 1) in positions that did not vary substantially between the experimental groups. One spot (framed by a black circle) was strikingly only present in hypertensive samples (Fig. 3B1), and was absent in all of the other experimental groups in normotensive animals (Fig. 3B2) a, animals with iridectomy (Fig. 3B3), and those treated with Ti (Fig. 3B3, B4), Ti/Tr (Fig. 3B5), Ti/D (Fig. 3B6), and Ti/B (Fig. 3B7). Subsequent MALDI-MS confirmed that the spot corresponded to cryβb2. Cryβb3 (framed by a circle) was present equally in all groups (Fig. 3B1–B7), demonstrating the reproducibility of the applied method.

## Confirmation with Western blotting and immunohistochemistry

Additional WB was performed for cryβb2, cryβb3, cryβL, cryβH, cryγ, cryμ, HSP-25, and HSP-70 on retinal samples to better characterize the changes in crystallin and HSP expression as seen through 2DE and MALDI-MS. Cryβb2, with a molecular mass of 23 kDa, was markedly up-regulated in the hypertensive retina ($7.4 \pm 1.1$-fold; $p < 0.001$), being only marginally present in the normotensive retina ($1.30 \pm 0.12$-fold), and nearly totally absent in retinal samples treated with Ti ($35.00 \pm 0.07$-fold), Ti/Tr ($20.0 \pm 0.1$-fold), Ti/D ($60.0 \pm 0.4$-fold), and Ti/B ($61.0 \pm 0.1$-fold; Fig. 4A, B). Cryβb3 expression did not differ significantly among the groups (Fig. 4C, D). Consistent with cryβb2, cryβL was strongly expressed in hypertensive samples ($7.2 \pm 1.8$-fold; $p < 0.001$), while it was only slightly expressed in all other groups (Fig. 4E, F). There were no marked changes in the expressions of either cryβH (Fig. 4G, H) or HSP-70 (Fig. 5A, B). Cryμ (Fig. 5C, D) and HSP-25 (Fig. 5E, F) were the most strongly expressed in the normotensive samples ($p < 0.001$). Cryγ expression resembled the expressions of cryβb2 and cryβL, showing markedly higher expression in hypertensive samples ($10.80 \pm 0.35$-fold; $p < 0.001$) than in the other groups (Fig. 5G, H).

To confirm and visualize cryβb up-regulation within the retinal tissue, immunohistochemical staining was performed on normotensive and hypertensive retinal slices. IHC revealed up-regulation of cryβb after IOP elevation relative to normotensive samples (Fig. 6A, B). The signal increased with the duration of exposure to elevated IOP (Fig. 6C). Cryβb signaling was higher at 28 days than at 7 days after IOP elevation, and cryβb expression was localized predominantly in the RGC layer of retinal slices (Fig. 6B, C), indicating that RGCs are mainly adversely affected by elevated IOP in glaucoma.

**Table 1.** Retinal proteins identified by two-dimensional gel electrophoresis and subsequent matrix-assisted laser desorption ionization mass spectrometry.

| No. | Protein | Potential function | MW/kDA |
|---|---|---|---|
| 1 | Glucose related-protein 78 | Cytosceleton | 78 |
| 2 | HSP 70 isoform 2 | Protein folding ATPase activity | 53 |
| 3 | Glucose related-protein 75 | Molecular chaperone | 73,6 |
| 4 | Glial fibrillary acidic protein | Cytosceleton | 50 |
| 5 | Enolase 2 | Carbohydrate transport, metabolism | 47 |
| 6 | ATP synthase beta subunit | ATP biosynthesis | 50,7 |
| 7 | Beta actin | Structural protein,cytoskeleton | 41,7 |
| 8 | Retinaldehyde-binding protein | Transport of retinalaldehyde | 44,5 |
| 9 | Kinase associated HSP 90 | Molecular chaperone | 44,4 |
| 10 | Crystalline mu | Amino acid transport, metabolism | 33,5 |
| 11 | Glucose-6-phosphatase isomerase | Carbohydrate transport, metabolism | 29 |
| 12 | Retinoidacid receptor responder protein | Type 2 membran protein | 29 |
| 13 | Recoverin | Regulation of rhodopsin | 23 |
| 14 | Class I beta tubulin | Tubulin, cytoskeleton | 45 |
| 15 | Synthaxin 2 | Epithelial morphogenesis | 33,3 |
| 16 | Phosphatydylethanolamin bindingprotein | Lipid and ATP binding | 20,7 |
| 17 | HSP 60 | Protein turnover, chaperonin | 61 |
| 18 | Enolase 1 | Glycolysis, lyase | 47 |
| 19 | Craniofacial dev. Protein 1, cyclin G1 | Cytochrome, craniofacial development | 34 |
| 20 | Calmodulin | Calcium-binding protein | 35 |
| 21 | Adaptor related protein complex3 | Intracellular trafficking and secretion | 34 |
| 22 | Malate dehydrogenase | Energy production and conversion | 36 |
| 23 | Proteasome | Inhibitor of apoptosis | 30 |
| 24 | Peroxiredoxin 6 | Thiol-specific antioxidant protein | 25 |
| 25 | ATP synthase delta subunit | ATP biosynthesis | 19 |
| 26 | Nucleoside diphosphate kinase B | Synthesis of nucleoside triphosphate | 18 |
| 27 | Carbonic anhydrase 1 | Hydration of carbon dioxide | 28 |
| 28 | Triose-phtosphat isomerase | Glycolysis | 28 |
| 29 | βb3 crystallin | Structural protein of the eye lens | 24 |
| 30 | Phosphoglycerate mutase | Glycolysis | 29 |
| 31 | Bb2 crystallin | Structural protein of the eye lens | 23 |
| 32 | Acetyl-coenzyme A dehydrogenase | Fatty acid, lipid metabolism | 24 |

The numbers in column 1 correspond to those given in Fig. 4. Column 4 lists the molecular mass of the respective protein. HSP = heat-shock protein.

## Microarrays and quantitative real-time polymerase chain reaction

To confirm that the change in the expression of crystallin is reflected at the mRNA level, microarray analysis and additional qRT-PCR were performed on normotensive samples as well as on samples at 4 weeks after IOP elevation. Harvesting of the retinal samples 4 weeks after IOP elevation (before the initiation of antihypertensive therapy) enabled us to detect whether crystallin mRNAs were up-regulated due to IOP and down-regulated due to antihypertensive treatment. Microarray analysis and qRT-PCR were conducted after reverse transcription of isolated RNA for cryαA, cryαB, cryβb1, cryβb2, cryβb3, and cryβb4. Compared with normotensive retinas, the gene activity in hypertensive retinas was up-regulated by four- to tenfold (Fig. 7). All data support the initial hypothesis that retinal crystallins, and in particular cryβb2,

are sensitive markers for detecting the pharmacological influences of drugs that are topically applied to reduce elevated IOP.

## Discussion

There are three principal findings from this study:

1. Prolonged IOP elevation modulates small HSPs, and in particular the pattern of expression of crystallin in the retina.
2. Pharmacological hypotensive treatments are effective at lowering IOP and consistently affect retinal cell metabolism including the regulation of distinctive crystallins to below baseline levels.
3. The beneficial effects on RGC survival of Ti/B, Ti/D, and Ti/Tr seem to operate independently of crystallin regulation.

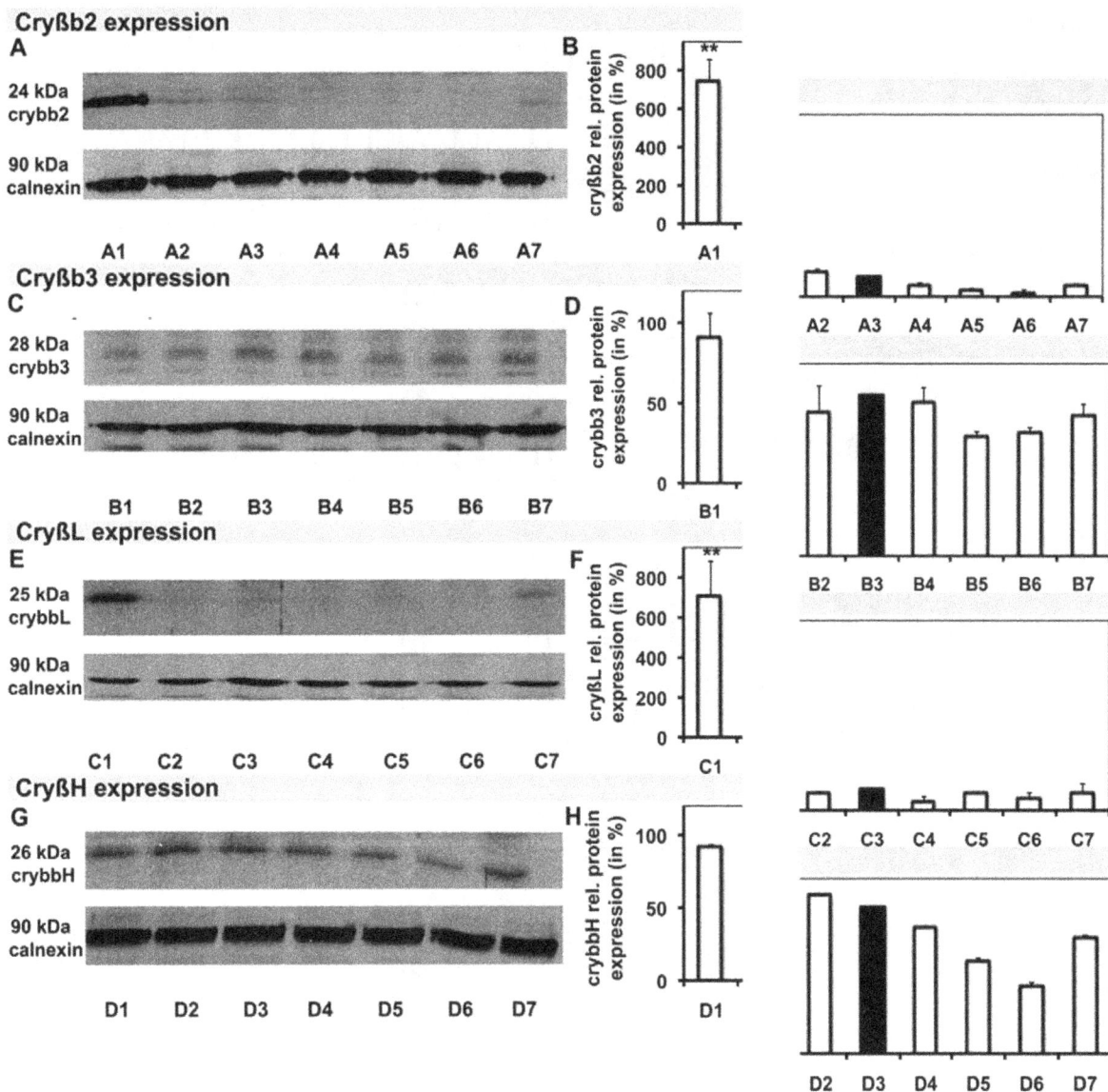

**Figure 4. Specific Western blot analysis and the correlated graph of the relative density of selected proteins, including the application controls.** A–G Blots of cryβb2 (**A**) cryβb3 (**C**), cryβL (**E**), and cryβH (**G**), and their correlated relative densities (**B, D, F**, and **H**, respectively), each with the corresponding control with calnexin. Hypertensive samples are demonstrated in **A1–D1**, normotensive samples in **A2–D2** and **A3–D3**, samples following Ti/B treatment in **A4–D4**, samples following Ti treatment in **A5–D5**, samples following Ti/Tr treatment in **A6–D6**, and samples following Ti/D treatment in **A7–D7**.

Elevated IOP plays a major role in RGC apoptosis, and lowering of IOP remains the mainstay of glaucoma treatment [2]. Reducing IOP often helps to slow the progression of degenerative changes in glaucoma. RGC loss may proceed despite normalization of IOP following effective IOP reduction and the absence of elevated IOP beforehand [3,5]. However, although elevated IOP is believed to make important contributions to optic-nerve and RGC damage, it is not the only risk factor involved, implying that further immunomodulatory and vascular factors are also crucial [5]. This finding has led to increasing interest in neuroprotective approaches.

Expanding on previous studies, we found that sustained elevation of IOP was correlated with changes in HSP expression. This may not be surprising since elevations in IOP have been shown to drive toxic metabolic changes within the retina, initiating

a self-propagating vicious circle of RGC degeneration [10], ultimately culminating in apoptosis [4]. There are significant positive correlations between RGC loss and change in IOP [32] and duration of elevated IOP [33], and IOP elevation can directly induce RGC death by apoptosis. RGC death after exposure to elevated IOP seems to take place in two phases: direct IOP-dependent RGC apoptosis followed by a second, slower phase involving neuron loss due to toxic and inflammatory effects of the primary degenerating neurons [31]. Inhibition of this second IOP-triggered self-propagating process of RGC degeneration may lead to new therapeutic approaches. Regulation of HSPs appears to reflect cellular attempts to resist an abnormal IOP.

To further scrutinize the molecular cascades initiated by elevations and reductions in IOP, we adopted the clinically well-proven therapy of topical application of IOP-lowering drugs. Daily

## Hsp 70 expression

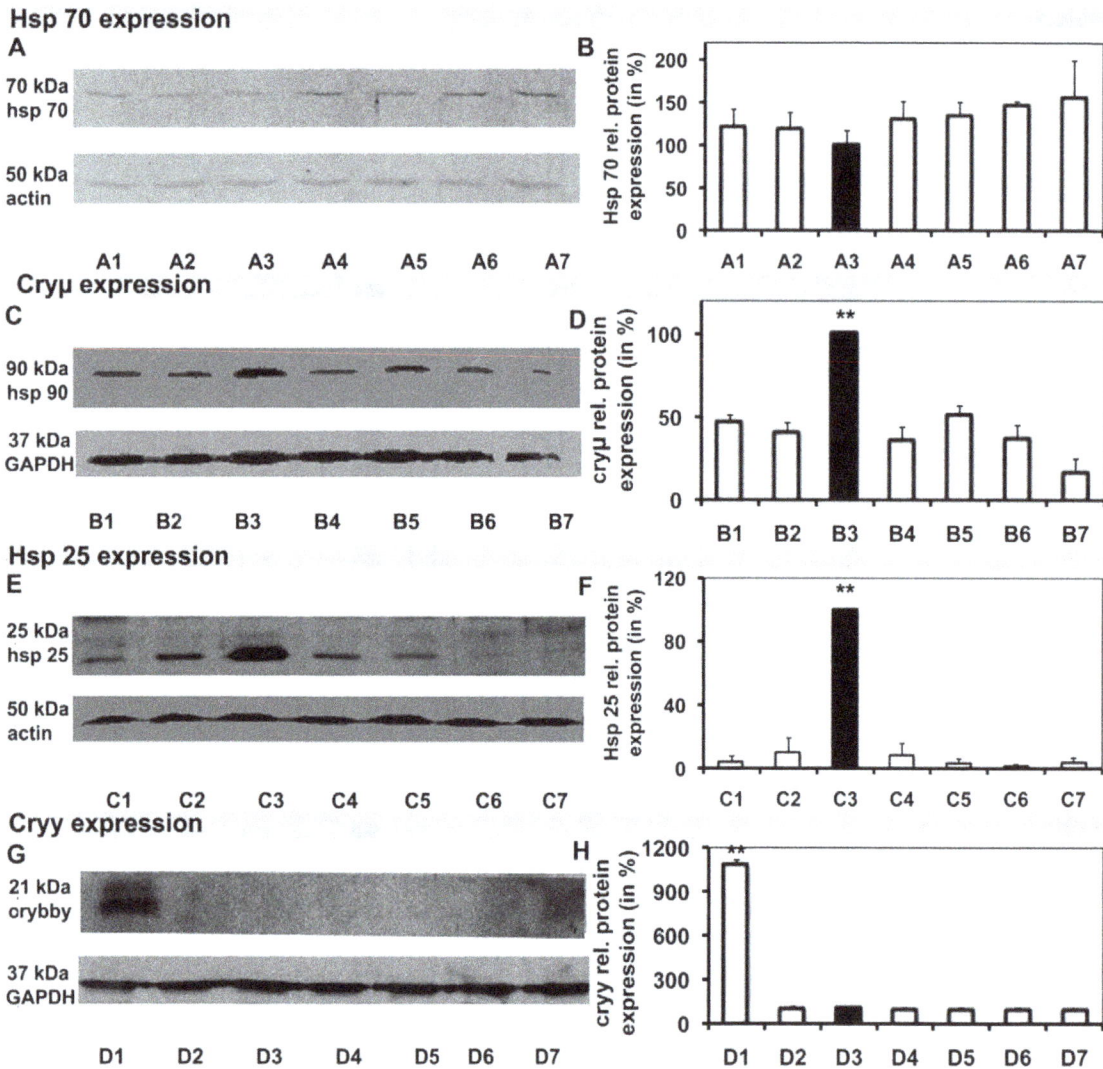

## Cryμ expression

## Hsp 25 expression

## Cryγ expression

**Figure 5. Specific Western blot analysis of selected proteins with the corresponding application controls.** The graphs next to them illustrate the relative protein densities. **A–H** Blots of heat-shock protein (HSP)-70 (**A**), HSP-90 (**C**), HSP-25 (**E**), and cryγ (**G**) and their relative densities (**B**, **D**, **F**, and **H**, respectively). Hypertensive samples are shown in **A1–D1**, normotensive samples in **A2–D2** and **A3–D3**, samples following Ti/B treatment in **A4–D4**, samples following Ti therapy in **A5–D5**, samples following Ti/Tr treatment in **A6–D6**, and samples following Ti/D treatment in **A7–D7**.

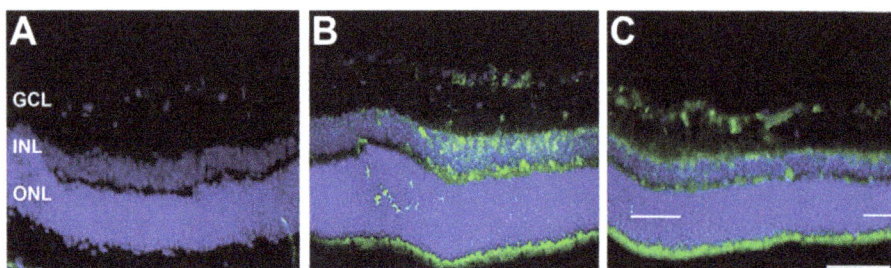

**Figure 6. Immunohistochemical analysis of crystallins.** Staining for cryβb (green) in a normotensive, sham-treated group (**A**), 7 days after induction of elevated IOP (**B**), and 28 days after induction of elevated IOP (**C**) in retinal slices. Cryβb staining revealed a distinctive up-regulation of cryβb after IOP elevation (**B**, **C**) relative to normotensive samples. Moreover, cryβb expression increased within the period of exposure to elevated IOP. The signal was more intense after 28 days (**C**) than after 7 days (**B**) of IOP elevation. Cryβb2 expression appeared predominantly in the RGC layer. Scale bar: 100 μm.

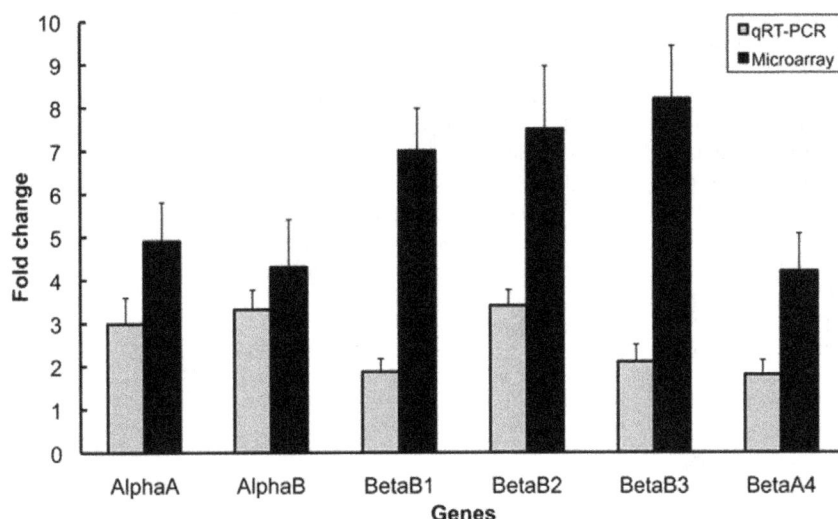

**Figure 7. Confirmation of crystallin expression at the gene level by microarray analysis and subsequent quantitative real-time polymerase chain reaction.** CryαA, cryαB, cryβb1, cryβb2, cryβb3, and cryβb4 were up-regulated due to elevated IOP at 8 weeks after IOP induction. The change **in** gene expression is expressed as the change relative to normotensive sham-treated retinas. The alterations in regulation of all six genes were statistically significant ($p < 0.001$).

topical medication is routinely performed in the clinical treatment of patients, and this produces crucial intraretinal responses that can be detected with sophisticated proteomic and genomic methods. We used an experimental animal model as a surrogate of glaucoma to detect the anticipated glaucomatous changes [18,20]. Our data showed the IOP-dependent regulation of small HSPs and crystallins at both the proteomic and mRNA levels. HSPs are a family of cellular chaperones that are defined according to their molecular masses (in kDa) as HSP-60, HSP-70, HSP-90, and small HSPs (a group with a molecular mass of 20–30 kDa).

Closely related in sequence, and subsummarized to the ubiquitous HSPs, are the crystallins, some of which display partial chaperoning functions [34]. Crystallins have long been considered as the structural proteins of the vertebrate lens [35], and in particular are synergistically responsible for refractive functions such as the preservation of lens transparency throughout life [36]. Crystallins have been localized in the nervous system and the retina, leading to advanced interest in their functions in extralenticular tissues [34,37–38].

The ubiquitous occurrence of crystallins in several tissues and cell types (including RGCs), and their homology and close relationship with the ubiquitous HSPs have led some of them to be classified as stress proteins, although they are also vital to normal tissue differentiation [36,37]. In this context, it is believed that the crystallins are temporarily differentially expressed within the rat retina after various forms of injury [12,39] indicating their involvement both in injury and in postinjury repair. For instance, the expression of cryαB is increased in various neurological disorders [40] such as Alexander's disease [41], Creutzfeld-Jakob disease, and Parkinson's disease [42]. The up-regulation of cryα, cryβ, and cryγ in the retina has been found consistently in gene expression studies after ischemia–reperfusion injury [43], light injury [44], and retinal tears [39], and in diabetic rats [45]. Crystallin regulation has recently been reported at the mRNA and protein levels in both hereditary and experimental models of glaucoma [12,19]. Cryβb expression is increased in the glaucomatous optic nerves of monkeys [46]. Interestingly, crystallin expression patterns shift due to the period of exposure to elevated

IOP, exhibiting down-regulation of crystallins at the mRNA level and up-regulation to control levels at 2 and 5 weeks after IOP elevation, respectively. It is assumed that crystallin transcription may be stimulated throughout RGC degeneration in response to IOP elevation or in response to the dynamics of elevated IOP, independent of RGC degeneration [12]. According to these findings, the marked up-regulation of crystallin mRNA and protein after IOP elevation and the subsequent down-regulation following antihypertensive treatment reflects the IOP-dependent regulation of crystallins.

According to our results, cryβb2 is expressed mainly in the RGCs, as presumed previously [12]. Three crystallins (cryβb2, cryβbL, and cryβbγ) were strikingly expressed in hypertensive samples compared to normotensive controls, and down-regulated to and below baseline levels following effective hypotensive treatment. On the other hand, the expressions of cryβb3, cryβbH, and HSP-70 remained unchanged, and those of cryμ and HSP-25 were significantly higher in normotensive samples, to become down-regulated after IOP elevation, and to remain down-regulated despite effective IOP lowering.

In addition to acting within neurons, HSPs induce immuno-modulatory cascades in glaucoma [16]. Titers of circulating antibodies against small HSPs are increased in the serum of glaucoma patients. Moreover, HSPs are considered to be associated with and responsible for increased RGC death. The functions of the immune system in glaucoma are probably surveillance and regulation, in which signaling pathways of the immune system regulate cell death in response to conditions that stressRGCs, such as elevated IOP or factors produced as a consequence thereof [47]. Whether those antibodies are produced primarily as autoantibodies or are released in response to enhanced expression of small HSPs due to elevated IOP remains unclear, since HSPs are known to have strong antigenetic potential [48–49]. The latter mechanism would require the release of cryβb into the plasma serum to induce an antigen reaction, which seems to be the case, at least for cryβb2. Cryβb2 can be released out of the cells into the culture medium and can be taken up by the cells again. Therefore cryββ2 presents as a molecule that trafficks between the cytosol and the extracellular space [13].

We found a drug-specific regulation of the pattern of crystallin expression and neuroprotective effects of antihypertensive treatments with Ti/Tr, Ti/D, and Ti/B that appear to be independent of each other. The drug components used in this study are assumed to be neuroprotective in various experiments, and the mechanisms involved have been established. In a manner unrelated to their β-adrenoreceptor blocking activity [50], β-adrenergic agonists reduce ligand-stimulated calcium and sodium influx into cells through direct interaction with L-type voltage-dependent calcium channels [51] and voltage-sensitive sodium channels [52]. α-2a agonists seem to inhibit glutamate and aspartate accumulation [53], up-regulate antiapoptotic genes such as *bcl-2* and *bcl-xl*, and produce neurotrophic factors, most evidently mediated through α-2a adrenoreceptor activation [54]. Prostaglandin $F_{2\alpha}$ analogues exert their neuroprotective effects via the retinal prostaglandin F receptor [55] by reducing the release of lactate dehydrogenase and through p44/p42 mitogen-activated protein kinase and caspase-3 inhibition [25]. Carbonic anhydrase inhibitors work by augmenting retrobulbar blood flow in glaucoma patients [56]. Our data show that antihypertensive treatment induces retinal metabolic changes and effectively reduces stress to neurons, as seen strikingly through the down-regulation of various crystallins.

In conclusion, our study shows that elevated IOP causes alterations at both the histopathological and proteomic levels, in accordance with previous reports. The novel findings of our study are the changes in the pattern of crystallin expression. We have also shown that antihypertensive treatment reverses specific IOP-induced alterations within the retina at the proteomic level. This effect is independent of the neuroprotective effects observed in our *in vivo* model, suggesting that the eye drops exert a direct effect on retinal metabolism. The significance of the marked regulation of small HSPs and crystallins, in particular due to neuronal degeneration following elevated IOP and antihypertensive treatment, merits further investigation.

## Acknowledgments

The authors are indebted to Dr. S. König (IFG, Münster) for help with protein identification, M. Wissing for technical assistance with immuno-histochemistry, M. Langkamp-Flock for technical help with Western blotting, and Dr. R. Naskar for providing the microarray data on crystallins.

## Author Contributions

Obtained permission from the ethics committee: ST. Designed experiments: VP. Conceived experiments: MS. Conceived and designed the experiments: VP MS ST. Performed the experiments: VP MS ST. Analyzed the data: VP MS ST. Contributed reagents/materials/analysis tools: VP MS. Wrote the paper: VP MS ST.

## References

1. Quigley HA (1996) Number of people with glaucoma worldwide. Br J Ophthalmol 80: 389–393.
2. Stone EM, Fingert JH, Alward WL, Nguyen TD, Polansky JR, et al (1997) Identification of a gene that causes primary open angle glaucoma. Science 275: 668–670.
3. Cockburn DM (1983) Does reduction of intraocular pressure (IOP) prevent visual field loss in glaucoma? Am J Optom Physiol Opt 60: 705–711.
4. Garcia-Valenzuela E, Shareef S, Walsh J, Sharma SC (1995) Programmed cell death of retinal ganglion cells during experimental glaucoma. Exp Eye Res 61: 33–44.
5. Hitchings RA (1995) Therapeutic rationale for normal-tension glaucoma. Curr Opin Ophthalmol 6: 67–70.
6. Quigley HA, Nickells RW, Kerrigan LA, Pease ME, Thibault DJ, et al (1995) Retinal ganglion cell death in experimental glaucoma and after axotomy occurs by apoptosis. Invest Ophthalmol Vis Sci 36: 774–786.
7. Dreyer EB, Zurakowski D, Schumer RA, Podos SM, Lipton SA (1996) Elevated glutamate levels in the vitreous body of humans and monkeys with glaucoma. Arch Ophthalmol 114: 299–305.
8. Caprioli J, Kitano S, Morgan JE (1996) Hyperthermia and hypoxia increase tolerance of retinal ganglion cells to anoxia and excitotoxicity. Invest Ophthalmol Vis Sci 37: 2376–2381.
9. Osborne NN, Wood JP, Chidlow G, Bae JH, Melena J, et al (1999) Ganglion cell death in glaucoma: what do we really know? Br J Ophthalmol 83: 980–986.
10. Schwartz M, Yoles E (2000) Self-destructive and self-protective processes in the damaged optic nerve: implications for glaucoma. Invest Ophthalmol Vis Sci 41: 349–351.
11. Quigley HA, McKinnon SJ, Zack DJ, Pease ME, Kerrigan-Baumrind LA, et al (2000) Retrograde axonal transport of BDNF in retinal ganglion cells is blocked by acute IOP elevation in rats. Invest Ophthalmol Vis Sci 41: 3460–3466.
12. Piri N, Song M, Kwong JM, Caprioli J (2007) Modulation of alpha and beta crystallin expression in rat retinas with ocular hypertension-induced ganglion cell degeneration. Brain Res 1141: 1–9.
13. Liedtke T, Schwamborn JC, Schröer U, Thanos S (2007) Elongation of axons during regeneration involves retinal crystallin beta b2 (crybb2). Mol Cell Proteomics 6: 895–907.
14. Tezel G, Seigel GM, Wax MB (1998) Autoantibodies to small heat shock proteins in glaucoma. Invest Ophthalmol Vis Sci 39: 2277–2287.
15. Salvador-Silva M, Ricard CS, Agapova OA, Yang P, Hernandez MR (2001) Expression of small heat shock proteins and intermediate filaments in the human optic nerve head astrocytes exposed to elevated hydrostatic pressure in vitro. J Neurosci Res 66: 59–73.
16. Grus FH (2010) Relationship between oxidatve stress and autoimmunity in glaucoma. Klin Monbl Augenheilkd 227: 114–119.
17. Joachim SC, Bruns K, Lackner KJ, Pfeiffer N, Grus FH (2007) Antibodies to alpha B-crystallin, vimentin, and heat shock protein 70 in aqueous humor of patients with normal tension glaucoma and IgG antibody patterns against retinal antigen in aqueous humor. Curr Eye Res 32: 501–509.
18. Mittag TW, Danias J, Pohorenec G, Yuan HM, Burakgazi E, et al (2000) Retinal damage after 3 to 4 months of elevated intraocular pressure in a rat glaucoma model. Invest Ophthalmol Vis Sci 41: 3451–3459.
19. Naskar R, Thanos S (2006) Retinal gene profiling in a hereditary rodent model of elevated intraocular pressure. Mol Vis 12: 1199–210.
20. Naskar R, Wissing M, Thanos S (2002) Detection of early neuron degeneration and accompanying microglial responses in the retina of a rat model of glaucoma. Invest Ophthalmol Vis Sci 43: 2962–2968.
21. Liu S, Zhang Y, Xie X, Hu W, Cai R, et al (2007) Application of two-dimensional electrophoresis in the research of retinal proteins of diabetic rat. Cell Mol Immunol 4: 65–70.
22. Wang YD, Wu JD, Jiang ZL, Wang YB, Wang XH, et al (2007) Comparative proteome analysis of neural retinas from type 2 diabetic rats by two-dimensional electrophoresis. Curr Eye Res 32: 891–901.
23. Saylor M, McLoon LK, Harrison AR, Lee MS (2009) Experimental and clinical evidence for brimonidine as an optic nerve and retinal neuroprotective agent: an evidence-based review. Arch Ophthalmol 127: 402–406.
24. Wood JP, Schmidt KG, Melena J, Chidlow G, Allmeier H, et al (2003) The beta-adrenoceptor antagonists metipranolol and timolol are retinal neuropro-tectants: comparison with betaxolol. Exp Eye Res 76: 505–516.
25. Nakanishi Y, Nakamura M, Mukuno H, Kanamori A, Seigel GM, et al (2006) Latanoprost rescues retinal neuro-glial cells from apoptosis by inhibiting caspase-3, which is mediated by p44/p42 mitogen-activated protein kinase. Exp Eye Res 83: 1108–1117.
26. Park HY, Lee NY, Kim JH, Park CK (2008) Intraocular pressure lowering, change of antiapoptotic molecule expression, and neuroretinal changes by dorzolamide 2%/timolol 0.5% combination in a chronic ocular hypertension rat model. J Ocul Pharmacol Ther 24: 563–571.
27. Hoyng PF, van Beek LM (2000) Pharmacological therapy for glaucoma: a review. Drugs 59: 411–434.
28. Thanos S, Naskar R, Heiduschka P (1997) Regenerating ganglion cell axons in the adult rat establish retinofugal topography and restore visual function. Exp Brain Res 114: 483–491.
29. O'Farrell PH (1975) High-resolution two-dimensional electrophoresis of proteins. J Biol Chem 250: 4007–4021.
30. Laemmli UK (1970) Cleavage of structural proteins during the assembly of the head of bacteriophage T4. Nature 227: 680–685.
31. Moore CG, Epley D, Milne ST, Morrison JC (1995) Long-term non-invasive measurement of intraocular pressure in the rat eye. Curr Eye Res 14: 711–717.
32. Levkovitch-Verbin H, Quigley HA, Martin KR, Valenta D, Baumrind LA, et al (2002) Translimbal laser photocoagulation to the trabecular meshwork as a model of glaucoma in rats. Invest Ophthalmol Vis Sci 43: 402–410.
33. Chauhan BC, Pan J, Archibald ML, LeVatte TL, Kelly ME, et al (2002) Effect of intraocular pressure on optic disc topography, electroretinography, and axonal loss in a chronic pressure-induced rat model of optic nerve damage. Invest Ophthalmol Vis Sci 43: 2969–2976.

34. Andley UP, Mathur S, Griest TA, Petrash JM (1996) Cloning, expression, and chaperone-like activity of human alphaA-crystallin. J Biol Chem 271: 31973–31980.

35. Graw J (1997) The crystallins: genes, proteins and diseases. Biol Chem 378: 1331–1348.

36. Berman ER (1994) Biochemistry of cataracts. In: Garner A, Klintworth GK (eds) Pathology of Ocular Diseases: a Dynamic Approach. Dekker, New York pp 533–590.

37. Sax CM, Piatigorsky J (1994) Expression of the alpha-crystallin/small heat-shock protein/molecular chaperone genes in the lens and other tissues. Adv Enzymol Relat Areas Mol Biol 69: 155–201.

38. Clayton RM, Thomson I, de Pomerai DI (1979) Relationship between crystallin mRNA expression in retina cells and their capacity to re-differentiate into lens cells. Nature 282: 628–629.

39. Vázquez-Chona F, Song BK, Geisert EE Jr (2004) Temporal changes in gene expression after injury in the rat retina. Invest Ophthalmol Vis Sci 45: 2737–2746.

40. Iwaki T, Wisniewski T, Iwaki A, Corbin E, Tomokane N, et al (1992) Accumulation of alpha B-crystallin in central nervous system glia and neurons in pathologic conditions. Am J Pathol 140: 345–356.

41. Head MW, Corbin E, Goldman JE (1993) Overexpression and abnormal modification of the stress proteins alpha B-crystallin and HSP27 in Alexander disease. Am J Pathol 143: 1743–1753.

42. Renkawek K, de Jong WW, Merck KB, Frenken CW, van Workum FP, et al (1992) Alpha B-crystallin is present in reactive glia in Creutzfeldt-Jakob disease. Acta Neuropathol 83: 324–327.

43. Yoshimura N, Kikuchi T, Kuroiwa S, Gaun S (2003) Differential temporal and spatial expression of immediate early genes in retinal neurons after ischemia-reperfusion injury. Invest Ophthalmol Vis Sci 44: 2211–2220.

44. Sakaguchi H, Miyagi M, Darrow RM, Crabb JS, Hollyfield JG, et al (2003) Intense light exposure changes the crystallin content in retina. Exp Eye Res 76: 131–133.

45. Kumar PA, Haseeb A, Suryanarayana P, Ehtesham NZ, Reddy GB (2005) Elevated expression of alphaA- and alphaB-crystallins in streptozotocin-induced diabetic rat. Arch Biochem Biophys 444: 77–83.

46. Furuyoshi N, Furuyoshi M, May CA, Hayreh SS, Alm A, et al (2000) Vascular and glial changes in the retrolaminar optic nerve in glaucomatous monkey eyes. Ophthalmologica 214: 24–32.

47. Tezel G, Yang J, Wax MB (2004) Heat shock proteins, immunity and glaucoma. Brain Res Bull 62: 473–480.

48. Young DB (1990) Stress proteins and the immune response. Antonie Van Leeuwenhoek 58: 203–208.

49. Young RA, Elliott TJ (1989) Stress proteins, infection, and immune surveillance. Cell 59: 5–8.

50. Zimmerman TJ (1993) Topical ophthalmic beta blockers: a comparative review. J Ocul Pharmacol 9: 373–384.

51. Melena J, Wood JP, Osborne NN (1999) Betaxolol, a beta1-adrenoceptor antagonist, has an affinity for L-type Ca2+ channels. Eur J Pharmacol 378: 317–322.

52. Chidlow G, Melena J, Osborne NN (2000) Betaxolol, a beta(1)-adrenoceptor antagonist, reduces Na(+) influx into cortical synaptosomes by direct interaction with Na(+) channels: Comparison with other beta-adrenoceptor antagonists. Br J Pharmacol 130: 759–766.

53. Donello JE, Padillo EU, Webster ML, Wheeler LA, Gil DW (2001) Alpha(2)-adrenoceptor agonists inhibit vitreal lutamate and aspartate accumulation and preserve retinal function after transient ischemia. J Pharmacol Exp Ther 296: 216–223.

54. Lai RK, Chun T, Hasson D, Lee S, Mehrbod F, et al (2002) Alpha-2 adrenoceptor agonist protects retinal function after acute retinal ischemic injury in the rat. Vis Neurosci 19: 175–185.

55. Davis TL, Sharif NA (1999) Quantitative autoradiographic visualization and pharmacology of FP-prostaglandin receptors in human eyes using the novel phosphor-imaging technology. J Ocul Pharmacol Ther 15: 323–336.

56. Martinez A, Sánchez-Salorio M (2009) A comparison of the long-term effects of dorzolamide 2% and brinzolamide 1%, each added to timolol 0.5%, on retrobulbar hemodynamics and intraocular pressure in open-angle glaucoma patients. J Ocul Pharmacol Ther 25: 239–248.

# 6

# Trabecular Meshwork Gene Expression after Selective Laser Trabeculoplasty

**Alberto Izzotti[1], Mariagrazia Longobardi[1], Cristina Cartiglia[1], Federico Rathschuler[2], Sergio Claudio Saccà[2]***

1 Department of Health Sciences, Faculty of Medicine, University of Genoa, Genoa, Italy, 2 Ophthalmology Unit, Department of Head/Neck Pathologies, St. Martino Hospital, Genoa, Italy

## Abstract

*Background:* Trabecular meshwork and Schlemm's canal are the tissues appointed to modulate the aqueous humour outflow from the anterior chamber. The impairment of their functions drives to an intraocular pressure increase. The selective laser trabeculoplasty is a laser therapy of the trabecular meshwork able to decrease intraocular pressure. The exact response mechanism to this treatment has not been clearly delineated yet. The herein presented study is aimed at studying the gene expression changes induced in trabecular meshwork cells by selective laser trabeculoplasty (SLT) in order to better understand the mechanisms subtending its efficacy.

*Methodology/Principal Findings:* Primary human trabecular meshwork cells cultured in fibroblast medium underwent selective laser trabeculoplasty treatment. RNA was extracted from a pool of cells 30 minutes after treatment while the remaining cells were further cultured and RNA was extracted respectively 2 and 6 hours after treatment. Control cells stored in incubator in absence of SLT treatment were used as reference samples. Gene expression was evaluated by hybridization on miRNA-microarray and laser scanner analysis. Scanning electron microscopic examination was performed on 2 Trabecular meshwork samples after SLT at 4th and 6th hour from treatment. On the whole, selective laser trabeculoplasty modulates in trabecular meshwork the expression of genes involved in cell motility, intercellular connections, extracellular matrix production, protein repair, DNA repair, membrane repair, reactive oxygen species production, glutamate toxicity, antioxidant activities, and inflammation.

*Conclusions/Significance:* SLT did not induce any phenotypic alteration in TM samples. TM is a complex tissue possessing a great variety of function pivotal for the active regulation of aqueous humour outflow from the anterior chamber. SLT is able to modulate these functions at the postgenomic molecular level without inducing damage either at molecular or phenotypic levels.

**Editor:** Christian Schönbach, Kyushu Institute of Technology, Japan

**Funding:** This study was supported by The Glaucoma Foundation (New York, United States of America). The funders had no role in study design, data collection and analysis, decision to publish, or preparation of the manuscript.

**Competing Interests:** The authors have declared that no competing interests exist.

* E-mail: sergio.sacca@hsanmartino.it

## Introduction

Glaucoma is a neurodegenerative multi-factorial disease affecting different target tissues: the lateral geniculate nucleus and the visual cortex in the central nervous system, [1] the optic nerve head in the retina, and the trabecular meshwork (TM) in the anterior chamber (AC) of the eye. In the majority of cases the glaucoma is accompanied by intraocular pressure increase that is the most important risk factor for the progression of disease [2]. All the pathogenic events leading to death of the retinal ganglion cells (RGCs) are not yet known with accuracy but it is established that TM play a major role in the glaucomatous pathogenic cascade. The concept that eye outflow system is a passive filter is outdated. Indeed Alvarado found that severe alterations occur in the cellular component and in the entire TM during POAG and ageing [3,4]. The same author shown that TM endothelial cells regulate aqueous outflow by actively releasing enzymes and cytokines that, upon binding to Schlemm's canal (SC) endothelial cells, increase transendothelial flow thereby facilitating the egress of aqueous humour [5]. TM endothelial cells secrete these factors in response

to stimuli such as mechanical stretching, laser irradiation, and pro-inflammatory cytokines [6,7]. In 1991 Saccà et al. [8,9] presented a new Argon Laser Trabeculoplasty (ALT) technique as applied to TM that took advantage of a very low power thus not creating burns in TM and being at the same time able to obtain a lasting effect of IOP decrease in subjects suffering from glaucoma (Figure 1). Some years later Latina et al. [10] employed a q-switched 532-nm neodymium (Nd):YAG laser to investigate the safety and efficacy of laser treatment. Laser parameters were set to selectively target pigmented TM cells without coagulative damage to the TM structure or nonpigmented cells. This technique was called "selective laser trabeculoplasty," (SLT) and decreased intraocular pressure by an amount similar to that achieved with standard trabeculoplasty [11]. Actually, SLT does not produce any anatomic alteration appreciable to microscope while ALT cause visible burns on TM (Figure 1). Anyway, SLT is equivalent to ALT in terms of IOP lowering at 1 year and is a safe and effective procedure for patients with open-angle glaucoma [12]. Indeed, the exact response mechanisms to this treatment has not been clearly delineated yet, even if it is known that energy laser has many

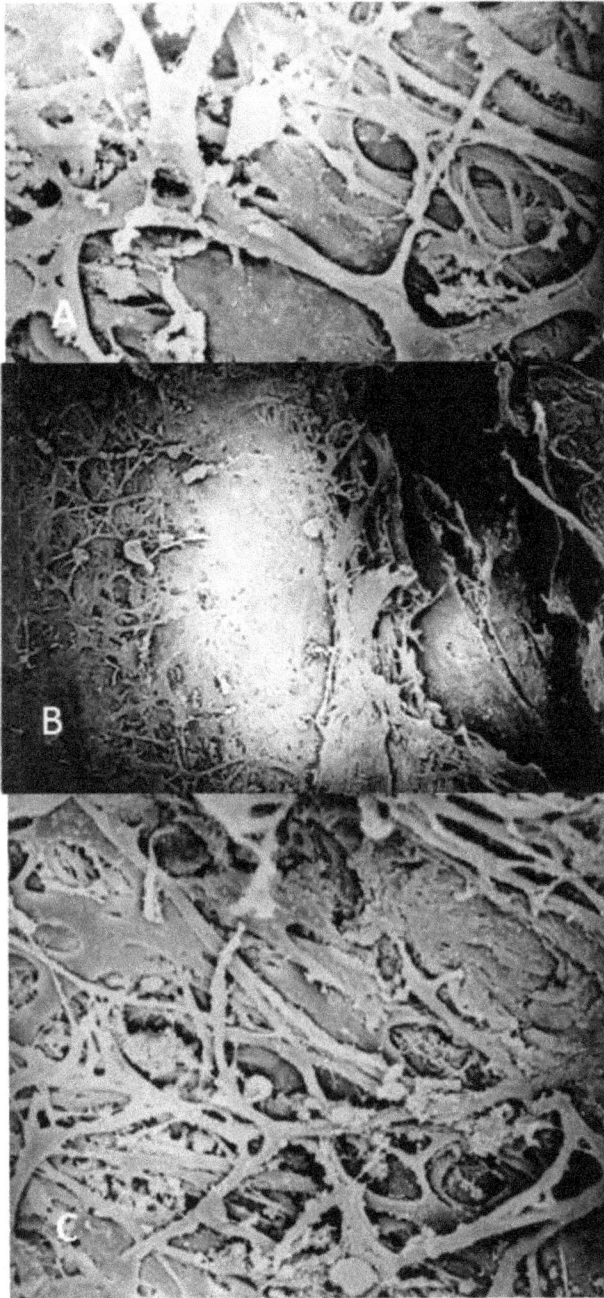

**Figure 1. Trabecular meschwork after SLT and ALT.** Scanning electron microscope photograph of the human sclerocorneal trabecular meshwork (magnification 2,000x in A and C, and 1,500x in B) 3 h (A) and 6 h (C) after SLT treatment. The architecture of TM is well conserved, showing intact trabecular beams (A,C). By comparison, following argon laser trabeculoplasty a coagulative damage with disruption of trabecular beams is well evident (B).

action of ALT or SLT is based on the release of cytokines and synthesis of matrix metalloprotease enzyme from TM cells induced by the heating effect of the laser and finally resulting in an increased turnover of the extracellular matrix [16,17].

The first "mechanical theory" stating that the laser application results in the local shrinkage of the meshwork, opening the intertrabecular spaces between the laser sites [18] has been nowadays neglected by most of the authors.

SLT applied on rabbit eyes increases in aqueous humour lipid peroxidase and free oxygen radicals levels [19]. Accordingly, it is conceivable that SLT induces a transient and moderate cell stress triggering cellular defences without coagulative damage to the TM [20]. In order to explore this hypothesis and gene-expression changes preceeding SLT effects, we performed the herein presented study aimed at studying the gene expression changes induced in TM cells by SLT.

The study adhered to the tenets of the Declaration of Helsinki and was approved by the Ethical Board of the Ophthalmologic Division.

## Results

SLT did not induce any phenotypic alteration in TM samples collected from corneal donors as evaluated by electron scanning microscopy either 3 h and 6 h after treatment (Fig. 1 a and c). By comparison, this lack of phenotypic effect is completely different from the remarkable tissue alterations induced by trabeculoplasty treatment in analogue sample after 3 h since treatment (Fig. 1 b). Conversely, SLT induced important changing at postgenomic level in TM cells.

SLT treatment induced a time-related change in the gene expression profile of TM cells. As evaluated by scatter plot such a change was well detectable starting since two hours after SLT treatment and persisted up to 6 hours (Fig. 2, upper panel). Changes of gene expression induced by SLT were time dependent, being mainly detectable after 2 and 6 hours since SLT exposure, and included both upregulation of genes expressed at low levels in Control (blue lines) and dowregulation of genes expressed at high level in Control (red lines) (Fig. 2, lower panel). The modulating effect on the global gene expression profile was pointed out by hierarchical cluster analysis demonstrating that gene expression profile of Control and SLT-treated TM cells after 30 min are similar and clustered together in the same dendrogram branch (Fig. 2, upper panel, left side). Conversely, gene expression profile of SLT-treated TM cells after 2 and 6 hours are remarkably different from Control being located in different branches of the dendrogram (Fig. 3, upper panel, right side). A similar situation was recorded by performing Principal Component Analysis of variance where Control and SLT-treated TM cells after 30 min (T0.5) are located in the same quadrant, while SLT-treated TM cells after 2 hours (T2) and 6 hours (T6) are located in different quadrants far away from Control (Fig. 3, lower panel).

Scatter plot analysis identified those genes up- or down-regulated by SLT after 30 min (T0.5), 2 hours (T2) and 6 hours (T6) (Fig. 4).

No effect was observed after 30 min since SLT treatment. Conversely, after 2 hours the number of genes changing their expression more than 2-fold as compared to controls accounted for 513, further rising up to 3,774 after 6 hours.

Out of the 94 genes spotted on the microarray activating cell death by apoptosis or necrosis no one significantly varied its expression as consequence of SLT. This finding demonstrates that, under our experimental conditions, SLT does not induce directly *per se* cell damage. This finding is in line with the lack of any

biological effects on TM depending on the magnitude of the energy used and the distance from the center of the irradiated zone [13]. One biologic response of the trabecular meshwork after laser trabeculoplasty is a change in the level of ongoing trabecular cell division [14]. This is the basis of the "repopulation theory" stating that laser would stimulate the repopulation of the meshwork with fresh trabecular cells, which may result in the formation of healthy TM [15]. The "biological theory" suggests that the mechanism of

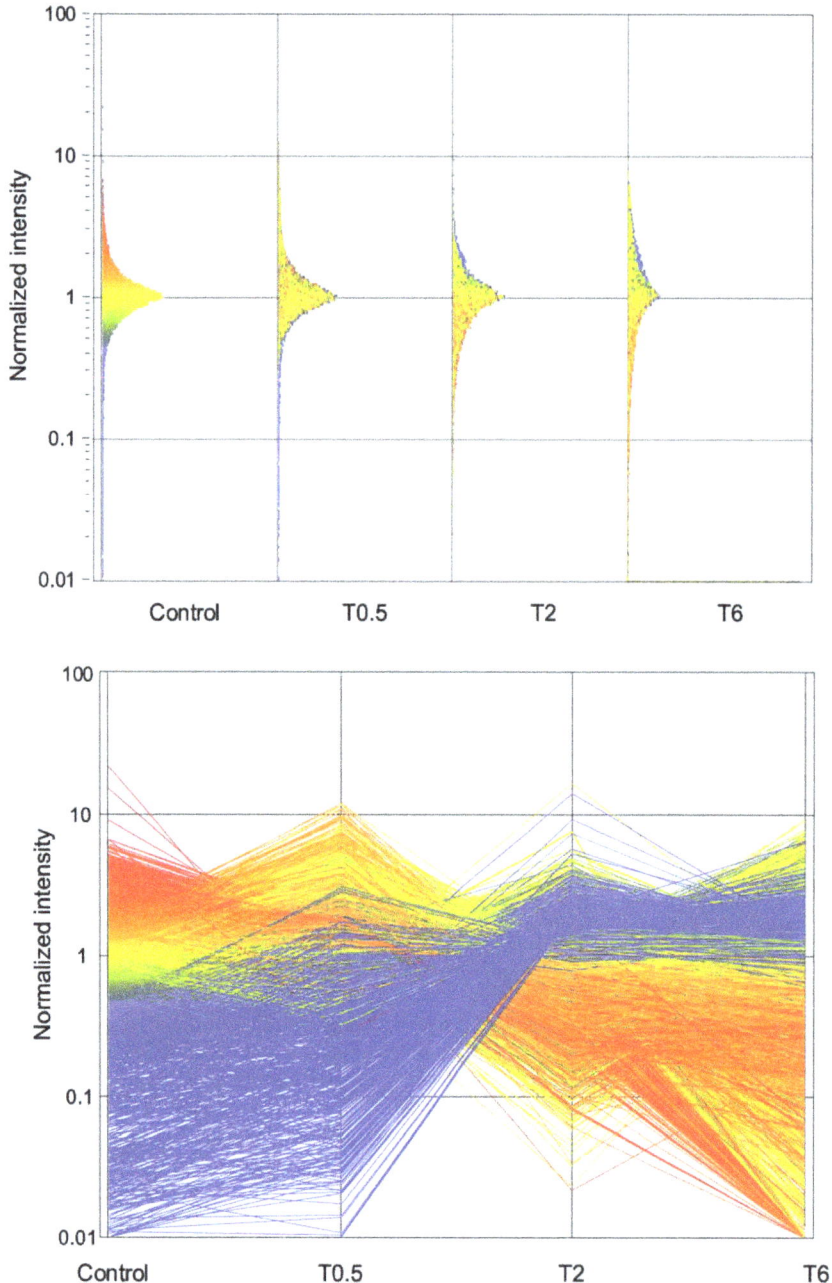

**Figure 2. Quantitative analysis of TM Gene expression after SLT.** Box plot (upper panel) and time course (lower panel) analyses of the expression of 18,401 genes in TM cells either unexposed (Control) or after various times (0.5, 2, and 6 hours) since SLT treatment. Box plot analysis report the level of expression of each gene (dot) located on vertical axis according to its level of expression expressed on a color scale referred to control (blue low expression, red high expression). Time course analysis reports the variation in the gene expression intensity for each analysed gene. Genes undergoing downregulation after SLT treatment as compared to control are indicated in blue, genes undergoing upregulation in red.

alteration in TM after 24 h since SLT treatment as ob served by electron microscopy (Fig. 1).

Among the many genes changing their expression, statistical support vector machine analysis identified 67 predictor genes specifically and significantly related with SLT treatment.

These genes, detailed in Table S1, online supporting information, are involved in various cell functions including cell motility, tissue integrity, cell membrane components, mitochondrion function, oxidative stress, DNA repair, glutamate metabolism, inflammation, and energy production.

Complete microarray data are available at GEO database (GEO number GSE29697) (http://www.ncbi.nlm.nih.gov/geo/).

## Discussion

Our work provides evidence at postgenomic level that TM actively modulates the aqueous humor outflow through a variety of molecular mechanisms that can be modulated by SLT.

### TM motility

Of the 67 genes modulated by SLT 7 (12%), encoding for activities involved in cell motility and contraction were upregulated by SLT indicating that this treatment enhance the contracting capacity of TM cells. The contractile function, cell shape, and cell adhesion properties of TM and SC cells have been

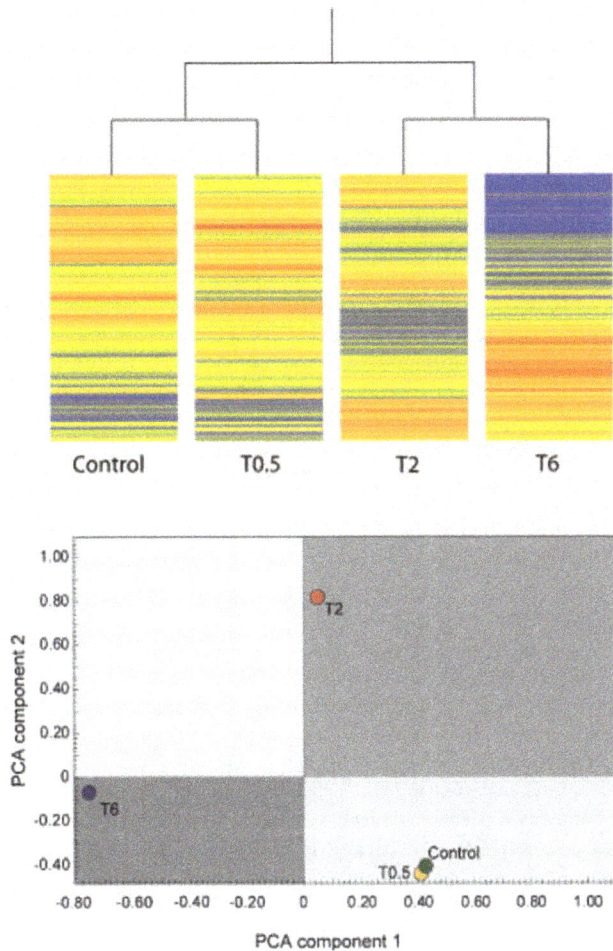

**Figure 3. Qualitative analysis of TM Gene expression before and after SLT.** Hierarchical cluster (upper panel) reporting gene expression profile as evaluated in TM cells before SLT (Control, left column) and at various times after SLT (0.5, 2, 6 h). Gene expression intensity is reported as color scale (blue low, red high). The same gene expression profile was compared among different experimental conditions (dots) by analyzing the two principal components of variance for each sample (PCA) (lower panel).

implicated widely in modulation of aqueous humor outflow through the conventional pathway [21,22]. Indeed, contraction of TM with its smooth muscle-like properties, decreases outflow, whereas relaxation increases this parameter [23]. This tissue has the ability to contract when exposed to appropriate stimulants [23], its property is important in helping regulate the outflow of aqueous humor [24]. Indeed, Trabecular meshwork cells express contractile elements such as smooth muscle $\alpha$-actin and myosin [25]. F-actin architecture in human outflow pathway cells in situ differs between normal and glaucoma eyes, glaucomatous tissue showing a more "disordered" actin architecture overall [26]. TM and its endothelial cells, as well as SC Schlemm's canal and the lining endothelial cells, undergo deformation and stretching with changes in intraocular pressure [5].

The above reported results could confirm the hypothesis of the "mechanical theory" of Wise and Witter [18], neverthenless also the "biological theory" [16,17] and the "repopulation theory" [15] are almost supported by our findings.

## Tissue integrity

Indeed, 15 out of the 67 genes (22%) modulated by SLT encoded for activities involved in maintaining TM tissue integrity. Among these, genes involved in adherence to basal membrane and intercellular connection and in extracellular matrix removal resulted up regulated. Conversely, SLT downregulated gene involved in the production of extracellular matrix. These mechanisms contributes to the maintenance of TM cellularity counteracting its decrease. It was demonstrated that a relative increase in the extracellular matrix/cells ratio is crucial for POAG progression [27]. IOP homeostasis, triggered by pressure changes or mechanical stretching of the TM, appears to involve the extracellular matrix turnover [28]. An upregulation of genes involved in repairing and removing damaged protein was observed. This finding indicate that SLT increase removal of oxidized proteins typically accumulating in degenerating and aged tissues [29].

## Cell membrane

Furthermore 8 out of 67 genes whose expression was affected by SLT treatment are cell membrane components. Genes encoding for activities involved in intracellular $Ca^{++}$ homeostasis were modulated by SLT. This finding probably reflects the SLT effect on mitochondrion (see below), which is the main intracellular $Ca^{++}$

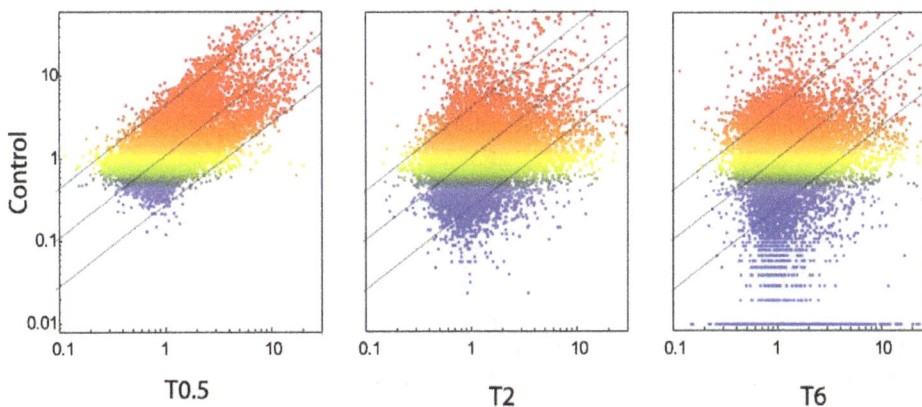

**Figure 4. Comparative analysis of TM Gene expression before and after SLT.** Scatter plot analysis comparing gene expression before (vertical axis, Control) and after SLT at various times (horizontal axis, 0.2, 2, 6 h). Gene expression intensity is reported as color scale referring to Control (blue low, red high). The diagonal lines indicate the 2-fold variation interval including genes whose expression did not change after SLT. Genes falling above these lines were downregulated, genes falling below these lines were upregulated more than 2-fold in their expression by SLT.

depot. Intracellular $Ca^{++}$ release is a pivotal step of the intrinsic apoptotic pathway. Thus this situation may be interpreted as a decreased trend towards apoptosis.

A study [30], examined the levels of Ca2+ in TM cells from POAG and nondiseased aged-matched individuals and demonstrated that both [Ca2+]c and [Ca2+]m were higher in POAG TM. POAG TM cells have defective mitochondrial function, which causes them to be abnormally vulnerable to $Ca^{2+}$ stress. The dysfunction in calcium regulation by these cells may contribute to the failure of this tissue to control IOP.

SLT treatment increased the expression of genes encoding for cell growth factor, aminoacids, and $Na^+$ uptake. On the whole these genes contribute to tissue integrity by stimulating cell growth and volume maintenance. SLC3A2, involved in the synthesis of nitric oxide, was upregulated. This indicates that SLT activates mechanisms contributing to the maintenance of TM integrity such as blood perfusion improvement, being nitric oxide able to increase vessel diameter and perfusion rate.

## Mitochondria

8 out of the 67 (12%) SLT-modulated genes were involved in mitochondrial functions. 7 of these genes, involved in ion transport and lipid peroxidation, were downregulated. This trend indicates a silencing of mitochondrial activities producing intracellular reactive oxygen species. However this situation does not result in energy shortage. In fact a gene (ATP5J) involved in ATP synthesis was upregulated.

## Energy production

Furthermore, among **6** genes involved in energy production (9% of 67), 3 genes, involved in glucose supply and anaerobic glycolysis, were upregulated. In parallel, 3 of these genes, involved in ATP consumption, were downregulated. These finding indicate that TM cells as a consequence of SLT exposure decrease energy consumption and increase energy production by anaerobic mechanisms. This balance results in the reduction of endogenous production of reactive oxygen species.

## Oxidative stress

8 out of 67 genes (10%) affected by SLT treatment are involved in response to oxidative stress and production of antioxidant activities. Upregulated antioxidant activities include glutathione, cyestine rich proteins, bilirubin metabolites, mitochondrial cytochrome. Two genes involved in removal of retinol derivatives were downregulated, suggesting that retinol metabolites too contribute to the increasing of the antioxidant status.

The role of reactive oxygen species in the pathogenicity of glaucoma is supported by increasing evidences [31]. Indeed, oxidative damage to the DNA of TM cells has been proved to be significantly higher in affected patients than in age-matched control subjects [32]. Oxidative damage and AH antioxidant defects mainly targets TM, which the most sensitive tissue of the anterior chamber to oxidative damage [33].

## DNA

Moreover an increased trend to DNA repair was observed. In fact among the 5 (7% of 67) genes involved in DNA repair and cell cycle, 2 involved in base repair and 1 inhibiting cell cycle were upregulated, while 3 inducing cell cycle progression were downregulated. This figure indicates a trend to cell cycle rate decrease paralleled by increased DNA repair.

Luna et al. [34] demonstrated that chronic oxidative stress may lead to increased synthesis and deposition of extracellular matrix in the TM and contribute to the elevation of intra-ocular pressure in glaucoma. Thus the trend toward oxidative damage reduction herein reported could act in synergism with the above underlined mechanisms of manteinance of the homeostasis between cells and extracellular matrix.

## Inflammation

All the 7 genes (10% out of 67) involved in inflammation and recruitment of inflammatory cells were downregulated after SLT treatment. This situation results in an immunosuppressive effect bearing relevance because inflammation has been proposed as a possible pathogenic step of POAG. These findings are in line with the ability of light to induce immunosuppression by modulating gene expression in exposed tissues [35]. Alvarado et al. [36] reported an increased expression of IL 8 in cultured TM cells treated with SLT. Unfortunately this data is not assessable in our study, the sequence of its gene not being present in our array. Furthermore Alvarado et al. recently demonstrated a monocyte recruitment in TM following SLT treatment [6] confirming a involvement of immunologic response to SLT treatment.

## Glutamate metabolism

3 out of the 67 genes modulated by SLT (4%) are involved in glutamate metabolism. This confirm a possible interaction between glutamate metabolism and the IOP in the optic nerve head where, in rabbits, the elevation of the IOP causes an increase in the glutamate levels [37]. Indeed, acute and transient intraocular hypertension induces neurodegenerative changes and the accompanying glial activation in the visual pathway. Brain changes may occur in parallel with the Retinal Ganglion Cells loss. Reactive glial cells in the brain may participate in the clearance of aberrantly released glutamate [38].

## TM gene expression

The expression of 9 genes (13%) characterizing neural tissue, as inferred from Swissprotein annotation, was well detectable expressed in TM cells and modulated by SLT treatment. These genes are identified by '*' in Table S1. This finding indicate that similarities at postgenomic levels exist between TM and other neural tissues recognized as POAG targets such as optic nerve head and geniculate ganglion. TM cells have a neuro-ectodermic origin, expressing, at least in part, a neural-like phenotype [39] TM cells derive from mesenchymal cells of the neural crest [40]. This may explains why the SLT increases also the genes expression of typical neural tissues, and further confirm the similarity between TM and neural tissue previously reported comparatively analyzing proteome in TM and optic nerve head [41,42,43]. Furthermore, neural proteins have been specifically detected in the aqueous humour of glaucomatous patients as resulting both from TM and optic nerve head damage and these molecules may be involved in the normal formation and function of these tissues [44].

The similarity between TM and neural tissue is important for glaucoma pathogenesis because they can share common pathogenic mechanisms. The herein reported results provide evidence that glutamate cytotoxic effects representing a major pathogenic element for nerve tissues targeted by glaucoma, are also important for TM homeostasis and may be modulated in TM by SLT treatment. A trend to decreasing TM cell to the adverse glutamate effects was detected. In fact, SLT decreased the expression of gene encoding for the NMDA glutamate receptors, which mediate glutamate induced cytotoxicity. In parallel, two genes encoding for enzymes involved in glutamate catabolism were upregulated.

On the whole SLT induces in TM cell motility, increased intercellular connections, decreased extracellular matrix production, protein repair, DNA repair, membrane repair, decreased reactive oxygen species production, decreased glutamate toxicity, increased antioxidant activities, and decreased inflammation. Nevertheless it has to be taken into account that the analysis of gene expression can give a broad quantity of data but not all of them will be actually effective in cell. As a matter of that Alvarado et al. [36] pointed out that only a small portion of the differentially expressed genes are actually involved in the SLT mediated effects. Further analyses of the SLT induced modulation of the mirnoma, in progress in our laboratory, will contribute to give a more detailed picture of the mechanisms subtending the SLT efficacy and will improve the understanding of the pathogenic events of POAG. Even if the mechanism underlying contraction or relaxation of TM cells *in vivo* is not clear, it is thought that a high IOP, can extend the trabecular beams, obtaining an increased exposure of endothelial cells in AH by increasing the surface of filtration [44] and a cytokines increase into the AC that then will increase flow across the SC [36]. If the IOP falls below the venous pressure, the surface of filtration decreases and the trabecular beams become flaccid, increasing the residence to the outflow of SC [36]. Extracellular matrix proteins contribute to the homeostatic modification of aqueous humor outflow resistance and are known to be upregulated or downregulated in response to mechanical stretching [45,46]. Our results indicate that SLT activate at least one gene encoding for a metalloprotease involved in extracellular matrix homeostasis (ADAMTS2). Other cellular changes may initially help to repair mechanical damage, and could eventually increase tissue rigidity and compromise the ability of the TM to maintain normal levels of outflow resistance [47]. TM cell adhesions, are not static structures but rather are dynamic – they come and go, vary in tightness, location, adhesivity – depending on what is going on in the environment of the cell [48]. SLT change this TM property, changing the proteins production not only structural that govern the TM functionality, in particular the assembly and disassembly of the junctions and the interactions of the cytokines that influencing the HA outflow between the TM and SC endothelium. Thus, the tri-dimensional architecture of human TM considerably increases the filtration surface, whose degeneration, resulting in the decay of HTM cellularity, causes IOP increase and triggers glaucoma pathogenesis [4]. According with Borras [41] model, the cells of the outflow pathway will initially respond to an IOP insult by triggering a defense mechanism through the activation of NF-kB. As the injury persists, as it is the case in a chronic disease, the increased activation of NF-kB will subsequently be followed by further activation of inflammatory cytokines that would then contribute to the cell damage observed in glaucoma. Particularly, chronic oxidative stress leads to the endogenous production of ROS by the mitochondria in TM cells, which in turn induces a sustained stress response characterized by activation of NF-κB and expression of inflammatory markers [49]. ROS present in AC can cause an error of replication of mtDNA determining a significant deletion of the mithocondria genome. The genome shorter replicates itself faster inducing the creation of mitochondria malfunctioning or inactive that causes an energy deficit and atrophy [50], farther mitochondria are key regulators of apoptosis [51]. The SLT lead the expression of distinct sets of genes that stimulates an improvement of TM perfomances, activating, as we have seen, genes concern the motility and the integrity of this tissue and trying to optimise the functioning of mitochondria in contrast to free radicals.

For instance, Bone morphogenetic proteins that controls multiple functions in a variety of cells are present in human optic nerve head (ONH) tissues, isolated ONH astrocytes, and Lamina Cribrosa cells [52], and can alter TGF-beta2 signaling in the TM and leads to increased ECM deposition and elevated IOP [43]. Our study confirm that glaucoma is associated with increased expression of genes that mediate axonal outgrowth, immune response, cell motility, neuroprotection, and ECM remodeling, and as glaucoma progresses, retinal ganglion cell axons may make a regenerative attempt to restore lost nerve cell contact [53]. Interestingly, some of the same genes have been reported to have an upregulated expression in the TM and lamina cribrosa cells treated with TGF, dexamethasone, mechanical stretch, or increased ocular pressure [22,41,42,43,45]. Furthermore, neural proteins have been specifically detected in the aqueous humour of glaucomatous patients as resulting both from TM and optic nerve head lamina cribrosa [39] in fact an increase in IOP resulted in morphological changes in the astrocytes [54], in a disturbances in axonal transport [55] and lead to a cytoskeletal damage in the prelaminar, lamina cribrosa, and postlaminar regions of the optic nerve, after 6 hours of raised IOP [56]. Under this light we can observe the gene expression correlated with glutamate metabolism. We know there is a way from AC and lamina cribrosa through the iris and the choroidal vessels posteriorly, [57], that may be related to glutamate receptor subunits regulating calcium fluxes, the specific pattern of neuronal vulnerability [58]. It is possible that Ionotropic glutamate receptor. L-glutamate acts as an excitatory neurotransmitter at many synapses in the central nervous system, bringing signals to the optic nerve head and leaving the vitreous relatively inert. Therefore the TM is to be considered as a organ that governs the flow from AC to SC whose functions are complex, and not unrelated to those of ciliary body whose physiopathologic meaning is now compared to a multifunctional neuroendocrine gland [59]. Anyway, it is to remember that both Aqueous Humour and plasma homocysteine levels were significantly increased in POAG, and this is a neurotoxin that induces apoptotic retinal ganglion cell death via stimulation of NMDA receptor, hence increased Hcy concentrations in AH and plasma might contribute to the optic nerve damage in POAG [60].

In conclusion SLT significantly increased the tonographic outflow facility and decreased IOP in patients with primary open angle glaucoma and ocular hypertension [61], thanks to trabecular gene-activations which involves a huge number of genes that affect mainly its metabolic functions and its micro environment. These protective effects occur without the induction of damage-related phenotypic alterations in treated TM specimens, as documented in Fig. 1.

For their absolute interest are those related to stress oxidative which confirm its pathogenetic importance [62], and those related to mitochondrial that confirm their primary role in TM function [63] and in the entire homeostasis of AC. The similarity between TM and neural tissue is important for glaucoma pathogenesis because they can share common pathogenic mechanisms. Indeed, herein reported results provide evidence that glutamate cytotoxic effects representing a major pathogenic element for nerve tissues targeted by glaucoma, are also important for TM homeostasis and may be modulated in TM by SLT treatment. Recently, our group has published a paper where it shows how the proteomic composition of aqueous humor reflects events of glaucoma pathogenesis [64]. In light of this presented results provide evidence that TM is a complex tissue possessing a great variety of function pivotal for the active regulation of aqueous humour outflow from the anterior chamber. SLT is able to modulate these function at postgenomic molecular level without inducing damage either at molecular of phenotypic level.

## Materials and Methods

### TM cell culture

Primary human TM cell line [HTM, ScienCell, San Diego, California: cat. n. 6590, see http://www.sciencellonline.com for details] were cultured in fibroblast medium (FM, ScienCell), 2% fetal bovine serum (FBS, ScienCell), fibroblast growth supplement (FGS, 1%, ScienCell) and penicillin/streptomycin solution (P/S, 1%, ScienCell) using poly-L-lysine-coated flasks having a 6 mm diameter. Cell were growth to semi confluence accounting for approximately $1 \times 10^5$ cell per well. When reaching semi-confluence cells underwent SLT treatment.

### Selective laser trabeculoplasty treatment

TM cells underwent SLT under similar conditions usually adopted for human subjects using a SLT laser system (Laserex Tango Ellex Medical Pty Ltd – Australia). Specific treatment conditions were Q-swithched frequency doubled with Nd:YAG laser at 532 nm.

Wavelength, energy settings at 0.5 mJ single pulse, pulse duration 3 nsec, and treatment spot size of 400 micron.

After treatment cells were immediately restored in incubator and then collected by scraping after 30 min (T0.5), 2 hours (T2), and 6 hours (T6). Control cells stored in incubator in absence of SLT treatment were used as reference samples.

Scanning electron microscopic examination (Siemens Elmiskop 101; Siemens AG, Berlin, Germany) were performed on 2 Trabecular meshwork samples after SLT at $4^{th}$ and $6^{th}$ hour from treatment (Figure 1). Immediately after laser light exposition, all samples were immersed in cold antioxidant chondroitin sulfate/dextran storage medium (Optisol, Chiron Vision, Irvine, California), coded blindly, and frozen at $-80°C$. Trabecular meshwork samples were collected from two corneal donors in collaboration with the Melvin Jones Eye Bank of Genoa, Italy.

### Gene expression analysis by cDNA microarray

The expression of 18,401 human genes was tested in SLT-treated cells by cDNA microarray. Custom microarray as made available from the Microarray Department-University of Amsterdam, were used. The whole list of spotted genes is available at the website http://www.micro-array.nl/libraries.html. Because of the poor amount of available cell extracted RNA underwent reverse transcription and pre-plateau amplification as previously reported [65].

All data is MIAME compliant and that the raw data has been deposited in a MIAME compliant database (e.g., ArrayExpress, GEO), as detailed on the MGED Society website http://www.mged.org/Workgroups/MIAME/miame.html

Purified RNA underwent reverse transcription and amplification using quantitative real-time PCR (qPCR) prior to probe synthesis for array hybridization. A particular retrotranscription protocol (SuperSMART, Clontech, Palo Alto, CA, USA) aimed at the introduction of a target sequence at 3′ and 5′ of the cDNA library was applied as follows: RNA was incubated with a mix of a target sequence-oligo(dT)-linked primer and a target sequence-oligo(dG)-linked at 72°C for 5 minutes then a master-mix solution was added containing reverse transcriptase and dNTPs mix. Samples were then incubated at 42°C for 90 minutes. Reaction was terminated by adding ethylenediamine-tetraacetic acid, mixture diluted in phosphate buffer and synthesized cDNA purified by column chromatography using a commercially available purification kit (QIAquick PCR purification kit, Qiagen, Chatsworth, CA, USA). A PCR mix, including the specific primer for the target sequences and the fluorescent tracers SYBR GREEN, was added to the purified cDNA. The PCR reaction was performed at 95°C ×1 minute, 50 amplification cycles at 95°C ×15 s, 65°C ×30 s and 68°C ×3 minutes. The amplification curve was observed in real time by recording fluorescence and the pre-plateau amplification cycle was identified for each sample. A second set of sample was amplified to the identified pre-plateau cycle using the same conditions without the fluorescent tracer. This procedure was applied to all samples in order to standardize the amplification process thus allowing reliable comparisons of microarray data among different samples. PCR reactions were performed in a thermocycler equipped with microvial rotating support (Rotorgene, Corbett Research, Mortlake, Australia).

2 ug of amplified cDNA, as purified by column chromatography, were converted in aminomodified probes performing a three cycle PCR using a PCR mix containing N-18 random primers, aminomodified dNTPs and Taq polymerase. The reaction was performed at 95°C ×5minutes, 94°C ×1 minute, 25°C ×90 s, 50°C ×10 minutes and 68°C ×5 minutes. Synthesized amino-modified oligo-nucleotides were purified by column chromatography and alcohol precipitation then labelled with fluorescent tracers Cy3 or Cy5 by incubation at room temperature in the dark for 90 minutes. Fluorescent oligonucleotides were precipitated by cold ethanol and sodium acetate, and then purified by column chromatography. The efficacy of the procedure was checked by spectrophotometric analysis measuring abosorbance at 550 (Cy3) and 650 (Cy5). Standardized amounts of labelled probes were hybridized on glass cDNA microarrays.

Probes were lyophilized, diluted in 4 ul of EDTA 10 mM and incubated at 95°C for 10 min. Hybridization solution (18 ul) was added and labelled probe mixed together to a final volume of 44 ul. Mixture was then transferred onto microarrays which were then covered with a coverslip and hybridized overnight at 50°C in a Hybridization Cassette (Life Technologies, Carlsbad, CA, USA). After 16 hours the microarrays were washed twice in a low stringency wash buffer (2X SSC, 0.5% SDS) and twice in a high stringency wash buffer (0.5X SSC, 0,5% SDS). Microarray were dried in centrifuge and signal acquired in a laser scanner (ScanArray, PerkinElmer, Waltham, MA,USA).

Data analysis was performed subtracting for each microarray the local spot background from raw spot intensity, log transformation, normalization per chip and per array (GeneSpring® software version 7.2, Agilent Technologies, Santa Clara, CA). Each gene was spotted in quadruplicate on the used microarray. Accordingly, results represent the mean among 4 data. Data generated for each mRNA were compared among the various experimental groups by volcano-plot analysis taking into account as thresholds of two-fold variation and statistical significance $P < 0.05$ as evaluated by ANOVA after Bonferroni multiple testing correction. Global mRNA expression profiles were compared by hierarchical cluster analysis (HC) and bidimensional principal component analysis of variance (PCA).

Gene function was inferred from annotation reported in gene databank (Weizmann Institute, www.genecards.org) and Swissprotein database (http://expasy.org/sprot/).

"Biological function of genes whose expression was modulate by SLT was inferred from data available on Swissprot (http://expasy.org/sprot/) and Weizmann Institute (http://www.genecards.org/) databases. Predictor genes were identified by statistical support vector machine analysis, which is a supervised learning methods that predicts, for each given input, which of possible classes the input is a member of identifying the most relevant genes affecting this classification".

## Acknowledgments

We are indebted to the Melvin Jones Eye Bank, Genoa, Italy, for supplying cadaver eyes. We thank Drs. Roberta Bertagno and Patrizia Romano, University of Genoa, Italy, for performing the electron microscope analyses.

## Author Contributions

Conceived and designed the experiments: AI SCS. Performed the experiments: FR CC ML. Analyzed the data: AI. Contributed reagents/materials/analysis tools: CC ML FR. Wrote the paper: AI SCS.

## References

1. Gupta N, Greenberg G, de Tilly LN, Gray B, Polemidiotis M, et al. (2009) Atrophy of the lateral geniculate nucleus in human glaucoma detected by magnetic resonance imaging. Br J Ophthalmol 93: 56–60.

2. Singh K, Shrivastava A (2009) Intraocular pressure fluctuations: how much do they matter? Curr Opin Ophthalmol 20: 84–87.

3. Alvarado J, Murphy C, Polansky J, Juster R (1984a) Studies on pathogenesis of primary open angle glaucoma: regional analyses of trabecular meshwork cellularity and dense collagen. In: Ticho U, David R, eds. Recent Advances in Glaucoma. Elsevier: Amsterdam. pp 3–8.

4. Alvarado JA, Murphy C, Juster R (1984b) Trabecular meshwork cellularity in primary open-angle glaucoma and nonglaucomatous normals. Ophthalmology 91: 564–579.

5. Alvarado JA, Alvarado RG, Yeh RF, Franse-Carman L, Marcellino GR, et al. (2005) A new insight into the cellular regulation of aqueous outflow: how trabecular meshwork endothelial cells drive a mechanism that regulates the permeability of Schlemm's canal endothelial cells. Br J Ophthalmol 89: 1500–1505.

6. Alvarado JA, Katz LJ, Trivedi S, Shifera AS (2010) Monocyte modulation of aqueous outflow and recruitment to the trabecular meshwork following selective laser trabeculoplasty. Arch Ophthalmol 128: 731–737.

7. Shifera AS, Trivedi S, Chau P, Bonnemaison LH, Iguchi R, et al. (2010) Constitutive secretion of chemokines by cultured human trabecular meshwork cells. Exp Eye Res 91: 42–47.

8. Sacca S, Rolando M, Traverso CE, Mochi B, Ciurlo G, et al. (1991b) An Alternative Laser treatment for open angle glaucoma associated with exfoliation syndrome. IGS Program, Jerusalem, Israel, August 18-22. 27 p.

9. Saccà SC, Rolando M, Mochi B, Murialdo U, Ciurlo G, et al. (1991) La trabeculoplastica ed il massaggio trabecolare: due tecniche parachirurgiche a confronto. Boll Ocul 70(suppl.5): 323–329.

10. Latina MA, Sibayan SA, Shin DH, Noecker RJ, Marcellino G (1998) Q-switched 532-nm Nd:YAG laser trabeculoplasty (selective laser trabeculoplasty): a multicenter, pilot, clinical study. Ophthalmology 105: 2082–2088.

11. Lanzetta P, Menchini U, Virgili G (1999) Immediate intraocular pressure response to selective laser trabeculoplasty. Br J Ophthalmol 83: 29–32.

12. Damji KF, Bovell AM, Hodge WG, Rock W, Shah K, et al. (2006) Selective laser trabeculoplasty versus argon laser trabeculoplasty: results from a 1-year randomised clinical trial. Br J Ophthalmol 90: 1490–1494.

13. Wood JP, Plunkett M, Previn V, Chidlow G, Casson RJ (2010) Rapid and delayed death of cultured trabecular meshwork cells after selective laser trabeculoplasty. Lasers Surg Med 42: 326–337.

14. Bylsma SS, Samples JR, Acott TS, Van Buskirk EM (1988) Trabecular cell division after argon laser trabeculoplasty. Arch Ophthalmol 106: 544–547.

15. Dueker DK, Norberg M, Johnson DH, Tschumper RC, Feeney-Burns L (1990) Stimulation of cell division by argon and Nd:YAG laser trabeculoplasty in cynomolgus monkeys. Invest Ophthalmol Vis Sci 31: 115–124.

16. Parshley DE, Bradley JM, Samples JR, Van Buskirk EM, Acott TS (1995) Early changes in MMPs and inhibitors after in vitro laser treatment to the trabecular meshwork. Curr Eye Res 14: 537–544.

17. Parshley DE, Bradley JM, Fish A, Hadaegh A, Samples JR, et al. (1996) Laser trabeculoplasty induces stromelysin expression by trabecular juxtacanalicular cells. Invest Ophthalmol Vis Sci 37: 795–804.

18. Wise JB, Witter SL (1979) Argon laser therapy for open angle glaucoma: a pilot study. Arch Ophthalmol 97: 319–322.

19. Guzey M, Vural H, Satici A, Karadede S, Dogan Z (2001) Increase of free oxygen radicals in aqueous humour induced by selective Nd:YAG laser trabeculoplasty in the rabbit. Eur J Ophthalmol 11: 47–52.

20. Cvenkel B (2004) One-year follow-up of selective laser trabeculoplasty in open-angle glaucoma. Ophthalmologica 218: 20–5.

21. Epstein DL, Roberts BC, Skinner LL (1997) Nonsulfhydryl-reactive phenoxyacetic acids increase aqueous humor outflow facility. Invest Ophthalmol Vis Sci 38: 1526–34.

22. Lutjen-Drecoll E (2005) Morphological changes in glaucomatous eyes and the role of TGFbeta2 for the pathogenesis of the disease. Exp Eye Res 81: 1–4.

23. Wiederholt M, Thieme H, Stumpff F (2000) The regulation of trabecular meshwork and ciliary muscle contractility. Progress in Retinal and Eye Research 19: 271–295.

24. Wiederholt M (1998) : Direct involvement of trabecular meshwork in the regulation of aqueous humor outflow. Current Opinion in Ophthalmology 9: 46–49.

25. De Kater AW, Spurr-Michaud SJ, Gipson IK (1990) Localization of smooth muscle myosin-containing cells in the aqueous outflow pathway. Invest Ophthalmol Vis Sci 31: 347–353.

26. Read AT, Chan DW, Ethier CR (2007) Actin structure in the outflow tract of normal and glaucomatous eyes. Exp Eye Res 84: 214–26.

27. Saccà SC, Izzotti A (2008) Oxidative stress and glaucoma: injury in the anterior segment of the eye. Prog Brain Res 173: 385–407.

28. Acott TS, Kelley MJ (2008) Extracellular matrix in the trabecular meshwork. Exp Eye Res 86: 543–61.

29. Izzotti A, Cartiglia C, Tanningher M, De Flora S, Balansky R (1999) Age-related increases of 8-hydroxy-2′-deoxyguanosine and DNA protein cross-link in mouse organs. Mutat Res (Genetic. Toxicol. Env. Mut.) 446: 215–223.

30. He Y, Ge J, Tombran-Tink J (2008) Mitochondrial defects and dysfunction in calcium regulation in glaucomatous trabecular meshwork cells. Invest Ophthalmol Vis Sci 49: 4912–4922.

31. Izzotti A, Bagnis A, Saccà SC (2006) The role of oxidative stress in glaucoma. Mutat Res 612: 105–114.

32. Izzotti A, Saccà SC, Cartiglia C, De Flora S (2003) Oxidative deoxyribonucleic acid damage in the eyes of glaucoma patients. Am J Med 114: 638–646.

33. Izzotti A, Saccà SC, Longobardi M, Cartiglia C (2009) Sensitivity of ocular anterior chamber tissues to oxidative damage and its relevance to the pathogenesis of glaucoma. Invest Ophthalmol Vis Sci 50: 5251–5258.

34. Luna C, Li G, Qiu J, Epstein DL, Gonzalez P (2009) Role of miR-29b on the regulation of the extracellular matrix in human trabecular meshwork cells under chronic oxidative stress. Mol Vis 15: 2488–2497.

35. Izzotti A, Cartiglia C, Longobardi M, Balansky RM, D'Agostini F, et al. (2004) Alterations of gene expression in skin and lung of mice exposed to light and cigarette smoke. FASEB J 18: 1559–1561.

36. Alvarado JA, Yeh RF, Franse-Carman L, Marcellino G, Brownstein MJ (2005) Interactions between endothelia of the trabecular meshwork and of Schlemm's canal: a new insight into the regulation of aqueous outflow in the eye. Trans Am Ophthalmol Soc 103: 148–162.

37. Okuno T, Oku H, Sugiyama T, Ikeda T (2006) Glutamate level in optic nerve head is increased by artificial elevation of intraocular pressure in rabbits. Exp Eye Res 82: 465–70.

38. Zhang S, Wang H, Lu Q, Qing G, Wang N, et al. (2009) Detection of early neuron degeneration and accompanying glial responses in the visual pathway in a rat model of acute intraocular hypertension. Brain Res 1303: 131–143.

39. Steely HT, Jr., English-Wright SL, Clark AF (2000) The similarity of protein expression in trabecular meshwork and lamina cribrosa: implications for glaucoma. Exp Eye Res 70: 17–30.

40. Cvekl A, Tamm ER (2004) Anterior eye development and ocular mesenchyme: new insights from mouse models and human diseases. Bioassays 26: 374–386.

41. Borras T (2003) Gene expression in the trabecular meshwork and the influence of intraocular pressure. Prog Retin Eye Res 22: 435–463.

42. Kirwan RP, Fenerty CH, Crean J, Wordinger RJ, Clark AF, et al. (2005) Influence of cyclical mechanical strain on extracellular matrix gene expression in human lamina cribrosa cells in vitro. Mol Vis 11: 798–810.

43. Wordinger RJ, Fleenor DL, Hellberg PE, Pang IH, Tovar TO, et al. (2007) Effects of TGF-beta2, BMP-4, and gremlin in the trabecular meshwork: implications for glaucoma. Invest Ophthalmol Vis Sci 48: 1191–1200.

44. Wordinger RJ, Agarwal R, Talati M, Fuller J, Lambert W, et al. (2002) Expression of bone morphogenetic proteins (BMP), BMP receptors, and BMP associated proteins in human trabecular meshwork and optic nerve head cells and tissues. Mol Vis 8: 241–250.

45. Vittal V, Rose A, Gregory KE, Kelley MJ, Acott TS (2005) Changes in gene expression by trabecular meshwork cells in response to mechanical stretching. Invest Ophthalmol Vis Sci 46: 2857–2868.

46. Keller KE, Kelley MJ, Acott TS (2007) Extracellular matrix gene alternative splicing by trabecular meshwork cells in response to mechanical stretching. Invest Ophthalmol Vis Sci 48: 1164–1172.

47. Luna C, Li G, Liton PB, Epstein DL, Gonzalez P (2009) Alterations in gene expression induced by cyclic mechanical stress in trabecular meshwork cells. Mol Vis 15: 534–544.

48. Kaufman PL (2008) Enhancing trabecular outflow by disrupting the actin cytoskeleton, increasing uveoscleral outflow with prostaglandins, and understanding the pathophysiology of presbyopia interrogating Mother Nature: asking why, asking how, recognizing the signs, following the trail. Exp Eye Res 86: 3–17.

49. Li G, Luna C, Liton PB, Navarro I, Epstein DL, et al. (2007) Sustained stress response after oxidative stress in trabecular meshwork cells. Mol Vis 13: 2282–2288.

50. Izzotti A, Sacca SC, Longobardi M, Cartiglia C (2010) Mitochondria loss and damage in the trabecular meshwork of primary open angle glaucomatous patients. Arch Ophth 128: 724–730.

51. Kroemer G, Reed JC (2000) Mitochondrial control of cell death. Nat Med 6: 513–519.
52. Zode GS, Clark AF, Wordinger RJ (2007) Activation of the BMP canonical signaling pathway in human optic nerve head tissue and isolated optic nerve head astrocytes and lamina cribrosa cells. Invest Ophthalmol Vis Sci 48: 5058–5067.
53. Kompass KS, Agapova OA, Li W, Kaufman PL, Rasmussen CA, et al. (2008) Bioinformatic and statistical analysis of the optic nerve head in a primate model of ocular hypertension. BMC Neurosci 9: 93–114.
54. Balaratnasingam C, Morgan WH, Bass L, Ye L, McKnight C, et al. (2008) Elevated pressure induced astrocyte damage in the optic nerve. Brain Res 1244: 142–154.
55. Gaasterland D, Tanishima T, Kuwabara T (1978) Axoplasmic flow during chronic experimental glaucoma. 1. Light and electron microscopic studies of the monkey optic nervehead during development of glaucomatous cupping. Invest Ophthalmol Vis Sci 17: 838–846.
56. Balaratnasingam C, Morgan WH, Bass L, Matich G, Cringle SJ, et al. (2007) Axonal transport and cytoskeletal changes in the laminar regions after elevated intraocular pressure. Invest Ophthalmol Vis Sci 48: 3632–3644.
57. Smith PJ, Samuelson DA, Brooks DE, Whitley RD (1986) Unconventional aqueous humor outflow of microspheres perfused into the equine eye. Am J Vet Res 47: 2445–53.
58. Hof PR, Lee PY, Yeung G, Wang RF, Podos SM, et al. (1998) Glutamate receptor subunit GluR2 and NMDAR1 immunoreactivity in the retina of macaque monkeys with experimental glaucoma does not identify vulnerable neurons. Exp Neurol 153: 234–241.
59. Coca-Prados M, Escribano J (2007) New perspectives in aqueous humor secretion and in glaucoma: the ciliary body as a multifunctional neuroendocrine gland. Prog Retin Eye Res 26: 239–262.
60. Roedl JB, Bleich S, Reulbach U, von Ahsen N, Schlötzer-Schrehardt U, et al. (2007) Homocysteine levels in aqueous humor and plasma of patients with primary open-angle glaucoma. J Neural Transm 114: 445–450.
61. Goyal S, Beltran-Agullo L, Rashid S, Shah SP, Nath R, et al. (2010) Effect of primary selective laser trabeculoplasty on tonographic outflow facility: a randomised clinical trial. Br J Ophthalmol 94: 1443–1447.
62. Sacca SC, Bolognesi C, Battistella A, Bagnis A, Izzotti A (2009) Gene-environment interactions in ocular diseases. Mutat Res 667: 698–117.
63. Osborne NN (2010) Mitochondria: Their role in ganglion cell death and survival in primary open angle glaucoma. Exp Eye Res 90: 750–757.
64. Izzotti A, Longobardi M, Cartiglia C, Saccà SC (2010) Proteome alterations in primary open angle glaucoma aqueous humor. J Proteome Res 9: 4831–8483.
65. Izzotti A, Pulliero A, Orcesi S, Cartiglia C, Longobardi M, et al. (2009) Interferon-related transcriptome alterations in the cerebro spinal fluid cells of Aicardi-Goutières patients. Brain Pathology 19: 650–660.

# 7

# The Heritability of Glaucoma-Related Traits Corneal Hysteresis, Central Corneal Thickness, Intraocular Pressure, and Choroidal Blood Flow Pulsatility

Ellen E. Freeman[1,2*,9], Marie-Hélène Roy-Gagnon[3,4,9], Denise Descovich[1], Hugues Massé[3], Mark R. Lesk[1,2]

1 Maisonneuve-Rosemont Hospital Research Center, Montreal, Quebec, Canada, 2 Department of Ophthalmology, University of Montreal, Montreal, Quebec, Canada, 3 CHU Sainte-Justine Research Center, University of Montreal, Montreal, Quebec, Canada, 4 Department of Social and Preventive Medicine, University of Montreal, Montreal, Quebec, Canada

## Abstract

**Purpose:** The purpose of this work was to investigate the heritability of potential glaucoma endophenotypes. We estimated for the first time the heritability of the pulsatility of choroidal blood flow. We also sought to confirm the heritability of corneal hysteresis, central corneal thickness, and 3 ways of measuring intraocular pressure.

**Methods:** Measurements were performed on 96 first-degree relatives recruited from Maisonneuve-Rosemont Hospital in Montreal. Corneal hysteresis was determined using the Reichert Ocular Response Analyser. Central corneal thickness was measured with an ultrasound pachymeter. Three measures of intraocular pressure were obtained: Goldmann-correlated and corneal compensated intraocular pressure using the Ocular Response Analyser, and Pascal intraocular pressure using the Pascal Dynamic Contour Tonometer. The pulsatility of choroidal blood velocity and flow were measured in the sub-foveolar choroid using single-point laser Doppler flowmetry (Oculix). We estimated heritability using maximum-likelihood variance components methods implemented in the SOLAR software.

**Results:** No significant heritability was detected for the pulsatility of choroidal blood flow or velocity. The Goldman-correlated, corneal compensated, and Pascal measures of intraocular pressure measures were all significantly heritable at 0.94, 0.79, and 0.53 after age and sex adjustment (p = 0.0003, p = 0.0023, p = 0.0239). Central corneal thickness was significantly heritable at 0.68 (p = 0.0078). Corneal hysteresis was highly heritable but the estimate was at the upper boundary of 1.00 preventing us from giving a precise estimate.

**Conclusion:** Corneal hysteresis, central corneal thickness, and intraocular pressure are all heritable and may be suitable as glaucoma endophenotypes. The pulsatility of choroidal blood flow and blood velocity were not significantly heritable in this sample.

**Editor:** Dana C. Crawford, Vanderbilt University, United States of America

**Funding:** This project was funded through a grant from the Canadian Glaucoma Clinical Research Council and the Canadian National Institute for the Blind, and also by the Fonds de Recherche en Ophtalmologie de l'Universite de Montreal. The funders had no role in study design, data collection and analysis, decision to publish, or preparation of the manuscript.

**Competing Interests:** The authors have declared that no competing interests exist.

* E-mail: eefreeman@gmail.com

9 These authors contributed equally to this work.

## Introduction

Most cases of open-angle glaucoma (including normal tension glaucoma) are probably multifactorial, involving multiple contributing genetic and environmental factors. Intermediate phenotypes, also called endophenotypes, are powerful tools in the search for genes contributing to multifactorial human diseases as they are likely to be more directly influenced by the genes than the resulting disease phenotype and they provide greater statistical power [1-4]. Phenotypes such as intraocular pressure and central corneal thickness may be suitable as endophenotypes in glaucoma since they are well-established risk factors for glaucoma [5,6]. In addition, ocular elasticity may play a major role in the susceptibility of the optic nerve to glaucoma [7]. As the cornea and the sclera together form the external wall of the eye and are formed of a continuous tissue of extracellular tissue[8], the mechanical properties of the cornea might be a good marker for those of the entire wall of the eye. Therefore, corneal hysteresis, or the biomechanical response of the cornea to a brief air impulse, may be another promising phenotype. Corneal hysteresis is, in fact, a risk factor for visual field damage [6,9] and the presence of glaucoma [10]. The pulsatility of choroidal blood flow, i.e. how choroidal blood flow changes with the pulse rate, is also a potential endophenotype for glaucoma given its relationship with glaucoma [11,12]. Only phenotypes that are heritable are useful endophenotypes in the search for genes contributing to a complex disease.

Genetic research of glaucoma-related traits has mainly focused on intraocular pressure and central corneal thickness, which have been found to be heritable in multiple studies [13–21]. No prior studies have assessed the heritability of the pulsatility of choroidal blood flow. One twin study has examined corneal hysteresis and found it to be heritable [22]. Twin studies are very valuable study designs but replication of heritability estimates using other study designs is warranted. Indeed, heritability estimation from twin studies involves assumptions that are difficult to verify and may not be representative of the general population [23]. Hence, additional research on the heritability of glaucoma-related phenotypes is needed. Therefore, our goal was to assess the heritability of several glaucoma-related traits including the pulsatility of choroidal blood flow for the first time in order to propel the search for genes likely to contribute to the susceptibility of the optic nerve to glaucoma.

## Materials and Methods

### Study Population

Participants were recruited from the ophthalmology clinics of Maisonneuve-Rosemont Hospital in Montreal, Quebec. A sample of 47 Caucasian people without glaucoma was recruited between July 2008 and November 2009 from a community-based screening program or from advertising flyers displayed at community events. Each person in the sample recruited at least one first-degree relative without glaucoma to also participate in the study giving 96 people overall (47 families including 29 parent-offspring pairs and 21 sibling pairs). The absence of glaucoma was determined by normal optic nerve appearance, normal optic nerve head morphology using Heidelberg Retina Tomography (HRT-2) imaging, normal automated visual field using frequency doubling technology (FDT 24-2), normal intraocular pressure (<21mmHg using Goldman tonometry), and normal gonioscopy. People who had undergone prior ocular surgery were excluded. Other exclusion criteria included the presence of ocular disease, cloudy ocular media, or inability to cooperate for the exams. Written informed consent was obtained from all participants. The research conformed to the tenets of the Declaration of Helsinki. The study was approved by the Ethics Committee at Maisonneuve-Rosemont Hospital.

### Data Collection

Participants underwent an hour long examination by a single observer (DD) to collect the data. In order to minimize the influence of diurnal variation, almost all participants were examined between 9am and noon. The Pascal Dynamic Contour Tonometer (DCT) was used to give a measure of intraocular pressure (IOP) that is independent of corneal thickness (SMT Swiss Microtechnology AG, Port, Switzerland). This device is used at the slit lamp but contains a pressure transducer that is placed into contact with the cornea and a wireless digital recording device. The Pascal DCT gave a measure of IOP (IOPp) measured in mmHg. The Ocular Response Analyzer (ORA) (Reichert Ophthalmic Instruments, Depew, NY), a device used to direct a burst of air at the cornea, was used to derive two applanation pressure measurements, one during the depression of the cornea and another during the recovery [24]. The average of these two measures gives the Goldmann-correlated IOP (IOPg) while the difference between these two measures gives corneal hysteresis. The corneal hysteresis measure allows the calculation of a corneal compensated IOP (IOPcc), which is less affected by properties of the cornea than other measures of tonometry. The pulsatility of choroidal blood flow was measured in the sub-foveolar choroid using single point laser Doppler flowmetry (Oculix) [25]. Central corneal thickness was measured with an ultrasound pachymeter (Reichert Ophthalmic Instruments, Depew, NY) taking the mean

of 50 consecutive measurements made during a single contact. Visual and ophthalmic exams were performed to confirm the absence of glaucoma or other ocular diseases and medical histories were reviewed for evidence of previous ocular surgery.

### Statistical Analysis

Data were used from one eye from each patient. The eye with the better visual acuity was used. If both eyes had the same visual acuity, the right eye was used. We performed heritability analyses using maximum likelihood variance components methods as implemented in the program SOLAR 26]. This approach can estimate heritability from families of arbitrary size and takes into account all relationships simultaneously by modeling the covariance among family members in terms of genetic proximity or kinship. Specifically, for a particular phenotype $y$, the value of $y$ for individual $i$ is modeled as $y_i = \mu + \sum \beta_j X_{ij} + g_i + e_i$, where $\mu$ is the mean of $y$, $X_{ij}$ is the $j$-th covariate with associated regression coefficient $\beta_j$; $g_i$ is an additive genetic effect normally distributed with mean 0 and variance $\sigma_g^2$, and $e_i$ is a random residual effect normally distributed with mean 0 and variance $\sigma_e^2$. Any non-additive genetic (such as dominance) and unmeasured non-genetic effects (as well as random errors) are incorporated into $e_i$. The narrow-sense heritability of the phenotype is estimated by the ratio of the variance attributable to additive genetic effects, $\sigma_g^2$, to the total phenotypic variance. We used likelihood-ratio tests to assess the significance of a parameter of interest by comparing the log-likelihood of the model in which the parameter is estimated to that of the model in which the parameter is fixed at zero 27]. We adjusted heritability estimates for age and sex. We also calculated heritability estimates from twice the regression coefficient of the offspring's trait value on the parent's trait value using the ROMPrev program 28] and from twice the sibling correlation coefficient 23]. Before performing the quantitative genetic analyses described above, we assessed the distributions of all traits and transformed them to approximate univariate normality when necessary. Only the pulsatility of choroidal blood flow was log-transformed. We assessed the impact of outliers on the estimates of heritability by examining the change in the estimates when extreme values were excluded. A p-value <0.05 was considered statistically significant. All analyses (except where noted above) were conducted using version 9.2 of the Statistical Analysis System programming language (SAS Institute, Cary, North Carolina, USA).

## Results

Out of the 47 families, there were 29 parent-offspring pairs and 21 sibling pairs. Forty-five families included only one pair (parent-offspring or sibling), one family included one parent and 2 children, and one family included a parent-offspring pair and the sibling of the parent. The mean age of the sample was 53 years old (SD = 15) and the sample was 60% female. Among parent-offspring pairs, the mean ages of the parents and offspring were 65 years old (SD = 11) and 39 years old (SD = 9), respectively. Parents were 76% female while offspring were 45% female. Among sibling pairs, the mean ages of the oldest and youngest sibling in the pair were 55 years old (SD = 13) and 51 years old (SD = 12), respectively. Older siblings were 67% female while younger siblings were 52% female. The mean values for the 7 glaucoma-related endophenotypes can be found in Table 1.

In variance components models, we found high heritability estimates for central corneal thickness, corneal hysteresis, and the 3 measures of intraocular pressure (Table 2). The heritability for central corneal thickness was 0.68 (SE = 0.26). For corneal

**Table 1.** Description of 7 glaucoma-related traits.

| Device | Glaucoma-Related Traits | Mean (SD) |
|---|---|---|
| Ultrasound Pachymeter | Central Corneal Thickness (μM) | 546.9 ± 34.9 |
| Reichart Ocular Response Analyzer | IOPcc (mmHg) | 16.6 ± 2.7 |
| | IOPg (mmHg) | 16.1 ± 3.5 |
| | Corneal Hysteresis (mmHg) | 10.4 ± 1.5 |
| Pascal DCT | IOPp (mmHg) | 16.8 ± 2.7 |
| Oculix | Pulsatility of Blood Velocity (kH2) | 0.35 ± 0.09 |
| | Pulsatility of Blood Flow (H2U) | 0.34 ± 0.10 |

IOPcc = corneal compensated intraocular pressure, IOPg = Goldmann-correlated intraocular pressure, IOPp = Pascal intraocular pressure.

hysteresis, the likelihood was maximized at the upper boundary constraint of 1.0 for the heritability estimate, indicating high heritability but not allowing precise estimation for this trait. Heritability estimates derived separately from parent-offspring regression and sibling correlations also reached the upper boundary of 1.0. Heritability estimates for the three measures of intraocular pressure were 0.94 (SE = 0.22) for IOPg, 0.79 (SE = 0.24) for IOPcc, and 0.53 (SE = 0.26) for IOPp.

We did not find that the pulsatility of choroidal blood flow measures were heritable as the velocity and flow heritability estimates were not significant and were less than 0.20 (Table 2).

Age and sex adjustment only slightly altered the heritability estimates (Table 2). In fact, age and sex did not explain a significant proportion of variance in the endophenotypes, except that corneal hysteresis was negatively associated with age (P = 0.001).

## Discussion

To our knowledge, no prior studies have examined the heritability of the pulsatility of choroidal blood flow. We did not find that the pulsatility of choroidal blood flow was heritable in our sample. Perhaps it is primarily determined by environmental factors. We do not think that poor reproducibility is the reason for the lack of heritability in our sample because we found in prior

research of 35 people that the pulsatility of choroidal blood velocity and flow were reproducible (intraclass correlation coefficient = 0.79 and 0.80, respectively) (Unpublished data).

Our results are consistent with previous studies indicating that several other glaucoma-related traits are heritable. Out of the 3 IOP measures, we found that IOPg had the highest heritability ($h^2 = 0.95$, SE = 0.22) compared to IOPcc ($h^2 = 0.79$, SE = 0.24) or IOPp ($h^2 = 0.55$, SE = 0.26). However, all three measures were strongly heritable. IOPg is affected by central corneal thickness, which itself is known to be heritable [6,16,18,20], while IOPcc and IOPp are independent of central corneal thickness. Furthermore, IOPg and IOPcc were measured using the ORA, which is a non-contact tonometer, while IOPp was measured using the DCT, which is a contact tonometer. Perhaps IOP measurements from a contact tonometer are influenced by other corneal factors that are not heritable thereby resulting in a lower heritability than the non-contact tonometers.

Our data support a high heritability for corneal hysteresis as shown by the estimate reaching the boundary of 1.0. An estimate of heritability at the boundary is not precise as no standard error can be obtained. However, although we are not able to precisely determine the estimate of heritability for corneal hysteresis, we can conclude that the heritability is high, which agrees with the findings of Carbonaro et al in their study of 264 twin pairs

**Table 2.** Heritability of 7 glaucoma-related traits.

| Device | Glaucoma-Related Traits | Unadjusted $h^2$ (SE) | P-value | Adjusted* $h^2$ (SE) | P-value |
|---|---|---|---|---|---|
| Ultrasound Pachymeter | Central Corneal Thickness | 0.65 (0.26) | 0.0097 | 0.68 (0.26) | 0.0078 |
| ORA | IOPcc | 0.79 (0.24) | 0.0021 | 0.79 (0.24) | 0.0023 |
| | IOPg | 0.95 (0.22) | 0.0002 | 0.94 (0.22) | 0.0003 |
| | Corneal Hysteresis | NA† | | NA† | |
| Pascal | IOPp | 0.55 (0.26) | 0.0187 | 0.53 (0.26) | 0.0239 |
| Oculix | Pulsatility of Blood Velocity | 0.02 (0.29) | 0.4666 | 0.10 (0.32) | 0.3813 |
| | Pulsatility of Blood Flow‡ | 0.20 (0.28) | 0.2409 | 0.16 (0.29) | 0.2922 |

*adjusted for age and sex.
† Estimate reached the upper boundary constraint of 1.
‡ Data were log-transformed to achieve normality.
ORA = Ocular Response Analyzer, IOPcc = corneal compensated intraocular pressure, IOPg = Goldmann-correlated intraocular pressure, IOPp = Pascal intraocular pressure.

($h^2 = 0.77$, 95% CI 0.70, 0.82) [22]. Further studies are needed to more precisely estimate the heritability of this trait in non-twin populations.

Our other results are consistent with prior literature in this research area. A study by Carbonaro *et al* also found that IOPg had the highest heritability compared to IOPp, IOPcc, and Goldmann applanation tonometry [13]. Prior studies of central corneal thickness also found it to be highly heritable [16,18,20]. For example, the Toh *et al* study, which examined 256 twin pairs, found a heritability of 0.95 [18]. Consistent with these heritability results, some genetic factors have been recently identified for central corneal thickness [29,30] and IOP [31].

Our study uses parent-offspring and sibling pairs to confirm the results of prior twin studies, which is important given the limitations of twin studies, including generalizability. It should be noted, however, that heritability estimates are population-specific due to possible differences in total, environmental, or genetic variance components of the trait. Hence, comparison between populations should be made carefully. Our study is also novel in its examination of the heritability of some new potential glaucoma endophenotypes. Indeed, no other researchers have presented the heritability of the pulsatility of choroidal blood flow or velocity and only one other study has examined corneal hysteresis [22].

A limitation of our study is that we used a convenience sample of people without glaucoma from the community. Therefore, our sample is not fully representative of the population. We also restricted our sample to Caucasian individuals since genetic factors and heritability may differ according to ethnicity and we did not have enough other ethnicities to study them separately. In addition, we excluded individuals with any previous ocular surgery, which may have also affected the representativeness of our sample but was necessary since ocular surgery may affect our outcomes. Also, our study had limited precision with standard errors of 0.2 to 0.3. Although we had adequate power (80%) to detect heritability estimates greater or equal to 0.60 as significantly different than zero, we were underpowered to detect a heritability of 0.20 as we saw for the pulsatility of choroidal blood flow. However, low heritability estimates indicate that the trait may not be a good endophenotype for genetic studies. Given the large environmental component of the trait variance, it would be difficult to find genes explaining variation in this trait. More studies of the pulsatility of choroidal blood flow and velocity are needed to determine their utility as glaucoma endophenotypes.

Our study provides further support that corneal hysteresis, intraocular pressure, and central corneal thickness are heritable and may be suitable endophenotypes in the search for genes for open-angle glaucoma. Conversely, the pulsatility of choroidal blood velocity and flow were not heritable in this sample and may therefore be more influenced by environmental factors.

## Author Contributions

Conceived and designed the experiments: EEF MHRG MRL. Performed the experiments: DD. Analyzed the data: MHRG HM. Contributed reagents/materials/analysis tools: ML. Wrote the paper: EEF MHRG ML.

## References

1. Gottesman II, Gould TD (2003) The endophenotype concept in psychiatry: etymology and strategic intentions. Am J Psychiatry 160: 636–645.
2. Goldman D, Ducci F (2007) Deconstruction of vulnerability to complex diseases: enhanced effect sizes and power of intermediate phenotypes. ScientificWorldJournal 7: 124–130.
3. Meyer-Lindenberg A, Weinberger DR (2006) Intermediate phenotypes and genetic mechanisms of psychiatric disorders. Nat Rev Neurosci 7: 818–827.
4. Wijsman EM, Amos CI (1997) Genetic analysis of simulated oligogenic traits in nuclear and extended pedigrees: summary of GAW10 contributions. Genet Epidemiol 14: 719–735.
5. Bahrami H (2006) Causal inference in primary open angle glaucoma: specific discussion on intraocular pressure. Ophthalmic Epidemiol 13: 283–289.
6. Congdon NG, Broman AT, Bandeen-Roche K, Grover D, Quigley HA (2006) Central corneal thickness and corneal hysteresis associated with glaucoma damage. Am J Ophthalmol 141: 868–875.
7. Sigal IA, Flanagan JG, Ethier CR (2005) Factors influencing optic nerve head biomechanics. Invest Ophthalmol Vis Sci 46: 4189–4199.
8. McBrien NA, Gentle A (2003) Role of the sclera in the development and pathological complications of myopia. Prog Retin Eye Res 22: 307–338.
9. De Moraes CV, Hill V, Tello C, Liebmann JM, Ritch R (2012) Lower corneal hysteresis is associated with more rapid glaucomatous visual field progression. J Glaucoma 21: 209–213.
10. Mangouritsas G, Morphis G, Mourtzoukos S, Feretis E (2009) Association between corneal hysteresis and central corneal thickness in glaucomatous and non-glaucomatous eyes. Acta Ophthalmol 87: 901–905.
11. Kochkorov A, Gugleta K, Katamay R, Flammer J, Orgul S (2010) Short-term variability of systemic blood pressure and submacular choroidal blood flow in eyes of patients with primary open-angle glaucoma. Graefes Arch Clin Exp Ophthalmol 248: 833–837.
12. Fuchsjager-Mayrl G, Wally B, Georgopoulos M, Rainer G, Kircher K, et al. (2004) Ocular blood flow and systemic blood pressure in patients with primary open-angle glaucoma and ocular hypertension. Invest Ophthalmol Vis Sci 45: 834–839.
13. Carbonaro F, Andrew T, Mackey DA, Spector TD, Hammond CJ (2008) Heritability of intraocular pressure: a classical twin study. Br J Ophthalmol 92: 1125–1128.
14. Chang TC, Congdon NG, Wojciechowski R, Munoz B, Gilbert D, et al. (2005) Determinants and heritability of intraocular pressure and cup-to-disc ratio in a defined older population. Ophthalmology 112: 1186–1191.
15. Charlesworth J, Kramer PL, Dyer T, Diego V, Samples JR, et al. (2010) The path to open-angle glaucoma gene discovery: endophenotypic status of intraocular pressure, cup-to-disc ratio, and central corneal thickness. Invest Ophthalmol Vis Sci 51: 3509–3514.
16. Landers JA, Hewitt AW, Dimasi DP, Charlesworth JC, Straga T, et al. (2009) Heritability of central corneal thickness in nuclear families. Invest Ophthalmol Vis Sci 50: 4087–4090.
17. Parssinen O, Era P, Tolvanen A, Kaprio J, Koskenvuo M, et al. (2007) Heritability of intraocular pressure in older female twins. Ophthalmology 114: 2227–2231.
18. Toh T, Liew SH, MacKinnon JR, Hewitt AW, Poulsen JL, et al. (2005) Central corneal thickness is highly heritable: the twin eye studies. Invest Ophthalmol Vis Sci 46: 3718–3722.
19. van Koolwijk LM, Despriet DD, van Duijn CM, Pardo Cortes LM, Vingerling JR, et al. (2007) Genetic contributions to glaucoma: heritability of intraocular pressure, retinal nerve fiber layer thickness, and optic disc morphology. Invest Ophthalmol Vis Sci 48: 3669–3676.
20. Zheng Y, Ge J, Huang G, Zhang J, Liu B, et al. (2008) Heritability of central corneal thickness in Chinese: the Guangzhou Twin Eye Study. Invest Ophthalmol Vis Sci 49: 4303–4307.
21. Zheng Y, Xiang F, Huang W, Huang G, Yin Q, et al. (2009) Distribution and heritability of intraocular pressure in chinese children: the Guangzhou twin eye study. Invest Ophthalmol Vis Sci 50: 2040–2043.
22. Carbonaro F, Andrew T, Mackey DA, Spector TD, Hammond CJ (2008) The heritability of corneal hysteresis and ocular pulse amplitude: a twin study. Ophthalmology 115: 1545–1549.
23. Falconer D, Mackay T (1996) Introduction to quantitative genetics. London: Addison Wesley Longman Limited.
24. Luce DA (2005) Determining in vivo biomechanical properties of the cornea with an ocular response analyzer. J Cataract Refract Surg 31: 156–162.
25. Polska E, Polak K, Luksch A, Fuchsjager-Mayrl G, Petternel V, et al. (2004) Twelve hour reproducibility of choroidal blood flow parameters in healthy subjects. Br J Ophthalmol 88: 533–537.
26. Almasy L, Blangero J (1998) Multipoint quantitative-trait linkage analysis in general pedigrees. Am J Hum Genet 62: 1198–1211.
27. Self S, Liang K (1987) Asymptotic properties of maximum likelihood estimators and likelihood ratio tests under nonstandard conditions. J Am Statist Assoc 82: 605–610.
28. Roy-Gagnon MH, Mathias RA, Fallin MD, Jee SH, Broman KW, et al. (2008) An extension of the regression of offspring on mid-parent to test for association and estimate locus-specific heritability: the revised ROMP method. Ann Hum Genet 72: 115–125.

29. Lu Y, Dimasi DP, Hysi PG, Hewitt AW, Burdon KP, et al. (2010) Common genetic variants near the Brittle Cornea Syndrome locus ZNF469 influence the blinding disease risk factor central corneal thickness. PLoS Genet 6: e1000947.

30. Ulmer M, Li J, Yaspan BL, Ozel AB, Richards JE, et al. (2012) Genome-Wide Analysis of Central Corneal Thickness in Primary Open-Angle Glaucoma Cases in the NEIGHBOR and GLAUGEN Consortia. Invest Ophthalmol Vis Sci 53: 4468–4474.

31. van Koolwijk LM, Ramdas WD, Ikram MK, Jansonius NM, Pasutto F, et al. (2012) Common genetic determinants of intraocular pressure and primary open-angle glaucoma. PLoS Genet 8: e1002611.

# 8

# The p53 Codon 72 PRO/PRO Genotype may be Associated with Initial Central Visual Field Defects in Caucasians with Primary Open Angle Glaucoma

Janey L. Wiggs[1]*, Alex W. Hewitt[2], Bao Jian Fan[1], Dan Yi Wang[1], Dayse R. Figueiredo Sena[1], Colm O'Brien[3], Anthony Realini[4], Jamie E. Craig[5], David P. Dimasi[5], David A. Mackey[6], Jonathan L. Haines[7], Louis R. Pasquale[1]

1 Department of Ophthalmology, Harvard Medical School, Massachusetts Eye and Ear Infirmary, Boston, Massachusetts, United States of America, 2 Centre for Eye Research Australia, University of Melbourne, Royal Victorian Eye and Ear Hospital, Melbourne, Australia, 3 School of Medicine and Medical Science, University College of Dublin, Dublin, Ireland, 4 Department of Ophthalmology, West Virginia University School of Medicine, Morgantown, West Virginia, United States of America, 5 Department of Ophthalmology, Flinders University, Flinders Medical Centre, Adelaide, Australia, 6 Centre for Ophthalmology and Visual Science, University of Western Australia, Lions Eye Institute, Perth, Australia, 7 Center for Human Genetics Research, Vanderbilt University School of Medicine, Nashville, Tennessee, United States of America

## Abstract

**Background:** Loss of vision in glaucoma is due to apoptotic retinal ganglion cell loss. While *p53* modulates apoptosis, gene association studies between *p53* variants and glaucoma have been inconsistent. In this study we evaluate the association between a *p53* variant functionally known to influence apoptosis (codon 72 Pro/Arg) and the subset of primary open angle glaucoma (POAG) patients with early loss of central visual field.

**Methods:** Genotypes for the p53 codon 72 polymorphism (Pro/Arg) were obtained for 264 POAG patients and 400 controls from the U.S. and in replication studies for 308 POAG patients and 178 controls from Australia (GIST). The glaucoma patients were divided into two groups according to location of initial visual field defect (either paracentral or peripheral). All cases and controls were Caucasian with European ancestry.

**Results:** The p53-PRO/PRO genotype was more frequent in the U.S. POAG patients with early visual field defects in the paracentral regions compared with those in the peripheral regions or control group ($p = 2.7 \times 10^{-5}$). We replicated this finding in the GIST cohort ($p = 7.3 \times 10^{-3}$, and in the pooled sample ($p = 6.6 \times 10^{-7}$) and in a meta-analysis of both the US and GIST datasets ($1.3 \times 10^{-6}$, OR 2.17 (1.58–2.98 for the PRO allele).

**Conclusions:** These results suggest that the p53 codon 72 PRO/PRO genotype is potentially associated with early paracentral visual field defects in primary open-angle glaucoma patients.

**Editor:** Anneke I. den Hollander, Radboud University Nijmegen Medical Centre, The Netherlands

**Funding:** This study was supported by National Institutes of Health/National Eye Institute grants: R01EY015872 (Wiggs), R01EY015473 (Pasquale), P30EY014104 (Wiggs), Research to Prevent Blindness (Wiggs, Pasquale, Realini), the Harvard Glaucoma Center of Excellence (Wiggs, Pasquale), The Massachusetts Lions Eye Research Fund (Wiggs, Pasquale), National Health & Medical Research Council Project grant 229960, the Ophthalmic Research Institute of Australia, and Glaucoma Australia. The funders had no role in study design, data collection and analysis, decision to publish, or preparation of the manuscript.

**Competing Interests:** The authors have declared that no competing interests exist.

* E-mail: janey_wiggs@meei.harvard.edu

## Introduction

Adult-onset primary open-angle glaucoma (POAG) is characterized by an irreversible degeneration of the optic nerve that is a common cause of blindness worldwide. POAG is phenotypically and genetically complex and it is likely that multiple genetic and environmental factors play a role in its etiology. Elevated intraocular pressure (IOP) is a major risk factor for optic nerve disease in glaucoma; however, most ocular hypertensive patients do not develop optic nerve degeneration [1] and a number of studies show that POAG patients can develop optic nerve disease despite IOPs in the normal range [2]. Randomized clinical trials, including the Collaborative Normal-tension Glaucoma Study report that lowering IOP does not always result in prevention of progressive visual loss [3]. Collectively these results suggest that some glaucoma patients have a greater susceptibility to optic nerve disease than others. The inherent optic nerve susceptibility exhibited by glaucoma patients may be influenced by a specific set of genetic and/or environmental risk factors, which could be new therapeutic targets for this disease.

Visual field defects in glaucoma patients frequently develop in the periphery and gradually extend to the central region. In a subset of patients the initial functional defect appears in the central visual field as a paracentral scotoma, representing a loss of the maculopapillary nerve fiber layer bundles. Glaucoma patients presenting with early-stage paracentral scotomas are more likely to have systemic risk factors for glaucoma (hypotension, migraine,

Raynaud's phenomenon, and sleep apnea) [4] are more likely to become blind from glaucoma [5] and have lower intraocular pressures than patients with initial defects in the periphery [4,6]. Together, these observations suggest that formation of paracentral scotomas at early stages of the disease characterizes a subtype of glaucoma, or glaucoma endophenotype, likely to be dependent on a specific set of genetic and environmental risk factors.

Loss of retinal ganglion cells in glaucoma is dependent on the balance of cellular pro-survival and pro-death pathways. Proteins that participate in these pathways are excellent candidates for factors that could influence the susceptibility of retinal ganglion cells to glaucoma-related apoptosis. One of the most important apoptotic regulatory proteins is the tumor suppressor protein p53, which responds to diverse cellular stresses to regulate cell cycle arrest, apoptosis, senescence, and DNA repair [7]. TP53 (coding for p53) is expressed in retinal ganglion cells under conditions that would stimulate apoptosis [8–10] and in an experimental model of glaucoma [11]. Family-based linkage studies have provided evidence for a glaucoma locus on chromosome 17 p that includes TP53 [12,13].

TP53 has a common DNA sequence polymorphism that results in either proline (p53-PRO) or arginine (p53-ARG) at amino-acid position 72 (dbSNP: rs1042522) in the p53 protein. This polymorphism occurs in the p53 proline-rich PXXP domain, which is necessary for the protein to fully induce apoptosis [14]. The proline and arginine variants significantly affect the biological activity of p53, although these effects are highly dependent on the conditions of the study. p53-PRO has increased apoptotic activity in cancer cells in hypoxic conditions [15] and is associated with age-dependent senescence in cultured fibroblasts [16]. p53-ARG increases transcriptional activity of apoptotic related genes in human osteosarcoma cell lines and has higher apoptotic activity in most tumor cells [17]. The apoptotic activity of the codon 72 variants in retinal ganglion cells or other cell types involved in glaucoma is not known.

The p53 codon 72 polymorphism has been studied previously as a risk factor for glaucoma and a consistent association has not been found [18–28]. The lack of consistent findings among these studies could be due to variable sample size, ascertainment methodologies, glaucoma case definitions, genotyping methods, and variation in genotypic and allelic frequencies related to population substructure. The p53-PRO allele is the ancestral allele in the African population, while the p53-ARG allele is much more common in European populations [29].

In this study we examine the association between POAG and the p53 codon 72 polymorphism in a Caucasian cohort of European ancestry from the United States and replicate our findings in an independent Caucasian cohort of European ancestry from Australia. The results of our study suggest that the p53-PRO/PRO genotype is potentially associated with a specific glaucoma endophenotype that includes paracentral scotoma formation at an early stage in the disease.

## Materials and Methods

### Participants

The tenets of Helsinki were adhered to and ethics approval was obtained from the Massachusetts Eye and Ear Infirmary (MEEI) institutional review board, and the ethics committees of the Royal Hobart Hospital and the Royal Victorian Eye and Ear Hospital. Written informed consent was obtained from all study participants at both the Massachusetts Eye and Ear Infirmary and the Royal Victorian Eye and Ear Hospital.

264 patients affected with adult onset primary open angle glaucoma (POAG) [64 patients affected with normal tension glaucoma (NTG) and 200 with HT-POAG ('high-tension'-POAG)], and 400 unaffected individuals were recruited from the Glaucoma Consultation Service and the Comprehensive Ophthalmology Service at the Massachusetts Eye and Ear Infirmary. An additional 308 unrelated people with POAG and 178 controls were recruited through the Glaucoma Inheritance Study in Tasmania (GIST). GIST is derived from a Caucasian population of European ancestry in southeastern Australia, and specific features of this glaucoma cohort have been described previously [23]. All participants had a complete ophthalmological examination, including funduscopic evaluation of the retina and slit-lamp evaluation of the lens. Any patient with retinal or lenticular pathology that could confound the visual field analysis was not included in this study. All of the study participants (all cases and all controls) from both the U.S. and GIST cohorts are Caucasian with reported European ancestry. The features of the cases and controls for both cohorts are presented in Table 1.

Only subjects older than 35 years of age were included in this analysis. HT-POAG was defined as an IOP greater than or equal to 22 mm Hg in both eyes, glaucomatous optic nerve damage in both eyes, and visual field loss in at least one eye. Normal tension glaucoma (NTG) patients had evidence of optic nerve disease and visual field defects with IOP less than 22 mm Hg. Intraocular pressure was measured with a Goldmann tonometer in the clinical setting during typical clinic hours (9 AM to 5 PM). The recorded IOP for each patient was the highest known IOP prior to

**Table 1.** Demographic features of the cases and controls.

| Cohort | Group | N | Female (%) | Age at diagnosis* (year) Range | Age at diagnosis* (year) Mean±SD | Maximum IOP (mm Hg) Range | Maximum IOP (mm Hg) Mean±SD |
|---|---|---|---|---|---|---|---|
| MEEI | All glaucoma | 264 | 51.5 | 32–86 | 61.3±11.3[‡] | 9–50 | 24.8±5.9[‡] |
| | HT-POAG | 200 | 47.5 | 32–86 | 61.4±11.3[‡] | 9–50 | 26.3±5.5[‡] |
| | NTG | 64 | 64.1[†] | 34–83 | 61.0±11.6[‡] | 13–21 | 17.9±2.2 |
| | PS | 67 | 59.7 | 32–83 | 60.0±11.2[‡] | 9–42 | 23.8±5.5[‡] |
| | NS | 147 | 52.4 | 34–86 | 62.0±11.4[‡] | 12–38 | 24.6±5.6[‡] |
| | Controls | 400 | 55.3 | 39–92 | 66.0±11.3 | 9–22 | 16.1+2.6 |
| GIST | All glaucoma | 308 | 60.7[‡] | 24–89 | 63.1±12.4 | 10–74 | 25.0+9.4 |
| | PS | 26 | 76.9 | 41–80 | 63.0±10.5 | 18–36 | 24.0+5.2 |
| | NS | 152 | 60.5 | 24–89 | 64.2±12.8 | 10–68 | 24.2+8.8 |
| | Controls | 178 | 70.2 | 17–95 | 65.7±22.3 | NA | NA |
| Pooled | All glaucoma | 572 | 56.5 | 24–89 | 62.2±11.9[‡] | | |
| | PS | 93 | 64.5 | 32–83 | 60.8±11.1[‡] | | |
| | NS | 299 | 56.5 | 24–89 | 63.1±12.1[‡] | | |
| | Controls | 578 | 59.9 | 17–95 | 65.9±15.5 | | |

*For controls, this refers to age at enrollment.
[†]p = 0.02 compared to POAG.
[‡]p<0.05 compared to controls.
Abbreviations: MEEI, Massachusetts Eye and Ear Infirmary; GIST, Glaucoma Inheritance Study in Tasmania; IOP, Intraocular pressure; HT-POAG, High-tension POAG; POAG, Primary Open Angle Glaucoma; NTG, Normal Tension Glaucoma; PS, Paracentral scotoma; NS, Nasal step/arcuate scotoma; NA, Not available; SD, standard deviation.

treatment. Controls had IOP less than 22 mmHg, normal optic nerves and no family history of glaucoma.

## Visual Field Scoring

The earliest reliable visual fields demonstrating reproducible defects on at least two independent tests were selected for each affected individual. For this analysis we only used Humphrey automated visual fields (Humphrey Instruments, San Leandro, California, USA) using either the Standard full threshold or Fast-Pac programs. To be included in the study the false positive and negative error rates were less than 20% and the fixation losses were less than 33%. Visual fields demonstrating advanced disease, or generalized depression (mean defect >12 dB) were not used for this analysis. The average pattern deviation in each of 6 regions of the visual field corresponding to the superior paracentral, inferior paracentral, superior nasal arcuate, inferior nasal arcuate, superior nasal step, and inferior nasal step were calculated for each individual (Figure 1). Patients were classified as having an early-stage paracentral scotoma (PS) if they had a focal mean pattern deviation score (PSD) in one of the paracentral regions (either superior or inferior) greater than 5 dB and also if the focal mean pattern deviation score, in at least one of the paracentral regions, was more than 5 dB greater than any other visual field region. Patients were classified as having nasal step/arcuate scotomas (NS) if one of the four possible nasal step or arcuate regions had a mean PSD greater than 5 dB and if one of the four possible regions was 5 dB greater than either of the paracentral regions. Individual eyes were scored independently, and one eye from each patient was used for the analysis. If both eyes qualified for the study, the eye demonstrating the earliest reproducible defect was chosen. 214 visual fields for the MEEI cohort and 178 visual fields for the GIST cohort met these criteria and were used for this analysis.

## Genotyping

DNA was extracted from either peripheral blood samples or mouthwash samples according to previously published protocols [30]. A region of exon 4 of the p53 gene containing the p53 codon 72 polymorphism was amplified and sequenced in all patients using an ABI310 automated sequencer and BIGDYE sequencing chemistry.

## Statistical Analysis

Association analysis was performed using PLINK [31]. Hardy-Weinberg equilibrium was assessed using the chi-squared test. Genotype and allele frequencies of the *TP53* codon 72 variant between patients with glaucoma and control subjects were compared using the Fisher's exact test. Age-adjusted OR and 95%CI were calculated using logistic regression after adjusting for age at diagnosis for patients with glaucoma and age at enrollment for control subjects. The heterogeneity of ORs between cohorts was evaluated using the Breslow-Day test. Meta-analysis was performed across cohorts assuming a fixed-effect. Multiple comparisons were corrected using the Bonferroni method.

## Results

Because previous studies suggested that p53 could contribute to the development of normal-tension glaucoma [4,32], we first evaluated the association of the p53 codon 72 polymorphism in the MEEI glaucoma cases with normal tension glaucoma (NTG) defined as IOP less than 22 at time of diagnosis, as well as in the MEEI POAG patients with IOPs at diagnosis equal to or greater than 22 (HT-POAG). The p53-PRO/PRO (proline/proline) genotype and proline allele was associated with NTG overall (p = 0.008 and 0.016 respectively), and nominally with POAG overall (NTG and HT-POAG combined) (p = 0.032 and 0.057 respectively) but not with HT-POAG (p = 0.26) in the MEEI sample (Table 2). Since the p53-PRO/PRO genotype showed more evidence of association with NTG in the MEEI sample and previous studies have suggested that NTG patients are more likely to develop paracentral visual field defects at an early stage of the disease [4,6], we examined the association between p53-PRO and early paracentral visual field defects in the overall POAG sample (both the NTG and HT-POAG patients).

We analyzed the earliest available visual fields that demonstrated a reliable significant defect (Figure 1) in the US cohort to assess the association between the p53 codon72 polymorphism and POAG stratified by pattern of visual field loss. 214 MEEI POAG patients had qualifying visual fields and of these 67 had early-stage paracentral defects. The p53-PRO/PRO genotype was more frequent in the paracentral (PS) group (0.22) than in the nasal step/arcuate (NS) group (0.04) or control group (0.05), p = $2.7 \times 10^{-5}$ (Table 3). The odds of the C allele at p53-PRO was over 2-fold higher in the PS group (p = $4.8 \times 10^{-4}$, age-adjusted OR 2.20, 95%CI [1.43–3.39]) than in controls.

To replicate this finding in a second independent sample we scored Humphrey visual fields for the GIST POAG cohort and evaluated the distribution of p53 alleles in the PS and NS groups. 178 GIST patients had qualifying visual fields and of these 26 had early-stage paracentral defects. In this sample the p53-PRO/PRO genotype was also more frequent in the PS group (0.23) compared with the NS group (0.05) and controls (0.07), (p = $7.3 \times 10^{-3}$), and the p53-PRO C allele was also more common in the PS group (p = $1.8 \times 10^{-3}$, age-adjusted OR 2.32, 95% CI [1.24–4.34]) (Table 3). After testing for heterogeneity we pooled the samples

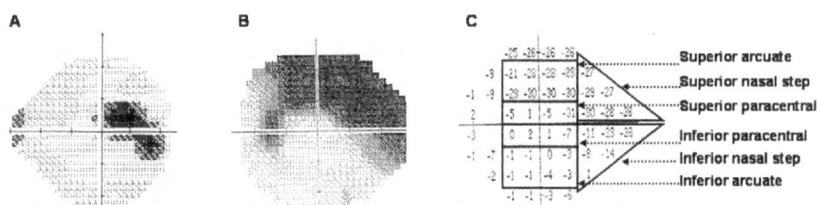

**Figure 1. Visual field scoring.** The average pattern standard deviation (PSD) in each of 6 regions of the visual field corresponding to the superior paracentral, inferior paracentral, superior nasal arcuate, inferior nasal arcuate, superior nasal step, and inferior nasal step were calculated for each individual. Patients were classified as having paracentral scotomas (PS) if they had a mean PSD in one of the paracentral regions greater than 5 dB and also if the mean PSD was more than 5 dB greater than any other visual field region. Patients were classified as having nasal step/arcuate scotomas (NS) if one of the four possible nasal step or arcuate regions had a mean PSD greater than 5 dB and if one of the four possible regions was 5 dB greater than either of the paracentral regions. The visual field in panel A is an example of a PS, and panel B an example of an NS visual field. The PSD plot in panel C corresponds to the visual field in panel B.

**Table 2.** Association of p53 codon 72 variant with NTG in the US (MEEI) cohort.

| Group | N | Genotype Frequency (%) | | | | Allele Frequency (%) | | | | |
|---|---|---|---|---|---|---|---|---|---|---|
| | | CC | CG | GG | $p^*$ | C | G | $p^*$ | OR (95%CI)[†] | Age-adjusted OR (95%CI)[†] |
| All glaucoma | 264 | 26 (9.9) | 120 (45.4) | 118 (44.7) | 0.032 | 172 (32.6) | 356 (67.4) | 0.057 | 1.27 (1.00–1.61) | 1.33 (1.03–1.73) |
| HT-POAG | 200 | 16 (8.0) | 91 (45.5) | 93 (46.5) | 0.26 | 123 (30.8) | 277 (69.3) | 0.28 | 1.16 (0.89–1.51) | 1.20 (0.90–1.59) |
| NTG | 64 | 10 (15.6) | 29 (45.3) | 25 (39.1) | 0.003 | 49 (38.3) | 79 (61.7) | 0.016 | 1.63 (1.10–2.40) | 1.88 (1.18–2.98) |
| Controls | 400 | 19 (4.8) | 183 (45.8) | 198 (49.5) | | 221 (27.6) | 579 (72.4) | | | |

*$p$ values are calculated using Fisher's exact test when compared to controls.
[†]OR and 95% CI are calculated using logistic regression when compared to controls.
Abbreviations: US, United States; MEEI, Massachusetts Eye and Ear Infirmary; POAG, Primary Open Angle Glaucoma; HT-POAG, High-tension glaucoma; NTG, Normal Tension Glaucoma.

and performed a meta-analysis. We found an overall association of the p53-PRO/PRO genotype with PS in the pooled sample ($p = 6.6 \times 10^{-7}$) and with the PRO allele in the meta-analysis ($1.3 \times 10^{-6}$, OR 2.17, 95% CI [1.58–2.98]). Stratification by gender prior to analysis showed statistically significant association between p53-PRO/PRO and paracentral scotoma formation in both males and females with a somewhat stronger association in males ($p = 1.1 \times 10^{-4}$ in males vs $p = 1.8 \times 10^{-3}$ in females; Table 4). For the p53-PRO/PRO genotype the sensitivity and specificity to detect early-stage paracentral scotoma formation in open angle glaucoma patients is 0.22 and 0.95 respectively with a positive predictive value of 0.6, and a negative predictive value of 0.80.

**Table 3.** Association of p53 codon 72 variants with paracentral scotomas (PS) in the US and GIST cohorts.

| | | N | Genotype Frequency (%) | | | | Allele Frequency (%) | | | | | | |
|---|---|---|---|---|---|---|---|---|---|---|---|---|---|
| | | | CC | CG | GG | $p^*$ | C | G | $p^*$ | OR (95%CI)[†] | Age-adjusted OR (95%CI)[†] | p-meta[‡] | Common OR (95%CI) |
| US | All glaucoma | 264 | 26 (9.9) | 120 (45.4) | 118 (44.7) | 0.034 | 172 (32.6) | 356 (67.4) | 0.057 | 1.27 (1.00–1.61) | 1.33 (1.03–1.73) | | |
| | PS | 67 | 15 (22.4) | 28 (41.8) | 24 (35.8) | $2.7\times10^{-5}$ | 58 (43.3) | 76 (56.7) | $4.8\times10^{-4}$ | 2.00 (1.37–2.91) | 2.20 (1.43–3.39) | | |
| | NS | 147 | 6 (4.1) | 68 (46.3) | 73 (49.6) | 0.99 | 80 (27.2) | 214 (72.8) | 0.94 | 0.98 (0.73–1.32) | 0.98 (0.70–1.36) | | |
| | Controls | 400 | 19 (4.8) | 183 (45.8) | 198 (49.5) | | 221 (27.6) | 579 (72.4) | | | | | |
| GIST | All glaucoma | 308 | 26 (8.4) | 118 (38.3) | 164 (53.3) | 0.25 | 170 (27.6) | 446 (72.4) | 0.11 | 1.29 (0.95–1.75) | 1.24 (0.91–1.67) | | |
| | PS | 26 | 6 (23.1) | 11 (42.3) | 9 (34.6) | $7.3\times10^{-3}$ | 23 (44.2) | 29 (55.8) | $1.8\times10^{-3}$ | 2.69 (1.48–4.91) | 2.32 (1.24–4.34) | | |
| | NS | 152 | 8 (5.3) | 60 (39.5) | 84 (55.2) | 0.36 | 76 (25.0) | 228 (75.0) | 0.52 | 1.13 (0.79–1.62) | 1.09 (0.75–1.57) | | |
| | Controls | 178 | 12 (6.7) | 57 (32.0) | 109 (61.2) | | 81 (22.8) | 275 (77.2) | | | | | |
| Pooled[‡] | All glaucoma | 572 | 52 (9.1) | 238 (41.6) | 282 (49.3) | 0.041 | 342 (29.9) | 802 (70.1) | 0.046 | 1.21 (1.01–1.45) | 1.21 (1.00–1.46) | 0.011 | 1.28 (1.06–1.54) |
| | PS | 93 | 21 (22.6) | 39 (41.9) | 33 (35.5) | $6.6\times10^{-7}$ | 81 (43.6) | 105 (56.4) | $2.9\times10^{-6}$ | 2.18 (1.59–3.00) | 2.23 (1.57–3.16) | $1.3\times10^{-6}$ | 2.17 (1.58–2.98) |
| | NS | 299 | 14 (4.7) | 128 (42.8) | 157 (52.5) | 0.90 | 156 (26.1) | 442 (73.9) | 0.99 | 1.00 (0.80–1.25) | 0.97 (0.76–1.24) | 0.74 | 1.04 (0.83–1.31) |
| | Controls | 578 | 31 (5.4) | 240 (41.5) | 307 (53.1) | | 302 (26.1) | 854 (73.9) | | | | | |

*$p$ values are calculated using Fisher's exact test when compared to controls.
[†]OR and 95% CI are calculated using logistic regression when compared to controls.
[‡]p-heterogeneity >0.05 (Breslow-Day test between cohorts). Meta-analysis assumed a fixed-effect, and common OR and 95%CI are calculated using the Mantel-Haenszel method.
Abbreviations: US, United States; GIST, Glaucoma Inheritance Study in Tasmania; PS, Paracentral Scotoma; NS, Nasal Step/Arcuate Scotoma.

**Table 4.** Association of p53 codon 72 variants with paracentral scotomas (PS) in the US and GIST cohorts stratified by gender.

| | | | | Genotype Frequency (%) | | | | Allele Frequency (%) | | | OR (95%CI)† | Age-adjusted OR (95%CI)† | p-meta‡ | Common OR (95%CI) |
|---|---|---|---|---|---|---|---|---|---|---|---|---|---|---|
| | | | N | CC | CG | GG | p* | C | G | p* | | | | |
| US | Male | PS | 27 | 7 (25.9) | 13 (48.2) | 7 (25.9) | 0.0010 | 27 (50.0) | 27 (50.0) | 0.0012 | 2.73 (1.52–4.89) | 3.15 (1.61–6.18) | | |
| | | Controls | 179 | 9 (5.0) | 78 (43.6) | 92 (51.4) | | 96 (26.8) | 262 (73.2) | | | | | |
| | Female | PS | 40 | 8 (20.0) | 15 (37.5) | 17 (42.5) | 0.0051 | 31 (38.8) | 49 (61.2) | 0.064 | 1.60 (0.98–2.63) | 1.68 (0.95–3.00) | | |
| | | Controls | 221 | 10 (4.5) | 105 (47.5) | 106 (48.0) | | 125 (28.3) | 317 (71.7) | | | | | |
| GIST | Male | PS | 6 | 3 (50.0) | 1 (16.7) | 2 (33.3) | 0.035 | 7 (58.3) | 5 (41.7) | 0.036 | 4.31 (1.26–14.74) | 2.27 (0.62–8.36) | | |
| | | Controls | 53 | 5 (9.4) | 16 (30.2) | 32 (60.4) | | 26 (24.5) | 80 (75.5) | | | | | |
| | Female | PS | 20 | 3 (15.0) | 10 (50.0) | 7 (35.0) | 0.041 | 16 (40.0) | 24 (60.0) | 0.018 | 2.36 (1.17–4.76) | 2.45 (1.18–5.11) | | |
| | | Controls | 125 | 7 (5.6) | 41 (32.8) | 77 (61.6) | | 55 (22.0) | 195 (78.0) | | | | | |
| Pooled‡ | Male | PS | 33 | 10 (30.3) | 14 (42.4) | 9 (27.3) | $1.1 \times 10^{-4}$ | 34 (51.5) | 32 (48.5) | $7.1 \times 10^{-5}$ | 2.98 (1.76–5.04) | 2.90 (1.62–5.21) | $2.8 \times 10^{-5}$ | 2.96 (1.75–5.01) |
| | | Controls | 232 | 14 (6.0) | 94 (40.5) | 124 (53.5) | | 122 (26.3) | 342 (73.7) | | | | | |
| | Female | PS | 60 | 11 (18.3) | 25 (41.7) | 24 (40.0) | 0.0018 | 47 (39.2) | 73 (60.8) | 0.0041 | 1.83 (1.22–2.74) | 1.89 (1.21–2.95) | 0.0034 | 1.82 (1.21–2.72) |
| | | Controls | 346 | 17 (4.9) | 146 (42.2) | 183 (52.9) | | 180 (26.0) | 512 (74.0) | | | | | |

*p values are calculated using Fisher's exact test when compared to controls.
†OR and 95%CI are calculated using logistic regression when compared to controls.
‡p-heterogeneity >0.05 (Breslow-Day test between cohorts). Meta-analysis assumed a fixed-effect, and common OR and 95% CI are calculated using the Mantel-Haenszel method.
Abbreviations: US, United States; GIST, Glaucoma Inheritance Study in Tasmania; PS, Paracentral Scotoma.

## Discussion

The results of this study suggest that the p53 codon 72 PRO/PRO genotype is potentially associated with early-stage paracentral visual field defects in patients with open-angle glaucoma. This is the first study to assess association of p53 with glaucoma subsets defined by visual field stratification. Our subgroup analysis could suggest that the previously observed inconsistent association between p53 codon 72 and glaucoma may reflect differences in the composition of the study cohorts with respect to early-onset paracentral cases due to differences in ascertainment methodologies and case definitions. The significant association between the p53 variant and paracentral visual loss among POAG cases vs controls that we discovered in our US cohort was confirmed in the Australian cohort. These results could point to another allele in linkage disequilibrium with the p53 codon 72 variant that is biologically significant; however, considering the known biological activity of the codon 72 polymorphism this possibility seems less likely.

The p53 codon 72 polymorphism influences apoptosis, and the apoptotic potential of the different forms of the protein is dependent on the cell type and cellular environment. p53 activity is determined by the mix of p53 activators and stimulators present in a particular cell type [33]. Stimulators and inhibitors bind specifically to the PXXP motif that contains the codon 72 polymorphic site, and p53-PRO binds both inhibitors and stimulators more efficiently than p53-ARG [30]. Depending on the relative amounts of inhibitors and stimulators the p53-PRO form may have more or less apoptotic activity than p53-ARG. *In vitro* studies using a variety of tumor cells have suggested that p53-ARG has more apoptotic activity than p53-PRO, including a more effective response to oxidative stress and more efficient translocation to the mitochondria [34]. However this relative increase in p53-ARG activity is due to increased activity of the p53 inhibitor iASPP (inhibitory member of the apoptosis-stimulating protein of p53), which reduces the activity of the p53-PRO form but not the p53-ARG form [33]. Interestingly, under conditions of low oxygen tension, the p53-PRO form induces more cell death in cancer cells than p53-ARG [15] and under these conditions the p53 stimulators may be more abundant rendering the p53-PRO form more active. Our results suggest that the p53-PRO has more apoptotic activity in glaucoma, which may reflect variable expression of p53 stimulators and inhibitors in cell types involved in the disease. The p53-PRO apoptotic potential could be enhanced by conditions creating low retinal oxygen tension such as sleep apnea, a condition previously demonstrated to be associated with initial paracentral scotoma formation in glaucoma [4].

Our results could suggest that the ganglion cells in the maculopapillary bundle are more susceptible to p53-mediated apoptosis. The maculopapillary bundle is recognized to be more susceptible to certain metabolic conditions (such as methyl alcohol toxicity) and genetic defects (such OPA1 mutations in dominant optic atrophy) that impair mitochondrial function [35]. The mitochondrial density is higher in the maculopapillary bundle [36] and these cells have higher levels of reactive oxygen species that may lower the apoptotic threshold. The maculopapillary bundle may be more vulnerable to the effects of UV light [37] which could influence mitochondrial function and lower the threshold for apoptosis in carriers of p53-PRO. Early-stage paracentral defects are more common in NTG patients [4] and NTG patients are more likely to have abnormalities of ocular blood flow [38] suggesting that ocular perfusion may also contribute to the increased susceptibility of p53 mediated apoptosis in the paracentral region.

The population frequencies of the PRO/PRO genotype support a role for the p53-PRO allele in glaucoma. p53-ARG is unique to humans, and while the arginine allele is the most common allele in Caucasian populations, the ancestral proline allele is the most common allele in African populations, an ethnic group known to have increased risk of glaucoma [39]. The PRO/PRO genotype is found in 47% of sub-Saharan Africans compared with 8% of European whites. The PRO/PRO genotype is also more common in Japanese (28%) than in European whites, a population with an increased prevalence of normal tension glaucoma [40].

Our results demonstrate a potential association between p53-PRO allele and early-stage paracentral scotoma formation in glaucoma. Several limitations of our study should be considered. First, the number of paracentral cases is low for a formal association study and it is possible that these results could be subject to type II statistical error. Furthermore, while we replicated our findings here, confirmation of these observations in additional datasets will be necessary before a formal association between p53 codon 72 alleles and paracentral scotoma can be established. Second, the low allele frequency and corresponding low sensitivity

indicates that testing for the p53-PRO/PRO genotype would not be useful as an overall glaucoma population screening test. The specificity of the association could help identify a subset of glaucoma patients who are at increased risk for early loss of central vision once a formal association is established. Third, these findings are limited to Caucasian patients with European ancestry and may not be generalizable to other populations. Finally, we found that the potential association between p53-PRO/PRO and paracentral scotoma is somewhat stronger in males than in females possibly suggesting that the contribution of p53-PRO is influenced by gender, however further study in other datasets would be required to confirm this observation.

Retinal ganglion cells that degenerate to cause central vision loss may be differentially susceptible to apoptosis and our results suggest that p53 is one protein that could influence this susceptibility. The regulation of glaucomatous ganglion cell apoptosis is clearly complex and it is likely that multiple genetic and environmental factors will contribute to this process. Recent studies have identified a number of genes, in addition to p53, with altered expression in glaucomatous ganglion cells [41,42]. Examining these genes and their respective pathways will help dissect the underlying genetic causes of early-stage paracentral scotoma formation in glaucoma. Identifying factors that influence the development of paracentral scotomas will be an important step toward preventing visual loss in patients with glaucoma.

## Author Contributions

Conceived and designed the experiments: JLW LRP. Performed the experiments: BJF DYW AWH DRFS DPD. Analyzed the data: BJF AWH JLH. Contributed reagents/materials/analysis tools: CO AR JEC DAM LRP JLW. Wrote the paper: JLW LRP JLH DAM AWH.

## References

1. Gordon MO, Beiser JA, Brandt JD, Heuer DK, Higginbotham EJ, et al. (2002) The Ocular Hypertension Treatment Study: baseline factors that predict the onset of primary open-angle glaucoma. Arch Ophthalmol 120: 714–720.

2. Cheng JW, Cai JP, Wei RL (2009) Meta-analysis of medical intervention for normal tension glaucoma. Ophthalmology 116:1243–1249.

3. Anderson DR, Drance SM, Schulzer M; Collaborative Normal-Tension Glaucoma Study Group (2003) Factors that predict the benefit of lowering intraocular pressure in normal tension glaucoma. Am J Ophthalmol 136: 820–829.

4. Park SC, De Moraes CG, Teng CC, Liebmann JM, Ritch R (2011) Initial Parafoveal Versus Peripheral Scotomas in Glaucoma: Risk Factors and Visual Field Characteristics. Ophthalmology 118: 1782–1789.

5. Deva NC, Insull E, Gamble G, Danesh-Meyer HV (2008) Risk factors for first presentation of glaucoma with significant visual field loss. Clin Experiment Ophthalmol 36: 217–221.

6. Kim NR, Hong S, Kim JH, Rho SS, Seong GJ, et al. (2011) Comparison of Macular Ganglion Cell Complex Thickness by Fourier-Domain OCT in Normal Tension Glaucoma and Primary Open-Angle Glaucoma. J Glaucoma Jan 22. [Epub ahead of print].

7. Viana RJ, Fonseca MB, Ramalho RM, Nunes AF, Rodrigues CM (2010) Organelle stress sensors and cell death mechanisms in neurodegenerative diseases. CNS Neurol Disord Drug Targets 9: 679–692.

8. Li Y, Schlamp CL, Poulsen GL, Jackson MW, Griep AE, et al. (2002) p53 regulates apoptotic retinal ganglion cell death induced by N-methyl-D-aspartate. Mol Vis 8: 341–350.

9. Umihira J, Lindsey JD, Weinreb RN (2002) Simultaneous expression of c-Jun and p53 in retinal ganglion cells of adult rat retinal slice cultures. Curr Eye Res 24: 147–159.

10. O'Connor JC, Wallace DM, O'Brien CJ, Cotter TG (2008) A novel antioxidant function for the tumor-suppressor gene p53 in the retinal ganglion cell. Invest Ophthalmol Vis Sci 49: 4237–4244.

11. Levkovitch-Verbin H, Dardik R, Vander S, Nisgav Y, Kalev-Landoy M, et al. (2006) Experimental glaucoma and optic nerve transection induce simultaneous upregulation of proapoptotic and prosurvival genes. Invest Ophthalmol Vis Sci 47: 2491–2497.

12. Wiggs JL, Allingham RR, Hossain A, Kern J, Auguste J, et al. (2000) Genome-wide scan for adult onset primary open angle glaucoma. Hum Mol Genet 9: 1109–1117.

13. Lemmelä S, Forsman E, Sistonen P, Eriksson A, Forsius H, et al. (2007) Genome-wide scan of exfoliation syndrome. Invest Ophthalmol Vis Sci 48: 4136–4142.

14. Dumont P, Leu J, Della Pietra AC, George DL, Murphy M (2003) The codon 72 polymorphic variants of p53 have markedly different apoptotic potential. Nat Genet 33: 357–365.

15. Sansone P, Storci G, Pandolfi S, Montanaro L, Chieco P, et al. (2007) The p53 codon 72 proline allele is endowed with enhanced cell-death inducing potential in cancer cells exposed to hypoxia. Br J Cancer 96: 1302–1308.

16. den Reijer PM, Maier AB, Westendorp RG, van Heemst D (2008) Influence of the TP53 codon 72 polymorphism on the cellular responses to X-irradiation in fibroblasts from nonagenarians. Mech Ageing Dev 129:175–182.

17. Toffoli G, Biason P, Russo A, De Mattia E, Cecchin E, et al. (2009) Effect of TP53 Arg72Pro and MDM2 SNP309 polymorphisms on the risk of high-grade osteosarcoma development and survival. Clin Cancer Res 15: 3550–3556.

18. Lin HJ, Chen WC, Tsai FJ, Tsai SW (2002) Distributions of p53 codon 72 polymorphism in primary open angle glaucoma. Br J Ophthalmol 86: 767–770.

19. Ressiniotis T, Griffiths PG, Birch M, Keers S, Chinnery PF (2004) Primary open angle glaucoma is associated with a specific p53 gene haplotype. J Med Genet 41: 296–298.

20. Daugherty CL, Curtis H, Realini T, Charlton JF, Zareparsi S (2009) Primary open angle glaucoma in a Caucasian population is associated with the p53 codon 72 polymorphism. Mol Vis 15: 1939–1944.

21. Fan BJ, Liu K, Wang DY, Tham CC, Tam PO, et al. (2010) Association of polymorphisms of tumor necrosis factor and tumor protein p53 with primary open-angle glaucoma. Invest Ophthalmol Vis Sci 51: 4110–4116.

22. Acharya M, Mitra S, Mukhopadhyay A, Khan M, Roychoudhury S, et al. (2002) Distribution of p53 codon 72 polymorphism in Indian primary open angle glaucoma patients. Mol Vis 8: 367–371.

23. Dimasi DP, Hewitt AW, Green CM, Mackey DA, Craig JE (2005) Lack of association of p53 polymorphisms and haplotypes in high and normal tension open angle glaucoma. J Med Genet 42: e55.

24. Silva RE, Arruda JT, Rodrigues FW, Moura KK (2009) Primary open angle glaucoma was not found to be associated with p53 codon 72 polymorphism in a Brazilian cohort. Genet Mol Res 8: 268–272.

25. Mabuchi F, Sakurada Y, Kashiwagi K, Yamagata Z, Iijima H, et al. (2009) Lack of association between p53 gene polymorphisms and primary open angle glaucoma in the Japanese population. Mol Vis 15: 1045–1049.

26. Saglar E, Yucel D, Bozkurt B, Ozgul RK, Irkec M, et al. (2009) Association of polymorphisms in APOE, p53, and p21 with primary open-angle glaucoma in Turkish patients. Mol Vis 15: 1270–1276.

27. Blanco-Marchite C, Sánchez-Sánchez F, López-Garrido MP, Iñigez-de-Onzoño M, López-Martínez F, et al. (2011) WDR36 and P53 gene variants and susceptibility to primary open-angle glaucoma: analysis of gene-gene interactions. Invest Ophthalmol Vis Sci 52: 8467–8478.

28. GuoY, Zhang H, Chen X, Yang X, Cheng W, et al. (2012) Association of TP53 polymorphisms with primary open angle glaucoma: A Meta-analysis. Invest Ophthalmol Vis Sci 12: 9818–9822.

29. Katkoori VR, Jia X, Shanmugam C, Wan W, Meleth S, et al. (2009) Prognostic significance of p53 codon 72 polymorphism differs with race in colorectal adenocarcinoma. Clin Cancer Res 15:2406–2016.

30. Fan BJ, Wang DY, Pasquale LR, Haines JL, Wiggs JL (2011) Genetic variants associated with optic nerve vertical cup-to-disc ratio are risk factors for primary open angle glaucoma in a US Caucasian population. Invest Ophthalmol Vis Sci 52: 1788–1792.

31. Purcell S, Neale B, Todd-Brown K, Thomas L, Ferreira MA, et al. (2000) PLINK: a tool set for whole-genome association and population-based linkage analyses. Am J Hum Genet 81: 559–575.

32. Golubnitschaja-Labudova O, Liu R, Decker C, Zhu P, Haefliger IO, et al. (2000) Altered gene expression in lymphocytes of patients with normal-tension glaucoma. Curr Eye Res 21: 867–876.

33. Bergamaschi D, Samuels Y, Sullivan A, Zvelebil M, Breyssens H, et al. (2006) iASPP preferentially binds p53 proline-rich region and modulates apoptotic function of codon 72-polymorphic p53. Nat Genet 38: 1133–1141.

34. Jeong BS, Hu W, Belyi V, Rabadan R, Levine AJ (2010) Differential levels of transcription of p53-regulated genes by the arginine/proline polymorphism: p53 with arginine at codon 72 favors apoptosis. FASEB J 24: 1347–1353.

35. Di Donato S (2009) Multisystem manifestations of mitochondrial disorders. J Neurol 256:693–710.

36. Yu Wai Man CY, Chinnery PF, Griffiths PG (2005) Optic neuropathies–importance of spatial distribution of mitochondria as well as function. Med Hypotheses 65:1038–1042.

37. Osborne NN, Kamalden TA, Majid AS, del Olmo-Aguado S, Manso AG, et al. (2010) Light effects on mitochondrial photosensitizers in relation to retinal degeneration. Neurochem Res 35:2027–2034.

38. Caprioli J, Coleman AL (2010) Blood Flow in Glaucoma Discussion. Blood pressure, perfusion pressure, and glaucoma. Am J Ophthalmol 149:704–712.

39. Racette L, Liebmann JM, Girkin CA, Zangwill LM, Jain S, et al. (2010) African Descent and Glaucoma Evaluation Study (ADAGES): III. Ancestry differences in visual function in healthy eyes. Arch Ophthalmol 128: 551–559.

40. Stein JD, Kim DS, Niziol LM, Talwar N, Nan B, et al. (2011) Differences in Rates of Glaucoma among Asian Americans and Other Racial Groups, and among Various Asian Ethnic Groups. Ophthalmology 118: 1031–1037.

41. Wang DY, Ray A, Rodgers K, Ergorul C, Hyman BT, et al. (2010) Global gene expression changes in rat retinal ganglion cells in experimental glaucoma. Invest Ophthalmol Vis Sci 51:4084–4095.

42. Guo Y, Cepurna WO, Dyck JA, Doser TA, Johnson EC, et al. (2010) Retinal cell responses to elevated intraocular pressure: a gene array comparison between the whole retina and retinal ganglion cell layer. Invest Ophthalmol Vis Sci 51: 3003–3018.

# 9

# Identifying Areas of the Visual Field Important for Quality of Life in Patients with Glaucoma

**Hiroshi Murata[1], Hiroyo Hirasawa[1], Yuka Aoyama[1], Kenji Sugisaki[1,2], Makoto Araie[1,3], Chihiro Mayama[1], Makoto Aihara[1,4], Ryo Asaoka[1]***

1 Department of Ophthalmology, University of Tokyo Graduate School of Medicine, Tokyo, Japan, 2 Tokyo Koseinenkin Hospital, Tokyo, Japan, 3 Kanto Central Hospital, The Mutual Aid Association of Public School Teachers, Tokyo, Japan, 4 Shirato Eye Clinic, Tokyo, Japan

## Abstract

*Purpose:* The purpose of this study was to create a vision-related quality of life (VRQoL) prediction system to identify visual field (VF) test points associated with decreased VRQoL in patients with glaucoma.

*Method:* VRQoL score was surveyed in 164 patients with glaucoma using the 'Sumi questionnaire'. A binocular VF was created from monocular VFs by using the integrated VF (IVF) method. VRQoL score was predicted using the 'Random Forest' method, based on visual acuity (VA) of better and worse eyes (better-eye and worse-eye VA) and total deviation (TD) values from the IVF. For comparison, VRQoL scores were regressed (linear regression) against: (i) mean of TD (IVF MD); (ii) better-eye VA; (iii) worse-eye VA; and (iv) IVF MD and better- and worse-eye VAs. The rank of importance of IVF test points was identified using the Random Forest method.

*Results:* The root mean of squared prediction error associated with the Random Forest method (0.30 to 1.97) was significantly smaller than those with linear regression models (0.34 to 3.38, p<0.05, ten-fold cross validation test). Worse-eye VA was the most important variable in all VRQoL tasks. In general, important VF test points were concentrated along the horizontal meridian. Particular areas of the IVF were important for different tasks: peripheral superior and inferior areas in the left hemifield for the 'letters and sentences' task, peripheral, mid-peripheral and para-central inferior regions for the 'walking' task, the peripheral superior region for the 'going out' task, and a broad scattered area across the IVF for the 'dining' task.

*Conclusion:* The VRQoL prediction model with the Random Forest method enables clinicians to better understand patients' VRQoL based on standard clinical measurements of VA and VF.

**Editor:** Bang V. Bui, Univeristy of Melbourne, Australia

**Funding:** The authors have no support or funding to report.

**Competing Interests:** The authors have declared that no competing interests exist.

* E-mail: rasaoka-tky@umin.ac.jp

## Introduction

Vision-related quality of life (VRQoL) can be defined as a person's satisfaction with their visual ability and how their vision impacts on their daily life [1]. In glaucoma patients, visual field (VF) loss [2–11] and reduced visual acuity (VA) [8–14] impact on VRQoL; however, these studies only investigated the influence of summary measures, such as mean deviation (MD), on VRQoL. Very few reports have attempted to identify the areas of the VF that are important for different daily tasks; Sumi et al. reported that retinal sensitivity in the lower hemifield within 5° of fixation, and better eye VA, play the most important role in VRQoL [15] while other studies have suggested the importance of other VF regions for specific tasks, such as driving [16] and postural stability [17]. Other reports have revealed that glaucomatous VF damage has an effect on hand-eye coordination [18], the likelihood of falling [19], the possibility of causing or being involved in a motor vehicle accident [19–23] (likely due to an inability to detect peripheral obstacles and hazards [16,21]), and the risk of fractures [24].

The two most significant measures of visual function, VA and VF sensitivity, are correlated in glaucoma patients [7], especially when glaucomatous damage affects the central VF [25,26]. Furthermore, VF sensitivities of neighboring test points are also correlated [27–29]; therefore, this spatial relationship should also be taken into account when analyzing the relationship between the VF and VRQoL. Nonetheless, most previous studies have investigated the impact of VA, and VF sensitivity in different regions of the VF, on VRQoL separately [9–15]. Indeed, previous studies have reported that the relationship between VRQoL and VF sensitivity attenuates when the relationship is adjusted for VA [8,10]. In the current study, we have used Breiman's 'Random Forest' machine learning algorithm [30] to predict VRQoL, and to identify the most important VF test points for a number of different daily tasks since this method can cope with highly correlated predictor variables. [31]. Indeed, the Random Forest algorithm has be used to explore interactions between different predictor variables[31–33]; thus, VA and VF sensitivity can be considered concurrently, and the spatial relationship between neighboring VF test points will not bias the results.

The purpose of this study is to generate a method to predict a glaucoma patient's VRQoL based on their VA and VF sensitivity, considering their inter-correlation, and to identify the areas of the VF most important for different daily tasks.

## Materials and Methods

The study was approved by the Research Ethics Committee of the Graduate School of Medicine and Faculty of Medicine at the University of Tokyo. Written consent was given by the patients for their information to be stored in the hospital database and used for research. This study was performed according to the tenets of the Declaration of Helsinki.

The subjects of the current study included 164 patients (86 males and 78 females) with glaucoma (85 patients with primary open-angle glaucoma, 72 patients with normal tension glaucoma, 4 patients with primary angle-closure glaucoma, and 3 patients with secondary open angle glaucoma). All of the study patients were recruited at the glaucoma clinic in the Hospital of the University of Tokyo. All patients enrolled in the study fulfilled the following criteria: (1) glaucoma was the only disease causing VF damage and/or VA impairment; (2) patients were followed for at least 6 months at the University of Tokyo Hospital. The VF was evaluated using the Humphrey Field Analyzer (Carl Zeiss Meditec, Dublin, CA) 30-2 Swedish Interactive Threshold Algorithm (SITA) standard program with reliable results: fixation losses $<25\%$, and false-positive error $<15\%$; false negative rate was not used, as a reliability criterion because it is has been shown to be positively correlated with the level of VF damage rather than patient attentiveness. [34]. All of the patients had a glaucomatous VF defect in at least one eye defined as three or more contiguous total deviation points at $p<0.05$, or two or more contiguous points at $p<0.01$, or a 10 dB difference across the nasal horizontal midline at two or more adjacent points, or MD worse than $-5$ dB [1]. VF damage was stable with medically- or surgically-controlled intraocular pressure for at least 2 years.

Characteristics of the study sample are summarized in **Table 1**. The mean ($\pm$ standard deviation) age of patients was $61.9\pm12.1$ years, ranging from 26 to 89 years. The MD of the better eye was $-13.1\pm9.3$ (range: $-31.4$ to 1.96) dB, while the MD of the worse eye was $-17.9\pm9.6$ (range: $-33.2$ to 0.4) dB. Mean best corrected VA in the logarithm of the minimum angle of resolution (logMAR) was $0.09\pm0.43$ (range: $-0.30$ to 2.6) in the better eye and $0.52\pm0.9$ (range: $-0.30$ to 2.8) in the worse eye.

**Table 1.** Patient demographics.

| | |
|---|---|
| Age, y, mean ± SD (range) | 61.9±12.1 (26 to 89) |
| Gender (male : Female) | 86:78 |
| MD of better eye, dB, mean ± SD (range) | −13.1±9.3 (−31.4 to 2.0) |
| MD of worse eye, dB, mean ± SD (range) | −17.9±9.6 (−33.2 to 0.4) |
| Visual acuity of better eye, mean ± SD (range) | 0.09±0.43 (−0.30 to 2.6) |
| Visual acuity of worse eye, mean ± SD (range) | 0.52±0.9 (−0.30 to 2.8) |
| Type of glaucoma (POAG, NTG, PACG, SOAG) | 85, 72, 4, 3 |

MD: mean deviation, SD: standard deviation, POAG: primary open-angle glaucoma, NTG: normal tension glaucoma, PACG: primary angle-closure glaucoma, and SOAG: secondary open angle glaucoma.

VRQoLwas assessed using the method developed by Sumi et. al. [15]. Briefly, the 'Sumi Questionnaire', written in Japanese, contains 30 questions regarding 7 tasks: legibility of letters ('letters'), legibility of sentences ('sentences'), walking, using public transportation ('going out'), dining, dressing, and additional miscellaneous activities ('miscellaneous') (see **Table 2**, note that questions have been translated into English for this article). The Sumi questionnaire also includes one question (question 7) regarding the difficulty in reading vertically, since this is the traditional way to read/write sentences in Japanese. Each question is associated with three possible responses, scored as follows; greatly disabled (2 points), slightly disabled (1 point), and not disabled (0 points). Mean score was calculated for each of the seven tasks to attain a visual disability index. The 'letters' and 'sentences' tasks were merged since these questions are closely related. The 'dressing' task was not analyzed because of the small number of questions (n = 2), but its score was used in the calculation of overall VRQoL. Within 3 months of visual disability assessment, we tested the VF in both eyes with a 5-minute rest between each eye examination.

To analyze the relationship between VF sensitivity at each test point and VRQoL, a binocular VF was calculated for each patient by merging a patient's monocular HFA VFs using the "best sensitivity" method (integrated VF (IVF)) [35–38]. In short, each point on a monocular VF has a spatially corresponding point on the VF of the fellow eye in binocular viewing. In the IVF, the sensitivity and TD at each point was calculated using the maximum raw sensitivity (dB) and best TD (least negative) value from each of the two overlapping points, as if the subject was viewing binocularly (**Figure 1** illustrates the numeric locations of all IVF test points).

The better- and worse-eyes were determined using the MD values (better-eye had less damaged MD). For the analysis of VA, logMAR was used.

The relationships between TD values, better-eye VA, worse-eye VA, TD values and age, and VRQoL scores were analyzed using the Random Forest method. The Random Forest algorithm is an ensemble classifier proposed by Breiman in 2001 [30], which consists of many decision trees and outputs the averaged value of all the individual trees. Each tree is constructed using a different bootstrap sample from the original data (bootstrapping is repeated until the sample size reaches the original sample size, allowing duplication). Thus, cross-validation is performed internally, removing the need for a separate cross-validation dataset to obtain an unbiased estimate of the test set error. Next, the optimal regression model is determined by a measure of model fitness to the data (mean-square error for linear regression). A particular merit of the Random Forest method is that any interaction or correlation between predictor variables can be taken into account. Subsequent partitioning of the data with a different predictor from the prior partition in the decision tree, which is the weak learner of the Random Forest method, represents an interaction effect, and consequently the decision tree can represent high order interactions. In addition, each predictor has less opportunity to compete against correlated predictors since each predictor is selected randomly for each stage of the learning process. As a result, predictors that might be overlooked with other methods can contribute to the prediction [31]. Squared prediction errors were estimated for each fold using the leave-one-out cross validation method [39] and then the root mean of the squared prediction error (RMSE) was calculated. In addition, we used a ten-fold cross validation test for comparing two models [40]. For this test, the original data was divided into ten subsets with equal numbers of patients in each subset; one subset was reserved as test data (to

**Table 2.** Questions included in the 'Sumi Questionnaire' (questions originally written in Japanese).

**Legibility of letters: letters**

1. Can you read the headlines of a newspaper? (Yes/With difficulty/No)

2. Can you read small print in a newspaper? (Yes/With difficulty/No)

3. Can you read words in a dictionary? (Yes/With difficulty/No)

4. Can you see the numbers in a telephone directory? (Yes/With difficulty/No)

5. Can you make out a fare table for trains and subways? (Yes/With difficulty/No)

**Sentences**

6. Do you have difficulty reading and writing? (No/Occasionally/Frequently)

7. When you write sentences in vertical lines, does it lean to either direction? (No/Occasionally/Frequently)

8. When you read, can you find the next line easily? (Yes/With difficulty/No)

**Walking**

9. Do you have difficulty walking because of your visual problems? (No/Occasionally/Frequently)

10. Can you take a walk by yourself? (Yes/With difficulty/No)

11. Do you misjudge traffic signals? (No/Occassionally/Frequently)

12. Do you bump into people or objects while walking? (No/Occasionally/Frequently)

13. Do you stumble on the stairs? (No/Occasionally/Frequently)

14. Do you fail to notice changes in the ground? (No/Occasionally/Frequently)

15. Do you fail to recognize your friends until they talk to you? (No/Occasionally/Frequently)

16. Do you fail to see people or cars approaching you from the side? (No/Occasionally/Frequently)

**Going out**

17. Do you have difficulty going out because of your visual problems? (No/Occasionally/Frequently)

18. Do you need somebody to accompany you to go to new places? (No/Preferably/Yes)

19. Can you get a cab by yourself? (Yes/With difficulty/No)

20. Do you have difficulty traveling by train? (No/Occasionally/Frequently)

21. Do you feel uneasy going out at night because of your visual problems? (No/Occasionally/Frequently)

**Dining**

22. Do you have difficulty dining because of your visual problems? (No/Occasionally/Frequently)

23. Do you drop food while dining because of your visual problems? (No/Occasionally/Frequently)

24. Do you spill tea while pouring into a cup? (No/Occasionally/Frequently)

25. Do you have difficulty using chopsticks? (No/Occasionally/Frequently)

**Dressing**

26. Do you ever button up clothing in the wrong order? (No/Occasionally/Frequently)

27. Can you see your face clearly in the mirror? (Yes/With difficulty/No)

**Miscellaneous**

28. Can you recognize people's faces on TV? (Yes/With difficulty/No)

29. Do you have difficulty finding objects dropped on the floor? (No/Occasionally/Frequently)

30. Do you have difficulty dialing the telephone? (No/Occasionally/Frequently)

calculate prediction errors), and models were generated using the remaining nine 'training data' subsets. This process was repeated ten times so that each of the ten subsets was used once as test data. The above procedure was repeated ten times in total so that the accuracy of each model was estimated 100 times. The differences in prediction errors between the two models were compared; Z-values with ten degrees of freedom were used to obtain p-values.

For comparison with the Random Forest method, a series of linear models were generated. VRQoLscores were regressed against a single predictor variable: (i) IVF MD; (ii) VA of better-eye; (iii) VA of worse-eye; and against multiple predictor variables: (iv) IVF TDs, and VAs of better- and worse-eyes (multiple linear regression).

The impact of reduced VA, and diminished VF sensitivity in different regions of the IVF, on each VRQoLtask was determined using the Random Forest 'Variable Importance' measure; this was calculated by randomly permuting a variable at each decision tree and measuring whether the squared errors decreased [30]. The rank of importance of IVF test points were identified for each VRQoL task and overall VRQoL.

All statistical analyses were carried out using the statistical programming language R (ver. 2.15.0, The R Foundation for Statistical Computing, Vienna, Austria) and the 'randomForest' package (ver. 4.6–6) [41].

|    |    |    |    | 1  | 2  | 3  | 4  |    |    |
|----|----|----|----|----|----|----|----|----|----|
|    |    | 5  | 6  | 7  | 8  | 9  | 10 |    |    |
|    | 11 | 12 | 13 | 14 | 15 | 16 | 17 | 18 |    |
| 19 | 20 | 21 | 22 | 23 | 24 | 25 | 26 | 27 | 28 |
| 29 | 30 | 31 | 32 | 33 | 34 | 35 | 36 | 37 | 38 |
| 39 | 40 | 41 | 42 | 43 | 44 | 45 | 46 | 47 | 48 |
| 49 | 50 | 51 | 52 | 53 | 54 | 55 | 56 | 57 | 58 |
|    | 59 | 60 | 61 | 62 | 63 | 64 | 65 | 66 |    |
|    |    | 67 | 68 | 69 | 70 | 71 | 72 |    |    |
|    |    |    | 73 | 74 | 75 | 76 |    |    |    |

**Figure 1. Integrated visual field test point locations.**

## Results

### Accuracy of Prediction of Vision-related Quality of Life

The RMSE associated with each model for each VRQoL task and overall VRQoL score are depicted in **Table 3**. Linear model prediction errors were smaller for the worse-eye VA compared with the better-eye VA, and significantly smaller for walking and going out tasks, and total VRQoL score (p-values were 0.33, 0.009, 0.02, 0.30, 0.07, for letters and sentences, walking, going out, dining, and total VRQoL, respectively). The RMSEs associated with the Random Forest method were significantly smaller than those by any other model for all tasks.

### Areas of the Visual Field Important for Vision-related Quality of Life

Worse-eye VA was the most important variable in all VRQoL tasks and for general VRQoL (**Table S1**). Better-eye VA was the third most important factor for all VRQoL tasks except walking (**Table S1**). IVF location 40 (see **Figure 1**) was the second most important variable for all tasks and general VRQoL (**Table S1**). Important VF test points varied, according to the task. The 26 most important VF test points (approximately one-third of all 76 points in the total VF) for each task are illustrated in **Figure 2**. To visualize the correspondence between the identified IVF test

locations and real life vision, IVF maps were superimposed onto photographs; distance to target was: 30 cm for the book as shown in **Figure 2a**, 5 m to the coffee shop flag as shown in **Figure 2b**, 5 m for the large information board shown in **Figure 2c**, and 40 cm for the plate of food shown in **Figure 2d**.

As suggested in **Figures 2a and 2b** and **Table S1 (online supplemental table)**, for the combined task of letters and sentences, and for the task of walking, important VF test points were concentrated along the horizontal meridian. In addition, test points in peripheral superior (10th, 11th, 13th and 20th important points) and inferior areas (5th and 21st important points) in the left hemifield were important for the letters and sentences task (**Figure 2a** and **Table S1**). For the task of walking, many test points ranked with high importance located in the peripheral, mid-peripheral and para-central inferior region (3rd, 4th, 6th, 9th, 13th and 14th important points) as well as test points along the horizontal meridian(**Figure 2b** and **Table S1**). For the task of going out, test points just beneath the horizontal meridian in the left and right hemifields and points in the peripheral superior region (2nd, 4th, 5th, 6th, 9th and 15th important points) were key points (**Figure 2c** and **Table S1**). For dining, important test points were scattered across the IVF, in addition to many test points along the horizontal meridian (**Figure 2d** and **Table S1**). The distribution of IVF test points important for overall VRQoL score was similar to that seen for the letters and sentences combined task (**Figure 2e**). Central test points within 5° of the fixation tended to be chosen as heavily important for the task of letters and sentences (4th, 9th and 14th important points) and walking (8th, 11th and 17th important points), but not for the task of going out and dining (only 18th and 20th important points, respectively) (**Figure 2** and **Table S1**).

## Discussion

In the current study, glaucoma patients' VRQoL was correlated with their IVF sensitivity and VA, and the Random Forest method yielded small prediction errors, compared to linear modeling approaches. We also identified the test points of the IVF that are most important for different daily tasks.

The linear model of worse-eye VA predicted VRQoL more accurately than the comparable models using better-eye VA or MD. Whether VA of better eye, or VA of worse eye, has a stronger influence on VRQoL remains controversial [7,9,11,15,42]. These previous reports investigated the influence of each index independently, however there is one study, that did analyze the VA of worse and better eyes simultaneously using multiple linear regression model and it has concluded that the VA of worse eye is more important for VRQoL [3]. Multiple linear regression does

**Table 3.** RMSE for each VRQoL task and overall VRQoL score.

| QoVL Task | VA (worse eye) | VA (better eye) | MD | MR | Random Forest |
|-----------|----------------|-----------------|-----|-----|---------------|
| 'Letters' and 'Sentences' | 0.98** | 1.03** | 0.94** | 1.38** | 0.84 |
| 'Walking' | 0.38** | 0.43** | 0.34** | 0.49** | 0.30 |
| 'Going out' | 0.40** | 0.46** | 0.42** | 0.54** | 0.32 |
| 'Dining' | 0.37* | 0.40** | 0.38* | 0.52** | 0.33 |
| Overall | 2.49** | 2.77** | 2.42** | 3.38** | 1.97 |

Each value is calculated as the absolute difference between predicted VRQoL score and the actual VRQoL score in the testing dataset in the leave-one-out cross validation. RMSE: root mean of the squared prediction error, VRQoL: vision-related quality of life, VA (worse-eye): visual acuity of the eye with worse mean deviation (MD), VA (better-eye): visual acuity of the eye with better MD, MR: Multiple regression with VA (better-eye), VA (worse-eye) and MD of IVF (Integrated Visual Field) (**: p<0.05, *: p<0.01, in comparison with Random Forest, ten fold cross validation).

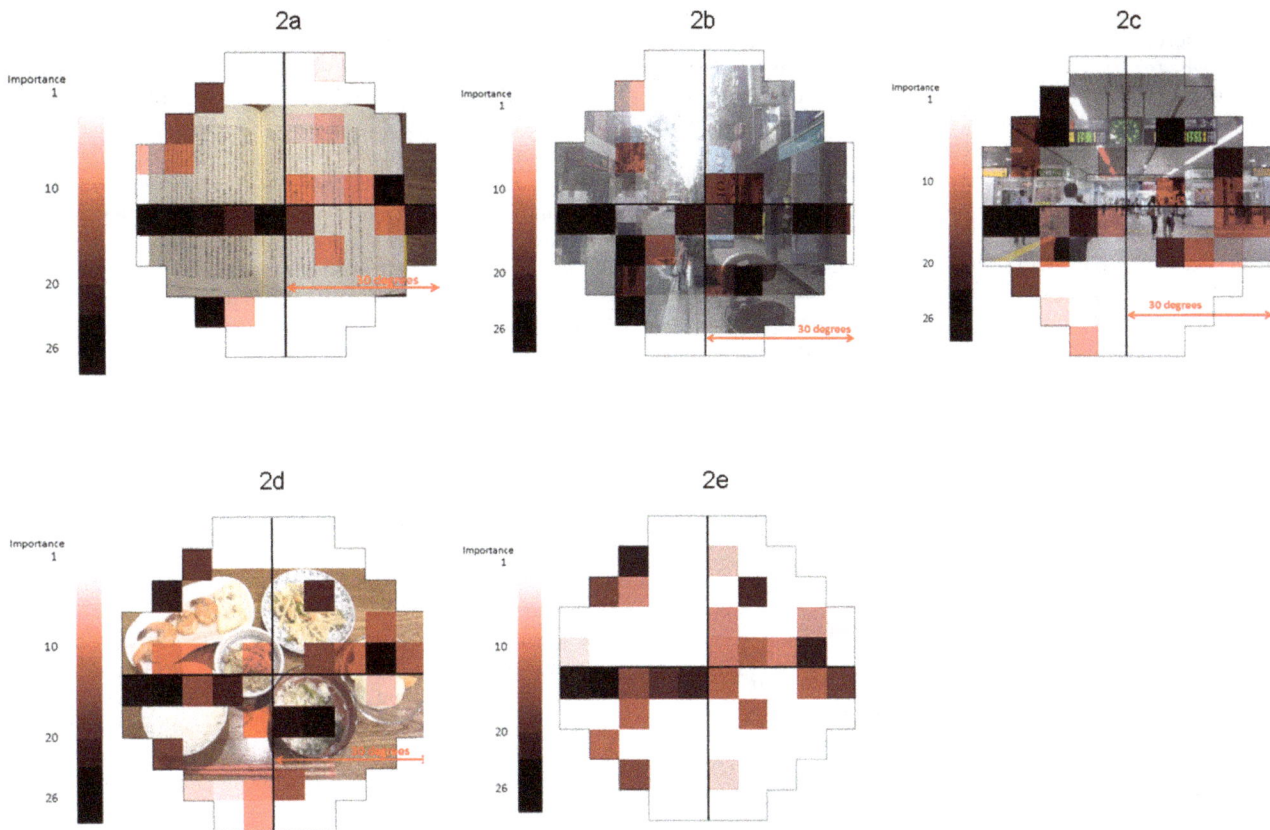

**Figure 2. Rank importance, where impairment at a point has a significant association with decreased vision-related quality of life.** The 26 important integrated visual field (IVF) test locations for each VRQoL task and overall VRQoL. IVF test points were superimposed onto an illustrative photograph corresponding to each task. The intensity of red increases according to the level of importance of each IVF test point. 1a: letters and sentences (viewing distance of 30 cm), 1b: walking (viewing distance of 5 m to the coffee shop flag, as viewed from the right hand side pavement, which is the walking direction in Japan), 1c: going out (viewing distance of 5 m to the information board), 1d: dining (viewing distance of 40 cm), 1e: total. Figure 2b has been edited to ensure anonymity of the people in it (the faces have been blurred) since written informed consent was not given.

not consider the influence of correlated predictor variables, and assumes independence; if this assumption is not valid, the importance of each variable is not accurately calculated. [43] For example, if two variables are closely related, the true influence of one of them will be masked by the other. Our results suggest that worse-eye VA tended to have a greater impact on VRQoL than better-eye VA; however, our results cannot be directly compared to previous reports because, in the current study, better- and worse-eye VA were defined using MD values, not VA directly.

The distribution of important test points for the total VRQoL score (**Figure 2e** and **Table S1**) became similar to that for combined letter and sentence task (**Figure 2a** and **Table S1**). One of the possible reasons for this similarity can be attributed to the large number of questionnaires in this task (eight in 30). In addition, difficulty with near vision tasks, such as reading, is a frequent complaint from visually-impaired persons [44], including glaucoma patients; moreover it was found to be the most important priority in glaucoma patients [45,46]. Sumi et al. reported that retinal sensitivity in the inferior hemifield within 5° of the fixation, and VA of better eye, are most closely correlated to a dissatisfaction regarding reading [15]. Our results also suggest that this area is important, however, other important test points were also identified in the peripheral region. Indeed there is a report which suggested even further peripheral region is important for reading; reading ability starts to deteriorate when

VF damage reaches to 50-degrees (with the II-4-e target in Goldmann perimetry)in patients with retinitis pigmentosa [47]. Our results suggest that it is very important to maintain VF sensitivity along the horizontal meridian, in particular in the left inferior hemifield, for the task of reading. In addition, test points in the inferior and superior peripheral regions in the left hemifield are also important (**Figure 2a** and **Table S1**). This finding is particularly interesting when we consider that Japanese literature is written in two directions: horizontally and vertically. When written horizontally, the first line begins at the top of the page, and each line is read left to right (exactly the same as English). When written vertically, the first line begins on the right hand side of the page, and is read top to bottom, and succeeding lines, to the left hand side, are then read in this manner. Thus, inferior and superior peripheral regions may play an important role in searching the next area of text when reading. In an eye movement tracking study, researchers found that in subjects reading 'Manga' (Japanese comics), which is written vertically, the eye fixation point moves rapidly from the bottom right hand side of the page to the top left hand side of the page, and restricting the viewing window to exclude these two areas resulted in reduced reading speeds [47,48]. Furthermore, these peripheral regions play an important role in searching when reading a large page, such as a newspaper. Also it is well known people carry out "search performance" using peripheral vision when they find out a place to focus [49]. Thus, it may be beneficial to be able to see the outer shape of a book or article before concentrating on the place to read, which may explain why the test points in the superior and inferior peripheral areas and left and right peripheral points along the horizontal meridian. Although the questionnaire used in the current study is identical to the one in Sumi et al. [15], the findings obtained were quite different with the most important VF test points distributed more widely across the IVF in our results. We propose that this may be attributed to our application of the Random Forest method in the current study, which can interpret IVF sensitivity and VA simultaneously, while not biasing the results.

Similarly to the combined task of letters and sentences, the IVF region along the horizontal meridian was also important for the task of walking. The test points in the central area within 5° of fixation were given high importance, however, interestingly, we found that there were many test points with higher importance rank in the peripheral and mid-peripheral areas in the inferior hemifield (**Figure 2b**) rather than the test points in the central region, in contrary to Sumi's report which suggested the central area is most important for this task. [15]. This may be because the visual function in the central area is compensated by VA, and so the key IVF locations are instead scattered in the inferior peripheral region. This finding is also in agreement with a previous study which suggested the importance of this area for postural stability [17]. Many reports have suggested that people with glaucoma walk more slowly than people without ocular disease [50,51]. Our results suggest that glaucoma patients with VF deterioration in the inferior peripheral area should be advised about walking problems. This is clinically important, because it has been reported that the risk of hip fractures is increased in glaucoma patients [52].

The task of 'going out' is unique to the Sumi questionnaire. This task mainly addresses the ability to find targets when travelling, such as information boards or tube maps at a train station, or a traffic signal when crossing a road. In metropolitan areas, such as Tokyo, it is very common to use public transportation rather than a private motor car, hence we would expect this particular task has a significant implication upon a person's quality of life. These targets usually need to be viewed from a long distance and are often located in a high position. With this in mind, it is very interesting that many test points in the upper peripheral and mid-peripheral IVF regions were selected as highly important, in addition to IVF points along the horizontal meridian and test points in the central area within 5° of the fixation were not selected with heavy importance which disagree with what reported by Sumi et al [15].

For the task of dining, IVF points along the horizontal meridian (left and right peripheral areas) and test points in the paracentral area in the inferior right hemifield were given high importance, as well as other peripheral areas. As shown in the **Figure 2d**, these test points overlap to rice bowl (1st, 4th, 7th, 10th, 12th, 17th and 19th important points), miso soup (2nd, 5th and 16th important points), main dish (7th and 19th), side dishes (6th, 9th, 11th, 19th, and 8th, 11th, 16th, and 3rd, 14th, 15th, 16th, 23rd important points) and chop sticks (13th, 21st, 24th and 25th important points). Interestingly this is not in agreement with Sumi et al. [15], where test points in the central area were selected as most important. In traditional Japanese dining, the rice bowl is held in the left hand. During eating, the rice bowl is repeatedly picked up and put down in one's left hand. This may explain why the selected IVF regions in **Figure 2d** are important for dining. In Western countries, we would expect that different IVF regions are more important, most likely the central area.

The VRQoL score observed for each different task is independent yet test point 40 was given the second highest importance for all of the tasks and overall VRQoL score as shown in Figure 2, and neighboring points were also given relatively high ranks. This suggests that test points just beneath the horizontal meridian in the left hemifield are important for many tasks in daily life and careful attention should be made when clinicians see patients with VF damage in this area.

Several classification tools, such as support vector machines, could also have been used for the purpose of this research. Previous reports support the use of the Random Forest method [53–55], however, future work is necessary to investigate which method is most appropriate to analyze the relationship between visual function and VRQoL. A limitation of the current study is that the Sumi Questionnaire does not include questions about driving. Outside of metropolitan areas like Tokyo, driving is an important feature of daily life, hence this task should be addressed in a future study. Another limitation in the current study is that we have merged the tasks of 'letters' and 'words' since the questions in these sections are very be similar in content, however, this has not been validated so this should be investigated in future. An important caveat of this study is that the most important VF test locations for different VRQoL tasks may be different in advanced glaucoma patients. A further study should be carried out in a sample of advanced glaucoma patients with a more constricted VF and damage near fixation, because more central areas (near fixation) of the VF could be more important in these patients. Conversely, the same study carried out in an early stage glaucomatous population would also be beneficial, because the deterioration of VRQoL in these patients may be attributed to different location areas of the VF.

## Conclusion

In conclusion, we have analyzed the relationship between VF sensitivity and VA, and VRQoL. The Random Forest method takes into account the interrelationships of the data and gives an accurate prediction of VRQoL. Most importantly, the model enables clinicians to better understand patients' VRQoL based on standard clinical measurements. Furthermore, VF test points critical for different daily tasks and VRQoL were identified. These results will help clinicians to concentrate on these regions when managing patients, and offer appropriate advice if these areas are damaged. These findings should be considered when welfare policy is decided by public administration, such as positioning information boards in a train station, and providing walking guides for the visually disabled. Moreover, this prediction system could be used to estimate VRQoL for the different tasks of daily life for a given patient, using only conventional VA and VF measurements.

## Supporting Information

**Table S1 The rank of the importance of integrated visual field (IVF) test points, visual acuities of better and worse eyes, gender and age.** The numbers represent the IVF test point locations (see Figure 1). VA (worse-eye): visual acuity of the eye with worse mean deviation (MD) and VA (better-eye): visual acuity of the eye with better MD.

## Author Contributions

Gave advice from the viewpoint of glaucoma specialist: YA KS M. Aihara CM M. Araie. Conceived and designed the experiments: RA HM. Performed the experiments: HH RA HM. Analyzed the data: HM RA. Contributed reagents/materials/analysis tools: HM RA HH. Wrote the paper: HM RA.

# References

1. Asaoka R, Crabb DP, Yamashita T, Russell RA, Wang YX, et al. (2011) Patients have two eyes!: binocular versus better eye visual field indices. Invest Ophthalmol Vis Sci 52: 7007–7011.

2. McKean-Cowdin R, Varma R, Wu J, Hays RD, Azen SP (2007) Severity of visual field loss and health-related quality of life. Am J Ophthalmol 143: 1013–1023.

3. Hyman LG, Komaroff E, Heijl A, Bengtsson B, Leske MC (2005) Treatment and vision-related quality of life in the early manifest glaucoma trial. Ophthalmology 112: 1505–1513.

4. Altangerel U, Spaeth GL, Rhee DJ (2003) Visual function, disability, and psychological impact of glaucoma. Curr Opin Ophthalmol 14: 100–105.

5. Nelson P, Aspinall P, Papasouliotis O, Worton B, O'Brien C (2003) Quality of life in glaucoma and its relationship with visual function. J Glaucoma 12: 139–150.

6. Ringsdorf L, McGwin G Jr, Owsley C (2006) Visual field defects and vision-specific health-related quality of life in African Americans and whites with glaucoma. J Glaucoma 15: 414–418.

7. Janz NK, Wren PA, Lichter PR, Musch DC, Gillespie BW, et al. (2001) Quality of life in newly diagnosed glaucoma patients : The Collaborative Initial Glaucoma Treatment Study. Ophthalmology 108: 887–897; discussion 898.

8. Odberg T, Jakobsen JE, Hultgren SJ, Halseide R (2001) The impact of glaucoma on the quality of life of patients in Norway. II. Patient response correlated to objective data. Acta Ophthalmol Scand 79: 121–124.

9. Sherwood MB, Garcia-Siekavizza A, Meltzer MI, Hebert A, Burns AF, et al. (1998) Glaucoma's impact on quality of life and its relation to clinical indicators. A pilot study. Ophthalmology 105: 561–566.

10. Parrish RK 2nd, Gedde SJ, Scott IU, Feuer WJ, Schiffman JC, et al. (1997) Visual function and quality of life among patients with glaucoma. Arch Ophthalmol 115: 1447–1455.

11. Gutierrez P, Wilson MR, Johnson C, Gordon M, Cioffi GA, et al. (1997) Influence of glaucomatous visual field loss on health-related quality of life. Arch Ophthalmol 115: 777–784.

12. Wilson MR, Coleman AL, Yu F, Bing EG, Sasaki IF, et al. (1998) Functional status and well-being in patients with glaucoma as measured by the Medical Outcomes Study Short Form-36 questionnaire. Ophthalmology 105: 2112–2116.

13. Varma R, Wu J, Chong K, Azen SP, Hays RD (2006) Impact of severity and bilaterality of visual impairment on health-related quality of life. Ophthalmology 113: 1846–1853.

14. West SK, Rubin GS, Broman AT, Munoz B, Bandeen-Roche K, et al. (2002) How does visual impairment affect performance on tasks of everyday life? The SEE Project. Salisbury Eye Evaluation. Arch Ophthalmol 120: 774–780.

15. Sumi I, Shirato S, Matsumoto S, Araie M (2003) The relationship between visual disability and visual field in patients with glaucoma. Ophthalmology 110: 332–339.

16. Crabb DP, Smith ND, Rauscher FG, Chisholm CM, Barbur JL, et al. (2010) Exploring eye movements in patients with glaucoma when viewing a driving scene. PLoS One 5: e9710.

17. Black AA, Wood JM, Lovie-Kitchin JE, Newman BM (2008) Visual impairment and postural sway among older adults with glaucoma. Optom Vis Sci 85: 489–497.

18. Kotecha A, O'Leary N, Melmoth D, Grant S, Crabb DP (2009) The functional consequences of glaucoma for eye-hand coordination. Invest Ophthalmol Vis Sci 50: 203–213.

19. Haymes SA, Leblanc RP, Nicolela MT, Chiasson LA, Chauhan BC (2007) Risk of falls and motor vehicle collisions in glaucoma. Invest Ophthalmol Vis Sci 48: 1149–1155.

20. Bowers A, Peli E, Elgin J, McGwin G Jr, Owsley C (2005) On-road driving with moderate visual field loss. Optom Vis Sci 82: 657–667.

21. Haymes SA, LeBlanc RP, Nicolela MT, Chiasson LA, Chauhan BC (2008) Glaucoma and on-road driving performance. Invest Ophthalmol Vis Sci 49: 3035–3041.

22. Ramulu P (2009) Glaucoma and disability: which tasks are affected, and at what stage of disease? Curr Opin Ophthalmol 20: 92–98.

23. McGwin G, Jr, Xie A, Mays A, Joiner W, DeCarlo DK, et al. (2005) Visual field defects and the risk of motor vehicle collisions among patients with glaucoma. Invest Ophthalmol Vis Sci 46: 4437–4441.

24. Coleman AL, Cummings SR, Ensrud KE, Yu F, Gutierrez P, et al. (2009) Visual field loss and risk of fractures in older women. J Am Geriatr Soc 57: 1825–1832.

25. Caprioli J, Spaeth GL (1984) Comparison of visual field defects in the low-tension glaucomas with those in the high-tension glaucomas. Am J Ophthalmol 97: 730–737.

26. Hitchings RA, Anderton SA (1983) A comparative study of visual field defects seen in patients with low-tension glaucoma and chronic simple glaucoma. Br J Ophthalmol 67: 818–821.

27. Zeyen TG, Zulauf M, Caprioli J (1993) Priority of test locations for automated perimetry in glaucoma. Ophthalmology 100: 518–522; discussion 523.

28. Lachenmayr BJ, Kiermeir U, Kojetinsky S (1995) Points of a normal visual field are not statistically independent. Ger J Ophthalmol 4: 175–181.

29. Suzuki Y, Araie M, Ohashi Y (1993) Sectorization of the central 30 degrees visual field in glaucoma. Ophthalmology 100: 69–75.

30. Breiman L (2001) Random Forests. Machine Learning 45: 5–32.

31. Strobl C, Boulesteix AL, Kneib T, Augustin T, Zeileis A (2008) Conditional variable importance for random forests. BMC Bioinformatics 9: 307.

32. Lunetta KL, Hayward LB, Segal J, Van Eerdewegh P (2004) Screening large-scale association study data: exploiting interactions using random forests. BMC Genet 5: 32.

33. Segal MR, Cummings MP, Hubbard AE (2001) Relating amino acid sequence to phenotype: analysis of peptide-binding data. Biometrics 57: 632–642.

34. Bengtsson B, Heijl A (2000) False-negative responses in glaucoma perimetry: indicators of patient performance or test reliability? Invest Ophthalmol Vis Sci 41: 2201–2204.

35. Viswanathan AC, McNaught AI, Poinoosawmy D, Fontana L, Crabb DP, et al. (1999) Severity and stability of glaucoma: patient perception compared with objective measurement. Arch Ophthalmol 117: 450–454.

36. Crabb DP, Viswanathan AC, McNaught AI, Poinoosawmy D, Fitzke FW, et al. (1998) Simulating binocular visual field status in glaucoma. Br J Ophthalmol 82: 1236–1241.

37. Crabb DP, Fitzke FW, Hitchings RA, Viswanathan AC (2004) A practical approach to measuring the visual field component of fitness to drive. Br J Ophthalmol 88: 1191–1196.

38. Nelson-Quigg JM, Cello K, Johnson CA (2000) Predicting binocular visual field sensitivity from monocular visual field results. Invest Ophthalmol Vis Sci 41: 2212–2221.

39. Japkowicz N (2011) Evaluating Learning Algorithms: A Classification Perspective. Cambridge, UK: Cambridge University Press.

40. Bouckaert RR (2003) Choosing Between Two Learning Algorithms Based on Calibrated Tests. Proc Int Conf Mach Learn: 51–58.

41. Liaw A, Wiener M (2002) Classification and Regression by randomForest. R News 2(3), 18–22.

42. Magacho L, Lima FE, Nery AC, Sagawa A, Magacho B, et al. (2004) Quality of life in glaucoma patients: regression analysis and correlation with possible modifiers. Ophthalmic Epidemiol 11: 263–270.

43. Maindonald J, Braun WJ (2010) Data analysis and graphics using R. An example-based approach (Cambridge Series in Statistical and Probabilistic Mathematics) 3rd edn. Cambridge, UK: Cambridge University Press.

44. Mangione CM, Berry S, Spritzer K, Janz NK, Klein R, et al. (1998) Identifying the content area for the 51-item National Eye Institute Visual Function Questionnaire: results from focus groups with visually impaired persons. Arch Ophthalmol 116: 227–233.

45. Aspinall PA, Johnson ZK, Azuara-Blanco A, Montarzino A, Brice R, et al. (2008) Evaluation of quality of life and priorities of patients with glaucoma. Invest Ophthalmol Vis Sci 49: 1907–1915.

46. Burr JM, Kilonzo M, Vale L, Ryan M (2007) Developing a preference-based Glaucoma Utility Index using a discrete choice experiment. Optom Vis Sci 84: 797–808.

47. Szlyk JP, Seiple W, Fishman GA, Alexander KR, Grover S, et al. (2001) Perceived and actual performance of daily tasks: relationship to visual function tests in individuals with retinitis pigmentosa. Ophthalmology 108: 65–75.

48. Ishii T, Igaki T, Kurata K, Omori T, Masuda N (2003) Toward an integrated methodology for the study of the mind. Annual Report of Grant-in-Aid for Scientific Research, Grant-in-Aid for Scientific Research (C) Tokyo, Japan: Japan Society for the Promotion of Science: 107–113.

49. Rosenholtz R, Huang J, Raj A, Balas BJ, Ilie L (2012) A summary statistic representation in peripheral vision explains visual search. J Vis 12.

50. Turano KA, Rubin GS, Quigley HA (1999) Mobility performance in glaucoma. Invest Ophthalmol Vis Sci 40: 2803–2809.

51. Friedman DS, Freeman E, Munoz B, Jampel HD, West SK (2007) Glaucoma and mobility performance: the Salisbury Eye Evaluation Project. Ophthalmology 114: 2232–2237.

52. White SC, Atchison KA, Gornbein JA, Nattiv A, Paganini-Hill A, et al. (2006) Risk factors for fractures in older men and women: The Leisure World Cohort Study. Gend Med 3: 110–123.

53. Maroco J, Silva D, Rodrigues A, Guerreiro M, Santana I, et al. (2011) Data mining methods in the prediction of Dementia: A real-data comparison of the accuracy, sensitivity and specificity of linear discriminant analysis, logistic regression, neural networks, support vector machines, classification trees and random forests. BMC Res Notes 4: 299.

54. Diaz-Uriarte R, Alvarez de Andres S (2006) Gene selection and classification of microarray data using random forest. BMC Bioinformatics 7: 3.

55. Douglas PK, Harris S, Yuille A, Cohen MS (2011) Performance comparison of machine learning algorithms and number of independent components used in fMRI decoding of belief vs. disbelief. Neuroimage 56: 544–553.

# 10

# Persistence, Spatial Distribution and Implications for Progression Detection of Blind Parts of the Visual Field in Glaucoma

**Francisco G. Junoy Montolio**[1,9], **Christiaan Wesselink**[1,9], **Nomdo M. Jansonius**[1,2]*

**1** Dept. of Ophthalmology, University Medical Center Groningen, University of Groningen, Groningen, The Netherlands, **2** Dept. of Epidemiology, Erasmus Medical Center, Rotterdam, The Netherlands

## Abstract

*Background:* Visual field testing is an essential part of glaucoma care. It is hampered by variability related to the disease itself, response errors and fatigue. In glaucoma, blind parts of the visual field contribute to the diagnosis but - once established – not to progression detection; they only increase testing time. The aims of this study were to describe the persistence and spatial distribution of blind test locations in standard automated perimetry in glaucoma and to explore how the omission of presumed blind test locations would affect progression detection.

*Methodology/Principal Findings:* Data from 221 eyes of 221 patients from a cohort study with the Humphrey Field Analyzer with 30–2 grid were used. Patients were stratified according to baseline mean deviation (MD) in six strata of 5 dB width each. For one, two, three and four consecutive <0 dB sensitivities in the same test location in a series of baseline tests, the median probabilities to observe <0 dB again in the concerning test location in a follow-up test were 76, 86, 88 and 90%, respectively. For <10 dB, the probabilities were 88, 95, 97 and 98%, respectively. Median (interquartile range) percentages of test locations with three consecutive <0 dB sensitivities were 0(0–0), 0(0–2), 4(0–9), 17(8–27), 27(20–40) and 60(50–70)% for the six MD strata. Similar percentages were found for a subset of test locations within 10 degree eccentricity (P>0.1 for all strata). Omitting test locations with three consecutive <0 dB sensitivities at baseline did not affect the performance of the MD-based Nonparametric Progression Analysis progression detection algorithm.

*Conclusions/Significance:* Test locations that have been shown to be reproducibly blind tend to display a reasonable blindness persistence and do no longer contribute to progression detection. There is no clinically useful universal MD cut-off value beyond which testing can be limited to 10 degree eccentricity.

**Editor:** Bang V. Bui, Univeristy of Melbourne, Australia

**Funding:** This research was supported by the University Medical Center Groningen and the foundation 'Stichting Nederlands Oogheelkundig Onderzoek', all in the Netherlands. The funders had no role in study design, data collection and analysis, decision to publish, or preparation of the manuscript.

**Competing Interests:** The authors have declared that no competing interests exist.

* E-mail: n.m.jansonius@umcg.nl

⑨ These authors contributed equally to this work.

## Introduction

Glaucoma is a progressive disease that may cause irreversible blindness. Monitoring of the disease with perimetry is an essential part of glaucoma care, unless patients have a short life expectancy and little glaucomatous damage. Variability hampers the use of perimetry in detecting small changes in visual function. In glaucoma, variability is presumably related to response errors, fatigue effects [1,2] and a flatter frequency-of-seeing curve in regions with a reduced sensitivity [3,4]. The development of the Swedish Interactive Threshold Algorithm (SITA) strategies for the Humphrey Field Analyzer (HFA) has partially resolved the fatigue issue by reducing the test time [5].

SITA reduces the test time, amongst others, by predicting the sensitivity in a test location from the sensitivity in neighboring test locations and by incorporating general knowledge on glaucomatous visual field patterns. However, SITA ignores an obvious other source of prior knowledge, being the previous test result. The use

of the previous test result can reduce test time [6,7] and test-retest variability [8]. To illustrate this, for a typical glaucomatous visual field, that is, a blind superior hemifield together with an intact inferior hemifield, the test time of SITA is about 1.5 times longer than for a normal field. Hence, to establish blindness in a test location takes twice as long as establishing a normal sensitivity – and thus a 33% test-time reduction should be possible by incorporating information from previous tests. This is in agreement with earlier findings [7]. To go one step further, if the superior hemifield would have been unresponsive on several consecutive occasions, it makes no sense to test it again: only the inferior hemifield needs to be tested to monitor the eye. Hence, a 67% test-time reduction would ultimately be possible in this case.

The aims of this study were (1) to describe the persistence and spatial distribution of blind test locations in standard automated perimetry in glaucoma and (2) to explore how the omission of presumed blind test locations would affect progression detection.

**Table 1.** Example of two patients as represented in the database, with two and eight test locations with a sensitivity of <0 dB in the fourth visual field, respectively.

| Patient | VF1 (dB) | VF2 (dB) | VF3 (dB) | VF4 (dB) | VF5 (dB) | VF6 (dB) | VF7 (dB) | VF8 (dB) | Position on VF | % <0 dB | Mean (dB) |
|---|---|---|---|---|---|---|---|---|---|---|---|
| 1 | 4 | 4 | 6 | <0 | 0 | 0 | 0 | 11 | 4 | 0 | 2.75 |
| 1 | <0 | <0 | <0 | <0 | <0 | 2 | <0 | 18 | 9 | 50 | 4.00 |
| 2 | 12 | 3 | 11 | <0 | <0 | <0 | 13 | 10 | 1 | 50 | 4.75 |
| 2 | 20 | 0 | 5 | <0 | <0 | <0 | 9 | 0 | 2 | 50 | 1.25 |
| 2 | <0 | <0 | <0 | <0 | <0 | 3 | <0 | <0 | 19 | 75 | −0.75 |
| 2 | 15 | 12 | <0 | <0 | 11 | <0 | <0 | 4 | 20 | 50 | 2.75 |
| 2 | 20 | 2 | <0 | <0 | <0 | 1 | <0 | <0 | 30 | 75 | −1.25 |
| 2 | 21 | <0 | 6 | <0 | 16 | <0 | <0 | 4 | 31 | 50 | 4.00 |
| 2 | 26 | 12 | 4 | <0 | 10 | 4 | 5 | 0 | 33 | 0 | 4.75 |
| 2 | <0 | 3 | <0 | <0 | <0 | 10 | <0 | <0 | 35 | 75 | 1.00 |

VF = visual field; columns VF1-VF4 refer to baseline, VF5-VF8 to follow-up; last two columns depict the data analysis as applied to the follow-up data (for details see text).

For the first aim, we determined the probability to observe a sensitivity below a certain value as a function of the number of preceding consecutive sensitivities below that value in the concerning test location. This was evaluated for <0, <5, <10 and <20 dB. The value <0 dB corresponds to the maximum stimulus intensity of the HFA perimeter; the values <5 and <10 dB approximately to the maximum stimulus intensities of the Octopus and Oculus perimeters, respectively. Subsequently, we compared the percentages of blind test locations between the regular standard automated perimetry 30–2 grid (with test locations up to 30 degree eccentricity) and the subset of test locations falling within the 10–2 grid (up to 10 degree eccentricity), as a function of disease stage as defined by the mean deviation (MD). The aim here was to determine a clinically useful MD cut-off value for preferring 10–2 testing over 30–2 testing in advanced glaucoma. After all, although glaucoma sometimes starts close to fixation [9,10], it is conceptually a disease affecting the peripheral visual field first and thus a transition from 30–2 to 10–2 testing would be the easiest way to avoid uninformative testing of unresponsive parts of the visual field in advanced disease. For the second aim, we studied the performance of an MD-based progression detection algorithm with and without assuming blind test locations as established at baseline to be blind in all follow-up fields.

## Methods

### Ethics Statement

The study protocol was approved by the ethics board of the University Medical Center Groningen. This board approved that for the current study no informed consent had to be obtained because the study comprised a retrospective anonymous analysis of visual field data collected during regular glaucoma care. To ensure a proper glaucoma diagnosis of the included patients, we limited the study population of this study to glaucoma patients that had been included in the Groningen Longitudinal Glaucoma Study (GLGS) in the past. In the GLGS, all glaucoma patients and glaucoma suspects who visited the glaucoma outpatient service of the University Medical Center Groningen between July 1, 2000, and June 30, 2001, and who provided informed consent were included in an observational study with conventional perimetry, frequency-

**Table 2.** Patient characteristics for all included 221 eyes of 221 patients and for the subset of 53 eyes of 53 patients with at least eight visual field tests and at least one test location showing a <0 dB sensitivity on four consecutive baseline tests (mean with standard deviation between brackets unless stated otherwise).

| | N = 221 | N = 53 |
|---|---|---|
| **Baseline** | | |
| Age (years) | 65.1 (12.3) | 65.1 (10.3) |
| Gender (% male) | 55.2 | 45.3 |
| Right eye (%) | 50.7 | 52.8 |
| Mean Deviation (median [interquartile range]; dB) | −7.0 (−14.5 to −3.0) | −14.7 (−18.7 to −10.9) |
| **Follow-up** | | |
| Follow-up duration (years) | 6.4 (1.2) | 6.9 (1.0) |
| Rate of progression (median [interquartile range]; dB/year) | −0.1 (−0.5 to +0.1) | −0.2 (−0.5 to 0.0) |
| Square root of the residual mean square of Mean Deviation (dB) | 1.1 (0.7) | 1.2 (0.7) |

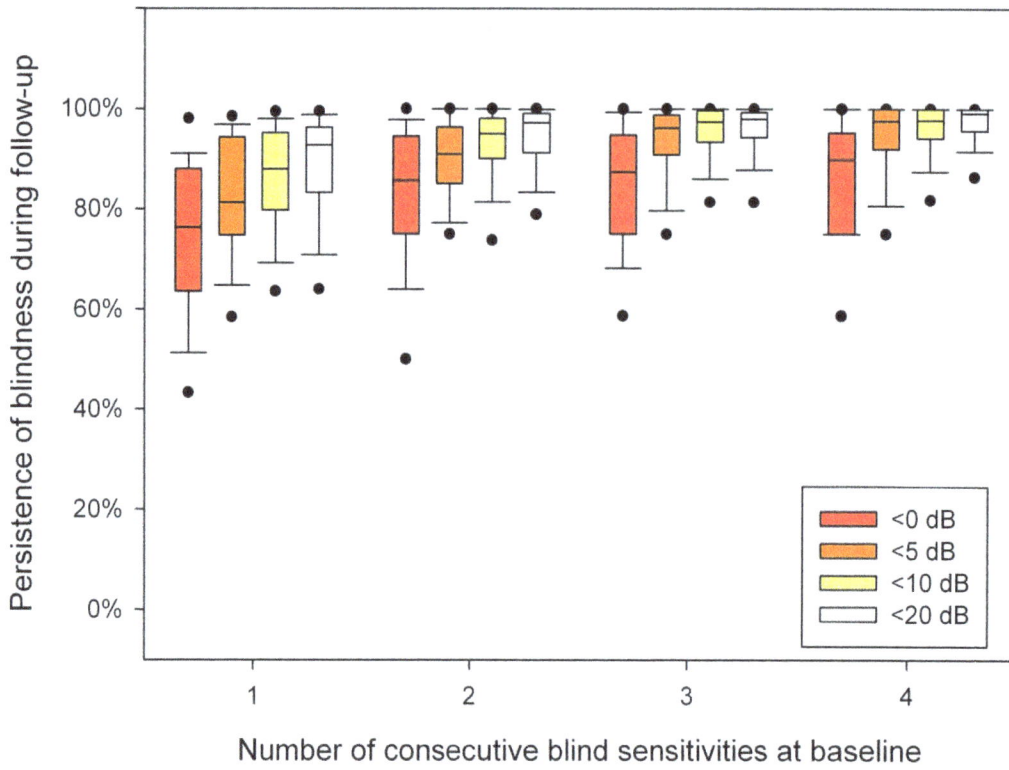

**Figure 1. Percentage of follow-up sensitivities being <0, <5, <10 and <20 dB as a function of the number of consecutive <0, <5, <10 and <20 dB baseline sensitivities.** Boxplots show median, interquartile range, and 5th, 10th, 90th and 95th percentiles.

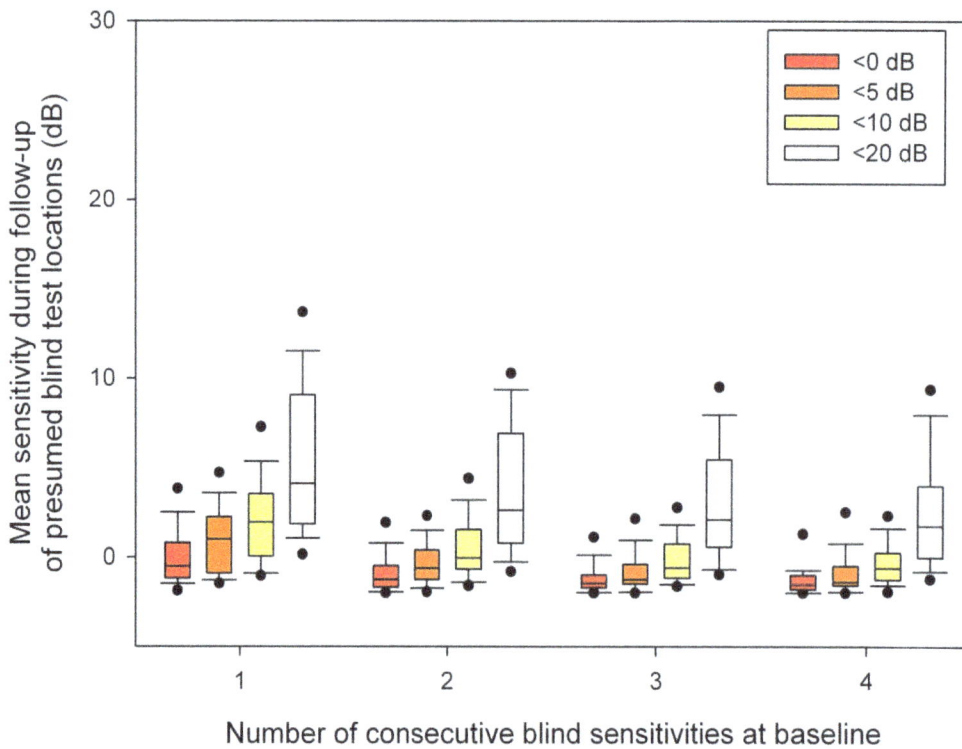

**Figure 2. Mean sensitivity during follow-up in test locations with 1, 2, 3 and 4 consecutive <0, <5, <10 and <20 dB baseline sensitivities.** Boxplots show median, interquartile range, and 5th, 10th, 90th and 95th percentiles.

**Table 3.** Analysis of variance with the number of consecutive tests showing blindness in a test location (N) and the definition of 'perimetrically blind' (B) as within-subject factors and the persistence of blindness as dependent variable.

| | df | MS | dfe | MSe | F | P |
|---|---|---|---|---|---|---|
| mean | 1 | 680.65 | 52 | 0.08460 | 8045 | <0.001 |
| N | 3 | 0.47354 | 156 | 0.00702 | 67 | <0.001 |
| B | 3 | 0.57498 | 156 | 0.01089 | 53 | <0.001 |
| N*B | 9 | 0.00547 | 468 | 0.00161 | 3 | <0.001 |

df = degrees of freedom; MS = mean squares (MS = SS/df with SS = sum of squares); dfe is df for error; MSe = mean squares for error.

doubling perimetry (FDT; Carl Zeiss Meditec AG, Jena, Germany) and laser polarimetry (GDx; Laser Diagnostic Technologies, San Diego, California, USA). Patients received written information at home at least two weeks before their regular care visit that was flagged as the baseline visit of the study. The receipt of the information and agreement to participate was checked verbally during the concerning visit. The aim of the study was explained; participation was voluntary and participation could be stopped also after having agreed to participate. The study essentially comprised the collection of regular care data obtained during regular visits and an additional FDT and GDx test embedded in a regular visit. FDT and GDx are non-invasive diagnostic tests with a very limited additional burden and no additional risk for the patient. The protocol of the original GLGS was approved by the department of Medical Technology Assessment of the University of Groningen. The original health technology assessment research question was if it was possible to replace, in glaucoma patients and/or glaucoma suspects, the lengthy and cumbersome conventional perimetry by FDT and/or GDx. The study followed the tenets of the Declaration of Helsinki.

## Study Population

Details of the GLGS have been described earlier [11,12]. In short, after the initial health technology assessment study described above, we continued performing conventional perimetry in glaucoma patients and moved to FDT/GDx in glaucoma suspects in our regular care. The GLGS continued as an ongoing anonymous gathering of all information from glaucoma patients and glaucoma suspects obtained during regular care. For the present study, we used data from a subpopulation of the GLGS cohort: patients had to have (1) glaucoma at baseline (for criteria see below) and (2) at least four (five with discarded learning test) standard automated perimetry tests (HFA; Carl Zeiss Meditec Inc., Dublin, CA).

## Perimetry

Perimetry was performed using the HFA 30–2 SITA fast strategy. For glaucoma, two consecutive, reliable tests had to have defects according to previously published criteria [11,12]. For being reproducible, defects had to be in the same hemifield and at least one depressed test point of these defects had to have exactly the same location on both tests. Moreover, defects had to be compatible with glaucoma and without any other explanation (for example, cataract, macular degeneration or lesions of the central visual pathways). Prior to these two tests, another test had to be made and this test was excluded to reduce the influence of

learning. During the follow-up period, perimetry was performed at a frequency of one test per year. In case of suspected progression or unreliable test results, clinicians could increase the frequency of testing. This was a subjective decision; no formal tools or rules were given (observational study design).

## Data analysis

One eye per patient was included. If both eyes met the above-described criteria, one eye was chosen randomly. For anatomical representation, all left-eye threshold data were converted to a right-eye format. Thresholds representing the blind-spot were excluded from the analysis, leaving 74 tests locations for analysis.

**Persistence of blindness.** For this analysis we only included patients who (1) performed at least eight tests and (2) had at least one test location showing a <0 dB sensitivity on four consecutive baseline tests (most stringent criterion for blindness). We defined four subgroups of test locations, based on the first four tests and named VF4<0, VF3-4<0, VF2-4<0 and VF1-4<0. A test location VF4<0 had to have a sensitivity of <0 dB in the fourth visual field test. A test location VF3-4<0 had to have a sensitivity of <0 dB in both the third and the fourth test, and so on. For VF4<0, the sensitivity of the test location in the third test may or may not be <0 dB. Hence, VF3-4<0 is a subset of VF4<0, and so on. We took the fourth test as a reference in order to be able to vary the number of baseline tests without the need of changing the selection of the four follow-up tests, which were the fifth to eighth test.

For all test locations with a sensitivity of <0 dB in the fourth test, we analyzed the corresponding sensitivities in the four follow-up tests. Outcome measures were (1) the percentage of follow-up tests showing a sensitivity of <0 dB and (2) the mean sensitivity. Here, test locations with <0 dB were set at -2 dB. This is the arbitrary interpretation of <0 dB as chosen by the manufacturer. For patients, the difference between 0 dB and <0 dB implies seeing the maximum light stimulus of the perimeter (0 dB) or not (<0 dB).

Test locations within a single subject cannot be considered independent. Therefore, to avoid that a few patients with many blind test locations would dominate the results, we first determined the averages and corresponding standard deviations of the outcome measures within each patient for each subgroup of test locations (VF4<0, VF3-4<0, VF2-4<0 and VF1-4<0). Subsequently, the averages were presented using nonparametric descriptive statistics and the standard deviations of the first outcome measure were averaged over all patients and presented as the "mean within-patient standard deviation".

Table 1 gives an example of two patients as represented in the database. These patients are present in the VF4<0 subgroup with two and eight test locations, respectively. The first patient is also present in the VF3-4<0, VF2-4<0 and VF1-4<0 subgroups, with one test location. The second patient is present in these subgroups with four, one and one test locations, respectively. For the first patient, blindness persistence was 25% for the VF4<0 subgroup and 50% for the VF3-4<0, VF2-4<0 and VF1-4<0 subgroups. For the second patient, this was 53, 69, 75 and 75% for the VF4<0, VF3-4<0, VF2-4<0 and VF1-4<0 subgroups, respectively.

The analyzes were repeated with blindness of a test location defined as a sensitivity of <5, <10 and <20 dB instead of <0 dB. The influence of the number of consecutive tests (1, 2, 3 or 4) showing blindness in a test location and the definition of blindness (<0, <5, <10 or <20 dB) on the persistence of blindness was analyzed with ANOVA, with the persistence of blindness (average

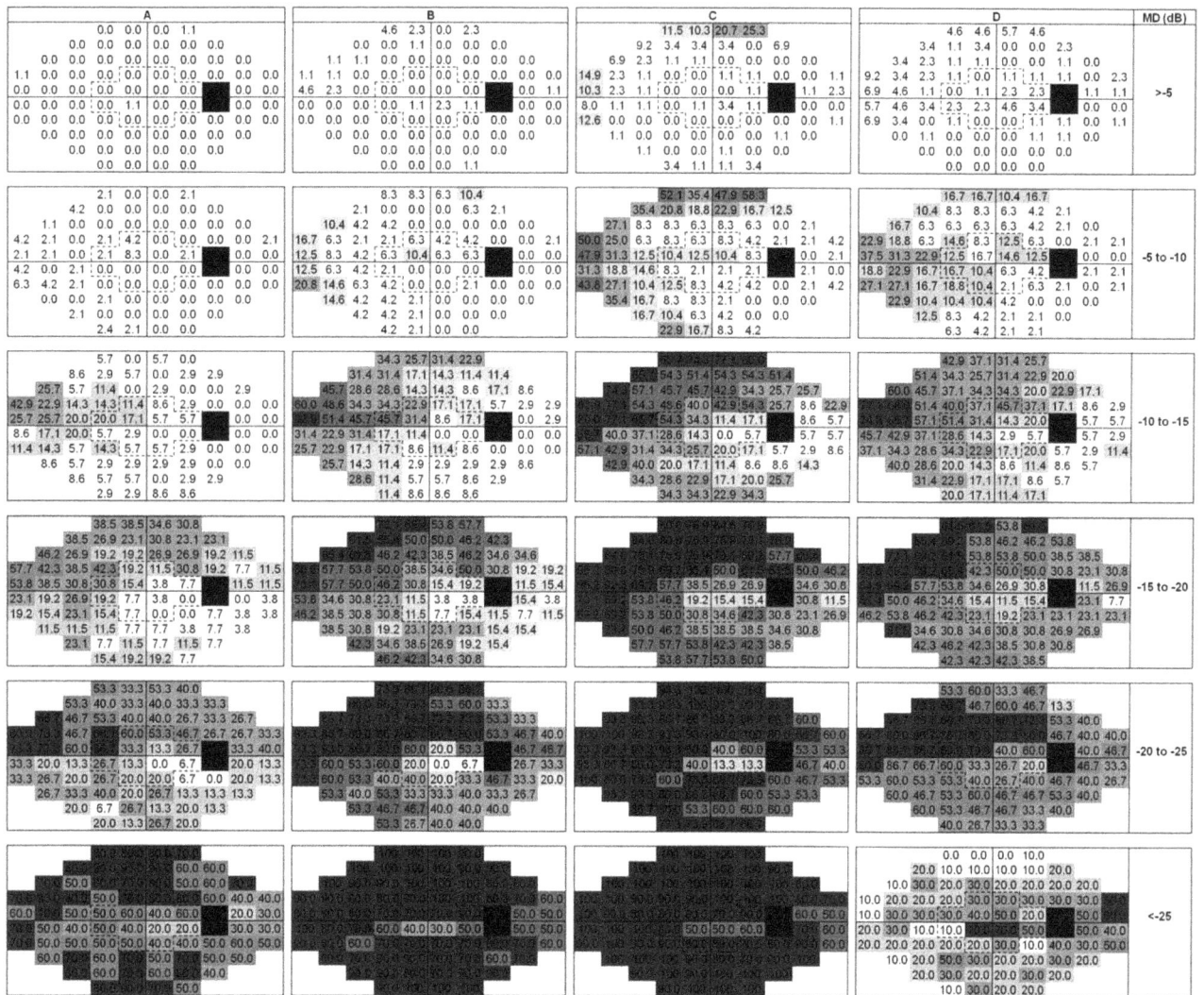

**Figure 3. Spatial distributions of test locations that met various criteria for blindness, as a function of baseline mean deviation (MD).** The criteria were three consecutive sensitivities of <0 (A), <10 (B) and <20 (C) dB, and being 'out of range' according to the Glaucoma Progression Analysis (GPA; D). Black squares are the blind spot; white squares are test locations flagged as blind in 0–10% of the patients. The remaining intermediate four gray scales denote, from light to dark, blindness in 10–20%, 20–40%, 40–60% and above 60% of the patients.

percentage of follow-up tests showing blindness in the concerning test locations) as the dependent variable.

**Spatial distribution of perimetrically blind test locations.** For this analysis, we included all patients who performed at least four tests. Patients were stratified according to baseline MD in six strata, being above -5 dB, from -5 to -10 dB, -10 to -15 dB, -15 to -20 dB, -20 to -25 dB en beyond -25 dB. We plotted the test locations considered blind based on their sensitivity history and calculated the percentages of these test locations, for all test locations of the 30-2 grid and for a subset laying within the 10-2 area. Percentages were compared with a nonparametric paired test (Wilcoxon).

A commonly used progression detection algorithm, the Glaucoma Progression Analysis (GPA) [13], has its own built-in criterion for blindness: a cross on the printout indicates that the test location is 'out of range' and not used for progression detection by the software. We compared – for all six MD strata - the spatial distributions and percentages of test locations flagged as 'out of range' by GPA with that of test locations considered blind based

on their sensitivity history. Percentages were compared using a nonparametric paired test (Wilcoxon).

**Influence of assuming blindness on progression detection.** If the sensitivity of a test location has been below a certain value on a number of consecutive tests, it might be an efficient approach to consider such a test location blind in all future tests – in glaucoma – without actually retesting it. This might result in a (slight) underestimation of the MD and thus might affect MD-based progression detection algorithms. To determine the influence of this approach on clinical decision making, we classified all included eyes as stable or progressing according to the MD-based Non-parametric Progression Analysis algorithm (NPA), with progression defined as at least possible progression at the end of the follow-up (NPA is based on a nonparametric ranking of MD values; for possible progression, the MDs of the last two tests have to be lower than the lower MD of two baseline tests) [12]. Subsequently, we repeated this after assuming test locations to be perimetrically blind based on their sensitivity history. Here, we excluded test locations from the

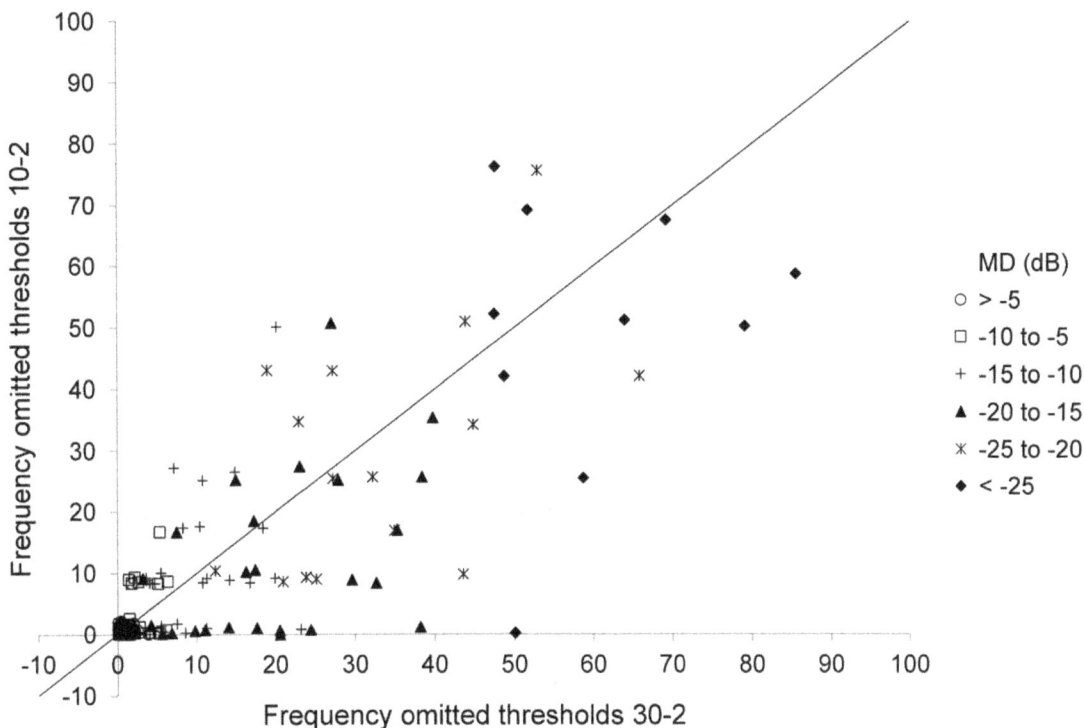

**Figure 4. Percentage of blind test locations according to the three consecutive <0 dB criterion for all test locations within the 30–2 grid (x-axis) versus a subset of test locations within the 10–2 grid (y-axis).** Symbols indicate stratification according to baseline mean deviation (MD) in six strata, being up to -5 dB, from -5 to -10 dB, -10 to -15 dB, 15 to 20 dB, -20 to -25 dB en beyond -25 dB. Noise with a standard deviation of 1% was added in order to avoid overlapping data points.

analysis if they were blind on the first three tests, according to four different definitions of blindness: <0, <5, <10 and <20 dB. For all four definitions, both classifications were compared with a McNemar test. Because the MD is an average weighed to test location eccentricity, and the weigh factors are unpublished, we applied the NPA criterion to the eccentricity-uncorrected average sensitivity of all test locations (mean sensitivity).

Calculations and statistical analyses were performed using SPSS Statistics 18.0 (SPSS Inc., Chicago, IL); the ANOVA was performed using MrF (http://psy.otago.ac.nz/miller/).

## Results

Table 2 shows the patient characteristics. Two-hundred-twenty-one patients were included of which 53 performed at least eight tests and had at least one test location showing a <0 dB sensitivity on four consecutive baseline tests. The average follow-up durations were 6.4 and 6.9 years, respectively, with median MD values at baseline of −7.0 and −14.7 dB.

Figure 1 shows the blindness persistence characteristics as a function of the number of consecutive baseline sensitivities below <0, <5, <10 and <20 dB. The boxplots visualize the between-patient variability; the corresponding mean within-patient standard deviations were, following the sequence of Fig. 1 from left to right, 25, 23, 21, 20, 16, 15, 13, 12, 14, 10, 9, 10, 13, 9, 9 and 8%. If the number of consecutive baseline tests on which a test location was blind increased, the probability of being blind during follow-up increased. The increase in blindness persistence appeared to saturate at three consecutive baseline sensitivities below the concerning value. Blindness persistence appeared to be highest for <10 and <20 dB and lowest for <0 dB. Table 3 shows that

blindness persistence depended significantly on both the number of consecutive tests showing blindness in a test location (P<0.001) and the definition of blindness (P<0.001). Figure 2 presents the corresponding mean sensitivity as recorded during the four follow-up tests in the presumed blind test locations.

Figure 3 illustrates the spatial distributions of test locations that met the requirement of three consecutive sensitivities of <0 (A), <10 (B) and <20 (C) dB, and that were 'out of range' according to the GPA (D), as a function of baseline MD. The number of blind test locations increased monotonically with MD for all criteria of blindness except for GPA; for GPA the number of test location flagged as 'out of range' decreased again with advanced glaucoma. As a consequence, significantly less sensitivities were 'out of range' according to GPA compared to blindness at <0 dB for baseline MD values below −25 dB (P<0.001), while the opposite was the case for all other strata (P<0.001). For the three consecutive <0 dB criterion (Figure 3A), the median (interquartile range) percentages of blind test locations were 0(0–0), 0(0–2), 4(0–9), 17(8–27), 27(20–40) and 60(50–70)% for the six MD strata.

Figure 4 presents a scatter plot showing the percentages of blind test locations according to the three consecutive <0 dB criterion for all test locations of the 30–2 grid versus a subset of 12 test locations located within the 10–2 grid. For the subset, the median (interquartile range) percentages of blind test locations were 0(0–0), 0(0–2), 6(4–11), 8(4–18), 23(13–48) and 50(40–70)% for the six MD strata. These percentages were similar to the corresponding percentages for the 30–2 grid (listed above) for all six MD strata (P = 0.32, 0.34, 0.11, 0.44, 0.17 and 0.23, respectively).

Figure 5 shows Venn diagrams indicating the number of eyes with at least possible progression at the end of the follow-up according to NPA versus NPA after removing all test locations that

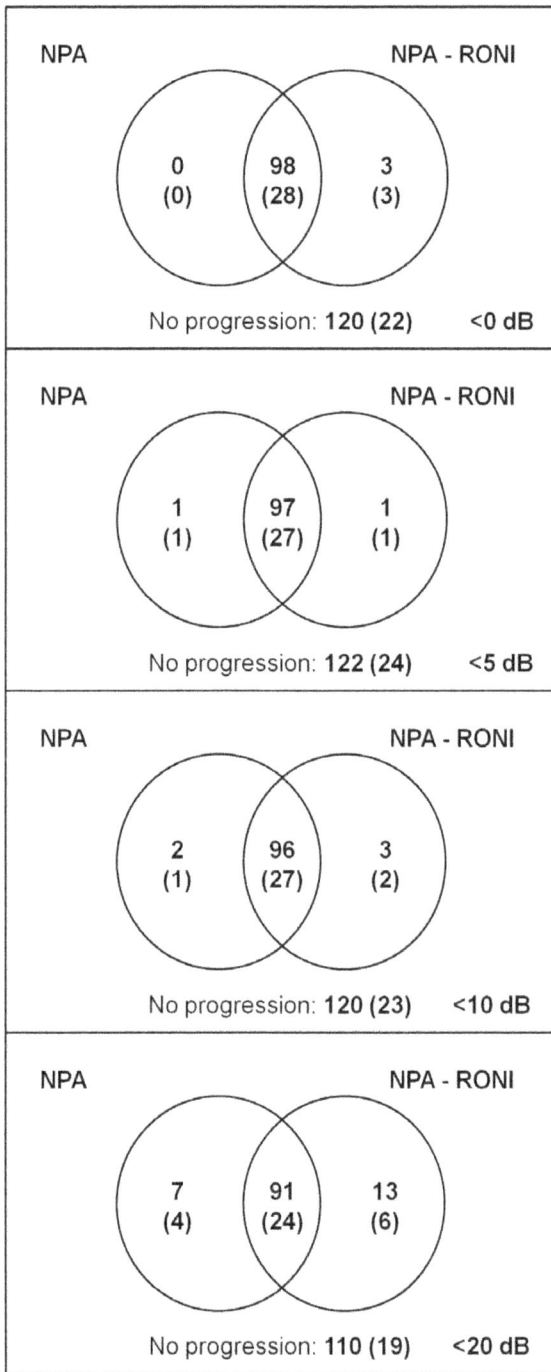

Figure 5. Venn diagrams showing progression according Nonparametric Progression Analysis (NPA) versus NPA after removing all test locations that were blind on the first three tests (NPA-RONI, where RONI is regions of no interest). Four different definitions of blindness were used: <0, <5, <10 and <20 dB. Results for all 221 subjects with results for the subset of 53 subjects between brackets.

were blind on the first three tests (NPA-RONI, where RONI is regions of no interest) for four different definitions of blindness: <0, <5, <10 and <20 dB. There was no significant difference between the classifications by both approaches (P = 0.25, P = 1.0, P = 1.0 and P = 0.26 for <0, <5, <10 and <20 dB, respectively).

Similar findings were done in the subset of 53 eyes (P = 0.25, P = 1.0, P = 1.0 and P = 0.75 for <0, <5, <10 and <20 dB, respectively).

## Discussion

Test locations with a sensitivity below a certain value on three consecutive occasions are unlikely to show a substantially higher sensitivity later on. Hence, if the concerning value corresponds to the maximum stimulus intensity of the perimeter used, these test locations do no longer contribute to progression detection. Omitting these locations from future tests will result in time saving without hampering progression detection. Obviously, the number of blind test locations (and thus the potential time saving) increases with increasing disease severity. Interestingly, the percentages of blind test locations appeared to be similar for 30–2 and 10–2 grids for all disease stages.

With the introduction of the SITA strategies in the late ninety's of the previous century, the examination time of standard automated perimetry decreased substantially [14]. Unfortunately, this advantage over the full-threshold strategy is largely lost in severe glaucoma. Older Octopus strategies and the German Adaptive Threshold Estimation (GATE) algorithm overcome this increase in test time by using information from previous test results to determine more appropriate starting values for the stair-case procedure [6,7]. We would suggest a further step by entirely omitting test locations that were shown to be blind at earlier occasions ('regions of no interest'). This enables more time saving but obviously limits the application of our approach to irreversible eye diseases. Leaving out test locations may seem crude, but this is what is actually done by clinicians who exchange the default 30–2 grid by a 10–2 grid in advanced glaucoma and by clinicians who rely on GPA for progression detection. Interestingly, GPA ignores even more test locations than we propose to do with our 'regions of no interest' approach (see below and Results section). As GPA leaves them out in the analysis phase only, however, no time saving is obtained.

The time gained by the suggested approach should be interpreted and weighed correctly. Obviously, if the time saving is compared to the total time spent in the hospital, the saving is negligible. However, not testing blind test locations refrains a patient with moderate or advanced glaucoma from long time periods in which he or she does not observe any stimulus but has to stay alert nonetheless. This should increase concentration, thus increasing the reliability of the test result. Second, long time periods without any visible stimulus increase patient frustration by emphasizing not seeing things. Third, the saved time can be used to study the remaining parts of the visual field in more detail without additional visits or costs. This can be done by either adding test locations or determining thresholds more accurately. Obviously, to allow for a reliable progression detection throughout the follow-up, only the test locations belonging to the original grid should contribute to the MD. The added test locations, however, may be analyzed separately and may yield important information [9,10].

A caveat of incorporating our regions-of-no-interest approach is that it may cause propagation of blindness through the visual field if applied to strategies that use some form of spatial smoothing (that is, do not determine a formal threshold in all individual test locations) in order to reduce test time (as possibly occurs in SITA). This will not occur in strategies that use neighboring sensitivities only for estimating a starting value for determining a threshold.

The classical picture of glaucoma deterioration is the development of visual field defects initially in the periphery, leaving vision

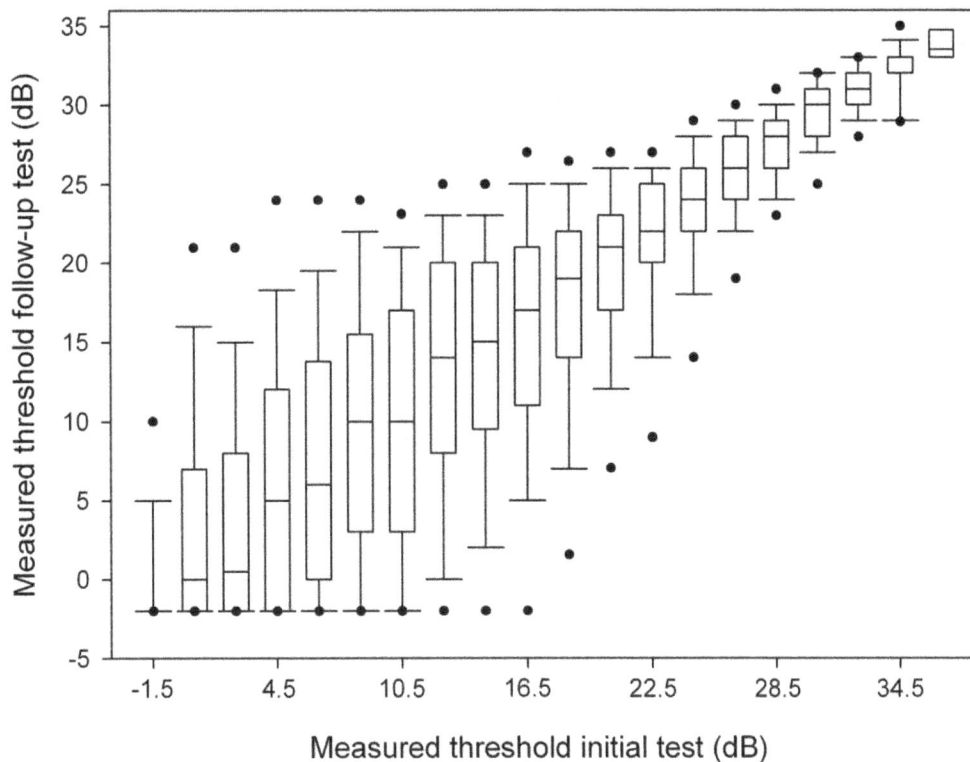

**Figure 6. Pointwise test-retest variability.** Data presented in strata of 2 dB, except for <0 dB which was set to -1.5 dB in one box. Boxplots show median, interquartile range, and 5th, 10th, 90th and 95th percentiles.

unaltered centrally until the latest stages of the disease. Albeit this picture has been challenged recently [9,10], the clinical translation of this picture is starting with 30–2 testing with a transition to 10–2 somewhere along the line - the easiest way to get rid of unresponsive parts of the visual field in advanced disease. One of the aims of this study was to develop a clinically useful guideline, that is, an MD cut-off value, for preferring 10–2 testing over 30–2 testing in advanced glaucoma. Interestingly, no such an MD value appeared to exist – the median percentage of blind test locations was essentially identical for 30–2 and 10–2 grids for all disease stages. With a closer look at our data, this corresponded to the three clinically well known patterns of visual field loss in severe glaucoma: (1) a central island without a peripheral (temporal) island, (2) a temporal island without a central island, and (3) both a central and a temporal island. This is also visible in Figure 4. Hence, in many patients a transition from 30–2 to 10–2 testing will never become an meaningful change. It is important to realize that we did not actually measure a 10–2 grid – a form of high spatial resolution perimetry [15,16] - but analyzed a subset of 30–2 test locations laying within the 10–2 area. Here, the assumption is that this can be considered a representative (unbiased) sample. Also, inclusion of a patient in this study implied the presence of 30–2 fields. This might have induced a selection bias, as patients with only a central island might be underrepresented because they were at baseline already monitored with 10–2 testing – and thus excluded. This is unlikely, however, as at the baseline of the GLGS Goldmann perimetry and not 10–2 testing was the default escape in advanced glaucoma [11] – suggesting an underrepresentation of temporal islands rather than of central islands in this study. To conclude, the transition from 30–2 to 10–2 testing should be individualized and the advantage of a more detailed monitoring of a central island should be weighed against the need of building a

new baseline and the loss of monitoring of any peripheral island. After all, it is not unlikely that progression in the periphery predicts future central loss.

Figure 3A-C actually depicts the "average" glaucoma progression pattern. Not unexpectedly, the glaucomatous deterioration starts nasal-superiorly. In agreement with the findings discussed in the paragraph above, both a central and a temporal island survived until the last MD stratum. With GPA, the number of test locations with a cross (indicating that the software ignores these location for progression detection) increases with disease progression up to an MD of about -20 dB but decreases beyond that point (Figure 3D). Although this pattern is identical to what is observed in the pattern deviation plot and is in agreement with the idea that GPA is based on pattern deviation analysis [17], it might mislead the clinician as it suggests erroneously that test locations that are actually blind are still monitored.

The absence of a response to the maximum stimulus intensity is not identical to blindness. The dynamic range of the perimeter can be increased by replacing stimulus size III by size V. Interestingly, this appears to reduce the test-retest variability [18–20]. Until now, however, the time-saving SITA strategy is not available for size V. Within a given stimulus size, it is not self-evidently beneficial to increase the dynamic range by increasing the maximum stimulus intensity. Although the well-known pointwise test-retest variability plot (for our data shown in Figure 6) suggests a reduced variability close to the maximum stimulus intensity, this is merely a floor effect. If we look in an alternative way to the same data (Figure 1), it might be the case that the extended dynamic range as used in HFA compared to Octopus and Oculus corresponds to a reduced reproducibility of blindness (Table 3). This is in line with the idea that a high test-retest variability is related to ganglion cell saturation [21], but requires further study.

The exclusion of test locations with a sensitivity of <0, <5 or <10 dB at baseline did not affect progression detection with NPA (Figure 5). Only for <20 dB some difference (albeit statistically not significant) appeared to occur. Here, progression according to NPA but not according to NPA-RONI might reflect deepening of existing defects (that is, test locations with a sensitivity already <20 dB at baseline); progression according to NPA-RONI but not according to NPA might be caused by a reduced variability in the calculated mean sensitivity for the RONI approach, which results in an increase in NPA sensitivity [22,23]. These observations are in line with the findings described in the previous paragraph. It might be possible that other progression detection algorithms would be affected differently. This requires further study.

Originally, the SITA fast strategy, as used in the GLGS, was considered a time-saving improvement of the SITA standard strategy and for that reason we adopted it in our study designed in 1999. Later it became clear that the strategies performed slightly different. Two studies reported a slightly higher sensitivity for SITA standard in comparison with SITA fast [24,25]; one study reported a higher sensitivity for SITA fast [26]. These differences –

if any – are not relevant to the current study. More relevant to the current study is the finding that SITA fast seems to have a higher test-retest variability in areas with a reduced sensitivity in comparison with SITA standard [27]. This tentatively suggests that blindness reproducibility might be better in SITA standard and thus our criterion – three consecutive <0 dB readings – should be applicable to SITA standard as well.

In conclusion, current perimetric strategies share the inconvenient property that test-time increases in advanced glaucoma, while a smaller residual visual field has to be tested. A more clever customizing to what has to be tested than a default change to 10–2 testing should allow for an improved and uninterrupted long-term monitoring of glaucoma patients with standard automated perimetry.

## Author Contributions

Conceived and designed the experiments: NMJ FGJM CW. Performed the experiments: FGJM CW. Analyzed the data: FGJM CW. Wrote the paper: FGJM NMJ CW.

## References

1. Bengtsson B, Heijl A (1998) Evaluation of a new perimetric threshold strategy, SITA, in patients with manifest and suspect glaucoma. Acta Ophthalmol Scand 76: 268–72.
2. Hudson C, Wild JM, O'Neill EC (1994) Fatigue effects during a single session of automated static threshold perimetry. Invest Ophthalmol Vis Sci 35: 268–80.
3. Chauhan BC, Tompkins JD, LeBlanc RP, McCormick TA (1993) Characteristics of frequency-of-seeing curves in normal subjects, patients with suspected glaucoma, and patients with glaucoma. Invest Ophthalmol Vis Sci 34: 3534–40.
4. Wall M (2004) What's new in perimetry. J Neuroophthalmol 24: 46–55.
5. Bengtsson B, Heijl A (1998) SITA fast, a new rapid perimetric threshold test: description of methods and evaluation in patients with manifest and suspect glaucoma. Acta Ophthalmol Scand 76: 431–7.
6. Fankhauser F, Spahr J, Bebie H (1977) Some aspects of the automation of perimetry. Surv Ophthalmol 22: 131–41.
7. Schiefer U, Pascual JP, Edmunds B, Feudner E, Hoffmann EM, et al. (2009) Comparison of the new perimetric GATE strategy with conventional full-threshold and SITA standard strategies. Invest Ophthalmol Vis Sci 50: 488–94.
8. Turpin A, Jankovic D, McKendrick AM (2007) Retesting visual fields: utilizing prior information to decrease test-retest variability in glaucoma. Invest Ophthalmol Vis Sci 48: 1627–34.
9. Schiefer U, Papageorgiou E, Sample PA, Pascual JP, Selig B, et al. (2010) Spatial pattern of glaucomatous visual field loss obtained with regionally condensed stimulus arrangements. Invest Ophthalmol Vis Sci 51: 5685–5689.
10. Hood DC, Raza AS, De Moraes CGV, Odel JG, Greenstein VC, et al. (2011) Initial arcuate defects within the central 10 degrees in glaucoma. Invest Ophthalmol Vis Sci 52: 940–946.
11. Heeg GP, Blanksma LJ, Hardus PL, Jansonius NM (2005) The groningen longitudinal glaucoma study. I: baseline sensitivity and specificity of the frequency doubling perimeter and the GDx nerve fibre analyser. Acta Ophthalmol Scand 83: 46–52.
12. Wesselink C, Heeg GP, Jansonius NM (2009) Glaucoma monitoring in a clinical setting: glaucoma progression analysis vs nonparametric progression analysis in the groningen longitudinal glaucoma study. Arch Ophthalmol 127: 270–4.
13. Leske MC, Heijl A, Hyman L, Bengtsson B (1999) Early manifest glaucoma trial: design and baseline data. Ophthalmology 106: 2144–53.
14. Bengtsson B, Olsson J, Heijl A, Rootzen H (1997) A new generation of algorithms for computerized threshold perimetry, SITA. Acta Ophthalmol Scand 75: 368–75.
15. Weber J, Schultze T, Ulrich H (1989) The visual field in advanced glaucoma. Int Ophthalmol 13: 47–50.
16. Westcott MC, McNaught AI, Crabb DP, Fitzke FW, Hitchings RA (1997) High spatial resolution automated perimetry in glaucoma. Br J Ophthalmol 81: 452–9.
17. Bengtsson B, Lindgren A, Heijl A, Lindgren G, Asman P, et al. (1997) Perimetric probability maps to separate change caused by glaucoma from that caused by cataract. Acta Ophthalmol Scand 75: 184–8.
18. Wall M, Kutzko KE, Chauhan BC (1997) Variability in patients with glaucomatous visual field damage is reduced using size V stimuli. Invest Ophthalmol Vis Sci 38: 426–35.
19. Wall M, Woodward KR, Doyle CK, Artes PH (2009) Repeatability of automated perimetry: a comparison between standard automated perimetry with stimulus size III and V, matrix, and motion perimetry. Invest Ophthalmol Vis Sci 50: 974–9.
20. Wall M, Woodward KR, Doyle CK, Zamba G (2010) The effective dynamic ranges of standard automated perimetry sizes III and V and motion and matrix perimetry. Arch Ophthalmol 128: 570–6.
21. Swanson WH, Sun H, Lee BB, Cao D (2011) Responses of primate retinal ganglion cells to perimetric stimuli. Invest Ophthalmol Vis Sci 52: 764–71.
22. Jansonius NM (2005) Bayes' theorem applied to perimetric progression detection in glaucoma: From specificity to positive predictive value. Graefe's Archive for Clinical and Experimental Ophthalmology 243: 433–437.
23. Wesselink C, Marcus MW, Jansonius NM (2011) Risk factors for visual field progression in in the groningen longitudinal glaucoma study: A comparison of different statistical approaches. J Glaucoma (e-pub ahead of print june 22, 2011).
24. Delgado MF, Nguyen NTA, Cox TA, Singh K, Lee DA, et al. (2002) Automated perimetry: a report by the american academy of ophthalmology. Ophthalmology 109: 2362–74.
25. Budenz DL, Rhee P, Feuer WJ, McSoley J, Johnson CA, et al. (2002) Sensitivity and specificity of the swedish interactive threshold algorithm for glaucomatous visual field defects. Ophthalmology 109: 1052–8.
26. Pierre-Filho Pde T, Schimiti RB, de Vasconcellos JP, Costa VP (2006) Sensitivity and specificity of frequency-doubling technology, tendency-oriented perimetry, SITA standard and SITA fast perimetry in perimetrically inexperienced individuals. Acta Ophthalmol Scand 84: 345–50.
27. Artes PH, Iwase A, Ohno Y, Kitazawa Y, Chauhan BC (2002). Properties of perimetric threshold estimates from full threshold, SITA standard, and SITA fast strategies. Invest Ophthalmol Vis Sci 43: 2654–9.

# 11

# Opposing Roles for Membrane Bound and Soluble Fas Ligand in Glaucoma-Associated Retinal Ganglion Cell Death

Meredith S. Gregory[1], Caroline G. Hackett[1], Emma F. Abernathy[1], Karen S. Lee[2], Rebecca R. Saff[3], Andreas M. Hohlbaum[2], Krishna-sulayman L. Moody[2,4], Maura W. Hobson[1,2], Alexander Jones[1], Paraskevi Kolovou[1], Saoussen Karray[5], Andrea Giani[6], Simon W. M. John[7], Dong Feng Chen[1], Ann Marshak-Rothstein[4*⑨], Bruce R. Ksander[1*⑨]

1 The Schepens Eye Research Institute, Department of Ophthalmology, Harvard Medical School, Boston, Massachusetts, United States of America, 2 Department of Microbiology, Boston University School of Medicine, Boston, Massachusetts, United States of America, 3 Department of Medicine, Harvard Medical School, Boston, Massachusetts, United States of America, 4 Department of Medicine, University of Massachusetts Medical School, Worcester, Massachusetts, United States of America, 5 Institut National de la Sante et de la Recherche Medicale (INSERM) Unite 580, Hopital Necker, Paris, France, 6 Massachusetts Eye and Ear Infirmary, Department of Ophthalmology, Harvard Medical School, Boston, Massachusetts, United States of America, 7 Howard Hughes Medical Institute, Jackson Laboratory, Bar Harbor, Maine, United States of America

## Abstract

Glaucoma, the most frequent optic neuropathy, is a leading cause of blindness worldwide. Death of retinal ganglion cells (RGCs) occurs in all forms of glaucoma and accounts for the loss of vision, however the molecular mechanisms that cause RGC loss remain unclear. The pro-apoptotic molecule, Fas ligand, is a transmembrane protein that can be cleaved from the cell surface by metalloproteinases to release a soluble protein with antagonistic activity. Previous studies documented that constitutive ocular expression of FasL maintained immune privilege and prevented neoangeogenesis. We now show that FasL also plays a major role in retinal neurotoxicity. Importantly, in both TNFα triggered RGC death and a spontaneous model of glaucoma, gene-targeted mice that express only full-length FasL exhibit accelerated RGC death. By contrast, FasL-deficiency, or administration of soluble FasL, protected RGCs from cell death. These data identify membrane-bound FasL as a critical effector molecule and potential therapeutic target in glaucoma.

**Editor:** Naj Sharif, Alcon Research, Ltd., United States of America

**Funding:** Funding sources: Lions Research Foundation (BRK), American Health Assistance Foundation (MSG), NEI EY016486 (BRK), NEI EY016145 (MSG), NCI CA90691 (AMR), EY11721 (SWMJ), the Glaucoma Foundation (BRK) and SWMJ is an investigator of the Howard Hughes Medical Institute. The funders had no role in study design, data collection and analysis, decision to publish, or preparation of the manuscript.

**Competing Interests:** The authors have declared that no competing interests exist.

* E-mail: ann.rothstein@umassmed.edu (AMR); bruce.ksander@schepens.harvard.edu (BRK)

⑨ These authors contributed equally to this work.

## Introduction

Glaucoma is one of the most common causes of blindness worldwide and, while there are many different forms of glaucoma that differ significantly in clinical presentation and disease progression, they all share a common endpoint which is the loss of retinal ganglion cells (RGCs) [1]. One of the most common forms of glaucoma, primary open angle glaucoma, is associated with increased intraocular pressure. However, patients with low or normal intraocular pressure can also develop glaucoma, indicating that mechanisms independent of elevated pressure contribute to the death of RGCs. In spite of extensive research, the pathobiology of glaucoma is poorly understood. Recent evidence indicates the loss of RGCs is due to apoptosis [2], nevertheless, the actual molecular mechanism that triggers apoptosis is controversial.

Data from clinical studies and animal models of induced elevated intraocular pressure (IOP) support the hypothesis that there is an inflammatory component to glaucoma and that TNFα contributes to disease progression. Elevated levels of TNFα have been detected in the aqueous humor and retinal layers of glaucoma patients with primary open angle, normal tension, and exfoliation glaucoma [3][4]. In addition, TNFα polymorphisms have been associated with primary open angle glaucoma in Japanese and Chinese populations [5,6]. Development of glaucoma also coincided with increased levels of TNFα and TNFα-inducible genes in laser induced rodent models of elevated IOP [7][8]. However, in this model, TNFα did not appear to directly induce cytolysis of RGCs, although it could be shown to activate microglia [7]. Moreover, a single injection of TNFα into the vitreous of eyes with normal pressure triggered the loss of RGCs. Together, these data indicate that ocular stress, such as elevated intraocular pressure, can trigger the release of TNFα, which in turn activates microglia to become neurotoxic for RGCs. However, the direct effector mechanism responsible for microglia mediated RGC neurotoxicity is not TNFα.

Fas Ligand (FasL) is one candidate that may link activation of microglia with the induction of apoptosis in RGCs. Fas Ligand

(FasL) is a 40 kDa type II transmembrane protein of the TNF family, originally identified by its capacity to induce apoptosis in Fas receptor positive cells [9] and mediate activation induced cell death in T cells [10]. FasL is expressed by activated T cells and constitutively expressed on ocular tissues where it is thought to contribute to the immune privileged status of the eye, either by inducing apoptosis of infiltrating inflammatory cells or by preventing neoangeogenesis [11]. In addition to its pro-apoptotic activity, FasL can also induce the release of proinflammatory cytokines [12,13,14]. Importantly, in a rat model of heat-shock protein-induced RGC degeneration, FasL+ autoreactive T cells have been implicated in the damage of Fas+ RGCs [15]. By contrast, RGC degeneration in the laser-induced ocular hypertension models does not appear to involve T cells. However, other cells of the innate immune system, notably macrophages and retinal microglia, can express FasL upon activation [16,17]. Thus FasL+ effector cells could be involved in T-independent destruction of RGCs. Such a pathogenic role for FasL appears to be in conflict with its purported role in immune privilege.

The diverse activities of FasL could result from functional differences in cell-bound vs soluble forms of the molecule, as is true for other TNF family members [18,19,20]. Moreover, FasL can be released from the cell by at least two mechanisms. FasL can be cleaved from the cell surface by metalloproteinases to produce a truncated soluble product derived from the extracellular domain (sFasL) [21]. In addition, cell lines and activated T cells have been reported to release full-length FasL in the form of microvesicles [22,23]. Both truncated sFasL and full-length vesicle-associated FasL can be detected as cell-free FasL by standard ELISA readouts, leading to some confusion as to the valency and functional activity of cell-free FasL. There is considerable data to suggest that murine sFasL is non-apoptotic and anti-inflammatory, and in some instances, sFasL has even been shown to antagonize the activity of mFasL. This is in contrast to an experimental form of FasL that corresponds to the entire extracellular domain [24,25]. On the other hand, sFasL bound to extracellular matrix proteins is cytotoxic and FasL has been localized to the extracellular matrix in the anterior chamber of the eye [26]. Thus, whether FasL accumulates in the ocular environment as full-length mFasL or truncated sFasL, matrix-associated or not, could influence its functional consequences. Remarkably, the relative levels of full-length and cleaved FasL in the eye have not been carefully evaluated.

Most direct functional comparisons of mFasL and sFasL have been carried out by using transfected cells that express only wild type FasL, mFasL or sFasL. In the current study, we have used FasL-deficient mice as well as mice from a gene-targeted line in which the FasL metalloproteinase cleavage sites were mutated to prevent cleavage of the membrane-bound protein. We have compared the ability of these mice to develop RGC degeneration following intraocular TNFα treatment and in a spontaneous model of glaucoma. Overall our data reveal a critical neurotoxic effector function for mFasL and neuroprotective function of sFasL.

## Results

### TNFα triggered loss of RGCs is dependent upon FasL

To examine the role of Fas/FasL interactions in the death of RGCs, we used the intravitreal TNFα injection model developed by Nakazawa et al (see **Figure 1A**) [7]. Recipients included a FasL knockout (KO) line, developed in our laboratory (**Figure**

S1). As the more commonly used point mutation encoded by the FasL$^{gld}$ locus does not completely eliminate Fas receptor engagement [27]. Groups of wild-type C57BL/6J (WT-B6) and FasL KO mice were given a single intravitreal injection of TNFα (1 ng/0.5 μl). As negative controls, mice were either untreated, or injected with normal saline. At four weeks post injection, retinal sections were stained with an anti-β-III-tubulin antibody to identify RGCs (**Figure 1 B–E**). The number of RGCs was determined quantitatively in representative retinal sections as described in the methods (**Figure 1F**). There was no significant difference in the number of RGCs between either untreated WT, WT mice given an intravitreal injection of saline, or untreated FasL KO mice. Therefore the absence of FasL did not have any spontaneous effect on the number of RGCs. However, consistent with previous studies, a single intravitreal injection of TNFα resulted in a significant loss of RGCs in the WT-B6 mice by four weeks post TNFα injection. By contrast, there was no loss of RGCs in TNFα treated FasL KO mice. We conclude from these experiments that FasL is required for the TNFα triggered loss of RGCs.

### ΔCS mice express only mFasL and maintain normal ocular histology

To examine the importance of sFasL in ocular homeostasis and RGC degeneration, we constructed a membrane-only FasL gene-targeted mouse in which the FasL metalloproteinase cleavage sites in exon 2 were mutated (**Figure S1**). This mouse line was designated as ΔCS. WT and ΔCS mice were tested for expression of mFasL and sFasL. Cell lysates and culture supernatants prepared from activated T cells were analyzed by Western blot. A 38 kDa mFasL band was detected in the WT lysate and a 27 kDa sFasL band was detected in the WT supernatant. By contrast, cell lysates from the ΔCS T cells contained more of the 38 kDa mFasL protein and the ΔCS supernatant contained no detectable sFasL (**Figure 2A**). Whole eye lysates were also prepared from WT and ΔCS mutant mice to test for ocular expression of mFasL and sFasL by Western blot (**Figure 2B**). Two mFasL bands (38 kD and 34 kD) were detected at low levels in whole eye lysates from WT mice. As an important specificity control, both mFasL bands were missing from eye lysates that were prepared from FasL knockout mice [27]. Therefore, the two bands most likely represent differential glycosylation, previously reported for mFasL [24,28,29]. In comparison to WT mice the expression of both the 38 kD and 34 kD mFasL bands were significantly increased in ΔCS mice (**Figure 2B and 2C**). It is important to note, that sFasL was not detected by Western blot in the whole lysates from WT mice, possibly reflecting clearance from the eye or instability of the soluble form.

Altogether, these data demonstrate that ΔCS mutant mice express increased levels of mFasL and no detectable sFasL. Importantly, the ΔCS mutant mice display no clinically detectable spontaneous systemic phenotype. Extensive histological studies of ocular tissues did not reveal any detectable spontaneous eye phenotype in either the anterior or posterior segment.

### Accelerated loss of RGCs in ΔCS mice

Groups of WT and ΔCS mice received a single intravitreal injection of TNFα (1 ng/0.5 μl) and 1 week later mice were euthanized and the eyes evaluated histologically for RGC degeneration (**Figure 2 D–H**). Untreated ΔCS and WT mice displayed no significant difference in the number of RGCs, indicating the ΔCS mutation had no visible effect on RGC development in healthy mice. As expected from the previous

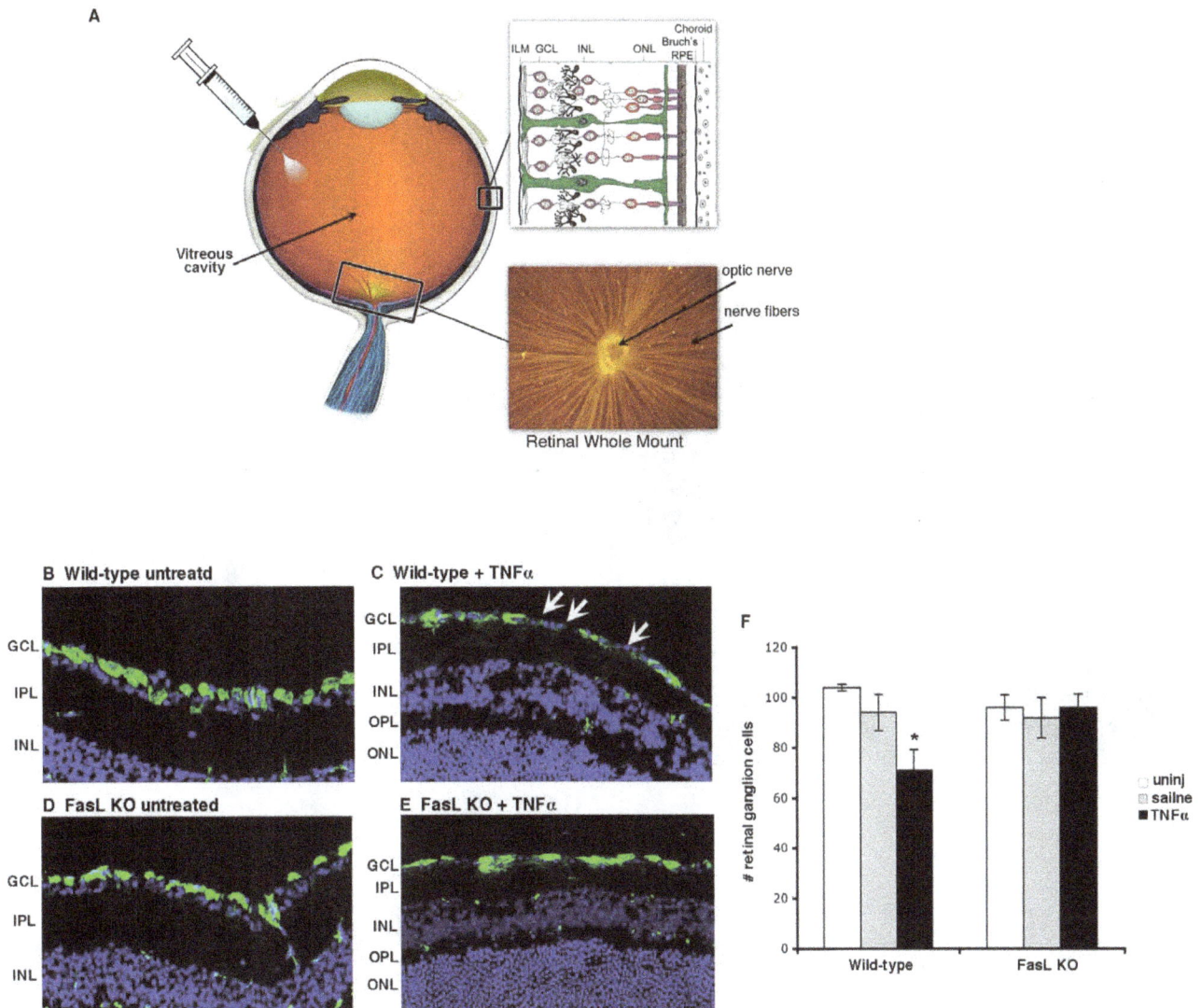

**Figure 1. FasL is required for the loss of RGCs following TNFα injection.** (A) Diagram of the cross section of an eye demonstrating: an intravitreal TNFα injection; the layers of the retina (ILM- inner limiting membrane, GCL- ganglion cell layer, INL- inner nuclear layer, ONL- outer nuclear layer); a retinal whole mount stained to identify the nerve fiber layer. (B–E) WT C57BL/6 or FasL KO mice were untreated or received intravitreal injections of saline or TNFα. Eyes were enucleated at 4 weeks and RGCs were identified in retinal sections using an anti-βIII-tubulin antibody (green) and TOPRO (blue nuclear stain). (F) All βIII-tubulin positive RGCs were counted in each retinal section and the average number RGCs per retinal section was calculated (10 sections per eye). N = 10 per treatment group. (* P<0.05).

work of Nakazawa [7], WT mice treated with TNFα did not display any significant loss of RGCs 1 week after administration; normally a reduction of RGCs in WT mice is not observed until 4 weeks after TNFα treatment. By contrast, there was a significant reduction in the number of RGCs in ΔCS mice treated with TNFα. Moreover, there was a small, but significant reduction in the number of RGCs in ΔCS mice that received an intravitreal saline injection. In this case, RGC loss is most likely due to a hypersensitive response to the modest release of TNFα that is triggered by the injection procedure. These data indicate that the increased expression of mFasL by microglia (or other effector cells), and/or the absence of sFasL in the ocular microenvironment, results in an accelerated loss of RGCs in response to TNFα.

To prove the ΔCS mutation accounted for the accelerated loss of RGCs via the Fas receptor, we intercrossed ΔCS mice with Fas-deficient lpr mice. B6/129$^{ΔCS/ΔCS\ lpr/lpr}$ and wild type littermates

expressing normal FasL and Fas were given intravitreal injections of either TNFα or normal saline. One week post TNFα injection, RGC degeneration was evaluated histologically. In Fas-deficient ΔCS mice, TNFα was unable to trigger the loss of RGCs (**Figure 2I**). Together these data prove that the accelerated loss of RGCs in TNFα injected ΔCS mice is dependent upon the Fas/FasL pathway.

## Loss of nerve fibers in the retina of ΔCS mice

Glaucoma is characterized not only by the loss of RGCs, but also by the loss of the their axons. The axonal loss is often visualized clinically as slit-like or wedge-shape defects in the retinal nerve fiber layer. To evaluate the effect of FasL triggered RGC death on axonal integrity, we examined the nerve fiber layer of WT and ΔCS mice in retinal whole mounts (**see diagram in Figure 1A**). There was no significant difference between the nerve fiber layers of WT and ΔCS mice that were either uninjected

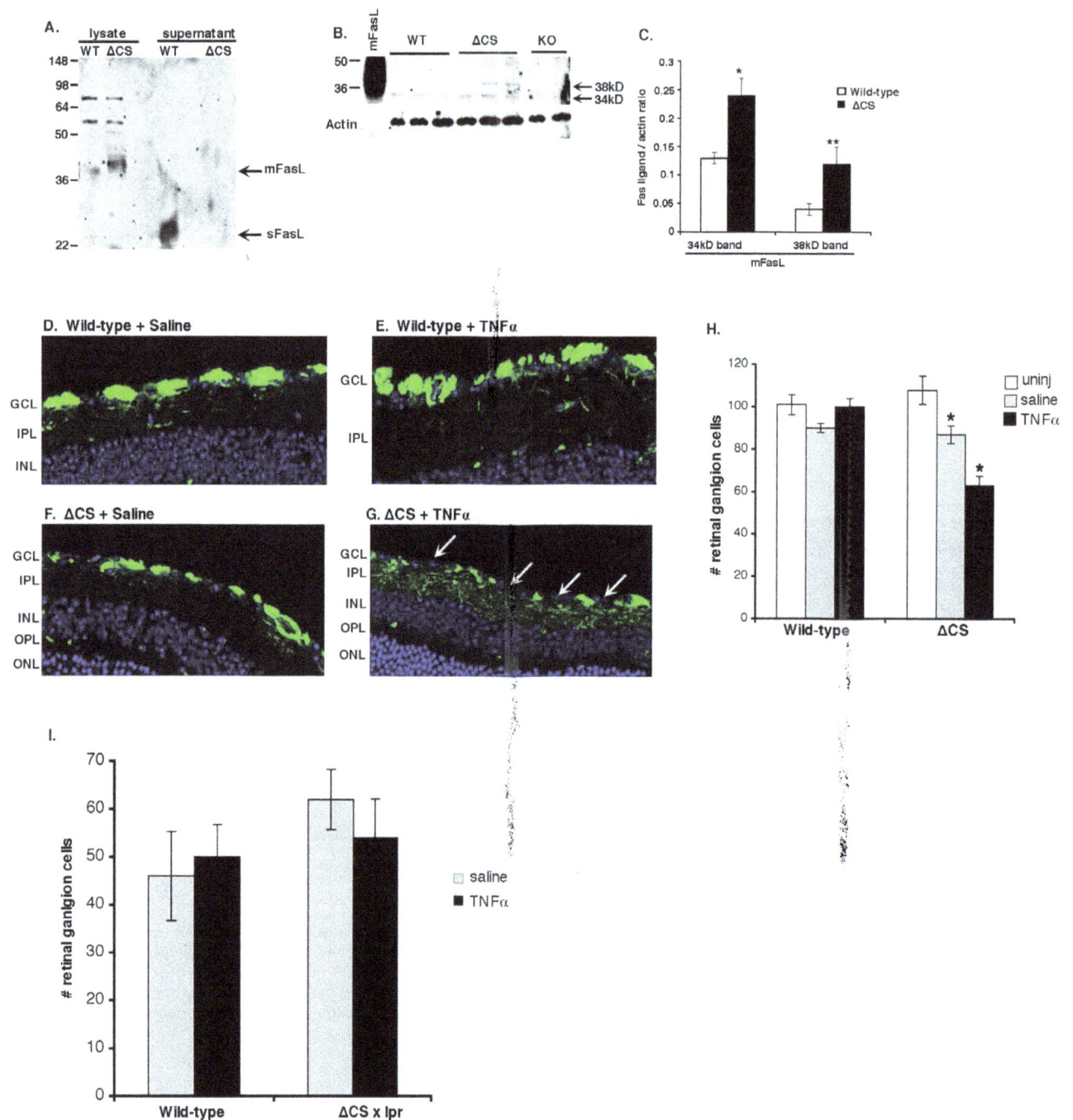

**Figure 2. Loss of RGCs in ΔCS mice is dependent upon the Fas/FasL pathway.** All Western blots displayed are representative of three independent experiments: (A) CD3 activated T cell lysates and supernatants, (B) whole eye lysates from individual eyes of: WT, ΔCS, and FasL KO mice, (C) densitometry of eye lysate Western blots (* and ** P<0.05), (D–G) WT or ΔCS mice received an intravitreal injection of saline, or TNFα. Retinal sections were obtained 7 days later and RGCs were stained with βIII-tubulin. Arrow heads highlight the loss of RGCs. (H) All βIII-tubulin positive RGCs were counted in each retinal section (5 sections per eye; 10 eyes per group) and the average number RGCs per retinal section was calculated. (I) WT or ΔCS×lpr mice received intravitreal injections of saline, or TNFα. The number of RGCs was determined 7 days later in retinal sections. Green = Beta tubulin III and blue = nuclear stain. N = 10 per treatment group. (* p>0.05).

(**Figure 3 A, B**), or administered an intravitreal injection of saline (data not shown). Moreover, WT mice treated with TNFα displayed a normal nerve fiber layer one week after treatment that was not significantly different from the untreated controls (**Figure 3C**). By contrast, at 1 week after treatment, the TNFα-treated ΔCS mice displayed a significant loss of nerve fibers (**Figure 3D**), with some mice displaying very few intact axons (**Figure 3E**). Axonal loss in the TNFα treated ΔCS mice was abrogated in B6/129$^{\Delta CS/\Delta CS\ lpr/lpr}$ mice that lacked a functional Fas receptor (**Figure 3F**). These data demonstrate that ΔCS mice exhibit accelerated loss of both the soma and axon in response to TNFα.

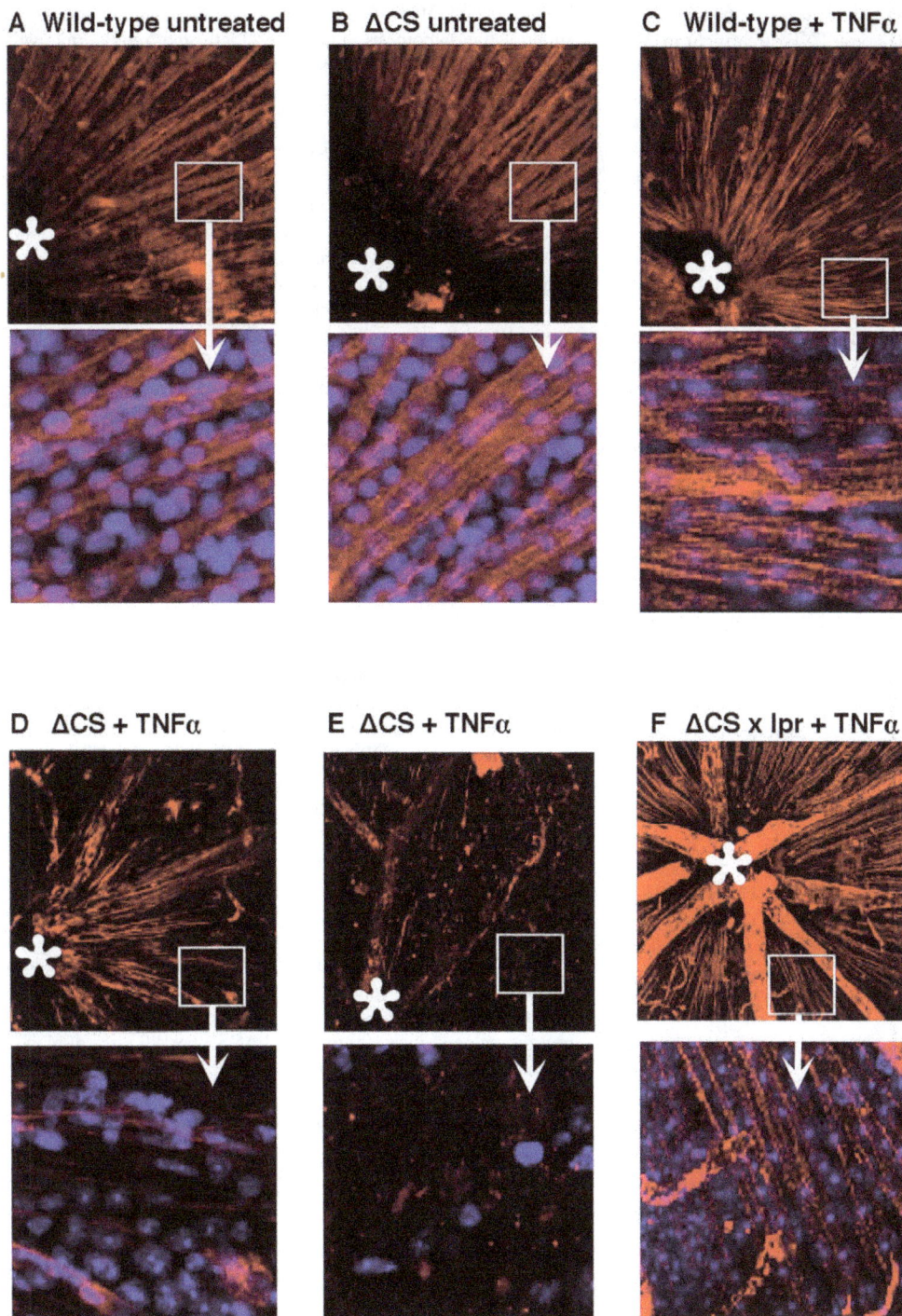

**Figure 3. The loss of retinal ganglion cell nerve fibers is accelerated in ΔCS mice.** WT, ΔCS, or ΔCS×lpr mice were either untreated, or received intravitreal TNFα. Seven days later the nerve fibers in retinal whole mounts were stained with SMi32 (anti-neurofilament antibody) and examined by confocal microscopy. (A) untreated WT retina, (B) untreated ΔCS retina, (C) WT+TNFα treated retina, (D and E) ΔCS+TNFα treated retina, (F) ΔCS×lpr+TNFα treated retina. Asterisks mark the optic nerve head, Red = SMi32, and blue = nuclear stain. The pictures presented are representative of individual mice (N = 10 for each group).

## Exogenous sFasL prevents the accelerated loss of RGC in ΔCS mice

We and others demonstrated previously that mFasL is proinflammatory and proapoptotic, while sFasL is anti-inflammatory and non-apoptotic [24]. To determine whether administration of recombinant sFasL could prevent the loss of RGCs in ΔCS mice,

TNFα treated ΔCS mice, ΔCS mice received an intravitreal injection of either sFasL alone (100 ng), TNFα alone (1 ng), or both sFasL and TNFα. At 7 days post injection, the eyes were evaluated for axonal degeneration in retinal whole mounts. No significant loss of nerve fibers was observed in either WT, or ΔCS mice treated with sFasL alone as compared with untreated WT and ΔCS mice (data not shown). As expected, a significant loss in nerve fibers was observed at 7 days post TNFα treatment in ΔCS mice compared to the untreated control mice (**Figure 4A, 4C**). However, intravitreal injection of recombinant soluble Fas ligand together with TNFα prevented the loss of nerve fibers (**Figure 4E**). It is important to note that the mouse recombinant sFasL used in these experiments corresponds with the physiological cleavage product (Pro 132 to Leu 279) and has weak or no cytolytic activity against A20 target cells.

Spectral domain optical coherence tomography (SD-OCT) provides a noninvasive method to assess the thickness of the retinal nerve fiber layer [30]. In the clinic, the retinal nerve fiber layer thickness is an essential measure for objective glaucoma assessment [31,32]. However, the use of SD-OCT to measure the retinal nerve fiber layer thickness in the mouse is a relatively new area of investigation. In the current study, SD-OCT was used to assess the retinal nerve fiber layer thickness prior to enucleation and preparation of retinal whole mounts. Sectorial areas containing retinal defects were identified in retinal whole mounts stained with SMI32 (**quadrant #1 in Figure 4A, 4C, and 4E**). The corresponding retinal areas were identified in the OCT-based en-face fundus reconstruction and nerve fiber thickness was assessed as described in the methods (**Figure 4B, 4D, and 4F**). SD-OCT measurements indicated a significant thinning of the nerve fiber layer in TNFα treated, but not TNFα+sFasL treated mice (**Figure 4G**). These data indicate that sFasL can block the neurotoxic effects of membrane FasL and prevent nerve fiber loss in ΔCS mice. Moreover, these date indicate that SD-OCT can be used as a non-invasive method to assess retinal nerve fiber layer thickness in mice.

### Retinal microglia express mFasL

Retinal tissue from TNFα treated WT and ΔCS mice were examined by immuno-histochemical staining for Fas and FasL to confirm that Fas+ target cells were present within the ganglion cell layer and to determine which cell types were potential FasL effector cells. As expected, Fas was highly expressed in the ganglion cell layer and the level of Fas was similar in TNFα treated WT and ΔCS mice (**Figure 5A**).

In contrast to Fas, FasL was expressed at much higher levels in ΔCS mice as compared to WT mice. Moreover, the most intense staining was observed in the ganglion cell layer, with some staining also observed in the inner nuclear layer (**Figure 5B**). Double staining for microglia (Iba1) and astrocytes (GFAP) clearly demonstrated that FasL expression in the ganglion cell layer was primarily restricted to retinal microglia (**Figure 5C**) and minimally, if at all, in astrocytes (**Figure 5D**). These data indicate that ΔCS retinal microglia express higher than normal levels of mFasL and/or that greater numbers of FasL+ microglial cells accumulate in the TNF-treated ΔCS retinae [33].

### RGCs are susceptible to mFasL induced apoptosis

We verified that the Fas+ human retinal ganglion cell line, RGC5, was susceptible to mFasL induced apoptosis using mFasL expressing microvesicles (**Figure S2**). To determine whether TNFα treatment of ΔCS mice triggered apoptosis of RGCs in vivo, ΔCS and WT mice were treated with TNFα and at 24 hrs post injection histological sections were stained with TUNEL and examined for apoptotic cells. No apoptotic cells were detected in sections from untreated WT or untreated ΔCS mice (data not shown). In addition, little to no apoptosis was observed in saline treated WT and ΔCS mice. However, a significant number of apoptotic cells were detected in the retinal ganglion cell layer of

TNFα treated ΔCS mice (**Figure 5 E, F**). Together these data support the hypothesis that TNFα activated retinal microglia express mFasL that triggers apoptosis of Fas receptor positive RGCs.

### mFasL induced retinal degeneration in a spontaneous model of glaucoma

DBA/2 mice spontaneously develop age-related elevated intraocular pressure due to mutations in the *Gpnmb* and *Tyrp1* genes that trigger iris stromal atrophy and pigment dispersion, respectively. This results in closure of the iridocorneal angle and elevated IOP by approximately 6–8 months of age, followed by the loss of RGCs and nerve fibers between 11 and 15 months [34,35]. To determine if mFasL also accelerates RGC degeneration in this spontaneous model of glaucoma, we backcrossed the ΔCS mutation onto the DBA/2J background. The 5th generation backcross mice were intercrossed to obtain ΔCS/ΔCS mice (DBA/2J- ΔCS), and a WT/WT littermate control group (DBA/2J-wt). Both the DBA/2J-wt and DBA/2J- ΔCS mice developed high intraocular pressure with age (**Figure 6A**), pigment dispersion (**Figure 6B**), an enlarged anterior chamber (**Figure 6C**), and angle closure (**Figure 6D**). The appearance of these symptoms was not significantly different from fully backcrossed DBA/2J mice as reported previously [34,35]. Thus the failure to cleave FasL in DBA/2J- ΔCS mice did not ameliorate these glaucoma-inducing phenotypes.

However, while there was no detectable loss of nerve fibers in 5 month old DBA/2J-wt mice, there was marked thinning of the nerve fibers in the DBA/2J- ΔCS mice (**Figure 6E** arrows), indicative of accelerated loss of axons. Previous extensive analysis of 12 month old DBA/2J mice by Jakobs and coworkers indicated that elevated intraocular pressure coincided with loss of *only* RGCs; no other retinal neurons were affected [36]. This is evident from the loss of cells in the ganglion cell layer in 12 month old DBA/2J-wt mice (**Figure 6F**, arrows). Unexpectedly, when the DBA/2J- ΔCS mice reached 12 months of age, they displayed not only a greater loss of ganglion cells and nerve fibers, but also extensive retinal degeneration in all layers of the retina (**Figure 6F**). This was not due to the presence of the ΔCS mutation alone, since 10 month old ΔCS B6×129 mice displayed normal retinal architecture and no loss of RGCs. Together, these data indicate that in a spontaneous elevated intraocular pressure model of glaucoma, mFasL is also highly neurotoxic.

### Discussion

Fas ligand is a potent pro-apoptotic molecule expressed by cytotoxic effector T and NK cells that is known for its ability to eliminate virally infected target populations, tumor cells, and autoreactive T and B cells [11]. However, persistent expression of FasL by Fas-deficient T cells in mice with Fas+ non-T cell populations can result in graft-vs-host-like disease [37], total elimination of wild type lymphocytes [38], or can even cause pulmonary fibrosis [39]. In addition, FasL has also been shown to rapidly induce the production of proinflammatory cytokines by a variety of Fas+ cell types and to promote T lymphocyte activation [13]. Therefore it is not surprising that expression of FasL on T and NK cells is tightly regulated either at the transcriptional level [40], by sequestration in cytoplasmic vesicles [41], or by metalloprotease cleavage [13].

Remarkably, in contrast to T cells and NK cells, FasL is constitutively expressed at sites of immune privilege, such as the eye. Ocular expression of FasL is thought to be required for the maintenance of immune privilege by limiting ocular inflamma-

## A. Untreated

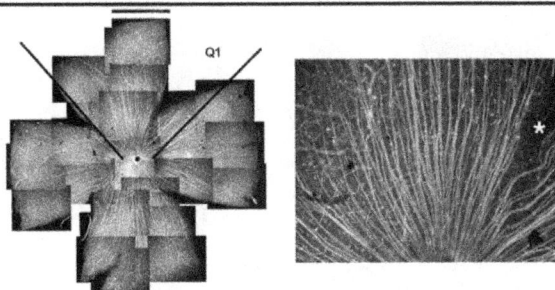

## B. Untreated

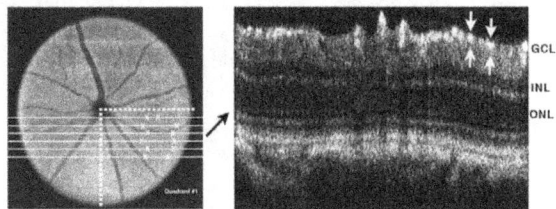

## C. TNFα only

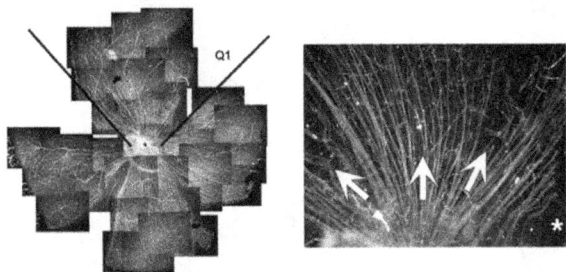

## D. TNFα only

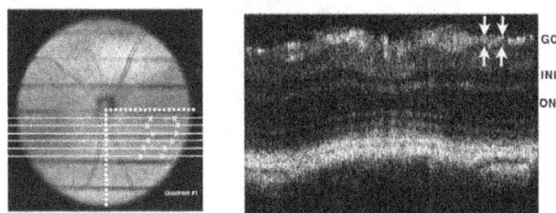

## E. TNFα + sFasL

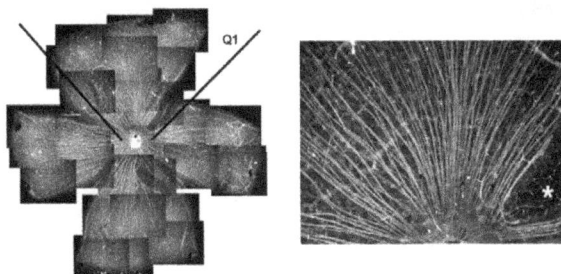

## F. TNFα + sFasL

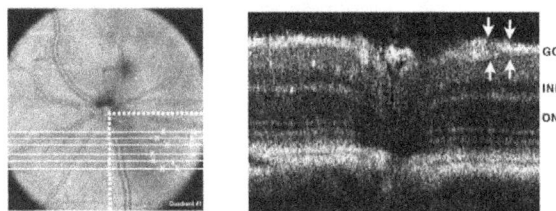

### G.

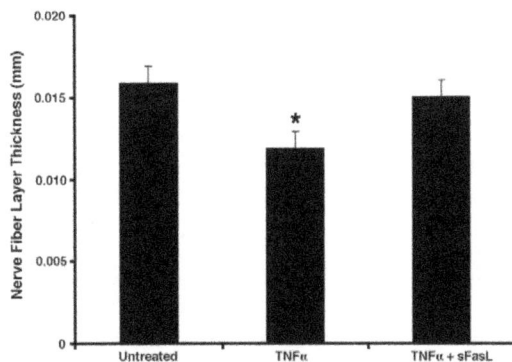

**Figure 4. sFasL protects retinal ganglion cell nerve fibers in ΔCS mice.** ΔCS mice were either untreated, or received intravitreal: TNFα (1 ng) alone, or TNFα+sFasL. Seven days later SD-OCT measurements were made and subsequently the nerve fibers in retinal whole mounts were stained with Smi32 (anti-neurofilament antibody). Displayed are a low power composite montage photograph of the entire Smi32 stained retina and a higher power (×20 magnification) of quadrant #1 (Q1). (A) untreated, (C) TNFα alone, and (E) TNFα+sFasL. Asterisks (*) indicate areas where retinas were dissected. Arrows highlight nerve fiber thinning. Pictures are representative of a single mouse from each group (N = 10 per group). The quadrant #1 was identified in the OCT en-face fundus reconstruction in (B) untreated, and (D) TNFα alone, and (F) TNFα+sFasL. Six sections within the quadrant were chosen and the nerve fiber thickness measured at two points in each section (identified by an X). A single OCT retinal section and the corresponding nerve fiber measurements are displayed. (G) A summary of the OCT measurements for each group (N = 3 per group; two experiments performed). (* p>0.05).

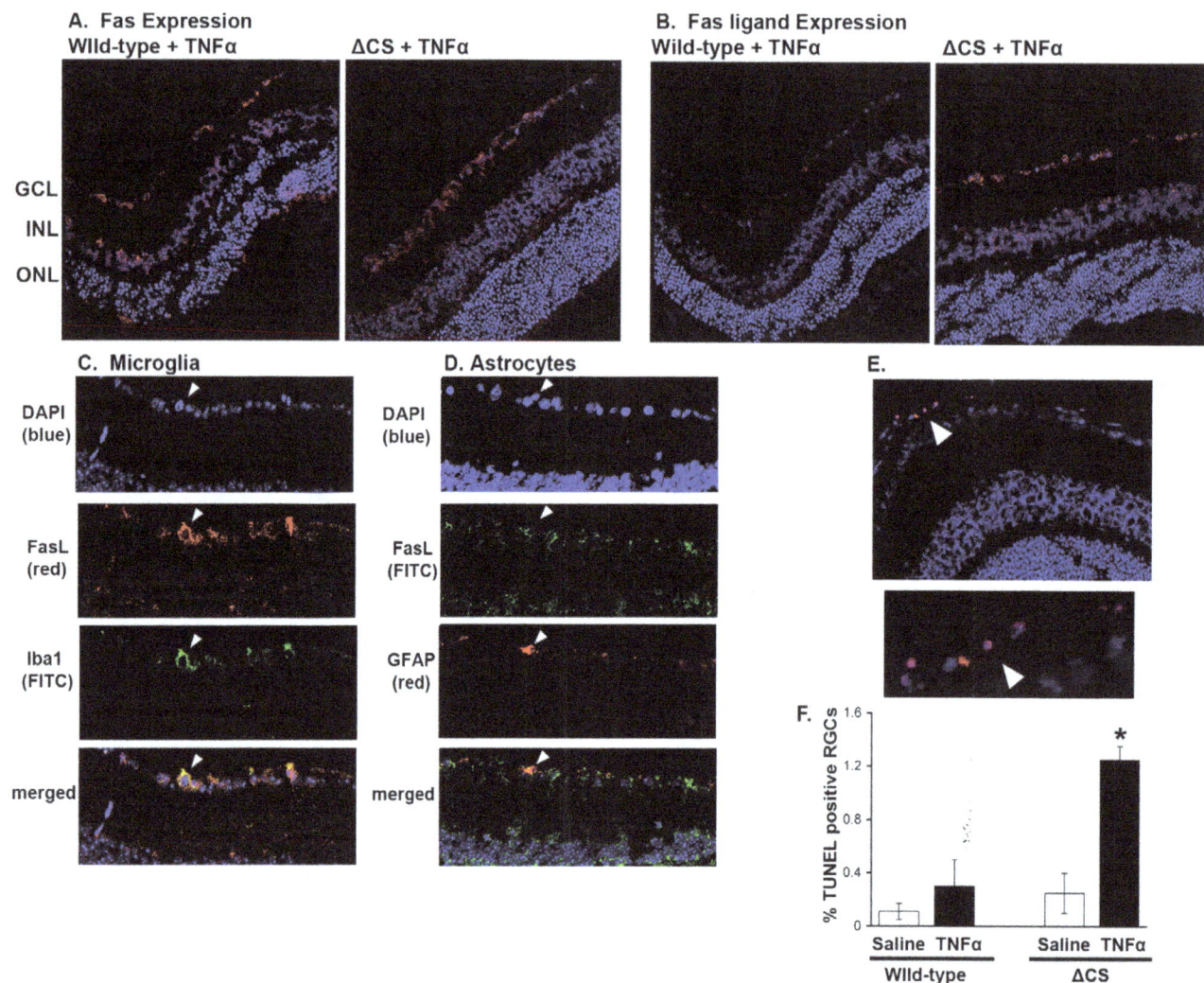

**Figure 5. Expression of Fas and FasL in the neural retina of WT and ΔCS mice.** Frozen retinal sections were prepared from WT and ΔCS mice that were either (i) untreated, or (ii) received a prior (7 days) intravitreal injection of TNFα. (A) Fas receptor expression using an anti Fas antibody (Red) and TOPRO (blue nuclear stain). (B) FasL expression using an anti FasL antibody (red) and TOPRO (blue nuclear stain). Identically treated retinal sections from FasL KO mice were used as a negative control. (C) Double staining for microglia (Iba1-green) and FasL (red) revealed retinal microglia (arrowhead) express FasL. (D) Double staining for astrocytes (GFAP-red) and FasL (green) revealed retinal astrocytes (arrowhead) were FasL negative. (E) Representative TUNEL staining in ΔCS mice at 24 hours post TNFα injection. Red = TUNEL, Blue = nuclear stain. GCL- ganglion cell layer; INL- inner nuclear layer; ONL- outer nuclear layer. (F) Percentages of TUNEL positive cells in the retina. (N = 5 per group). (* p>0.05). See also Figure S2.

tion [42] and/or neoangeogenesis [43]. Consistent with this notion, FasL deficient mice develop a more severe inflammatory response in a murine model of acquired ocular taxoplasmosis [44]. Natural expression of ocular FasL (i) promotes engraftment of allogeneic corneal transplants by inducing apoptosis of infiltrating Fas+ activated T cells [42], and (ii) prevents suture induced neovascularization by inducing apoptosis of vascular endothelial cells [45]. By contrast, FasL-deficient mice present with increased corneal graft rejection and suture induced neovascularization [45,46]. More recent studies, however, reveal an apparent paradox in FasL function within the ocular environment, where ocular expression of membrane-bound FasL actually promotes immunoreactivity. For example: (i) over expression of non-cleavable FasL in the cornea triggers accelerated transplant rejection [47], and (ii) tumor cells that express a membrane-only form of FasL induce a severe ocular inflammatory response [48] Moreover, a number of studies have shown that the soluble form of FasL antagonizes the functional

outcome of membrane-bound FasL [24,25,49], while others reported that sFasL could bind to ocular matrix proteins and thereby acquire potent apoptotic activity [26]. Thus it is unclear how immune privileged sites regulate FasL activity and control its potentially dangerous effects related to inflammation and apoptosis of host tissues.

As previously documented [50] and confirmed in the current report, whether or not a mouse either fails to express FasL, or over expresses membrane-bound FasL, does not appear to affect ocular development or normal lymphocyte homeostasis. Since numerous cell types in the eye constitutively express Fas, the functional outcome of Fas engagement must be constrained, either by cytokines present in the ocular microenvironment, such as TGFβ [51], and/or by some other mechanism. Based on our characterization of the ΔCS mFasL mice, we propose that cleavage of the membrane form of FasL is a critical factor in the regulation of ocular FasL activity in the immune privileged environment of the eye.

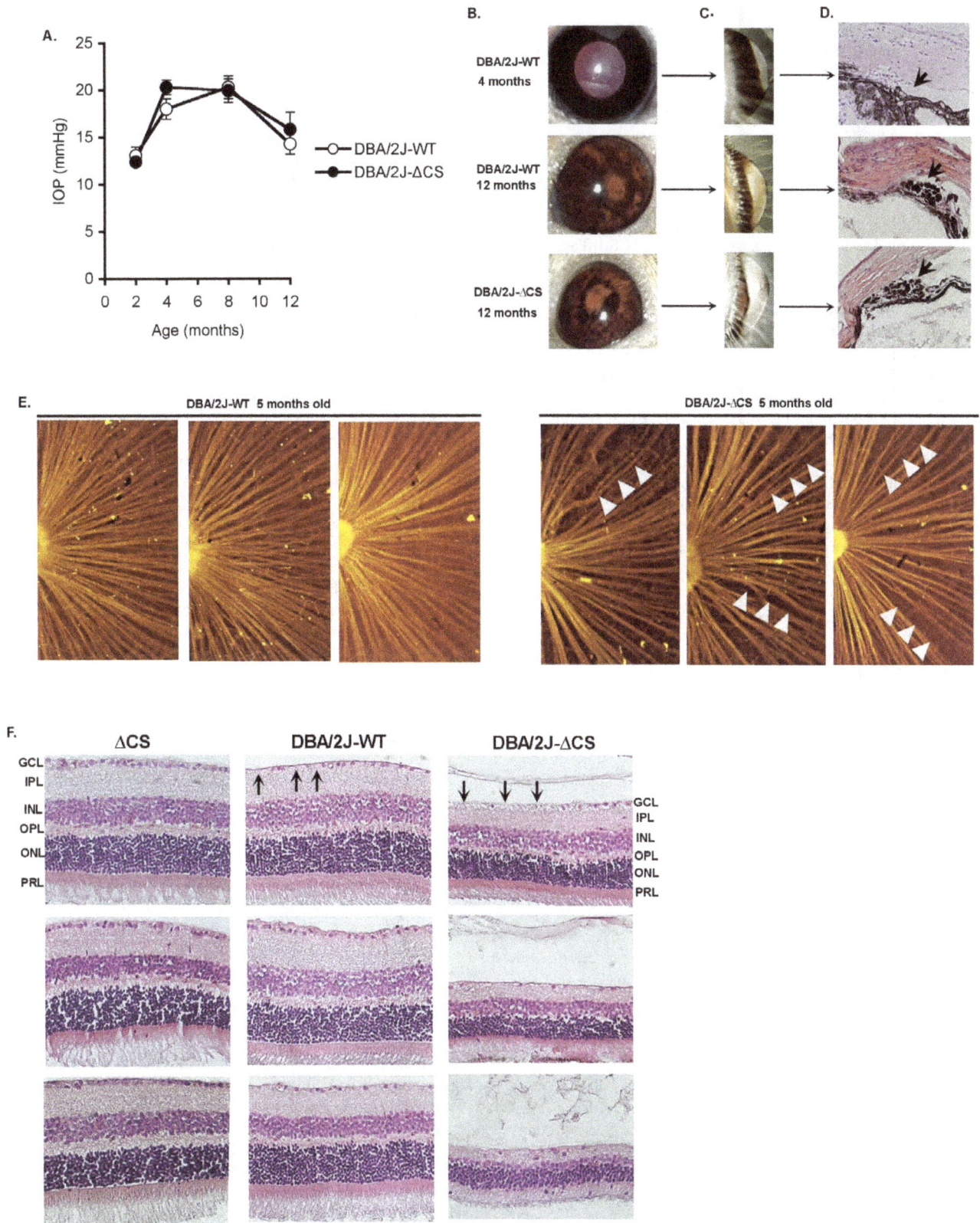

**Figure 6. mFasL induced retinal degeneration in DBA/2J mice.** The ΔCS mutation was backcrossed to DBA/2J mice (DBA/2J-ΔCS) and compared with littermate controls (DBA/2J-WT). (A) intraocular pressure (IOP) (N≥10 mice per group; mean +/− SEM). DBA/2J-WT and DBA/2J-ΔCS (12 mons old) were compared with young (4 mons old) DBA/2J mice for: (B) pigment dispersion and iris atrophy, (C) size of the anterior chamber, and (D) H&E sections of the iridocorneal angle revealing pigment laden cells (arrow) blocking the aqueous outflow pathway. (E) retinal whole mounts stained with Smi32 (anti-neurofilament antibody); arrows identify thinning of the nerve fibers. (F) H&E stained retinal sections from: B6×129 ΔCS mice (10 mons old), DBA/2J-WT (12 mons old), and DBA/2J-ΔCS (12 mons old). The pictures presented are representative of individual mice in each group (N = 10).

While it is well established that FasL is constitutively expressed in the eye, little is known about the extent of cleavage. Cell-free FasL has been identified by ELISA in the ocular fluids of the eye [52,53]. However, the ELISA assay can not distinguish cleaved sFasL from full-length FasL released from the cell in the form of microvesicles [22]. These studies have been further confounded by irrelevant cross-reactivities of many of the commercially available FasL-specific antibodies. In the current study we rigorously compared whole cell lysates from wild type, ΔCS, and FasL KO mice for FasL expression using a highly specific anti-peptide rabbit antiserum for Western blot analysis [24]. The ΔCS mFasL mice express a gene-targeted form of FasL in which the major cleavage sites were mutated to render the molecule resistant to metallo-proteinases. While we were able to distinguish clearly two bands corresponding to full-length FasL in lysates from ΔCS mice, we could barely detect a comparable band in lysates derived from wild type mice. Thus it appears that most ocular FasL is cleaved under normal physiological conditions. Our inability to detect sFasL in the eye lysates from WT mice may reflect increased clearance or instability of the soluble form.

There is general agreement that RGCs die via apoptosis in glaucoma, although the molecular events underlying RGC loss are still debated. The participation of glial cells in the death of RGCs was demonstrated in work from Nakazawa and colleagues linking increased intraocular pressure with a rapid upregulation of retina-associated TNFα and subsequent activation of microglia in the optic nerve head [7]. While both TNFα and activated microglia were required for the death of RGCs, the direct cytotoxic effector mechanism remained unclear. TNFα is detected by 2 receptors; engagement of TNFR1 is thought to trigger apoptosis and engagement of TNFR2 is thought to trigger the Akt signaling cascade and promote survival. TNFR2-deficient, but not TNFR1-deficient mice fail to exhibit RGCs loss following experimentally induced elevated intraocular pressure or TNFα injection, consistent with the premise that TNFα indirectly promotes RGC death [7]. A potential role for FasL, another TNF family member, in glaucoma was suggested by immunohistological examination of the retina in a rat model of glaucoma indicating an increased expression of FasL on microglia in the glaucomatous retina [17].

In the current study we clearly demonstrate that FasL-deficient mice are resistant to TNFα-triggered loss of RGCs subsequent to intravitreal injection. Moreover, TNFα treated ΔCS mice displayed a more rapid loss of retinal ganglion cells and nerve fibers (1 week in ΔCS mice versus 4 weeks in wild type mice). Our observations were not limited to TNFα treated mice. Using the spontaneous DBA/2J model of glaucoma [35], we again observed a significant increase and acceleration in the loss of RGCs and nerve fibers in mice expressing the ΔCS mutation. Unexpectedly, we also observed a dramatic degeneration in all layers of the retina in 12 month old DBA/2J-ΔCS mice. While it is generally accepted that retinal damage in glaucoma patients is restricted to the ganglion cells, there are reports of damage to other types of retinal cells [54]. Taken together, these studies establish the membrane-bound form of FasL as a key neurotoxic effector molecule in glaucoma and suggest that cleavage of FasL is important in protecting retinal tissue from extensive degeneration.

Based on our immunohistological examination of the retina, we further concluded that FasL expression in the retina was predominantly associated with microglial cells and not astrocytes. Prior studies had demonstrated that brain microglia express FasL [55], and therefore it was not surprising to find that retinal microglial cells also expressed FasL. In addition, the neurotoxic effects of FasL in the brain had been previously described in a model of chronic idiopathic demyelinating polyneuropathy, where macrophage-mediated demyelination was shown to be dependent upon FasL mediated death of Schwann cells [56]. Together these data support the hypothesis that RGC-neurotoxic FasL is expressed by retinal microglia. Whether the increased expression of FasL in the retina of TNFα treated mice reflects increased migration of FasL+ microglial cells to the retina and/or increased level of FasL expression/cell remains to be determined. Letellier et al recently demonstrated that FasL triggers migration of Fas+ macrophages and neutrophils into the site of spinal cord injury via activation of the Syk kinase [33]. Importantly, the increased migration triggered via FasL resulted in increased inflammation and tissue damage at the injury site, indicating that FasL triggered migration is a new mechanism by which FasL can trigger destructive inflammation. Whether FasL triggered migration is due to the membrane and/or soluble form of FasL is unknown.

Our data also have important implications for the role of sFasL in glaucoma. The most straightforward explanation for the accelerated loss of RGCs in ΔCS versus WT mice is that greater expression of membrane-bound FasL causes more extensive RGC death. However, we also found that sFasL could antagonize the activity of mFasL and, in the context of glaucoma, be neuroprotective. The opposing activities of membrane and soluble FasL further suggest that FasL cleavage is a major mechanism for limiting the neurotoxic activity of FasL in the eye and raises the intriguing possibility that TNFα may in fact regulate FasL cleavage. The cleavage of FasL is mediated primarily by MMPs (MMP7 and MMP3) as well as TIMPs that are the major endogenous regulators of MMP activities [57]. Both MMPs and TIMPs are expressed by retinal microglia, RGCs, and their axons [58]. Therefore, changes in MMP and/or TIMP expression triggered by TNFα or other factors induced by elevated IOP may be critical in regulating the ratio of soluble to membrane FasL expressed by microglia during glaucoma. In conclusion, our data indicate the enhancement of FasL cleavage and/or forced expression of sFasL may have therapeutic applications in preventing RGC apoptosis in glaucoma.

## Materials and Methods

### Ethics Statement

All animals were treated according to the Association for Research in Vision and Ophthalmology Resolution on the Use of Animals in Research. The Schepens IACUC committee approved all procedures under protocols #S223-1211 and # S230-0312.

### Animals

To examine the importance of sFasL in ocular homeostasis and RGC degeneration, we constructed a FasL-deficient mouse line (designated as FasL KO) and a membrane-only FasL gene-targeted mouse line (this cleavage site deleted-mouse line was designated as ΔCS). The details of how these mice were produced are described in the supplemental data (Figure S1). The ΔCS founder mice were crossed to C57BL/6 mice for one generation and then intercrossed for the TNFα studies. Wild-type littermates were used as WT controls. A second group of mice were backcrossed to DBA/2J mice (Jackson Laboratories), and then intercrossed for in vivo analysis. Assessment of the ΔCS×DBA/2J and wild-type DBA/2J littermates was performed at the fifth generation backcross. FasL knockout mice were described previously [27].

### Intravitreal injections

The intravitreal injection, just posterior to the limbus-parallel conjunctival vessels, were described previously. Mice received a

0.5 µl intravitreal injection of TNF-α (Millipore/Chemicon) (1 ng/0.5 µL of sterile saline) or saline alone. Some mice received recombinant murine soluble FasL alone (R & D Systems) (100 ng/ 0.5 µl sterile physiological saline) or in combination with the TNFα (100 ng sFasL/1 ng TNFα/0.5 µl sterile physiological saline). The mouse recombinant sFasL corresponds with the physiological cleavage product (Pro 132 to Leu 279) and has weak or no cytolytic activity against A20 target cells.

## Quantitation of retinal ganglion cells

Enucleated eyes were fixed and cryostat sections (8 µm) sections were blocked in 2.5% BSA/0.3% triton in PBS, followed by incubation with a RGC specific primary antibody, anti-βIII-tubulin (TU-20, Millipore), a biotinylated secondary antibody, and Cy2-conjugated streptavidin (Jackson Immuno research). Nuclei were counterstained with To-pro-3 (Molecular Probes). The total number of β-III-tubulin/To-Pro-3 double positive retinal ganglion cells were counted throughout the entire RGC layer of each section. A total of 10 sections were analyzed per eye (10 eyes analyzed per group). The sections were taken through the central globe of each eye.

## Retinal whole mounts

Neural retina was isolated, fixed, and incubated with an anti-neurofilament antibody (SMi32, Covance) for 3 days at 4°C followed by a Rhodamine (TRITC)-conjugated secondary antibody for 2 days at 4°C. Nuclei were counter stained with To-Pro-3 (Molecular Probes, Eugene, OR). Following staining, the retinas were mounted RGC layer side up and examined by confocal microscopy (Leica Microsystems; Wetzlar, Germany).

## Western blots

Protein lysates were prepared from whole eyes (excluding the lens) and splenic T cells stimulated with plate-bound anti-CD3. Proteins were separated on 12% Tris-glycine gels (Invitrogen, Carlsbad, CA), and transferred onto polyvinylidene difluoride membranes (Invitrogen, Carlsbad, CA). The membranes were probed for Fas ligand using a polyclonal rabbit anti-Fas ligand antibody [24] followed by a goat anti-rabbit-IIRP secondary antibody (Santa Cruz Biotechnology, Santa Cruz, CA). L5178Y-R tumor transfectants served as positive controls for membrane and soluble FasL.

## Immunofluorescent staining

Immunofluorescent staining was performed on frozen retinal cross sections using primary antibodies to astrocytes (Cy3-conjugated GFAP, Jackson ImmunoResearch), microglia (Iba1, Santa Cruz Technology Inc), FasL (C178 and N20, Santa Cruz technology Inc), and Fas receptor (C20 Santa Cruz technology Inc). The secondary antibody for Iba1, FasL, and Fas was a Cy3-conjugated anti-rabbit. In all cases, isotyped matched antibodies served as negative controls and To-Pro-3 (Molecular Probes, Eugene, OR) was used to stain all nucleated cells.

**SD-OCT (Spectral Domain Optical Coherence Tomography).** Optical coherence tomography was performed using a SD-OCT system (Bioptigen Inc., Durham, NC) at day 7 after intravitreal TNFα injection. A volume analysis was performed, using 100 horizontal, raster, and consecutive B-scan lines, each one composed by 1200 A-scans. The volume size was 1.6×1.6 cm. The software was able to generate the en-face fundus image using the reflectance information obtained from the OCT sections (volume intensity projection), so that the point-to-point correlation between OCT and fundus position was possible and accurate.

**In vivo quantification of retinal nerve fiber layer thickness.** Sectorial areas containing retinal defects were identified in the retinal whole mount images and the corresponding retinal areas were identified in the OCT-based en-face fundus reconstruction. This was achieved by aligning the two images using the retinal vessels shape and position. Within the OCT images passing through these areas, six sections from each eye were randomly chosen and used by a masked operator to assess the retinal nerve fiber layer thickness. For the measurements, the caliper tool provided by the Bioptigen software was used in 2 different, and randomly chosen positions on the same image. The retinal nerve fiber layer thickness was defined as the interval between the inner and outer boundary of the most internal retinal hyper-reflective layer visualized in the OCT image. Measurement was avoided in OCT points that corresponded to retinal vessels.

## RGC apoptosis

Apoptotic cells were identified in 8 µm frozen retinal sections using a TUNEL In Situ Cell Death detection Kit (TMR red, Roche Applied Science) and sections were mounted using DAPI pan-nuclear stain (Vectashield). Following staining, the ratio of TUNEL positive to total DAPI positive cells was calculated in 6 visual fields at 100× magnification. These calculations were repeated in 3 sections per experimental eye with at least 5 animals per group per time point.

## Intraocular (IOP) measurements

IOP was measured using a TonoLab tonometer (Colonial Medical Supply, Espoo, Finland) and performed as previously described [34].

## Statistics

Where normally distributed, the data were analyzed with an unpaired $t$ test with a $P$ value of $<0.05$ as the basis for rejection of the null hypothesis. Statistical analysis and graphing were performed using Microsoft Excel.

## Supporting Information

**Figure S1 Production of the mutant mice.** (A) Targeting vectors designed to delete the 2 cleavage sites (AA 124/125 and AA 127/128) located in exon 2 [59,60] were constructed from a 129/OLA P1 genomic clone (Genomesystems Inc, St. Louis) and used to transfect 129 ES cells. Appropriately targeted cells were subsequently transfected with the pMC-Cre expression vector to remove the neo cassette [62]. (B) In the Cre-FasL construct, 8 residues (121–128) were deleted from exon 2. This mutation resulted in a splicing error and frameshift mutation, thereby creating a FasL-deficient strain, referred to in the text as FasL KO. By contrast, the ΔCS construct replaced the 4 residues that bracket the 2 potential cleavage sites (designated by the asterisks in the 4 black boxes). These exchange mutations ($124_{Ser \to Thr}$, $125_{PHe \to Leu}$, $127_{Lys \to Arg}$, and $128_{Gln \to Asn}$) eliminated the cleavage sites within the full-length protein and prevented the cleavage of FasL to produce the soluble form of FasL. (C) RNA was isolated from activated CD8+ T cells from FasL KO, heterozygous, and wild-type mice. RT-PCR was performed using primers (designated by arrows) to amplify the region spanning exon 1, exon 2, and exon 3. The results demonstrated that wild-type mice expressed a 473 bp fragment indicating all 3 exons are present, while knockout mice expressed only a 427 bp fragment indicating the loss of exon 2. As expected, the heterozygous mice expressed both products. (D) CD8+ T cells were isolated from the spleen and lymph node of:

WT, FasL KO heterozygous, and FasL KO homozygous mice. T cells were activated with anti-CD3, and analyzed for FasL expression by FACS analysis. Activated CD8+ T cells from wild-type mice displayed significant levels of FasL, while heterozygous mice displayed a significant reduction in FasL. Activated CD8+ T cells from FasL KO mice displayed no detectable staining over the isotype control antibody, indicating no FasL was expressed on these cells. Similar data was obtained with activated CD4+ T cells (data not shown). (E) Phenotypically, the FasL knock-out mice present with significantly greater splenomegally and lymphadenopathy than *gld/gld* mice.

## Figure S2  Apoptosis of RGCs is induced by mFasL in vitro.

RGC5 cells were differentiated in a 96 well microplates ($1.5 \times 10^3$ cells per well) as previously described [61]. After differentiation the media was removed and complete DMEM was added. Control vesicles or mFasL vesicles prepared as previously described [13] were added at various dilutions to differentiated RGC5 cells and at incubated at 37°C for 16 hours. Cell viability was assessed using the standard 3-[4,5-dimethylthiazol-2-yl]-2,5-diphenyltetrazolium (MTT) reduction assay. (A) The immortalized RGC-5 cell line was differentiated in vitro and treated with microvesicles expressing membrane-only FasL (mFasL) or no FasL (neo) at increasing concentrations 1:100, 1:20, 1:7. The MTT cytotoxicity assay was used to measure viability and revealed significant loss of viability only in RGCs incubated with mFasL microvesicles. * p>0.05 and ** p>0.01 as compared to media alone.

## Acknowledgments

We would like to thank Marie Ortega and Jennifer Wendtland for their excellent assistance with animal breeding and Don Pottle for technical assistance with Confocal Analysis.

## Author Contributions

Conceived and designed the experiments: BRK AM-R MSG. Performed the experiments: MSG CGH EFA KSL RRS AMH K-sLM MWH AJ PK AG. Analyzed the data: MSG AG BRK AMR. Contributed reagents/materials/analysis tools: SK SWMJ. Wrote the manuscript: MSG AM-R BRK. Consulted on experimental design: SWMJ DFC.

## References

1. Kwon YH, Fingert JH, Kuehn MH, Alward WLM (2009) Primary open-angle glaucoma. N Engl J Med 360: 1113–1124.
2. McKinnon SJ (1997) Glaucoma, apoptosis, and neuroprotection. Current Opinion in Ophthalmology 8: 28–37.
3. Sawada H, Fukuchi T, Tanaka T, Abe H (2010) Tumor necrosis factor-alpha concentrations in the aqueous humor of patients with glaucoma. Invest Ophthalmol Vis Sci 51: 903–906.
4. Tezel G, Li LY, Patil RV, Wax MB (2001) TNF-alpha and TNF-alpha receptor-1 in the retina of normal and glaucomatous eyes. Invest Ophthalmol Vis Sci 42: 1787–1794.
5. Funayama T, Ishikawa K, Ohtake Y, Tanino T, Kurosaka D, et al. (2004) Variants in optineurin gene and their association with tumor necrosis factor-alpha polymorphisms in Japanese patients with glaucoma. Invest Ophthalmol Vis Sci 45: 4359–4367.
6. Lin HJ, Tsai FJ, Chen WC, Shi YR, Hsu Y, et al. (2003) Association of tumour necrosis factor alpha -308 gene polymorphism with primary open-angle glaucoma in Chinese. Eye (Lond) 17: 31–34.
7. Nakazawa T, Nakazawa C, Matsubara A, Noda K, Hisatomi T, et al. (2006) Tumor necrosis factor-alpha mediates oligodendrocyte death and delayed retinal ganglion cell loss in a mouse model of glaucoma. J Neurosci 26: 12633–12641.
8. Yang Z, Quigley HA, Pease ME, Yang Y, Qian J, et al. (2007) Changes in gene expression in experimental glaucoma and optic nerve transection: the equilibrium between protective and detrimental mechanisms. Invest Ophthalmol Vis Sci 48: 5539–5548.
9. Kagi D, Vignaux F, Ledemann B, Burki K, Depraetere V, et al. (1994) Fas and perforin pathways as major mechanisms of T cell-mediated cytotoxicity. Science 265: 528–530.
10. Ju S-T, Panka DJ, Cui H, Ettinger R, El-Khatib M, et al. (1995) Fas (CD95)/FasL interactions required for programmed cell death after T-cell activation. Nature 373: 444–448.
11. Lee HO, Ferguson TA (2003) Biology of FasL. Cytokine Growth Factor Rev 14: 325–335.
12. Rescigno M, Piguet V, Valzasina B, Lens S, Zubler R, et al. (2000) Fas engagement induces the maturation of dendritic cells (DCs), the release of interleukin (IL)-1beta, and the production of interferon gamma in the absence of IL-12 during DC-T cell cognate interaction: a new role for Fas ligand in inflammatory responses. J Exp Med 192: 1661–1668.
13. Hohlbaum AM, Gregory MS, Ju S-T, Marshak-Rothstein A (2001) Fas ligand engagement of resident peritoneal macrophages in vivo induces apoptosis and the production of neutrophil chemotactic factors. J Immunol 167: 6217–6224.
14. Park SM, Schickel R, Peter ME (2005) Nonapoptotic functions of FADD-binding death receptors and their signaling molecules. Curr Opin Cell Biol 17: 610–616.
15. Wax MB, Tezel G, Yang J, Peng G, Patil RV, et al. (2008) Induced autoimmunity to heat shock proteins elicits glaucomatous loss of retinal ganglion cell neurons via activated T-cell-derived fas-ligand. J Neurosci 28: 12085–12096.
16. Apte RS, Richter J, Herndon J, Ferguson TA (2006) Macrophages inhibit neovascularization in a murine model of age-related macular degeneration. PLoS Med 3: e310.
17. Ju KR, Kim HS, Kim JH, Lee NY, Park CK (2006) Retinal glial cell responses and Fas/FasL activation in rats with chronic ocular hypertension. Brain Res 1122: 209–221.
18. Bazzoni F, Beutler B (1996) The tumor necrosis factor ligand and receptor families. N Engl J Med 334: 1717–1725.
19. Perez C, Albert I, DeFay K, Zachariades N, Gooding L, et al. (1990) A nonsecretable cell surface mutant of tumor necrosis factor (TNF) kills by cell-to-cell contact. Cell 63: 251–258.
20. Sherry B, Cerami A (1988) Cachectin/tumor necrosis factor exerts endocrine, paracrine, and autocrine control of inflammatory responses. J Cell Biol 107: 1269–1277.
21. Tanaka M, Suda T, Takahashi T, Nagata S (1995) Expression of the soluble form of the human Fas ligand in activated lymphocytes. EMBO J 14: 1129–1135.
22. Jodo S, Xiao S, Hohlbaum AM, Strehlow D, Marshak-Rothstein A, et al. (2001) Apoptosis-inducing membrane vesicles: a novel agent with unique properties. J Biol Chem 276: 39938–39944.
23. Bossi G, Griffiths GM (2005) CTL secretory lysosomes: biogenesis and secretion of a harmful organelle. Semin Immunol 17: 87–94.
24. Hohlbaum AH, Moe S, Marshak-Rothstein A (2000) Opposing effects of transmembrane and soluble Fas ligand expression on inflammation and tumor cell survival. J Exp Med 191: 1209–1219.
25. Suda T, Hashimoto H, Tanaka M, Ochi T, Nagata S (1997) Membrane Fas ligand kills human peripheral blood T lymphocytes, and soluble Fas ligand blocks the killing. J Exp Med 186: 2045–2050.
26. Aoki K, Kurooka M, Chen JJ, Petryniak J, Nabel EG, et al. (2001) Extracellular matrix interacts with soluble CD95L: retention and enhancement of cytotoxicity. Nat Immunol 2: 333–337.
27. Karray S, Kress C, Cuvellier S, Hue-Beauvais C, Damotte D, et al. (2004) Complete loss of Fas ligand gene causes massive lymphoproliferation and early death, indicating a residual activity of gld allele. J Immunol 172: 2118–2125.
28. Martinez-Lorenzo MJ, Alava MA, Gamen S, Kim KJ, Chuntharapai A, et al. (1998) Involvement of APO2 ligand/TRAIL in activation-induced death of Jurkat and human peripheral blood T cells. Eur J Immunol 28: 2714–2725.
29. Powell WC, Fingleton B, Wilson CL, Boothby M, Matrisian LM (1999) The metalloproteinase matrilysin proteolytically generates active soluble Fas ligand and potentiates epithelial cell apoptosis. Curr Biol 9: 1441–1447.
30. Kim JS, Ishikawa H, Sung KR, Xu J, Wollstein G, et al. (2009) Retinal nerve fibre layer thickness measurement reproducibility improved with spectral domain optical coherence tomography. Br J Ophthalmol 93: 1057–1063.
31. Schuman JS, Hee MR, Puliafito CA, Wong C, Pedut-Kloizman T, et al. (1995) Quantification of nerve fiber layer thickness in normal and glaucomatous eyes using optical coherence tomography. Arch Ophthalmol 113: 586–596.
32. Wollstein G, Schuman JS, Price LL, Aydin A, Stark PC, et al. (2005) Optical coherence tomography longitudinal evaluation of retinal nerve fiber layer thickness in glaucoma. Arch Ophthalmol 123: 464–470.
33. Letellier E, Kumar S, Sancho-Martinez I, Krauth S, Funke-Kaiser A, et al. (2010) CD95-Ligand on Peripheral Myeloid Cells Activates Syk Kinase to Trigger Their Recruitment to the Inflammatory Site. Immunity 32: 240–252.
34. Anderson MG, Libby RT, Mao M, Cosma IM, Wilson LA, et al. (2006) Genetic context determines susceptibility to intraocular pressure elevation in a mouse pigmentary glaucoma. BMC Biol 4: 20.
35. Anderson MG, Smith RS, Hawes NL, Zabaleta A, Chang B, et al. (2002) Mutations in genes encoding melanosomal proteins cause pigmentary glaucoma in DBA/2J mice. Nat Genet 30: 81–85.

36. Jakobs T, Libby R, Ben Y, John S, Masland R (2005) Retinal ganglion cell degeneration is topological but not cell type specific in DBA/2J mice. J Cell Biol 171: 313–325.

37. Theofilopoulos AN, Balderas RS, Gozes Y, Aguado MT, Hang L, et al. (1985) Association of lpr gene with graft-vs-host disease-like syndrome. J Exp Med 162: 1–18.

38. Nemazee D, Guiet C, Buerki K, Marshak-Rothstein A (1991) B lymphocytes from the autoimmune-prone mouse strain MRL/lpr manifest an intrinsic defect in MRL/lpr <-> DBA/2 chimeras. J Immunol 147: 2536–2539.

39. Hao Z, Hampel B, Yagita H, Rajewsky K (2004) T cell-specific ablation of Fas leads to Fas ligand-mediated lymphocyte depletion and inflammatory pulmonary fibrosis. J Exp Med 199: 1355–1365.

40. Kavurma MM, Khachigian LM (2003) Signaling and transcriptional control of Fas ligand gene expression. Cell Death Differ 10: 36–44.

41. He JS, Ostergaard HL (2007) CTLs contain and use intracellular stores of FasL distinct from cytolytic granules. J Immunol 179: 2339–2348.

42. Griffith TS, Brunner T, Fletcher SM, Green DR, Ferguson TA (1995) Fas-ligand induced apoptosis as a mechanism of immune privilege. Science 270: 1189–1192.

43. Ferguson TA, Apte RS (2008) Angiogenesis in eye disease: immunity gained or immunity lost? Semin Immunopathol 30: 111–119.

44. Hu MS, Schwartzman JD, Yeaman GR, Collins J, Seguin R, et al. (1999) Fas-FasL interaction involved in pathogenesis of ocular toxoplasmosis in mice. Infect Immun 67: 928–935.

45. Stuart PM, Pan F, PLambeck S, Ferguson TA (2003) FasL-Fas interactions regulate neovascularization in the cornea. Invest Ophthalmol Vis Sci 44: 93–8.

46. Stuart PM, Griffith TS, Usui N, Pepose J, Yu X, et al. (1997) CD95 ligand (FasL)-induced apoptosis is necessary for corneal allograft survival. J Clin Invest 99: 396–402.

47. Sano Y, Yamada J, Ishino Y, Adachi W, Kawasaki S, et al. (2002) Non-cleavable mutant Fas ligand transfection of donor cornea abrogates ocular immune privilege. Exp Eye Res 75: 475–483.

48. Gregory MS, Repp A, Hohlbaum AM, Marshak-Rothstein A, Ksander BR (2002) Membrane Fas ligand activates innate immunity and terminates ocular immune privilege. J Immunol 2002: 2727–2735.

49. Shudo K, Kinoshita K, Imamura R, Fan H, Hasumoto K, et al. (2001) The membrane-bound but not the soluble form of human Fas ligand is responsible for its inflammatory activity. Eur J Immunol 31: 2504–2511.

50. O' Reilly LA, Tai L, Lee L, Kruse EA, Grabow S, et al. (2009) Membrane-bound Fas ligand only is essential for Fas-induced apoptosis. Nature 461: 659–663.

51. Ohta K, Yamagami S, Taylor AW, Streilein JW (2000) IL-6 antagonizes TGF-beta and abolishes immune privilege in eyes with endotoxin-induced uveitis. Invest Ophthalmol Vis Sci 41: 2591–2599.

52. Sotozono C, Sano Y, Suzuki T, Tada R, Ikeda T, et al. (2000) Soluble Fas ligand expression in the ocular fluids of uveitis patients. Curr Eye Res 20: 54–57.

53. Sugita S, Taguchi C, Takase H, Sagawa K, Sueda J, et al. (2000) Soluble Fas ligand and soluble Fas in ocular fluid of patients with uveitis. Br J Ophthalmol 84: 1130–1134.

54. Lei Y, Garrahan N, Hermann B, Becker DL, Hernandez MR, et al. (2008) Quantification of retinal transneuronal degeneration in human glaucoma: a novel multiphoton-DAPI approach. Invest Ophthalmol Vis Sci 49: 1940–1945.

55. Taylor DL, Jones F, Kubota ES, Pocock JM (2005) Stimulation of microglial metabotropic glutamate receptor mGlu2 triggers tumor necrosis factor alpha-induced neurotoxicity in concert with microglial-derived Fas ligand. J Neurosci 25: 2952–2964.

56. Dace DS, Khan AA, Stark JL, Kelly J, Cross AH, et al. (2009) Interleukin-10 overexpression promotes Fas-ligand-dependent chronic macrophage-mediated demyelinating polyneuropathy. PLoS One 4: e7121.

57. Vargo-Gogola T, Crawford HC, Fingleton B, Matrisian LM (2002) Identification of novel matrix metalloproteinase-7 (matrilysin) cleavage sites in murine and human Fas ligand. Arch Biochem Biophys 408: 155–161.

58. Agapova OA, Ricard CS, Salvador-Silva M, Hernandez MR (2001) Expression of matrix metalloproteinases and tissue inhibitors of metalloproteinases in human optic nerve head astrocytes. Glia 33: 205–216.

59. Vargo-Gogola T, Crawford HC, Fingleton B, Matrisian LM (2002) Identification of novel matrix metalloproteinase-7 (matrilysin) cleavage sites in murine and human Fas ligand. Arch Biochem Biophys 408: 155–161.

60. Tanaka M, Itai T, Adachi M, Nagata S (1998) Downregulation of Fas ligand by shedding. Nat Med 4: 31–36.

61. Tchedre KT, Yorio T (2008) sigma-1 receptors protect RGC-5 cells from apoptosis by regulating intracellular calcium, Bax levels, and caspase-3 activation. Invest Ophthalmol Vis Sci 49: 2577–2588.

62. Gu H, Zou YR, Rajewsky K (1993) Independent control of immunoglobulin switch recombination at individual switch regions evidenced through Cre-loxP-mediated gene targeting. Cell 73: 1155–1164.

# 12

# Glaucomatous Patterns in Frequency Doubling Technology (FDT) Perimetry Data Identified by Unsupervised Machine Learning Classifiers

**Christopher Bowd**[1]*, **Robert N. Weinreb**[1], **Madhusudhanan Balasubramanian**[1], **Intae Lee**[1], **Giljin Jang**[1,2], **Siamak Yousefi**[1], **Linda M. Zangwill**[1], **Felipe A. Medeiros**[1], **Christopher A. Girkin**[3], **Jeffrey M. Liebmann**[4,5], **Michael H. Goldbaum**[1]

1 Hamilton Glaucoma Center, Department of Ophthalmology, University of California, San Diego, La Jolla, California, United States of America, 2 School of Electrical and Computer Engineering, Ulsan National Institute of Science and Technology, Ulsan, South Korea, 3 Department of Ophthalmology, University of Alabama at Birmingham, Birmingham, Alabama, United States of America, 4 Department of Ophthalmology, New York University School of Medicine, New York, New York, United States of America, 5 New York Eye and Ear Infirmary, New York, New York, United States of America

## Abstract

*Purpose:* The variational Bayesian independent component analysis-mixture model (VIM), an unsupervised machine-learning classifier, was used to automatically separate Matrix Frequency Doubling Technology (FDT) perimetry data into clusters of healthy and glaucomatous eyes, and to identify axes representing statistically independent patterns of defect in the glaucoma clusters.

*Methods:* FDT measurements were obtained from 1,190 eyes with normal FDT results and 786 eyes with abnormal FDT results from the UCSD-based Diagnostic Innovations in Glaucoma Study (DIGS) and African Descent and Glaucoma Evaluation Study (ADAGES). For all eyes, VIM input was 52 threshold test points from the 24-2 test pattern, plus age.

*Results:* FDT mean deviation was −1.00 dB (S.D. = 2.80 dB) and −5.57 dB (S.D. = 5.09 dB) in FDT-normal eyes and FDT-abnormal eyes, respectively (p<0.001). VIM identified meaningful clusters of FDT data and positioned a set of statistically independent axes through the mean of each cluster. The optimal VIM model separated the FDT fields into 3 clusters. Cluster $N$ contained primarily normal fields (1109/1190, specificity 93.1%) and clusters $G_1$ and $G_2$ combined, contained primarily abnormal fields (651/786, sensitivity 82.8%). For clusters $G_1$ and $G_2$ the optimal number of axes were 2 and 5, respectively. Patterns automatically generated along axes within the glaucoma clusters were similar to those known to be indicative of glaucoma. Fields located farther from the normal mean on each glaucoma axis showed increasing field defect severity.

*Conclusions:* VIM successfully separated FDT fields from healthy and glaucoma eyes without *a priori* information about class membership, and identified familiar glaucomatous patterns of loss.

**Editor:** Pedro Gonzalez, Duke University, United States of America

**Funding:** This work was supported by NIH EY022039, EY020518, NIH EY011008, NIH EY014267, NIH EY019869, NIH EY021818, and an unrestricted grant from Research to Prevent Blindness, Eyesight Foundation of Alabama, Corinne Graber Research Fund of the New York Glaucoma Research Institute. The authors also would like to acknowledge funding from Alcon Laboratories, Allergan, and Pfizer in the form of glaucoma medications at no cost to study participants to which they are prescribed. The funders had no role in study design, data collection and analysis, decision to publish, or preparation of the manuscript.

**Competing Interests:** The authors have read the journal's policy and declare the following conflicts. R.N. Weinreb: Provision of equipment used for research by Heidelberg Engineering GmbH, Nidek, Optovue Inc., Topcon Medical Systems Inc. Consultant for Carl Zeiss Meditec. L.M. Zangwill: Provision of equipment used for research by Carl Zeiss Meditec, Heidelberg Engineering GmbH, Optovue Inc., Topcon Medical Systems Inc. F.A. Medeiros: Provision of equipment used for research by Carl Zeiss Meditec, Heidelberg Engineering GmbH, Topcon Medical Systems Inc. J.M. Liebmann: Provision of equipment used for research by Carl Zeiss Meditec, Diopsys Corp., Heidelberg Engineering GmbH, Optovue Inc., Topcon Medical Systems Inc. Consultant for Diopsys Corp., Optovue Inc., Topcon Medical Systems.

* E-mail: cbowd@ucsd.edu

## Introduction

A number of previous studies have used supervised machine-learning techniques to separate healthy from glaucomatous eyes successfully, based on visual function and optical imaging data. [1–20] In several instances, machine-learning classifiers (MLCs) have outperformed commercially available software-generated parameters at this task. [6–8,15,18] Supervised MLCs are trained with labeled examples of class membership (e.g., healthy or glaucoma), preferably based on a teaching label other than the test being assessed. [8] For example the presence of glaucomatous optic neuropathy (GON) can indicate which eyes have glaucoma when assessing visual field-based MLCs, and the presence of visual field defects can indicate which eyes have glaucoma when assessing optical imaging-based MLCs. [21] The MLCs then "learn" to separate healthy and glaucomatous eyes in a training set and the performance (i.e., diagnostic accuracy) of each MLC is assessed on a separate test set not used during training (often using k-fold cross validation, holdout method, or bootstrapping).

An alternate class of MLCs, based on unsupervised learning, also has been employed to identify healthy and glaucomatous eyes, based on visual field data. [22–24] Unsupervised learning is a technique that discerns how the data are organized by learning to separate data into statistically independent groups by cluster analysis, or into representative axes by component analysis, without a priori information regarding class membership. For instance, component analysis can decompose data by projecting multidimensional data onto n axes that meaningfully represent the data.

Independent component analysis (ICA) [25] is an unsupervised classification method that reveals a single set of independent axes underlying sets of random variables. ICA has proven highly successful for noise reduction in a wide range of applications. [26–28] However, there are data distributions where components are nonlinearly related or clustered such that they are difficult to describe by a single ICA model, for example, perimetric visual field results from a mixture of healthy and glaucomatous eyes. In these cases, nonlinear mixture model ICA can extend the linear ICA model by learning multiple ICA models and weighting them in a probabilistic (i.e., Bayesian) manner. [25] The ICA mixture model learns the number of clusters and orients statistically independent axes within each cluster. The variational Bayesian framework helps to capture the number of axes in the local axis set and reduces computational complexity. [29] The amalgamation of all these processes is the unsupervised variational Bayesian independent component analysis-mixture model (henceforth, called VIM).

We previously applied VIM to standard automated perimetry (SAP) results from glaucoma patients. Each axis identified by VIM represented a glaucomatous visual field defect pattern, and the severity of that pattern was organized from mild to advanced along each axis. Although identified automatically using mathematical techniques and no human input, VIM for SAP data identified patterns that were similar to those known to be indicative of glaucoma based on decades of expert visual field assessment [24].

Frequency Doubling Technology (FDT) stimuli test the responses of a subset of all available retinal ganglion cells that have different temporal and spatial summation properties compared to those tested using SAP. [30] It is currently undetermined if FDT perimetry data can similarly be organized by VIM into meaningful patterns and axes. The purpose of this study is to determine if VIM can separate a set of normal and glaucomatous FDT fields into acceptable clusters of normal and glaucomatous eyes and to determine if this technique can identify axes representing statistically independent patterns of defect within the glaucoma clusters. If independent axes are identifiable within each glaucoma cluster, future work could use severity changes along the axes composing these clusters to describe glaucomatous progression in FDT data [31].

## Methods

### Study Participants

Individuals included in the current study were participants in the University of California, San Diego (UCSD)-based Diagnostic Innovations in Glaucoma Study (DIGS) and African Descent and Glaucoma Evaluation Study (ADAGES, which also includes participants from University of Alabama, Birmingham, UAB; and New York Eye and Ear Infirmary, NYEE). In total, FDT results from 1,976 eyes of 1,136 individuals were studied.

Each study participant underwent a comprehensive ophthalmologic evaluation including review of medical history, best-corrected visual acuity testing, slit-lamp biomicroscopy, intraocular pressure measurement with Goldmann applanation tonometry, gonioscopy, dilated fundus examination with a 78 diopter lens, simultaneous stereoscopic optic disc photography (TRC-SS, Topcon Instruments Corp. of America, Paramus, NJ), and SAP using the 24-2 SITA Standard test strategy (Humphrey Field Analyzer II, Carl Zeiss Meditec, Dublin, CA). To be included in the study, participants had to have a best-corrected acuity better than or equal to 20/40, spherical refraction within ±5.0 D and cylinder correction within ±3.0 D at baseline, and open angles on gonioscopy. Eyes with non-glaucomatous optic neuropathy, uveitis or coexisting retinal disease that could affect visual fields were excluded.

This research followed the tenets of the Declaration of Helsinki and Health Insurance Portability and Accountability Act guidelines. All study participants provided written informed consent and the UCSD, UAB, and NYEE Human Research Protection Programs approved all methodology.

### Frequency Doubling Technology (FDT) Perimetry Testing

Each participant was tested using FDT with the Humphrey Matrix (24-2 test pattern) FDT Visual Field Instrument (Carl Zeiss Meditec, Dublin, California, USA) with Welch-Allyn technology (Skaneateles Falls, New York, USA) using the Zippy Estimation by Sequential Testing (ZEST) thresholding algorithm. [32,33] FDT measures the contrast necessary to detect vertical grating targets that undergo counter-phase flicker. Each target subtends 5 degrees of visual angle and has a spatial frequency of 0.5 cycle/degree and counter phases with a temporal frequency of 18 Hz. The test is based on the frequency-doubling illusion and is a sensitive way to measure glaucomatous visual field loss. In addition, the variability of FDT Matrix measurements is less affected by disease-related decreases in sensitivity than the variability of SAP measurements. [34] The details of this test have been described elsewhere [35].

For the purpose of assessing the specificity and sensitivity of VIM-defined clusters, FDT Matrix results from each study eye were classified as within normal limits (i.e., healthy based on FDT results, 1,190 eyes) or abnormal [786 eyes with FDT Glaucoma Hemifield Test (GHT) outside of normal limits or Pattern Standard Deviation ≤5%], based on the instrument's normative database. All FDT results were reliable, defined as false positives, fixation losses and false negatives ≤33%. Mean reliability results were 2.86%, 5.51% and 1.61% for false positives, fixation losses and false negatives, respectively.

Previous studies using unsupervised classifiers to identify patterns of visual field defect in glaucoma eyes used glaucomatous optic neuropathy (GON), as determined by stereophotograph assessment, as an indicator of disease. [23,24] Because some eyes with GON have normal appearing visual fields and some eyes with abnormal visual fields do not have glaucomatous optic neuropathy, and since the goal of this study was to understand the structure of the data rather than diagnosis, in particular to find axes that represented visual field patterns within the data, we considered that the truth values used to validate the clusters that best separated glaucoma and normal eyes should be based on FTD visual field results instead of GON. We hypothesized that clusters that best separated healthy and glaucoma results would lead to the axes within the clusters that best represented the visual field patterns within the clusters.

FDT mean deviation was −1.00 dB (S.D. = 2.80 dB) in FDT-normal eyes and −5.57 dB (S.D. = 5.09 dB) in FDT-abnormal eyes, respectively (one-tailed t-test, p<0.001). Individuals providing abnormal FDT results in at least one eye were slightly, but significantly, older than individuals providing normal FDT results from both eyes (55.9 years, S.D. = 15.3 years versus 50.0 years, S.D. = 14.7 years, respectively, two-tailed t-test p<0.001).

### Variational Bayesian Independent Components Analysis Mixture Model (VIM) Description

This technique has been described in varying degrees of detail previously, by our collaborators and by us. [22–24,36,37] As described above, VIM is an amalgamation of multiple ICA models weighted in a probabilistic manner. This combination allows the unsupervised identification of independent clusters of data, each containing statistically independent axes of information. In the current study, VIM training was based on the absolute sensitivity values from each of the 52 visual field test points (excluding blind-spot points) and age (a total of 53 dimensions) from all FDT tests (1,976 in total).

First, several candidate VIM models were created using two to five possible Gaussian clusters, with a maximum of 10 or 20 possible axes per cluster and three, six or eight possible mixture components. These candidate VIM models were repeated with 30 random initializations to avoid finding a locally optimal solution. Thus, a total of 720 VIM models were created (4 trial clusters, 2 axis choices per cluster, 3 mixture component sets, and 30 random initializations), and each model was subjected to 500 iterations of training (a sufficiently high number of iterations, arbitrarily specified, to identify model convergence) in an attempt to identify the models that provided the highest specificity versus sensitivity trade-off (defined with a specificity goal of 0.90). Figure 1 shows the initial specificity and sensitivity (prior to 500 iterations of retraining) of all 720 models tested, and shows the two "best" models.

The single best model (#202 with the highest specificity versus sensitivity trade-off) maximized specificity and sensitivity using three clusters, each including a maximum of 20 axes. The optimal number of axes within each cluster was manually chosen based on the previously described process of finding the "knee" points. [38]

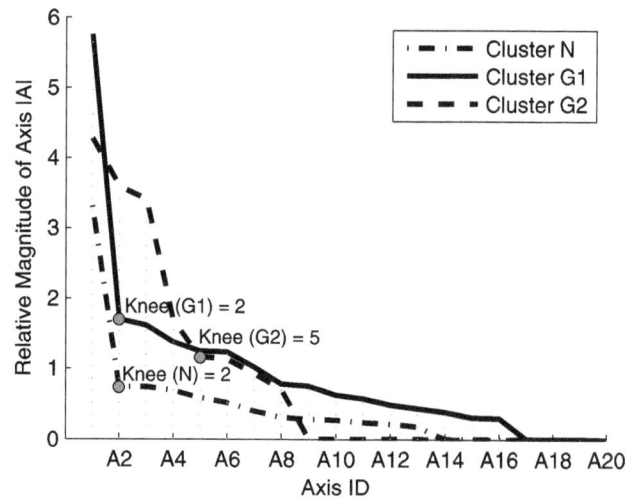

**Figure 2. Plot of axis contribution of variational Bayesian independent component analysis mixture (VIM) (Y) versus number of axes (X).** Axes beyond the knee point were removed, leaving 2 axes each for Clusters 1 and 2 and 5 axes for Cluster 3. The best VIM model was retrained 500 times, constrained to the reduced number of axes.

Knee points were chosen by ranking the axes in each cluster based on their length/magnitudes and including the number of axes with the largest relative magnitudes and excluding axes with less significant magnitudes. Figure 2 shows the axes manually selected for each cluster.

The optimal (i.e., best) version of model #202 contained three clusters, C1, C2 and C3, composed of two, two and five axes, respectively. This version was retrained 500 times to determine the final best specificity and sensitivity of the model.

### Results

The optimal VIM model (#202) had an initial specificity of 0.887 and sensitivity of 0.817 (Figure 1). After 500 iterations of retraining, the specificity and sensitivity improved to 0.931 and sensitivity of 0.828, respectively.

The three clusters identified by the best VIM model were one cluster composed mainly of normal FDT fields and two independent clusters composed mainly of abnormal (i.e., glaucomatous) fields. The primarily normal cluster (called cluster $N$) was composed of 1,109 normal fields (89%) and 135 abnormal fields (11%). The first "glaucoma" cluster (called cluster $G1$) was composed of 474 abnormal fields (85%) and 81 normal fields (15%) and the second glaucoma cluster ($G2$) was composed of 177 abnormal fields and 0 normal fields. Table 1 shows the number of normal and abnormal FDT fields assigned to each cluster.

Recall that cluster $N$ was represented by two axes; cluster $G1$ was represented by two axes and cluster $G2$ was represented by five axes. VIM projects visual fields along each axis, and the location of the projection on the axis indicates disease severity. The further away in the positive direction a field projection is from the cluster mean, the more severe the visual field defect. Increased distance in the negative direction represents a defect less severe than the mean defect, along a given axis.

Figure 3 shows generated FDT fields and age on VIM axes ±2 standard deviations from the cluster mean for each of the two axes that compose cluster $N$. The color scale simulates a total deviation plot (FDT defined total deviation at each test point with red

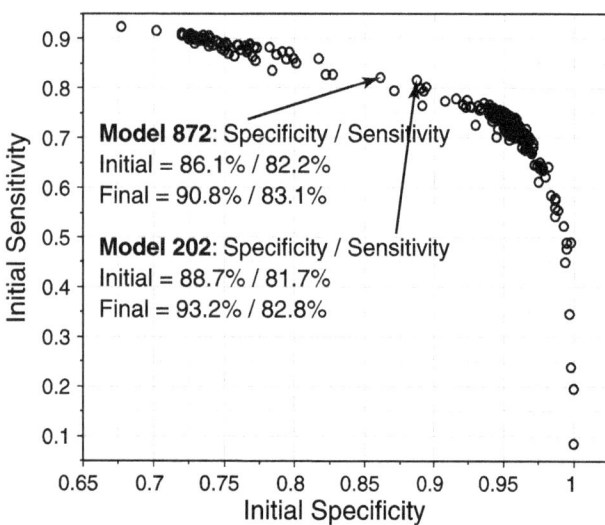

**Figure 1. Scatter plot showing sensitivity (Y) and specificity (X) of each of 720 variational Bayesian independent component analysis mixture (VIM) models created from FDT Matrix threshold sensitivities (52 inputs, plus age).** Results for the two best models (defined subjectively with a goal of 0.90 specificity and a maximum sensitivity) are shown.

**Table 1.** Number of normal and abnormal FDT fields assigned to each VIM-identified cluster. Overall specificity was 0.931 and sensitivity was 0.828.

| FDT field results | Cluster N | Cluster G1 | Cluster G2 |
|---|---|---|---|
| Normal (n = 1,190) | 1,109 (89%) | 81 (15%) | 0 (0%) |
| Abnormal (n = 786) | 139 (11%) | 474 (85%) | 177 (100%) |
| Total (n = 1,976) | 1,244 | 555 | 177 |

FDT = Frequency Doubling Technology perimetry, VIM = variational Bayesian independent component analysis mixture model.

indicating decreases in sensitivity and green indicating increases in sensitivity, relative to the 53-dimensional normal cluster mean), with the values also expressed for each visual field location. Predictably, both of them appear as normal, or close to normal, fields because 89% of the actual FDT fields clustered there are normal, and the 11% of fields from glaucoma eyes differed little in appearance to the fields from normal eyes. The actual fields closest to *Axis 1* form a set composed of 657 fields, 592 of which are normal and 65 of which are abnormal. The fields closest to *Axis 2* form a set composed of 587 fields, 517 of which are normal and 70 of which are abnormal.

Figure 4 shows generated FDT fields and age on VIM axes ±2 standard deviations from the mean of the normal cluster N for each of the two axes that represent cluster *G1*. Regarding visual field patterns generated at +2 standard deviations from the cluster means (i.e., significant, moderate defects), *Axis 1* appears to represent primarily moderate superior hemifield defects and *Axis 2*

appears to represent primarily moderate inferior hemifield defects (i.e., both are altitudinal defects), both with diffuse loss in the opposing hemifield. The actual fields closest to *Axis 1* form a set composed of 293 fields, 240 of which are abnormal and 53 of which are normal. The set for *Axis 2* is composed of 262 fields, 234 of which are abnormal and 28 of which are normal.

Figure 5 shows generated FDT fields and age on VIM axes ±2 standard deviations from the mean of the normal cluster N for each of the five axes that represent cluster *G2*. Regarding visual fields placed +2 standard deviations from the cluster means, *Axis 1* appears to represent diffuse moderate visual field loss and the fields closest to this axis form a set composed of 39 fields, all of which are abnormal. *Axis 2* and *Axis 3* appear to represent more severe superior nasal and inferior nasal defects, respectively. The set of fields closest to *Axis 2* is composed of 39 fields, and the set of fields closest *Axis 3* is composed of 38 fields (all abnormal). *Axis 4* (41 fields, all abnormal) has the pattern of an "arrowhead" shaped defect, similar to the pattern observed using the VIM technique to identify patterns of visual field defect in SAP data. [38] Likely, this defect pattern represents combined superior and inferior nasal step defects. Finally, *Axis 5* within this cluster (20 fields, all abnormal) appears to represent a diffuse pattern of loss, primarily localized superiorly.

## Discussion

The variational Bayesian independent component analysis mixture model employed in this study to identify clusters of FDT Matrix visual fields discriminated between normal and abnormal fields with high specificity and sensitivity, without any *a priori* information regarding class membership. We believe this is important because mathematical techniques were used to define

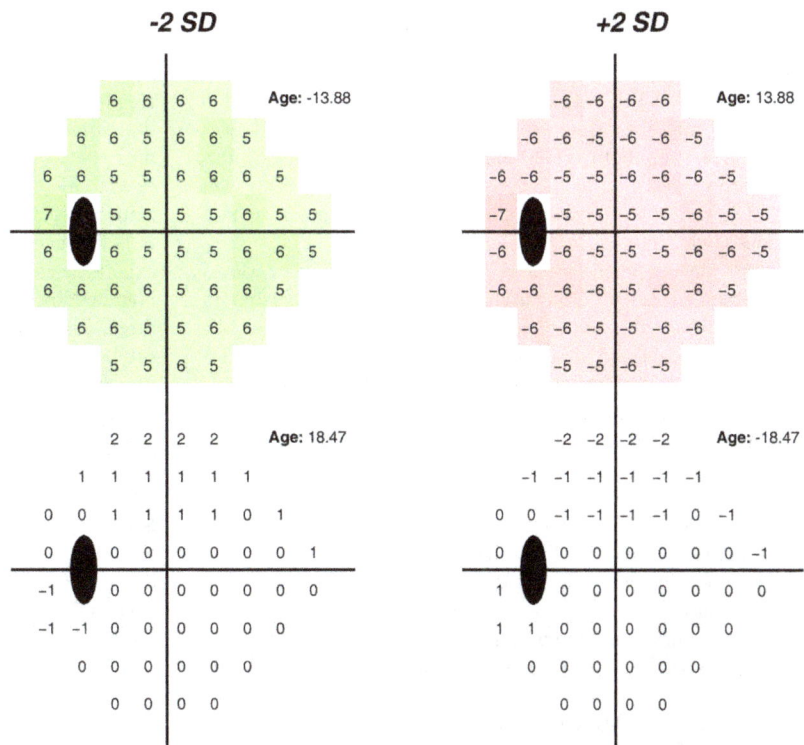

**Cluster N, Axis A1**
(Total fields assigned = 657; normals = 592; abnormals = 65)

**Cluster N, Axis A2**
(Total fields assigned = 587; normals = 517; abnormals = 70)

**Figure 3. Color-coded displays simulating total deviation plots along with age at −2 and +2 standard deviations of each axis from the centroid of Cluster N, that was composed primarily of normal FDT fields.** *Axis 1* and *Axis 2* appear normal or near normal. Numerical values shown are simulated total deviation values at each corresponding test point.

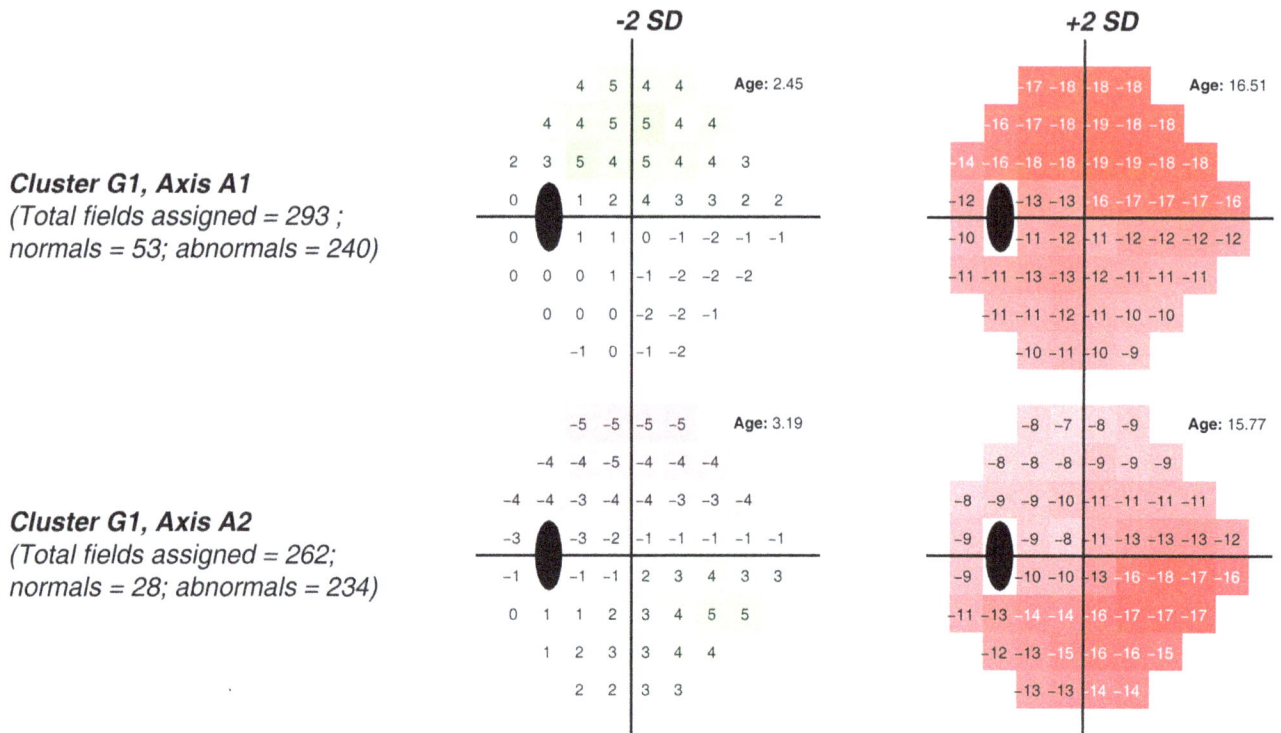

**Figure 4. Color-coded displays simulating total deviation plots along with age at −2 and +2 standard deviations of each axis from the centroid of the normal Cluster _N_, that was composed primarily of abnormal FDT fields.** _Axis 1_ appears to represent primarily moderate superior hemifield defects and _Axis 2_ appears to represent primarily moderate inferior hemifield defects (i.e., both are altitudinal defects), both showing less severe, diffuse loss in the opposing hemifield.

clusters with no human input (i.e., FDT fields were not sorted by a trained perimetry expert). In addition, patterns of FDT visual field loss generated on the VIM axes were similar to the patterns uncovered by VIM with SAP reported in previous studies [23,24,38], and the visual fields closest to the individual axes were similar for both FDT and SAP data. To allow this comparison, eyes used in the current study are a subset of eyes with FDT exams within six months of the SAP exams used in a previous study.

As an unsupervised learning classifier, VIM relies on a probabilistic measure of the likelihood of class membership to identify normal and abnormal clusters instead of relying on labeling of normal and abnormal visual field "templates" against which classifiers are trained by supervised learning and later tested. Although VIM was not designed specifically to segregate normal and abnormal visual fields, the FDT clusters created by VIM from the structure of the data yielded clusters that classified normal and glaucoma fields with specificity and sensitivity similar to that accomplished by supervised machine learning techniques, using data labeled with the class identity. [7,8,11,15].

Eleven percent of eyes (n = 135) assigned to the VIM normal field (i.e., cluster _N_) were abnormal based on our criteria (they had GHT outside of normal limits or PSD p≤5%, of these 89% were abnormal based on GHT alone). Upon inspection of Matrix printouts, most of these eyes had mild to moderate scattered decreases in thresholds across the visual field with no apparent pattern of defect (i.e., they appeared somewhat noisy), so they likely did not fit into a specific, identifiable glaucoma cluster. They were, however, outside normal limits when compared to the FDT normative database. Conversely, 15% of the eyes (n = 80) in glaucoma cluster _G₁_ were within normal limits based on the FDT normative database. Upon inspection of Matrix printouts, many eyes had mild, scattered decreases in thresholds, although a hypothetical reason for misclassification was not obvious. These results are not wholly unexpected, because the VIM technique described herein does not rely on results from the FDT normative database to identify patterns of defect.

The identifiable patterns of defect (i.e., axes) within each glaucoma cluster generally resembled those that have been shown to be indicative of glaucoma in SAP tests, based on many years of expert assessment. [39–43] The optimal number of clusters obtained by _post hoc_ analysis of the VIM applied to FDT was three, as it was for SAP [38]; the members of the clusters were similar for FDT and for SAP, the number of axes in each cluster was the same for FDT and for SAP [38], and the visual field patterns represented by the axes were similar for FDT and for SAP. The latter observation may not be surprising because recent evidence suggests that the assumed target cells for FDT testing (magnocellular ganglion cells) are sensitive to both FDT-like stimuli and SAP-like stimuli [44] (although see [45]). For both FDT and for SAP, the visual field patterns uncovered by VIM resembled those discovered by human perimetry experts over decades of experience (as previously mentioned). For instance, VIM identified diffuse and altitudinal defects of different severities, in addition to nasal step-like defects (e.g., _G₂_, _Axis 4_) within the glaucoma clusters.

Age is a significant risk factor of glaucoma and its progression. To study how the age of study eyes influenced the defect patterns identified and generated by the VIM algorithm, we ran the VIM algorithm with the age parameter input set to zero for all study eyes. The VIM model generated without age provided a similar diagnostic accuracy and defect patterns. Therefore, it was evident

**Cluster G2, Axis A1**
*(Total fields assigned = 39; normals = 0; abnormals = 39)*

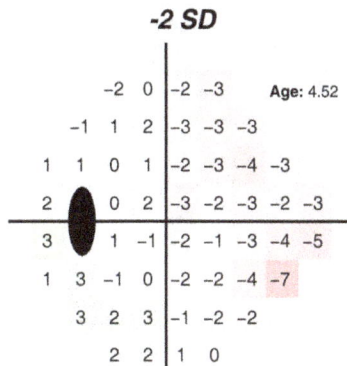

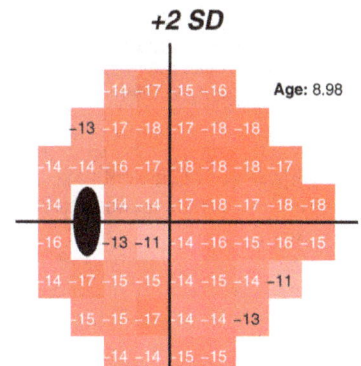

**Cluster G2, Axis A2**
*(Total fields assigned = 39; normals = 0; abnormals = 39)*

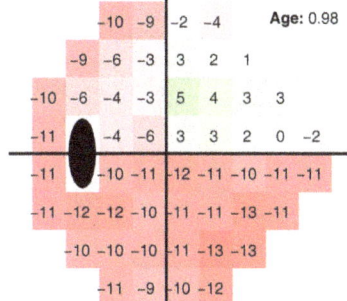

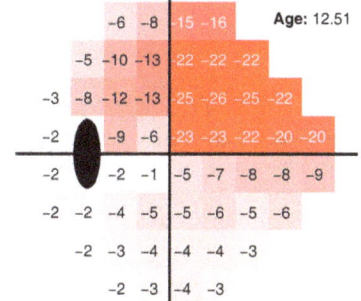

**Cluster G2, Axis A3**
*(Total fields assigned = 38; normals = 0; abnormals = 38)*

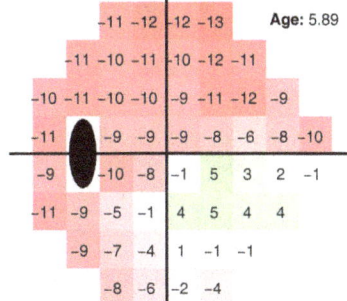

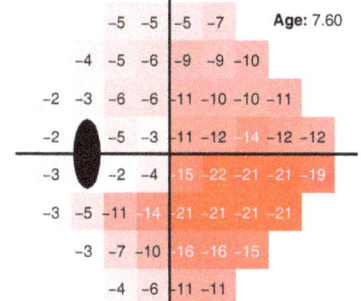

**Cluster G2, Axis A4**
*(Total fields assigned = 41; normals = 0; abnormals = 41)*

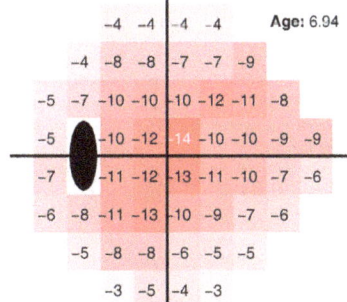

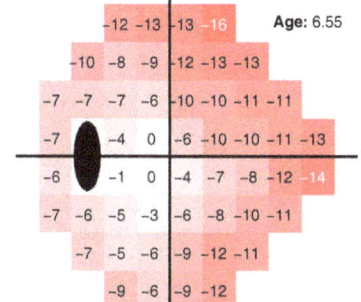

**Cluster G2, Axis A5**
*(Total fields assigned = 20; normals = 0; abnormals = 20)*

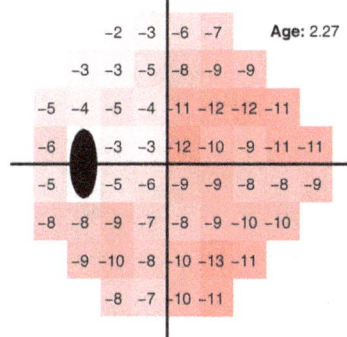

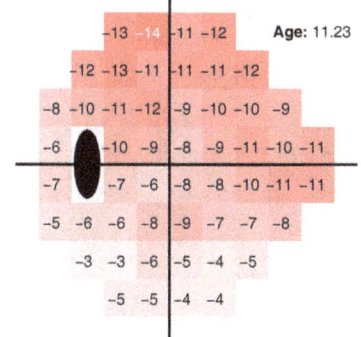

**Figure 5. Color-coded displays simulating total deviation plots along with age at −2 and +2 standard deviations of each axis from the centroid of normal Cluster N, that was composed entirely of abnormal FDT fields.** *Axis 1* appears to represent diffuse moderate visual field loss. *Axis 2* and *Axis 3* appear to represent more severe superior nasal and inferior nasal defects, respectively. *Axis 4* appears to represent combined superior and inferior nasal step defects, and *Axis5* appears to represent a diffuse pattern of loss, primarily localized superiorly.

that age did not significantly affect or bias how the FDT defect patterns were identified and automatically generated by the VIM algorithm.

Although the specificity and sensitivity of VIM-discovered clusters were very good relative to the result of the FDT test (within normal limits versus abnormal), cluster assignment did not always agree with characteristics of the optic nerve and retinal nerve fiber layer, as assessed by masked stereoscopic photograph assessment. This is not unexpected, because several studies have shown a disagreement between classification by visual function and structural assessments (e.g., [46]). This disagreement likely is attributable, in part, to the sensitivity of the tests used and the variability in results, particularly for masked stereophotograph assessment, which is a subjective process. The variability in appearance of healthy optic discs makes this task difficult even with significant training, particularly in the cases of borderline (i.e., suspected glaucoma) discs. A *post-hoc* examination of agreement between VIM-defined clusters and the presence of glaucomatous optic neuropathy (GON, defined based on masked assessment by two independent graders, adjudicated by a third if agreement was not observed) showed that in cluster $\mathcal{N}$ (the "normal cluster", n = 1,244; Table 1), 67 (5%) eyes had apparent GON and 136 (11%) eyes had FDT results outside normal limits. Both methods classified as abnormal 10 of the same eyes in this cluster; suggesting misclassification by either method likely was due to the presence of early disease (because agreement between methods usually is better in advanced disease, when defects using both methods are expected). Within the "glaucoma" clusters ($G_1$ and $G_2$), 278 (38%) eyes had apparent GON and 649 (89%) had abnormal FDT results.

In previous studies [22,23,38], VIM applied to SAP created an environment for the development of machine learning methods for detecting progression of glaucomatous field defect. [31] Since the outcome of VIM applied to FDT data was similar to that of SAP, the expectation is that the outcome of VIM analysis of FDT data likewise will be a good environment for analyzing glaucomatous progression.

In summary, VIM was applicable to FDT data. The outcome of the VIM process with FDT data was similar to the outcome with SAP data. Even without foreknowledge of the diagnosis of normal or glaucoma, unsupervised learning analyzing the internal structure of the data yielded separation of normal and glaucomatous eyes as well as can be achieved with supervised learning with foreknowledge of the diagnosis. Variational Bayesian independent component analysis mixture model can find statistically different visual field patterns similar to those identified by human experts. The axis representation of the internal structure of the data arranges mild to severe orientation of each pattern of visual field defect, thus permitting analysis for progression of disease. VIM, both for FDT and SAP, likely provides a good environment for the development of machine learning methods for detecting progression.

## Author Contributions

Conceived and designed the experiments: CB MB IL GJ MHG. Performed the experiments: RNW LMZ FAM CAG JML. Analyzed the data: CB MB IL GJ SY. Wrote the paper: CB MB MHG. Provided critical comments/suggestions for revision and final approval of the manuscript: RNW LMZ FAM CAG JML.

## References

1. Goldbaum MH, Sample PA, White H, Colt B, Raphaelian P, et al. (1994) Interpretation of automated perimetry for glaucoma by neural network. Invest Ophthalmol Vis Sci 35: 3362–3373.
2. Spenceley SE, Henson DB, Bull DR (1994) Visual field analysis using artificial neural networks. Ophthalmic Physiol Opt 14: 239–248.
3. Brigatti L, Hoffman D, Caprioli J (1996) Neural networks to identify glaucoma with structural and functional measurements. Am J Ophthalmol 121: 511–521.
4. Uchida H, Brigatti L, Caprioli J (1996) Detection of structural damage from glaucoma with confocal laser image analysis. Invest Ophthalmol Vis Sci 37: 2393–2401.
5. Lietman T, Eng J, Katz J, Quigley HA (1999) Neural networks for visual field analysis: how do they compare with other algorithms? J Glaucoma 8: 77–80.
6. Bowd C, Chan K, Zangwill LM, Goldbaum MH, Lee TW, et al. (2002) Comparing neural networks and linear discriminant functions for glaucoma detection using confocal scanning laser ophthalmoscopy of the optic disc. Invest Ophthalmol Vis Sci 43: 3444–3454.
7. Chan K, Lee TW, Sample PA, Goldbaum MH, Weinreb RN, et al. (2002) Comparison of machine learning and traditional classifiers in glaucoma diagnosis. IEEE Trans Biomed Eng 49: 963–974.
8. Goldbaum MH, Sample PA, Chan K, Williams J, Lee TW, et al. (2002) Comparing machine learning classifiers for diagnosing glaucoma from standard automated perimetry. Invest Ophthalmol Vis Sci 43: 162–169.
9. Hothorn T, Lausen B (2003) Bagging tree classifiers for laser scanning images: a data- and simulation-based strategy. Artif Intell Med 27: 65–79.
10. Zangwill LM, Chan K, Bowd C, Hao J, Lee TW, et al. (2004) Heidelberg retina tomograph measurements of the optic disc and parapapillary retina for detecting glaucoma analyzed by machine learning classifiers. Invest Ophthalmol Vis Sci 45: 3144–3151.
11. Bengtsson B, Bizios D, Heijl A (2005) Effects of input data on the performance of a neural network in distinguishing normal and glaucomatous visual fields. Invest Ophthalmol Vis Sci 46: 3730–3736.
12. Bowd C, Medeiros FA, Zhang Z, Zangwill LM, Hao J, et al. (2005) Relevance vector machine and support vector machine classifier analysis of scanning laser polarimetry retinal nerve fiber layer measurements. Invest Ophthalmol Vis Sci 46: 1322–1329.
13. Burgansky-Eliash Z, Wollstein G, Chu T, Ramsey JD, Glymour C, et al. (2005) Optical coherence tomography machine learning classifiers for glaucoma detection: a preliminary study. Invest Ophthalmol Vis Sci 46: 4147–4152.
14. Bowd C, Chiou C, Hao J, Racette L, Zangwill L, et al. (2006) Relevance vector machine for combining HRT II and SWAP results for discriminating between healthy and glaucoma eyes. Acta Ophthalmol Scand (Abstracts) 84: 569.
15. Bizios D, Heijl A, Bengtsson B (2007) Trained artificial neural network for glaucoma diagnosis using visual field data: a comparison with conventional algorithms. J Glaucoma 16: 20–28.
16. Bowd C, Hao J, Tavares IM, Medeiros FA, Zangwill LM, et al. (2008) Bayesian machine learning classifiers for combining structural and functional measurements to classify healthy and glaucomatous eyes. Invest Ophthalmol Vis Sci 49: 945–953.
17. Grewal DS, Jain R, Grewal SP, Rihani V (2008) Artificial neural network-based glaucoma diagnosis using retinal nerve fiber layer analysis. Eur J Ophthalmol 18: 915–921.
18. Townsend KA, Wollstein G, Danks D, Sung KR, Ishikawa H, et al. (2008) Heidelberg Retina Tomograph 3 machine learning classifiers for glaucoma detection. Br J Ophthalmol 92: 814–818.
19. Racette L, Chiou CY, Hao J, Bowd C, Goldbaum MH, et al. (2010) Combining functional and structural tests improves the diagnostic accuracy of relevance vector machine classifiers. J Glaucoma 19: 167–175.
20. Wroblewski D, Francis BA, Chopra V, Kawji AS, Quiros P, et al. (2009) Glaucoma detection and evaluation through pattern recognition in standard automated perimetry data. Graefes Arch Clin Exp Ophthalmol 247: 1517–1530.
21. Bowd C, Lee I, Goldbaum MH, Balasubramanian M, Medeiros FA, et al. (2012) Predicting glaucomatous progression in glaucoma suspect eyes using relevance vector machine classifiers for combined structural and functional measurements. Invest Ophthalmol Vis Sci 53: 2382–2389.
22. Sample PA, Chan K, Boden C, Lee TW, Blumenthal EZ, et al. (2004) Using unsupervised learning with variational bayesian mixture of factor analysis to

identify patterns of glaucomatous visual field defects. Invest Ophthalmol Vis Sci 45: 2596–2605.

23. Goldbaum MH (2005) Unsupervised learning with independent component analysis can identify patterns of glaucomatous visual field defects. Trans Am Ophthalmol Soc 103: 270–280.

24. Goldbaum MH, Sample PA, Zhang Z, Chan K, Hao J, et al. (2005) Using unsupervised learning with independent component analysis to identify patterns of glaucomatous visual field defects. Invest Ophthalmol Vis Sci 46: 3676–3683.

25. Lee TW, Lewicki MS, Sejnowski TJ (2000) ICA mixture models for unsupervised classification of non-Gaussian classes and automatic context switching in blind signal separation. IEEE Trans PAMI 22: 1078–1089.

26. Kiviluoto K, Oja E (1998) Independent component analysis for parallel financial time series; Tokyo, Japan. 895–898.

27. Makeig S, Jung TP, Sejnowski TJ (1996) Independent Component Analysis of Electroencephalographic Data. Advances in Neural Information Processing Systems. Cambridge, MA: MIT Press. 145–151.

28. Skillicorn D (2006) Social network analysis via matrix decompositions. In: Popp R, Yen J, editors. Emergent Information Technologies and Enabling Policies for Counter-Terrorism: IEEE, Inc. 331–347.

29. McKay D (1995) Probable networks and plausible predictions - A review of practical Bayesian methods for supervised neural netwrks. Network: Computation in Neural Systems. 469–505.

30. Sample PA, Bosworth CF, Blumenthal EZ, Girkin C, Weinreb RN (2000) Visual function-specific perimetry for indirect comparison of different ganglion cell populations in glaucoma. Invest Ophthalmol Vis Sci 41: 1783–1790.

31. Goldbaum MH, Lee I, Jang G, Balasubramanian M, Sample PA, et al. (2012) Progression of patterns (POP): A machine classifier algorithm to identify glaucoma progression in visual fields. Invest Ophthalmol Vis Sci 53: 6557–6567.

32. Turpin A, McKendrick AM, Johnson CA, Vingrys AJ (2002) Performance of efficient test procedures for frequency-doubling technology perimetry in normal and glaucomatous eyes. Invest Ophthalmol Vis Sci 43: 709–715.

33. Turpin A, McKendrick AM, Johnson CA, Vingrys AJ (2002) Development of efficient threshold strategies for frequency doubling technology perimetry using computer simulation. Invest Ophthalmol Vis Sci 43: 322–331.

34. Wall M, Woodward KR, Doyle CK, Artes PH (2009) Repeatability of automated perimetry: a comparison between standard automated perimetry with stimulus size III and V, matrix, and motion perimetry. Invest Ophthalmol Vis Sci 50: 974–979.

35. Racette L, Medeiros FA, Zangwill LM, Ng D, Weinreb RN, et al. (2008) Diagnostic accuracy of the Matrix 24–2 and original N-30 frequency-doubling technology tests compared with standard automated perimetry. Invest Ophthalmol Vis Sci 49: 954–960.

36. Chan K, Lee TW, Sejnowski T (2002) Variational learning of clusters of under complete nonsymmetric independent components. J Mach Learn Res 3: 99–114.

37. Choudrey RA, Roberts SJ (2003) Variational mixture of Bayesian independent component analyzers. Neural Comput 15: 213–252.

38. Goldbaum MH, Jang GJ, Bowd C, Hao J, Zangwill LM, et al. (2009) Patterns of glaucomatous visual field loss in sita fields automatically identified using independent component analysis. Trans Am Ophthalmol Soc 107: 136–144.

39. Armaly MF (1971) Visual field defects in early open angle glaucoma. Trans Am Ophthalmol Soc 69: 147–162.

40. Drance SM (1969) The early field defects in glaucoma. Invest Ophthalmol 8: 84–91.

41. Drance SM (1972) The glaucomatous visual field. Br J Ophthalmol 56: 186–200.

42. Heijl A, Lundqvist L (1984) The frequency distribution of earliest glaucomatous visual field defects documented by automatic perimetry. Acta Ophthalmol (Copenh) 62: 658–664.

43. Keltner JL, Johnson CA, Cello KE, Edwards MA, Bandermann SE, et al. (2003) Classification of visual field abnormalities in the ocular hypertension treatment study. Arch Ophthalmol 121: 643–650.

44. Swanson WH, Sun H, Lee BB, Cao D (2011) Responses of primate retinal ganglion cells to perimetric stimuli. Invest Ophthalmol Vis Sci 52: 764–771.

45. Maddess T (2011) Frequency-doubling technology and parasol cells. Invest Ophthalmol Vis Sci 52: 3759; author reply 3759–3760.

46. De Moraes CG, Liebmann JM, Ritch R, Hood DC (2012) Understanding disparities among diagnostic technologies in glaucoma. Arch Ophthalmol 130: 833–840.

# 13

# Endothelin B Receptors Contribute to Retinal Ganglion Cell Loss in a Rat Model of Glaucoma

**Alena Z. Minton[1], Nitasha R. Phatak[1], Dorota L. Stankowska[1], Shaoqing He[1], Hai-Ying Ma[2], Brett H. Mueller[2], Ming Jiang[2], Robert Luedtke[2], Shaohua Yang[2], Colby Brownlee[1], Raghu R. Krishnamoorthy[1]***

1 Department of Cell Biology and Anatomy, University of North Texas Health Science Center, Fort Worth, Texas, United States of America, 2 Department of Pharmacology and Neuroscience, University of North Texas Health Science Center, Fort Worth, Texas, United States of America

## Abstract

Glaucoma is an optic neuropathy, commonly associated with elevated intraocular pressure (IOP) characterized by optic nerve degeneration, cupping of the optic disc, and loss of retinal ganglion cells which could lead to loss of vision. Endothelin-1 (ET-1) is a 21-amino acid vasoactive peptide that plays a key role in the pathogenesis of glaucoma; however, the receptors mediating these effects have not been defined. In the current study, endothelin B (ET$_B$) receptor expression was assessed in vivo, in the Morrison's ocular hypertension model of glaucoma in rats. Elevation of IOP in Brown Norway rats produced increased expression of ET$_B$ receptors in the retina, mainly in retinal ganglion cells (RGCs), nerve fiber layer (NFL), and also in the inner plexiform layer (IPL) and inner nuclear layer (INL). To determine the role of ET$_B$ receptors in neurodegeneration, Wistar-Kyoto wild type (WT) and ET$_B$ receptor-deficient (KO) rats were subjected to retrograde labeling with Fluoro-Gold (FG), following which IOP was elevated in one eye while the contralateral eye served as control. IOP elevation for 4 weeks in WT rats caused an appreciable loss of RGCs, which was significantly attenuated in KO rats. In addition, degenerative changes in the optic nerve were greatly reduced in KO rats compared to those in WT rats. Taken together, elevated intraocular pressure mediated increase in ET$_B$ receptor expression and its activation may contribute to a decrease in RGC survival as seen in glaucoma. These findings raise the possibility of using endothelin receptor antagonists as neuroprotective agents for the treatment of glaucoma.

**Editor:** Steven Barnes, Dalhousie University, Canada

**Funding:** This work was supported by a National Glaucoma Research grant from the American Health Assistance Foundation (AHAF) and by funding from National Eye Institute (1RO1EY019952) to RRK. The funders had no role in study design, data collection and analysis, decision to publish, or preparation of the manuscript.

**Competing Interests:** The authors have declared that no competing interests exist.

\* E-mail: Raghu.Krishnamoorthy@unthsc.edu

## Introduction

Glaucoma is an optic neuropathy with a world-wide incidence of nearly 60.5 million patients, characterized by optic nerve degeneration, apoptosis of retinal ganglion cells (RGCs), and corresponding visual field defects, which could lead to blindness [1–3]. Glaucoma and other neurodegenerative diseases have several points of similarities, such as axonal degeneration, selective loss of neuron populations (RGCs selectively undergo apoptosis) [4–8], and glial activation [9]. Elevated intraocular pressure (IOP) is a major risk factor in primary open-angle glaucoma (POAG), which accounts for the majority of glaucoma patients. Apart from its well-known IOP related effects, glaucoma is recognized as a heterogeneous group of multifactorial neurodegenerative diseases with varying etiologies and clinical presentations. Hence, multiple hypotheses have been proposed to explain the pathophysiology of glaucoma, including mechanical stress of elevated IOP, disruption of retrograde transport of neurotrophins [6], ocular ischemia [10–12] glutamate-induced excitotoxicity [13], and oxidative stress [14–16]. Currently, the mainstay of glaucoma treatment is a IOP-lowering drug. However, reduction of IOP can only slow RGC loss and optic nerve damage, but cannot completely prevent further degeneration [17,18]. Hence, understanding molecular mechanisms contributing to RGC death can lead to the development of more effective treatments for glaucoma patients [19].

Corroborative evidence from several laboratories suggests that endothelin-1 (ET-1), a vasoactive peptide, has neurodegenerative effects in glaucoma [20–22]. However, the exact mechanisms underlying ET-1's actions remain to be elucidated. Studies have shown that ET-1 concentrations are significantly increased in the aqueous humor (AH) of patients with POAG and in animal models of glaucoma [23–25]. Both peribulbar and intravitreal administration of ET-1 has been found to produce axon loss and RGC death [26–30].

ET-1 exerts its functions via binding to two classes of G-protein coupled receptors, namely endothelin A (ET$_A$) and endothelin B (ET$_B$) receptors, both of which are abundantly expressed in various ocular tissues [21,31,32]. In animal models of glaucoma, studies have shown that there is an increase in ET$_B$ receptor mRNA expression in rat retinas as early as 1 day following IOP elevation and persisted up to 8 weeks of ocular hypertension [33]. Another study [34] demonstrated an increased frequency of ET$_B$ receptor immunolocalization in human glaucomatous optic nerves, compared to those of age-matched controls. Previous work from our laboratory suggests that the $ET_B$ receptor could be a key mediator of ET-1's neurodegenerative effects following intravitreal administration of ET-1 [30]. The purpose of this study was to analyze $ET_B$ receptor expression in the retinas of rats with elevated IOP and to determine if RGC loss is attenuated in $ET_B$ receptor-deficient transgenic rats.

## Results

### Elevation of intraocular pressure produced an upregulation of $ET_B$ receptors in rat retinas

Previous studies from our laboratory suggested the involvement of $ET_B$ receptors in several cellular pathways contributing to neurodegeneration of RGCs [20,25,30]. In the present study, we sought to determine whether there are any changes in the $ET_B$ receptor expression in rat retinas following IOP elevation for 2 and 4 weeks. Briefly, Brown Norway rats were used to elevate IOP in one eye while the corresponding contralateral eye served as control. Rats were sacrificed after 2 and 4 weeks of IOP elevation and retina sections were obtained from rat eyes. Immunohisto-chemical analysis of retinal sections from adult Brown Norway rats showed an increased immunostaining for $ET_B$ receptors primarily in the nerve fiber layer (NFL) and ganglion cell layer (GCL) in retinas of rats with IOP elevation for 2 weeks (white arrows, Figure 1B), compared to those of the contralateral control eyes. Increased immunostaining for $ET_B$ receptors was also observed in inner plexiform layer (IPL), and outer plexiform layer (OPL) in retinas of rats with IOP elevation for 2 weeks, compared to those of the contralateral control eyes (Fig. 1B). A modest increase in immunostaining for $ET_B$ receptors was also seen in the inner nuclear layer (INL) after 2 weeks of IOP elevation. Four weeks of IOP elevation also resulted in an increase in $ET_B$ receptor expression primarily in the NFL, GCL, IPL, and OPL in retinas of rats with IOP elevation, as compared to control (Fig. 1D). The increase in $ET_B$ receptor expression was similar to that seen after 2 weeks of IOP elevation (Fig. 1B). Based upon values of fluorescence intensities (using the Image J software) obtained from confocal images of retinal sections, there a 2.59 fold increase in $ET_B$ receptor immunostaining after 2 weeks of IOP elevation and a 2.52 fold increase after 4 weeks of IOP elevation. Interestingly, robust staining for the $ET_B$ receptor was also observed in the INL following 4 weeks of IOP elevation.

To ascertain that an increase in $ET_B$ receptor expression occurred in RGCs after IOP elevation, an immunostaining for $ET_B$ receptors was performed on retinal sections from Fluoro-Gold (FG) labeled rats. Briefly, retinal ganglion cells of adult male Brown Norway rats were retrogradely labeled with FG, following which IOP was elevated in one eye [35]. After maintaining the rats for 2 weeks following IOP elevation, the animals were sacrificed, retina sections were obtained and immunostained for $ET_B$ expression. An increased immunostaining for $ET_B$ receptor was observed mainly in retrogradely labeled RGCs in the RGC layer in IOP elevated eyes, compared to the corresponding control eyes (Figure 2B). This provides further confirmation for increased $ET_B$ receptor expression in RGCs following IOP elevation in rats.

### $ET_B$ receptor binding activity was increased in retinas of rats with elevated IOP

Since an increase in $ET_B$ proteins was observed by immuno-staining in IOP elevated rat retinas, further confirmation was made by receptor binding assays using radiolabeled ET-1. In preliminary experiments $^{125}$I-labeled ET-1 was found to bind to rat retinal membrane (3 µg of protein) in a linear pattern. The

$ET_A$ receptor antagonist, BQ-610, yielded a Ki value of 16.3 nM in competitive binding assays using rat retinal membranes. This experimental Ki is very close to the Ki value (20 nM) provided for BQ-610 by the manufacturer (Peninsula Lab Inc. Belmont, CA, USA). Based on the Ki value, BQ-610 was used at a concentration of 200 nM in the receptor binding assays Three individual binding assays were performed to plot endothelin receptor binding sites in the presence of 0.2–2 nM of $^{125}$I-ET-1, 1 µM of unlabeled ET-1 and 200 nM of BQ-610. The number of binding sites, Bmax (fmol/mg), of total endothelin receptors ($ET_A$ and $ET_B$ receptors) and $ET_B$ receptors was calculated for retinas from elevated IOP and contralateral eyes using unweighted linear regression analysis after normalization to the amount of protein by the method of Scatchard [36]. Total specific endothelin receptor binding (Bmax values) in retinal membranes from IOP-elevated eyes increased 2.7-, 1.5- and 1.7-fold respectively (from three independent binding assays) compared to the binding in the contralateral eye (Figure 3B). There was a significant ($p<0.05$) mean 1.9-fold increase in the total specific endothelin receptor binding activity (Bmax values) in the IOP elevated eyes, compared to the contralateral eyes (Table 1). On the other hand, there was no significant change in the binding affinity (reflected by the Kd values) for the total endothelin binding between control and elevated IOP eyes (Table 2). Specific $ET_B$ receptor binding (Bmax values) was increased 4.8-, 3.3- and 2.2-fold in the IOP-elevated eye, compared to the corresponding contralateral eye (Figure 3B). There was a significant ($p<0.05$) mean 3.3-fold increase in specific $ET_B$ receptor binding in IOP elevated eyes, compared to control eyes (Table 1). The Kd values for the specific $ET_B$ receptor binding were not significantly different between control and IOP elevated eyes (Table 2). The results indicate that number of endothelin receptors was increased in the retina from IOP-elevated eye, and in particular $^{125}$I-ET-1 binding to $ET_B$ receptors was even higher in IOP elevated eyes, compared to contralateral eyes.

### Retinal ganglion cell loss was attenuated in $ET_B$ receptor-deficient transgenic rats after 4 weeks of IOP elevation

IOP elevation in the Morrison rat model of glaucoma has been shown to result in a significant increase in TUNEL-positive RGCs, axonal loss, and gliosis [37–39]. However, the key contributors to RGC death are not completely understood. The endothelin family of peptides has recently gained prominence for their neurodegen-erative effects in the retina [28,30,40]; however, the receptors mediating these effects have not been identified. To determine the involvement of $ET_B$ receptors in neurodegenerative effects, RGCs of wild type (WT) and $ET_B$ receptor-deficient transgenic rats (KO) were retrogradely labeled with FG, following which IOP elevation was carried out and maintained for 4 weeks (Figure 4A). After sacrificing the animals, retinal flat mounts were obtained and RGC survival was assessed by counting viable RGCs (Figure 4B) in three eccentricities (E1, E2 and E3) within each retinal quadrant (Figure 4C). The loss of RGCs due to IOP elevation was computed by calculating the ratio of RGC counts between left (IOP elevated) and right (control) eye for each eccentricity. The ratio of RGC counts between left and right eye for each eccentricity was then compared between WT and KO rats (Figure 4D). Interestingly, the ratios of RGC counts between left and right eye were significantly higher in KO rats in the first two eccentricities (E1 and E2), compared to those of the WT rats (Figure 4D). The ratio of RGCs counts between left and right eyes was also higher in the third eccentricity of the KO rats; however, it did not attain statistical significance (Figure 4D). These results demonstrate that the $ET_B$ receptor may play a causative role in RGC death

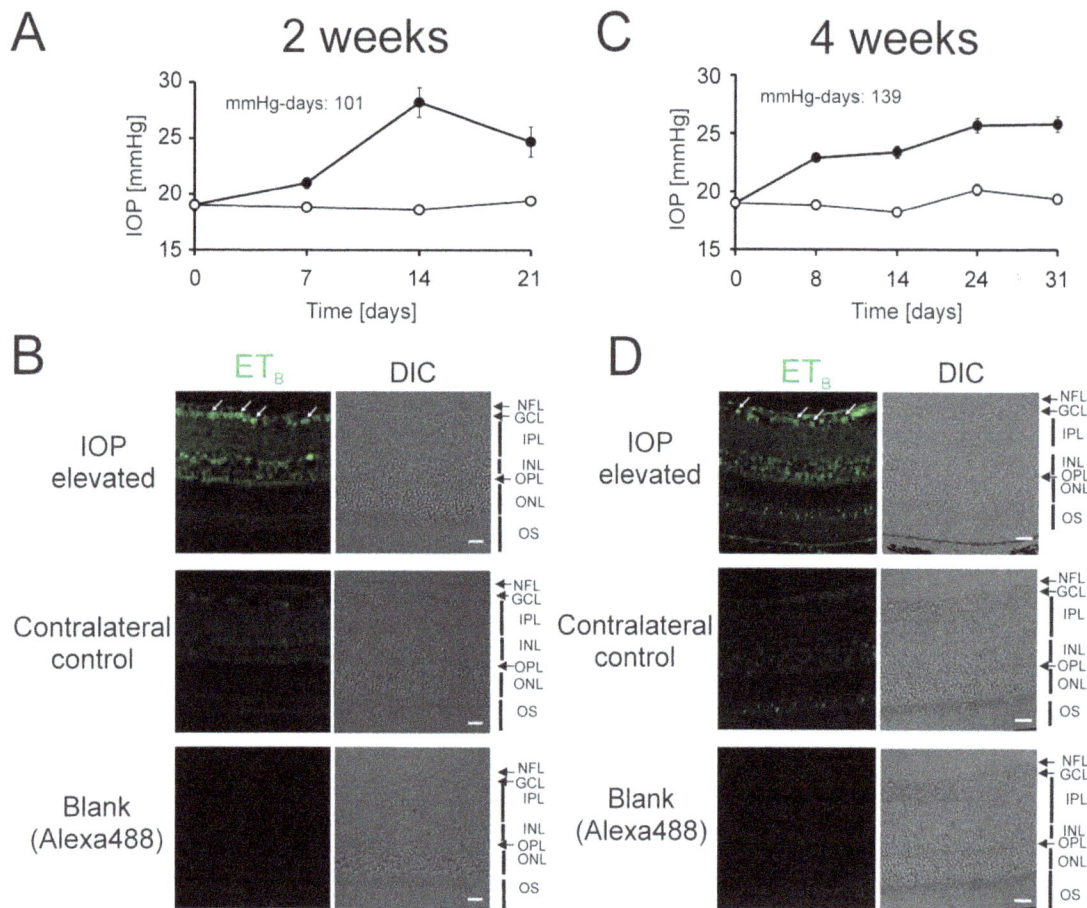

**Figure 1. IOP elevation produced a marked increase in ET$_B$ receptor expression in rat retinas.** Representative IOP elevation profile for 2 weeks (**A**) and 4 weeks (**C**) in adult Brown Norway rats. IOP was elevated in one eye (closed circles), while the other eye served as a contralateral control eye (open circles). The experiment was carried out in six Brown Norway rats for 2 weeks and seven Brown Norway rats for 4 weeks of IOP elevation. IOP values were plotted as mean $\pm$ SEM. Retinal sections from 2 weeks (**B**) and 4 weeks (**D**) IOP elevated rat eyes were immunostained for ET$_B$ receptor expression (green fluorescence) using a custom made rabbit polyclonal ET$_B$ receptor specific antibody. White arrows indicate RGCs in which an increase in immunostaining for ET$_B$ receptors was observed. Retinal sections in which the primary antibody incubation was omitted are labeled as blank and showed minimal fluorescence. NFL, nerve fiber layer; GCL, ganglion cell layer; IPL, inner plexiform layer; OPL, outer plexiform layer; INL, Inner Nuclear Layer; OPL, Outer Plexiform Layer; OS, Rod Outer Segment. Scale bar indicates 20 μm.

following elevation of IOP, and blocking this receptor may aid in neuroprotection of RGCs.

## Axonal integrity was maintained in ET$_B$-deficient rats after IOP elevation

Since a significant protection of RGCs was observed in KO rats subjected to IOP elevation, compared to WT rats, optic nerve axonal integrity was assessed in these animals. IOP was elevated in one eye of WT and KO rats, while the corresponding contralateral eye served as control [35]. After IOP elevation, rats were maintained for 4 weeks, sacrificed and optic nerve sections were obtained and stained with paraphenylenediamine (PPD). As seen in Figure 5, an increased staining with PPD was observed in optic nerve sections from IOP elevated WT rats. In addition, disruption of axon bundles, increased gliosis and glial scar formation was seen in the optic nerve sections from WT rats following IOP elevation. In contrast, optic nerve sections from IOP elevated KO rats showed a better preservation of axon morphology (Figure 5). Glial scarring was less prominent in KO rats compared to that seen in WT rats following IOP elevation. Optic nerve grading was done by masked observers essentially according to the method described

by Chauhan et al. (2006). Grade 0 was assigned to optic nerves with no damage with all the nerve bundles intact, while grades 3 and 6 correspond to nearly 30% and 60% of mean damage. The analysis indicated that there was no appreciable difference between the integrity of optic nerve between contralateral control eyes of the WT and KO rats (graded 1 to 2). However, the optic nerve sections from IOP elevated KO rat eyes showed lesser damage (graded 2 to 3) compared to optic nerves from the IOP elevated WT rats (graded 3 to 4). These observations suggest that lack of ET$_B$ receptor activation could have protective effects on the axons of the optic nerve in addition to preventing RGC loss.

## ET-1 treatment produced increased cell death in cultured primary retinal ganglion cells

Primary cultures of RGCs were isolated and were first tested by immunocytochemistry to determine if they express ET$_B$ and ET$_A$ receptors. Immunostaining for ET$_B$ and ET$_A$ receptors was observed both in the soma and neurites of cultured primary RGCs (Figure 6A, B). Immunocytochemical analysis of primary RGCs in which the primary antibody was excluded (Blank) showed minimal staining indicating that there was no appreciable

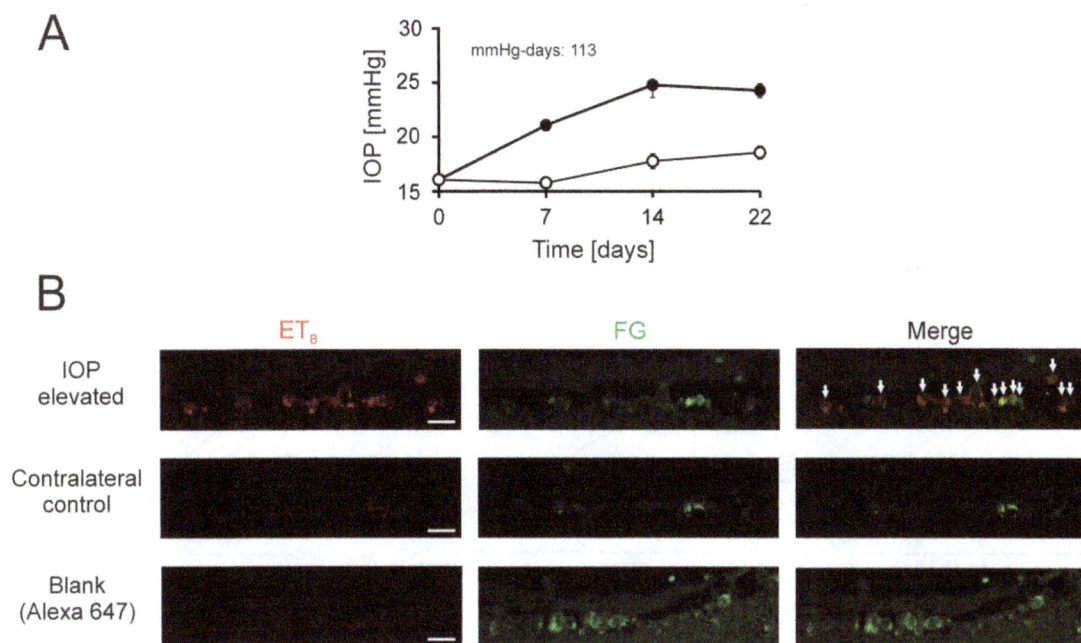

**Figure 2. Increased ET$_B$ receptor immunostaining in Fluoro-Gold labeled retinal ganglion cells following IOP elevation in rats. A.** Representative IOP elevation profile for 2 weeks in adult Brown Norway rats. Adult male Brown Norway rats (n = 3) were subjected to retrograde labeling using Fluoro-Gold (FG) to fluorescently label RGCs. IOP elevation was carried out in one eye in these rats and maintained for 2 weeks, while the companion eye served as a contralateral control. **B.** Immunohistochemical staining with a ET$_B$ receptor antibody was done using retinal sections from IOP elevated eyes and their corresponding contralateral control eyes and detected with an Alexa 647 conjugated secondary antibody. Fluorescence images were taken in a confocal microscope and merged images of the ET$_B$ immunofluorescence with FG was obtained (Merge). Scale bar indicates 20 μm.

non-specific binding of the Alexa647 conjugated secondary antibody (Figure 6C). To determine if endothelin receptor activation could promote death of RGCs, primary RGCs grown on coverslips were treated with two different concentrations of ET-1 (10 nM and 100 nM) or with the ET$_B$ receptor agonist, ET-3 (100 nM). Another group of RGCs grown on coverslips that did not undergo any treatment served as controls. Following the treatments, a mixture of green-fluorescent calcein-AM (indicative of intracellular esterase activity of viable cells) and red-fluorescent ethidium homodimer-1 (EtHD) (indicative of loss of plasma membrane integrity of dead cells) was added to assess the viability and death of the cells respectively. As seen in figure 7A, untreated RGCs had good morphology as evidenced by multiple neurites from each cell and forming a network of synaptic connections with neighboring cells. The cells were brightly stained with calcein-AM (green fluorescence) indicating that they were viable. There were also some EtHD stained cells (Mean ± SEM: 27±1.7% of cells) indicative of cell death in the untreated cells, possibly due to loss of trophic support in these cells. In cells treated with 10 nM ET-1 there was a decrease in staining with calcein AM and a withdrawal of neurites from many cells. The number of EtHD stained cells, indicative of cell death significantly increased in the 10 nM ET-1 treated cells (Mean ± SEM: 41±2.7% of cells), compared to the controls. The cell viability was further exacerbated in primary RGCs when treated with 100 nM ET-1. These cells exhibited fewer processes, compared to the 10 nM treatment, and nuclei were found to be more condensed indicative of apoptotic changes (Figure 7A). Moreover, RGCs treated with 100 nM ET-1 showed significantly higher EtHD staining (Mean ± SEM: 43±4.2% of cells), compared to untreated control cells (Figure 7B). Primary RGCs treated with the ET$_B$ receptor agonist, ET-3, demonstrated almost complete withdrawal of neurites and also showed

significantly higher number of EtHD staining indicative of cell death, compared to controls (Mean ± SEM: 43±2.9% of cells) (Figure 7B). These results suggest that ET-1 acting predominantly through the ET$_B$ receptor promotes cell death of RGCs.

## ET-1 treatment promoted cell death via apoptosis in primary retinal ganglion cells

Since ET-1 treatment produced increased cell death of primary retinal ganglion cells, further experiments were carried out to ascertain if this occurred through an apoptotic mechanism. To test this, primary RGCs were isolated from post natal day 3–7 rat pups, seeded on 12 mm coverslips and allowed to attach and grow for 1 week. The RGCs were either untreated or treated with ET-1 (10 nM), ET-1 (100 nM) or ET-3 (100 nM) for 24 hr. After the treatments, cells were fixed with 4% paraformaldehyde for 25 min at 4°C and TUNEL assays were carried out to detect apoptotic cell death using a commercially available kit from Promega (Madison, WI, USA) as per the manufacturer's instructions. As seen in Figure S1, RGCs treated with a reaction mix in which the TdT enzyme was excluded (negative control) showed no staining whereas cells treated with DNAse I to introduce artificial strand breaks (positive control) yielded a robust TUNEL positive reaction, ensuring the validity of the TUNEL assay. Untreated RGCs showed minimal staining for TUNEL positive cells, indicating that there was no appreciable apoptotic cell death in the untreated RGCs (Figure 8). However, in both 10 nM and 100 nM ET-1 treatment increased TUNEL labeling was observed, indicative of apoptosis (Figure 8). The most intense TUNEL labeling was observed in primary RGCs treated with the ET$_B$ receptor agonist, ET-3, suggesting that the ET$_B$ receptor could be a key mediator of apoptosis in RGCs (Figure 8).

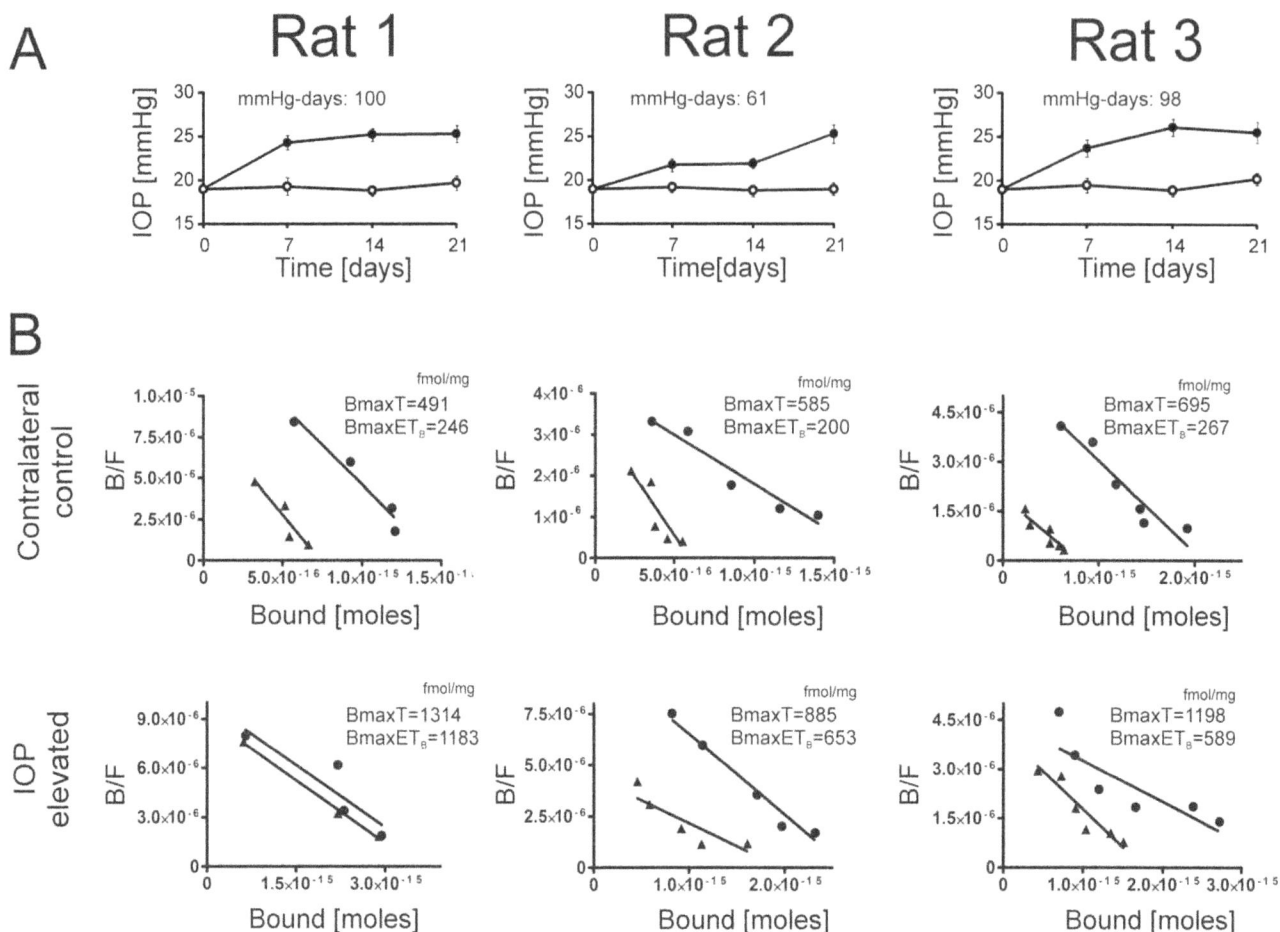

**Figure 3. ET$_B$ receptor binding activity was increased in retinas of IOP elevated Brown Norway rats. A.** IOP elevation profile in adult male Brown Norway rats. IOP was elevated in one eye (treated eye: closed circles), while the other eye served as the contralateral control eye (open circles). The experiment was carried out in three Brown Norway rats (n = 3) represented by Rat 1, Rat 2, and Rat 3. **B.** Scatchard plots of binding of [125]I-ET-1 to rat retinal membranes from contralateral control and IOP elevated eyes. Data points represent the means of triplicate binding reactions (Circles represent total endothelin receptor binding, while triangles represent ET$_B$ receptor binding). Three individual binding experiments were performed using contralateral control eyes from three rats (Rat 1, Rat 2, and Rat 3). Bmax (fmol/mg) representing total number of binding sites are indicated in the plots. B/F represents the ratio of bound to free radioactive ET-1 ligand. Binding assays for both control and elevated IOP eyes were carried out concurrently using the same conditions.

## Discussion

An accumulating body of evidence suggests the involvement of ET-1 [20,21,41–43] and ET$_B$ receptors [25,30,33,34,42,44–46] in the pathogenesis of glaucoma, however a causal link of ET$_B$ receptors to neurodegeneration has not been clearly established.

The endothelin family is comprised of three endothelin isoforms, namely ET-1, ET-2, and ET-3, each of which is

encoded by different genes [47,48]. ET-1 is the most studied isoform, which is constitutively synthesized and secreted from several tissues. Originally purified and characterized from vascular endothelial cells [49], ET-1 has been shown to be present in several tissues and organs including the eye [50–52] and brain [53,54]. The normal physiological role of ET-1 in the central nervous system remains to be understood. However, studies have demonstrated that ET-1 is a key player in various neurodegen-

**Table 1.** Bmax values (fmol/mg) for endothelin receptor binding.

|                                    | Rat No. 1 | Rat No. 2 | Rat No. 3 | Mean ± SD    |
|------------------------------------|-----------|-----------|-----------|--------------|
| Control (Total Binding)            | 491       | 585       | 695       | 590±83.4     |
| Control (ET$_B$ receptor binding)  | 246       | 200       | 267       | 238±28       |
| Elevated IOP (Total Binding)       | 1314      | 885       | 1198      | 1132±181*    |
| Elevated IOP (ET$_B$ receptor binding) | 1183  | 653       | 589       | 808±266*     |

*indicates statistical significance (p<0.05) by Student's t-test.

**Table 2.** Kd values (pM) for endothelin receptor binding.

| | Rat No. 1 | Rat No. 2 | Rat No. 3 | Mean ± SD |
|---|---|---|---|---|
| Control (Total Binding) | 103 | 419 | 358 | 293±136.87 |
| Control (ET$_B$ receptor binding) | 86 | 177 | 414 | 225±138.26 |
| Elevated IOP (Total Binding) | 395 | 253 | 798 | 482±230.8 |
| Elevated IOP (ET$_B$ receptor binding) | 390 | 443 | 432 | 421±22.8 |

erative conditions, including Alzheimer's disease, retinal degeneration and glaucoma [22,40,55,56]. In Parkinson's disease, the Parkin-associated endothelin receptor-like receptor (Pael-R) has been shown to induce unfolded protein response (UPR)-mediated cell death [57]. Nevertheless, the detailed mechanisms underlying ET-1's neurodegenerative effects remain to be elucidated.

ET-1 exerts its functions via binding to two classes of G-protein coupled receptors, ET$_A$ and ET$_B$ [21,31,32]. The two receptors have different affinities for the different endothelin peptides. The ET$_A$ receptor has equal affinity for ET-1 and ET-2 peptides, but much lower affinity for ET-3 (ET$_A$: ET-1 = ET-2 » ET-3), while the ET$_B$ receptor has equal affinity for all the three endothelin

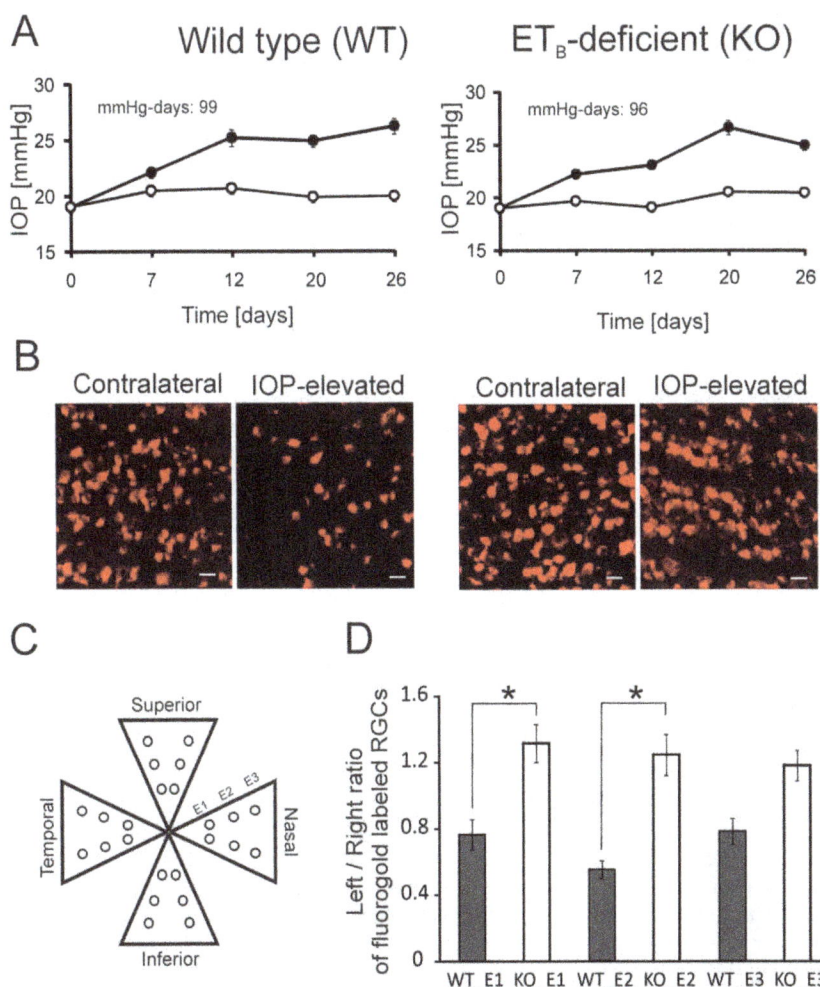

**Figure 4. RGC loss following IOP elevation was attenuated in KO rats compared to WT rats. A.** IOP elevation profile in WT and KO rats. Following FG labeling, IOP was elevated in one eye (closed circles), while the other eye served as the contralateral control eye (open circles). IOP values are plotted as mean ± SEM. **B.** Fluorescent images of retrograde labeled retinal ganglion cells in contralateral and IOP elevated retinas from WT and KO rats. **C.** Scheme for analysis of RGC counts in three eccentricities (E1, E2 and E3) in four quadrants of retinal flat mounts. **D.** Plot of ratio of Fluoro-gold labeled RGCs between left (IOP elevated) and right (contralateral) eyes in different eccentricities. The ratio was compared between WT and KO rats for three eccentricities (E1, E2 and E3). A significant increase in RGC survival was observed in KO rats (n = 4) as compared to WT rats (n = 3). Bars represent mean ± SEM. * indicates significance (p<0.05) by ANOVA on ranks followed by pair-wise multiple comparisons (Dunn's method). Scale bar indicates 20 μm.

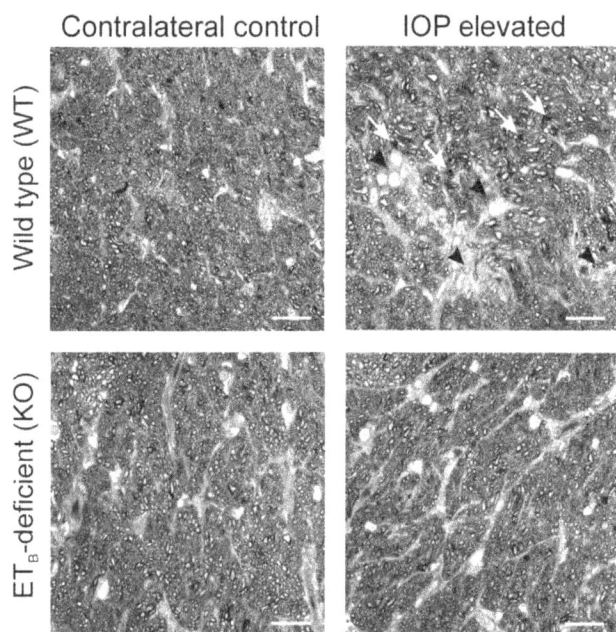

**Figure 5. Survival of optic nerve axons in KO rats, compared to WT rats following IOP elevation.** IOP was elevated in one eye of WT and KO rats, while the other eye served as corresponding contralateral control. The rats were maintained for 4 weeks following IOP elevation. Rats were sacrificed and optic nerve sections were stained with paraphenylenediamine. Dark spots (white arrows) indicate dying/degenerating axons. Glial scar formation (black arrow heads) was more abundant in WT rats, compared to KO rats in IOP elevated eyes. Scale bar indicates 20 µm.

peptides ($ET_B$: ET-1 = ET-2 = ET-3). Thus, ET-3 could be used as an $ET_B$ receptor agonist. Clinical studies have found increased levels of ET-1 in aqueous humor of primary open angle glaucoma patients [58] and increased circulating levels of ET-1 in normal tension glaucoma patients [59]. ET-1 concentrations were also found to be elevated in exfoliation syndrome (the production and progressive accumulation of a fibrillar extracellular material in many ocular tissues) [60,61]. $ET_A$-like receptor binding sites have been identified in the retina and choroidal blood vessels [31]. In contrast, $ET_B$-like receptor-binding sites were primarily found in the neural and glial components of the retina [32,62]. Studies have demonstrated that primary cultures of human trabecular meshwork, ciliary muscle, and ciliary nonpigmented epithelial cells predominately express the $ET_A$ receptor [62].

Since $ET_B$ receptor expression increases at very early time points of IOP elevation (when no appreciable loss of RGCs occurs) [33], it could play a causative role in neurodegeneration in glaucoma. Interestingly, we found a profound increase in $ET_B$ receptor expression in the nerve fiber layer (NFL) and ganglion cell layer (GCL) in retinas of rats with IOP elevation for 2 weeks, compared to those of the contralateral control eye (Fig. 1B) and this elevation in $ET_B$ receptor expression was maintained up to 4 weeks of IOP elevation. Since RGCs are located in the GCL along with displaced amacrine cells [63–65], it is important to distinguish between these two cell populations to conclude that changes in $ET_B$ receptor expression occur primarily in RGCs in IOP elevated eyes. An increased staining of $ET_B$ receptors was observed mainly in the FG labeled RGCs in the RGC layer after IOP elevation for 2 weeks (Figure 2B). We also observed an increase in the expression of $ET_B$ receptors in the inner plexiform layer (IPL) and

outer plexiform layer (OPL) in retinas of rats with IOP elevation for 2 weeks, in comparison to contralateral control eye (Fig. 1B). It is known that IPL is the layer where the bipolar cell axons form synapses with dendrites of the ganglion and amacrine cells, whereas OPL contains projections of rods and cones [66]. Interestingly, increased staining for $ET_B$ receptors was observed in the inner nuclear layer (INL) following 4 weeks of IOP elevation INL, which is composed the cell bodies of the bipolar, horizontal, and amacrine cells (Figure 1D). The significance of upregulation of $ET_B$ receptors in these retinal layers is currently unclear, however these cell types do not undergo pathological changes in glaucoma.

Receptor-binding assays using [125]I-ET-1 showed a preferential upregulation of $ET_B$ receptors in the retina following IOP elevation. A significant increase in the Bmax values (indicative of number of receptor binding sites) for $ET_B$ receptor binding was observed without a significant increase in the corresponding Kd values (indicative of receptor affinity), which is a classic pharmacological measure of upregulation of receptor expression. $ET_B$ receptors function as clearance receptors and play a critical role in maintaining normal levels of ET-1 [67,68]. It is possible that expression of $ET_B$ receptors is increased in response to elevation of ET-1 concentrations following IOP elevation. Increased expression of $ET_B$ receptors was also detected at the level of the optic nerve head in animal models, as well as in glaucoma patients [25,30,34]. In animal models of photoreceptor degeneration, another member of the endothelin family, ET-2, was found to be elevated and accompanied by more than 10-fold increase in $ET_B$ expression primarily in the glial cells in the retina [40].

In glaucoma, RGCs are selectively lost via apoptosis [7,69–73], while other retinal neurons are largely unaffected. However, the key contributors to RGC death have not been completely identified. To assess RGC viability in vivo, we used retrograde labeling with FG, which has been shown to label 98.4% and 97.8% of the RGCs in albino and pigmented rats, respectively [74]. Using this method followed by IOP elevation, it was found that four weeks of IOP elevation in WT rats produced a significant loss of RGCs. In contrast, loss of RGCs was significantly attenuated ($p < 0.05$) in the first two eccentricities in retinas of KO rats, compared to those of WT rats. Apart from RGCs, neuroprotective effects were also observed in the axons of KO rats in comparison to WT rats following IOP elevation. Considering the robust neuroprotection observed in KO rats, it is possible that $ET_B$ receptor activation in multiple cell types (including lamina cribrosa, RGCs and optic nerve head astrocytes) may be contributing to neurodegeneration in glaucoma. Thus, blocking $ET_B$ receptors could have additive neuroprotective effects due to the involvement of $ET_B$ receptors in pathological changes in several tissues in glaucoma.

Using primary RGCs, it was found that ET-1 treatment at two different concentrations (10 and 100 nM) produced a significant increase in cell death, suggesting that ET-1 acting through its receptors produces neurodegenerative effects. Since ET-3, an $ET_B$ receptor agonist, produced a similar extent of cell death as seen with ET-1 (which acts on both $ET_A$ and $ET_B$ receptors), it is possible most of endothelin-1 mediated degenerative effects on RGCs occur through the $ET_B$ receptors. Using the TUNEL assay, it was found that the mode of cell death by ET-1 treatment was via apoptosis in primary RGCs. The $ET_B$ receptors appeared to play a key role in apoptotic cell death of RGCs since the most intense TUNEL labeling was observed in primary RGCs treated with an $ET_B$ receptor agonist (ET-3) (Figure 8). In a recent study, bosentan treatment (which blocks both $ET_A$ and $ET_B$ receptors) was shown to protect against axonal degeneration in the DBA/2J mouse

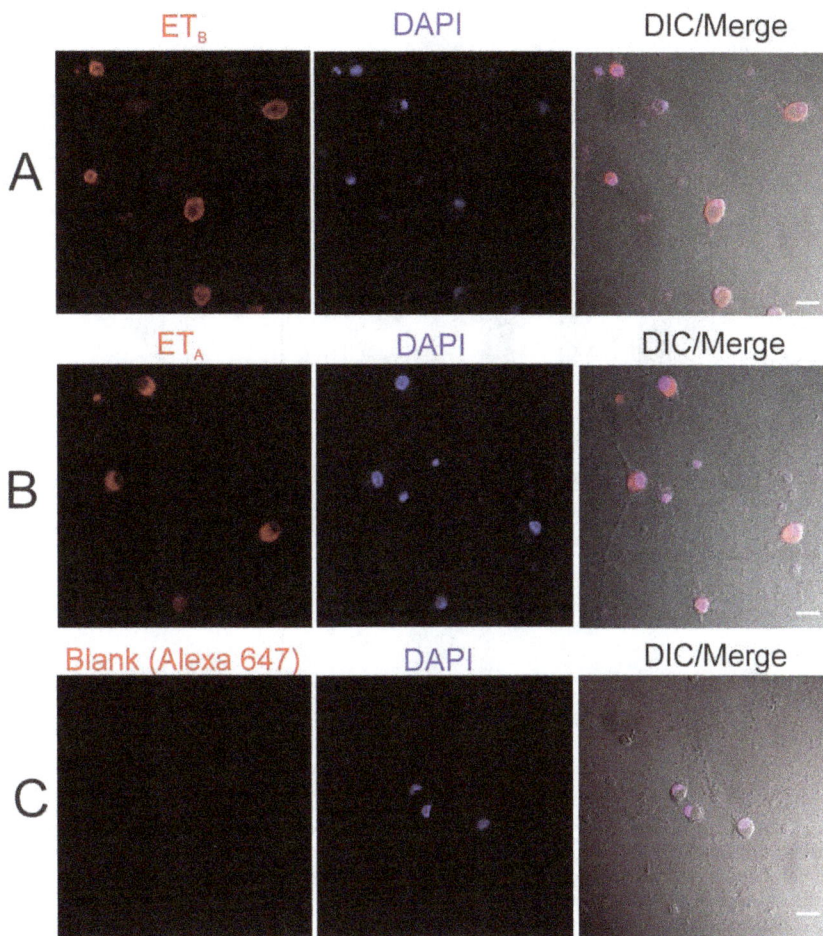

**Figure 6. Immunocytochemical analysis of endothelin receptor expression in primary rat retinal ganglion cells (RGCs).** Primary rat RGCs were isolated from post-natal day 3–7 rat pups and immunocytochemical analysis of (**A**) $ET_B$ and (**B**) $ET_A$ expression was performed using a custom-made $ET_B$ antibody and a commercially available $ET_A$ antibody. The immunostaining was detected using corresponding Alexa 647 conjugated secondary antibodies. (**C**) A negative control immunostaining (Blank) in which the primary antibody was omitted showed minimal staining. Cells were counterstained with DAPI to detect cell nuclei. Scale bar indicates 20 μm.

model of glaucoma, suggesting that some of the degenerative effects could also occur through the $ET_A$ receptor [75].

In conclusion, we have found that upregulation of $ET_B$ receptors in RGCs occurs at early stages in the Morrison's ocular hypertension rodent model of glaucoma, and may contribute to the death of RGCs. Endothelin receptor antagonists could be promising candidates for neuroprotection in glaucoma.

## Materials and Methods

### Animals

All animal experiments were performed in accordance with the Association for Research in Vision and Ophthalmology (ARVO) policy on the Use of Animals in Vision Research, and all protocols were reviewed and approved by the institutional animal care and use committee (IACUC) at the University of North Texas Health Science Center. Adult male retired breeder Brown Norway (Rattus norvegicus) rats (200–350 g) were purchased from Charles River (Wilmington, MA). Wistar-Kyoto $ET_B$ receptor-deficient transgenic rats (KO) (a kind gift from Dr. Masashi Yanagisawa, UT Southwestern Medical Center, Dallas, Texas) were maintained in the vivarium at the UNT Health Science Center. The rats were rescued transgenic $ET_B$-deficient spotting lethal

($^{TG}ET_B{}^{sl/sl}$) rats. The parental heterozygous spotting lethal strain carries a naturally occurring deletion in the first exon of the $ET_B$ receptor gene that completely abrogates expression of a functional $ET_B$ receptor. Deletion of the $ET_B$ receptor in rats is lethal beyond the first few weeks after birth due to aganglionic intestinal obstruction. However, the $ET_B$ receptor-deficient transgenic rats used in this study had been rescued by tissue-specific expression of the $ET_B$ receptor in the intestine, mediated by the dopamine-β-hydroxylase promoter linked to a functional $ET_B$ transgene, which directs $ET_B$ expression specifically to the intestine. This allows for normal development of the enteric nervous system; thus, preventing neonatal lethality in these $ET_B$-deficient rats [76]. Heterozygous breeding pairs were used to produce offsprings typically with a Mendelian ratio of genotypes. We performed routine genotyping of rat pups to ensure the genotypes of the WT and KO rats that were used in these studies. Rats were maintained under constant low illumination (90 lux).

### Retrograde labeling with Fluoro-Gold (FG)

Retrograde labeling of RGCs was carried out in WT and KO rats as described earlier [77]. The animals were anesthetized with intraperitoneal injection (i.p.) of an anesthesia cocktail comprising of 50 mg/ml ketamine, 5 mg/ml xylazine and 1 mg/ml acepro-

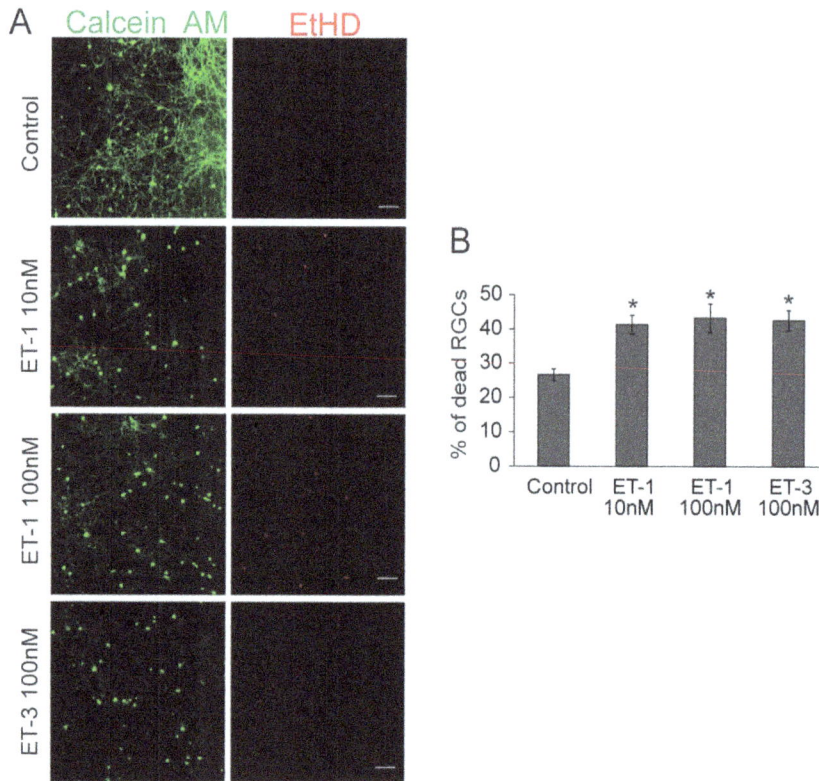

**Figure 7. Live-dead assay of primary RGCs treated with endothelins. A.** Primary retinal ganglion cells were obtained from post-natal day 3–7 rat pups and seeded on coverslips. The cells were either untreated (control) or treated with 10 nM ET-1, 100 nM ET-1 or 100 nM ET-3 for 24 hrs. Following the treatments, a mixture of calcein AM (green fluorescence indicating living cells) and Ethidium homodimer (EtHD) (red fluorescence indicating dead cells) was added and cell viability assessed. **B.** Plot of percentage of dead cells after treatment of primary RGCs with ET-1 (10 nM), ET-1 (100 nM) and ET-3 (100 nM). The plot represents the average of three independent experiments and bars represent mean ± SEM. * indicates statistical significance (p<0.05) by Kruskal-Wallis One Way ANOVA on Ranks followed by Dunn's multiple comparison. Scale bar indicates 100 μm.

mazine (100 μl/100 g body weight) and placed into a stereotaxic frame (Tujunga, CA, USA) to secure the cranium. Double injections of FG (Denver, CO, USA), were carried out using two sets of stereotaxic coordinates: (i) anterior posterior (AP) = 5.8, ML = +1.3, DV = 3.5 and (ii) AP = 5.8, ML = −1.3, DV = 3.5 from the bregma. For each injection, approximately 3 μl of FG (2% solution in isotonic saline) were injected using a 10 μl Hamilton syringe (Reno, NV, USA) at a rate of 1 μl/min. Following recovery for 2 weeks, IOP was elevated in one eye of each rat by injection of hypertonic saline through episcleral veins [35].

## Morrison's ocular hypertension model of glaucoma in rats

The procedure of Morrison et al. (1997) was used to elevate IOP in rats [35]. Initial studies were carried out in male Brown Norway retired breeder rats to study the effect of elevated IOP on expression of $ET_B$ receptors in the retina. To test the role of $ET_B$ receptors in neurodegeneration, wild type and $ET_B$ receptor-deficient transgenic rats were used after IOP elevation. Animals were maintained on a reduced constant light environment of 90 lux for a minimum of 3 days prior to surgery for elevating IOP. Daily IOP measurements using a Tonolab tonometer (Icare Finland Oy, Espoo, Finland), conducted on the conscious animals after slight sedation with intramuscular (i.m.) administration of acepromazine. On the day of the surgery, animals were anesthetized with an i.p. injection of a standard rat cocktail

consisting of ketamine, xylazine, and acepromazine. One eye of each animal was injected with 1.8 M hypertonic saline via an episcleral vein, while the contralateral eye served as a control. A micro glass needle was inserted into the episcleral vein and approximately 50 μl of hypertonic saline was injected with a force sufficient to blanch the aqueous plexus. This procedure produces scarring of the trabecular meshwork with a resultant rise in IOP and damage to the optic nerve [35]. The rats were sacrificed by overdose with pentobarbital (administered first intraperitoneal and then intracardial) at two different time points (2 and 4 weeks) following IOP elevation.

## IOP measurements

IOP was measured in conscious animals using Tonolab tonometer (iCare, Finland). Rats were slightly sedated by an intramuscular injection of acepromazine (2 mg/kg) and IOP measurements were taken 2 to 5 min after the injection. During each IOP measurement session, ten average readings from control and IOP-elevated eyes were obtained. A plot of mean IOP versus time was carried out and IOP exposure was calculated as the number of mmHg days by performing a separate "area-under the curve" (AUC) integration of IOP over the days of exposure for the treated and control eye in each rat [78]. The integral IOP value of the control eye was subtracted from the integral value of the IOP-elevated eye to give the "IOP-integral difference" which was expressed as mmHg days.

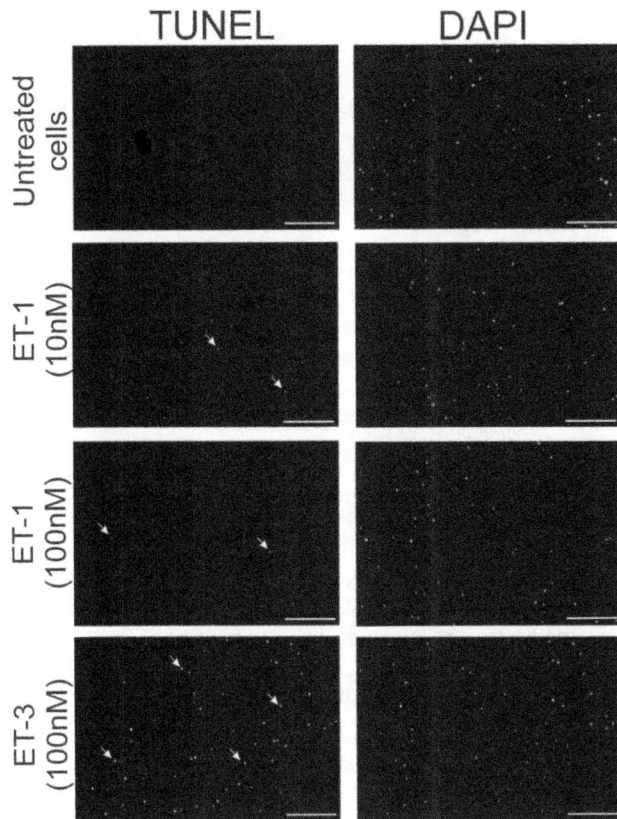

**Figure 8. TUNEL assay of primary RGCs treated with endothelins.** Primary RGCs were either untreated or treated with ET-1 (10 nM), ET-1 (100 nM) or ET-3 (100 nM) and TUNEL assays were carried out to detect apoptosis. The left vertical panel (TUNEL) indicates fluorescent images from cells incorporating fluorescinated dUTP indicative of apoptosis. The right vertical panel (DAPI) shows stained nuclei using DAPI. Scale bar indicates 200 μm.

## Quantification of RGC survival

Retrograde labeling of retinal ganglion cells using FG was carried out in rats as described by Husak et al. (2000). Two weeks following retrograde labeling, IOP was elevated in the left eye, while the right eye served as the contralateral control eye. After IOP elevation for 4 weeks, rats were sacrificed using intraperitoneal injection of pentobarbital (120 mg/kg), and the orientation of each eye was marked. Eyes were enucleated and immersion-fixed in 4% paraformaldehyde (PFA) (Phillipsburg, NJ, USA) in 0.1 M sodium phosphate, pH 7.2, for 3 h at room temperature. The retinas were dissected and flat-mounted in fluorosave reagent (Calbiochem, USA). Fluorescent images of the retinal flat mounts were taken using a Zeiss LSM 510 META confocal microscope.

FG-labeled cells were manually counted by a blinded observer using fluorescent images obtained from the confocal microscope. Each retina was divided into four quadrants: superior, inferior, nasal, and temporal. Six pictures were taken at 40× magnification in each retinal quadrant. Briefly, the number of RGCs was counted in a blinded manner in 6 areas per retinal quadrant at three different eccentricities (E1, E2 and E3) located at 2/6, 4/6, and 5/6 of the radius of the retina from the optic nerve head respectively (Figure 4C). A total of 24 pictures were taken from each retina. The number of FG-labeled RGC was counted as relatively round somata with dendritic processes from a slide-projected image with 0.37 to 0.53 mm$^2$ area of the retina. The

spindle-shaped, FG-positive microglia could be easily recognized from these photographs and were not counted. RGC survival was expressed as a ratio of the counts in the elevated IOP eye to that of the contralateral control eye, for the same eccentricity.

## Immunohistochemistry

Retinal sections from Brown Norway rats were subjected to immunohistochemical detection of $ET_B$ receptor expression essentially as described by Krishnamoorthy et al. [30]. Briefly, five-micron saggital retinal sections through the optic nerve head were de-paraffinised in xylene (Fisher Scientific, NJ, USA), re-hydrated using a descending series of ethanol washes. Following permeabilization with 0.1% Triton X-100 and blocking with 5% Donkey serum and 5% BSA in PBS, retinal sections were treated with primary antibodies: custom made rabbit anti-$ET_B$ (Antibody Research Corporation, St. Charles, MO) diluted 1:200 (7.5 μg/ml), and incubated for 1 h at room temperature. Secondary incubation for 1 hr was carried out with a 1:1000 dilution of the appropriate secondary antibody conjugated with Alexa 488 (Molecular Probes, Eugene, OR). Retinal sections in which the primary antibody incubation was excluded served as blanks and were used to assess non-specific staining by the secondary antibody. Fluorescence images were taken in a Zeiss LSM 510 META confocal microscope.

## Receptor Binding Assays

IOP was elevated in the left eye of Brown Norway rats by the method of Morrison et al. (1997), while the corresponding right eye served as contralateral control. After maintaining the rats with elevated IOP for 2 weeks, they were sacrificed and retinas were isolated form left and right eyes. The retinas were homogenized in a solution of 1× TBS (50 mM Tris.HCl, pH 7.4 and 150 mM NaCl) containing protease inhibitors and plasma membrane fractions were isolated by centrifugation at 100, 000 g.

Approximately 3 μg of membrane protein from rat retinas were used for each binding reaction. $^{125}$I-ET-1 (NEN Life Science Products Inc., Boston, MA, USA) binding was performed in polypropylene tubes in a total assay volume of 90 μl containing 30 μl of $^{125}$I-ET-1 (ranged from 0.2 to 2 nM), 30 μl of membrane fraction and 30 μl of competition reagent (either cold ET-1 or $ET_A$ receptor antagonist) or buffer at 37°C for 1 hr. Binding was terminated by adding 5 ml of cold wash buffer (10 mM Tris.HCl pH 7.4 containing 150 mM NaCl) and binding solution was rapidly vacuum filtered through glass fiber filters (No. 30, Schleicher and Schuell Keene, NH, USA). Filters were washed twice with 5 ml of wash buffer and the bound radioactivity was quantitated in a gamma counter. Non-specific binding was assessed by determining filter-bound radioactivity in the presence of 1 μM unlabeled ET-1 (Bachem, Torrance, CA, USA) after addition of $^{125}$I-ET-1. The binding of $ET_A$ receptor was determined by measuring the decrease in binding in the presence of 200 nM of BQ-610 ($ET_A$ receptor antagonist) (Peninsula Lab Inc. Belmont, CA, USA). $ET_B$ receptor binding was defined as the total specific $^{125}$I-ET-1 binding minus the amount of $ET_A$ receptor binding. Estimates of maximum number of binding sites ($B_{max}$) were obtained using unweighted linear regression analysis of data transformed by the method of Scatchard [36].

## Live-Dead Assay for primary RGC viability

Primary cultures of rat retinal ganglion cells were prepared using a two-step panning procedure [79]. Briefly, post-natal 3–7 day old Sprague Dawley rat pups (30 pups from 3 litters) (Charler River, Wilmington, MA) were euthanized, and the retinas were placed in 4.5 units/mL of papain solution (Worthington, Lakewood, NJ) to dissociate the tissue. This was followed by incubation of cells for 10 min with a rabbit anti-macrophage antibody (Cedarlane, Burlington, Onatario, Canada). After that cell suspensions were incubated in a 150-mm Petri dish coated with a goat anti-rabbit IgG (H+L chain) antibody (Jackson ImmunoResearch, West Grove, PA) for 30 minutes. Cells that did not adhere to the 150-mm dish were then transferred to a 100-mm dish coated with anti-Thy1.1 antibody (from hybridoma T11D7; American Type Culture Collection, Rockville, MD) for 45 minutes. Cells were then trypsinized off (1250 units/mL) (Sigma-Aldrich, St. Louis, MO) the petri dish and plated on coverslips coated with mouse-laminin (Trevigen Inc., Gaithersburg, MD). Then, cells were cultured in a serum free defined media containing BDNF (50 ng/mL) (Peprotech, Rocky Hill, NJ), CNTF (10 ng/mL) (Peprotech, Rocky Hill, NJ), and forskolin (5 ng/mL) (Sigma-Aldrich, St. Louis, MO). Cells were incubated at 37°C in a humidified atmosphere of 10% $CO_2$ and 90% air.

After 1 week in culture, primary RGCs were viable and showed good neurite outgrowth. Primary RGCs grown on coverslips were either untreated (control) or were treated with ET-1(10 nM and 100 nM) or ET-3 (100 nM) for 24 hr. The cells were treated with a mixture of green-fluorescent calcein-AM (to indicate intracellular esterase activity of living cells) and red-fluorescent ethidium homodimer-1 (EtHD) (indicative of dead cells) was added to assess the viability of the cells (Live/Dead® Viability/Cytotoxicity Kit, Eugene, OR, USA). Eight images were taken for each treatment condition, in a Zeiss LSM 510 META confocal microscope and the number of viable and dead cells was counted using the imageJ software. The number of dead cells were expressed as a percentage of total cells in each field of view and mean values of percent of dead cells for each treatment condition was calculated. Statistical analyses were performed by One Way ANOVA to determine if there was a significant increase in cell death in various treatment groups in comparison to the untreated control group.

## Paraphenylenediamine (PPD) staining

IOP elevation was carried out in WT and KO rats [35]. The rats were maintained for 4 weeks after IOP elevation, following which they were sacrificed, eyes enucleated and optic nerves were excised 2 mm posterior to the globe. The optic nerves were fixed with 2% paraformaldehyde, 2.5% glutaraldehyde in 0.1 M sodium cacodylate buffer for 3 hrs at room temperature. After osmification and embedding in epon, optic nerve cross sections were obtained and stained with 1% paraphenylenediamine for 10 min at room temperature by a modification of a published protocol [80]. Images were taken in a Zeiss LSM 510 META confocal microscope. The images were graded in a blinded manner by five individuals giving a score ranging from 0 to 9 by a modification of the method [81]. The grades assigned to each treatment group were compared to determine if there were neuroprotective/neurodegenerative changes between the different groups.

## TUNEL assay for detection of apoptosis

Primary RGCs were isolated from postnatal day 3–7 rat pups using a two step panning procedure (78) and seeded on 12 mm coverslips. The cells were allowed to attach and grow for 1 week till they displayed good neurite outgrowth. The RGCs were either untreated or treated with ET-1 (10 nM), ET-1 (100 nM) or ET-3 (100 nM) for 24 hr. Following treatments, the RGCs on coverslips were fixed with 4% formaldehyde in PBS for 25 min at 4°C. TUNEL assays were carried out using the DeadEnd Fluorometric TUNEL System (Promega, Madison, WI) by the manufacturer's instructions. Briefly, the cells were permeabilized in 0.2% Triton X-100 in PBS for 5 min followed by two washes with PBS. A negative control reaction was carried out by incubating one coverslip of RGCs with fluorescein-12-dUTP in the absence of TdT enzyme. Another coverslip was treated with DNase I enzyme to introduce DNA cleavage prior to the incubation with the reaction mix. The labeling reaction was carried out by incubating with a mixture of fluorescein-12-dUTP and terminal deoxynucleotidyl transferase (TdT) at for 60 min at 37°C. Following the incubation, the cells were washed with PBS and incubated with 4′ 6 Diamidino-phenylindole dichloride (DAPI) to stain nuclei. The TUNEL positive cells were detected by incorporation of fluorescein and fluorescent images were taken in an EVoS microscope.

## Supporting Information

**Figure S1   Experimental controls for TUNEL assay of primary RGCs.** Primary RGCs were either untreated (top horizontal panel) or treated with DNAse I as a positive control (middle horizontal panel). TUNEL assay was carried out using a combination of terminal deoxynucleotidyl transferase (TdT) and fluorescein-12-dUTP. Another set of RGCs were subjected to the negative control reaction by treatment with fluorescein-12-dUTP alone, with the exclusion of TdT (lower horizontal panel). The left vertical panel (TUNEL) indicates fluorescent images from cells incorporating fluorescein-12-dUTP indicative of apoptosis. The right vertical panel (DAPI) shows stained nuclei using DAPI. Scale bar indicates 400 μm.

## Acknowledgments

The authors thank Dr. Thomas Yorio for several useful discussions, insightful comments and suggestions on the manuscript. The technical assistance of Ms. Michelle Taylor in receptor binding assays is gratefully acknowledged. We also thank Mr. Yong Park for help with the primary culture of retinal ganglion cells.

## Author Contributions

Conceived and designed the experiments: AZM SH BHM RL RRK. Performed the experiments: AZM NRP H-YM SH BHM DLS MJ RRK. Analyzed the data: AZM SH BHM DLS RL CB RRK. Contributed reagents/materials/analysis tools: RL SY. Wrote the paper: AZM SH BHM RRK.

## References

1. Quigley HA (1996) Number of people with glaucoma worldwide. Br J Ophthalmol 80: 389–393.
2. Quigley HA, Broman AT (2006) The number of people with glaucoma worldwide in 2010 and 2020. Br J Ophthalmol 90: 262–267.
3. Gupta N, Yucel YH (2007) Glaucoma as a neurodegenerative disease. Curr Opin Ophthalmol 18: 110–114.
4. Quigley HA, Addicks EM (1980) Chronic experimental glaucoma in primates. II. Effect of extended intraocular pressure elevation on optic nerve head and axonal transport. Invest Ophthalmol Vis Sci 19: 137–152.
5. Quigley HA, Addicks EM, Green WR (1982) Optic nerve damage in human glaucoma. III. Quantitative correlation of nerve fiber loss and visual field defect in glaucoma, ischemic neuropathy, papilledema, and toxic neuropathy. Arch Ophthalmol 100: 135–146.
6. Quigley HA (1995) Ganglion cell death in glaucoma: pathology recapitulates ontogeny. Aust N Z J Ophthalmol 23: 85–91.
7. Quigley HA, Nickells RW, Kerrigan LA, Pease ME, Thibault DJ, et al. (1995) Retinal ganglion cell death in experimental glaucoma and after axotomy occurs by apoptosis. Invest Ophthalmol Vis Sci 36: 774–786.
8. Kerrigan LA, Zack DJ, Quigley HA, Smith SD, Pease ME (1997) TUNEL-positive ganglion cells in human primary open-angle glaucoma. Arch Ophthalmol 115: 1031–1035.

9. Varela HJ, Hernandez MR (1997) Astrocyte responses in human optic nerve head with primary open-angle glaucoma. J Glaucoma 6: 303–313.

10. Begg IS, Drance SM (1971) Progress of the glaucomatous process related to recurrent ischaemic changes at the optic disc. Exp Eye Res 11: 141.

11. Hayreh SS (1971) Posterior ciliary arterial occlusive disorders. Trans Ophthalmol Soc U K 91: 291–303.

12. Cioffi GA (1996) Care guidelines and optic nerve assessment. J Glaucoma 5: A12.

13. Vorwerk CK, Lipton SA, Zurakowski D, Hyman BT, Sabel BA, et al. (1996) Chronic low-dose glutamate is toxic to retinal ganglion cells. Toxicity blocked by memantine. Invest Ophthalmol Vis Sci 37: 1618–1624.

14. Levin LA (1999) Direct and indirect approaches to neuroprotective therapy of glaucomatous optic neuropathy. Surv Ophthalmol 43 Suppl 1: S98–101.

15. Osborne NN (2008) Pathogenesis of ganglion "cell death" in glaucoma and neuroprotection: focus on ganglion cell axonal mitochondria. Prog Brain Res 173: 339–352.

16. Kong GY, Van Bergen NJ, Trounce IA, Crowston JG (2009) Mitochondrial dysfunction and glaucoma. J Glaucoma 18: 93–100.

17. Cockburn DM (1983) Does reduction of intraocular pressure (IOP) prevent visual field loss in glaucoma? Am J Optom Physiol Opt 60: 705–711.

18. Chauhan BC, Drance SM (1992) The relationship between intraocular pressure and visual field progression in glaucoma. Graefes Arch Clin Exp Ophthalmol 230: 521–526.

19. Almasieh M, Wilson AM, Morquette B, Cueva Vargas JL, Di Polo A (2012) The molecular basis of retinal ganglion cell death in glaucoma. Prog Retin Eye Res 31: 152–181.

20. Yorio T, Krishnamoorthy R, Prasanna G (2002) Endothelin: is it a contributor to glaucoma pathophysiology? J Glaucoma 11: 259–270.

21. Chauhan BC (2008) Endothelin and its potential role in glaucoma. Can J Ophthalmol 43: 356–360.

22. Rosenthal R, Fromm M (2011) Endothelin antagonism as an active principle for glaucoma therapy. Br J Pharmacol 162: 806–816.

23. Tezel G, Kass MA, Kolker AE, Becker B, Wax MB (1997) Plasma and aqueous humor endothelin levels in primary open-angle glaucoma. J Glaucoma 6: 83–89.

24. Kallberg ME, Brooks DE, Garcia-Sanchez GA, Komaromy AM, Szabo NJ, et al. (2002) Endothelin 1 levels in the aqueous humor of dogs with glaucoma. J Glaucoma 11: 105–109.

25. Prasanna G, Hulet C, Desai D, Krishnamoorthy RR, Narayan S, et al. (2005) Effect of elevated intraocular pressure on endothelin-1 in a rat model of glaucoma. Pharmacol Res 51: 41–50.

26. Orgul S, Cioffi GA, Wilson DJ, Bacon DR, Van Buskirk EM (1996) An endothelin-1 induced model of optic nerve ischemia in the rabbit. Invest Ophthalmol Vis Sci 37: 1860–1869.

27. Cioffi GA, Sullivan P (1999) The effect of chronic ischemia on the primate optic nerve. Eur J Ophthalmol 9 Suppl 1: S34–36.

28. Chauhan BC, LeVatte TL, Jollimore CA, Yu PK, Reitsamer HA, et al. (2004) Model of endothelin-1-induced chronic optic neuropathy in rat. Invest Ophthalmol Vis Sci 45: 144–152.

29. Lau J, Dang M, Hockmann K, Ball AK (2006) Effects of acute delivery of endothelin-1 on retinal ganglion cell loss in the rat. Exp Eye Res 82: 132–145.

30. Krishnamoorthy RR, Rao VR, Dauphin R, Prasanna G, Johnson C, et al. (2008) Role of the ETB receptor in retinal ganglion cell death in glaucoma. Can J Physiol Pharmacol 86: 380–393.

31. MacCumber MW, D'Anna SA (1994) Endothelin receptor-binding subtypes in the human retina and choroid. Arch Ophthalmol 112: 1231–1235.

32. Stitt AW, Chakravarthy U, Gardiner TA, Archer DB (1996) Endothelin-like immunoreactivity and receptor binding in the choroid and retina. Curr Eye Res 15: 111–117.

33. Yang Z, Quigley HA, Pease ME, Yang Y, Qian J, et al. (2007) Changes in gene expression in experimental glaucoma and optic nerve transection: the equilibrium between protective and detrimental mechanisms. Invest Ophthalmol Vis Sci 48: 5539–5548.

34. Wang L, Fortune B, Cull G, Dong J, Cioffi GA (2006) Endothelin B receptor in human glaucoma and experimentally induced optic nerve damage. Arch Ophthalmol 124: 717–724.

35. Morrison JC, Moore CG, Deppmeier LM, Gold BG, Meshul CK, et al. (1997) A rat model of chronic pressure-induced optic nerve damage. Exp Eye Res 64: 85–96.

36. Scatchard G (1949) Equilibrium in non-electrolyte mixtures. Chem Rev 44: 7–35.

37. McKinnon SJ, Lehman DM, Kerrigan-Baumrind LA, Merges CA, Pease ME, et al. (2002) Caspase activation and amyloid precursor protein cleavage in rat ocular hypertension. Invest Ophthalmol Vis Sci 43: 1077–1087.

38. Schlamp CL, Johnson EC, Li Y, Morrison JC, Nickells RW (2001) Changes in Thy1 gene expression associated with damaged retinal ganglion cells. Mol Vis 7: 192–201.

39. Chauhan BC, Pan J, Archibald ML, LeVatte TL, Kelly ME, et al. (2002) Effect of intraocular pressure on optic disc topography, electroretinography, and axonal loss in a chronic pressure-induced rat model of optic nerve damage. Invest Ophthalmol Vis Sci 43: 2969–2976.

40. Rattner A, Nathans J (2005) The genomic response to retinal disease and injury: evidence for endothelin signaling from photoreceptors to glia. J Neurosci 25: 4540–4549.

41. Prasanna G, Narayan S, Krishnamoorthy RR, Yorio T (2003) Eyeing endothelins: a cellular perspective. Mol Cell Biochem 253: 71–88.

42. Rao VR, Krishnamoorthy RR, Yorio T (2007) Endothelin-1, endothelin A and B receptor expression and their pharmacological properties in GFAP negative human lamina cribrosa cells. Exp Eye Res 84: 1115–1124.

43. Prasanna G, Krishnamoorthy R, Yorio T (2011) Endothelin, astrocytes and glaucoma. Exp Eye Res 93: 170–177.

44. Wang X, LeVatte TL, Archibald ML, Chauhan BC (2009) Increase in endothelin B receptor expression in optic nerve astrocytes in endothelin-1 induced chronic experimental optic neuropathy. Exp Eye Res 88: 378–385.

45. Resch H, Karl K, Weigert G, Wolzt M, Hommer A, et al. (2009) Effect of dual endothelin receptor blockade on ocular blood flow in patients with glaucoma and healthy subjects. Invest Ophthalmol Vis Sci 50: 358–363.

46. Murphy JA, Archibald ML, Chauhan BC (2010) The role of endothelin-1 and its receptors in optic nerve head astrocyte proliferation. Br J Ophthalmol 94: 1233–1238.

47. Rubanyi GM, Polokoff MA (1994) Endothelins: molecular biology, biochemistry, pharmacology, physiology, and pathophysiology. Pharmacol Rev 46: 325–415.

48. Good TJ, Kahook MY (2010) The role of endothelin in the pathophysiology of glaucoma. Expert Opin Ther Targets 14: 647–654.

49. Yanagisawa M, Kurihara H, Kimura S, Tomobe Y, Kobayashi M, et al. (1988) A novel potent vasoconstrictor peptide produced by vascular endothelial cells. Nature 332: 411–415.

50. MacCumber MW, Ross CA, Glaser BM, Snyder SH (1989) Endothelin: visualization of mRNAs by in situ hybridization provides evidence for local action. Proc Natl Acad Sci U S A 86: 7285–7289.

51. MacCumber MW, Jampel HD, Snyder SH (1991) Ocular effects of the endothelins. Abundant peptides in the eye. Arch Ophthalmol 109: 705–709.

52. Wollensak G, Schaefer HE, Ihling C (1998) An immunohistochemical study of endothelin-1 in the human eye. Curr Eye Res 17: 541–545.

53. Lee ME, de la Monte SM, Ng SC, Bloch KD, Quertermous T (1990) Expression of the potent vasoconstrictor endothelin in the human central nervous system. J Clin Invest 86: 141–147.

54. MacCumber MW, Ross CA, Snyder SH (1990) Endothelin in brain: receptors, mitogenesis, and biosynthesis in glial cells. Proc Natl Acad Sci U S A 87: 2359–2363.

55. Nie XJ, Olsson Y (1996) Endothelin peptides in brain diseases. Rev Neurosci 7: 177–186.

56. Torbidoni V, Iribarne M, Ogawa L, Prasanna G, Suburo AM (2005) Endothelin-1 and endothelin receptors in light-induced retinal degeneration. Exp Eye Res 81: 265–275.

57. Imai Y, Soda M, Inoue H, Hattori N, Mizuno Y, et al. (2001) An unfolded putative transmembrane polypeptide, which can lead to endoplasmic reticulum stress, is a substrate of Parkin. Cell 105: 891–902.

58. Lepple-Wienhues A, Becker M, Stahl F, Berweck S, Hensen J, et al. (1992) Endothelin-like immunoreactivity in the aqueous humour and in conditioned medium from cultured ciliary epithelial cells. Curr Eye Res 11: 1041–1046.

59. Cellini M, Possati GL, Profazio V, Sbrocca M, Caramazza N, et al. (1997) Color Doppler imaging and plasma levels of endothelin-1 in low-tension glaucoma. Acta Ophthalmol Scand Suppl: 11–13.

60. Sugiyama T, Moriya S, Oku H, Azuma I (1995) Association of endothelin-1 with normal tension glaucoma: clinical and fundamental studies. Surv Ophthalmol 39 Suppl 1: S49–56.

61. Koliakos GG, Konstas AG, Schlotzer-Schrehardt U, Hollo G, Mitova D, et al. (2004) Endothelin-1 concentration is increased in the aqueous humour of patients with exfoliation syndrome. Br J Ophthalmol 88: 523–527.

62. Tao W, Prasanna G, Dimitrijevich S, Yorio T (1998) Endothelin receptor A is expressed and mediates the [Ca2+]i mobilization of cells in human ciliary smooth muscle, ciliary nonpigmented epithelium, and trabecular meshwork. Curr Eye Res 17: 31–38.

63. Drager UC, Olsen JF (1981) Ganglion cell distribution in the retina of the mouse. Invest Ophthalmol Vis Sci 20: 285–293.

64. Perry VH (1981) Evidence for an amacrine cell system in the ganglion cell layer of the rat retina. Neuroscience 6: 931–944.

65. Jeon CJ, Strettoi E, Masland RH (1998) The major cell populations of the mouse retina. J Neurosci 18: 8936–8946.

66. Rodieck RW (1973) The vertebrate retina; principles of structure and function. San Francisco,: Freeman. x, 1044 p.

67. Fukuroda T, Fujikawa T, Ozaki S, Ishikawa K, Yano M, et al. (1994) Clearance of circulating endothelin-1 by ETB receptors in rats. Biochem Biophys Res Commun 199: 1461–1465.

68. Dupuis J, Goresky CA, Fournier A (1996) Pulmonary clearance of circulating endothelin-1 in dogs in vivo: exclusive role of ETB receptors. J Appl Physiol 81: 1510–1515.

69. Berkelaar M, Clarke DB, Wang YC, Bray GM, Aguayo AJ (1994) Axotomy results in delayed death and apoptosis of retinal ganglion cells in adult rats. J Neurosci 14: 4368–4374.

70. Garcia-Valenzuela E, Shareef S, Walsh J, Sharma SC (1995) Programmed cell death of retinal ganglion cells during experimental glaucoma. Exp Eye Res 61: 33–44.

71. Kermer P, Ankerhold R, Klocker N, Krajewski S, Reed JC, et al. (2000) Caspase-9: involvement in secondary death of axotomized rat retinal ganglion cells in vivo. Brain Res Mol Brain Res 85: 144–150.

72. Watanabe M, Fukuda Y (2002) Survival and axonal regeneration of retinal ganglion cells in adult cats. Prog Retin Eye Res 21: 529–553.

73. Weishaupt JH, Diem R, Kermer P, Krajewski S, Reed JC, et al. (2003) Contribution of caspase-8 to apoptosis of axotomized rat retinal ganglion cells in vivo. Neurobiol Dis 13: 124–135.

74. Salinas-Navarro M, Mayor-Torroglosa S, Jimenez-Lopez M, Aviles-Trigueros M, Holmes TM, et al. (2009) A computerized analysis of the entire retinal ganglion cell population and its spatial distribution in adult rats. Vision Res 49: 115–126.

75. Howell GR, Macalinao DG, Sousa GL, Walden M, Soto I, et al. (2011) Molecular clustering identifies complement and endothelin induction as early events in a mouse model of glaucoma. J Clin Invest 121: 1429–1444.

76. Gariepy CE, Williams SC, Richardson JA, Hammer RE, Yanagisawa M (1998) Transgenic expression of the endothelin-B receptor prevents congenital intestinal aganglionosis in a rat model of Hirschsprung disease. J Clin Invest 102: 1092–1101.

77. Husak PJ, Kuo T, Enquist LW (2000) Pseudorabies virus membrane proteins gI and gE facilitate anterograde spread of infection in projection-specific neurons in the rat. J Virol 74: 10975–10983.

78. McKinnon SJ, Lehman DM, Tahzib NG, Ransom NL, Reitsamer HA, et al. (2002) Baculoviral IAP repeat-containing-4 protects optic nerve axons in a rat glaucoma model. Mol Ther 5: 780–787.

79. Barres BA, Silverstein BE, Corey DP, Chun LL (1988) Immunological, morphological, and electrophysiological variation among retinal ganglion cells purified by panning. Neuron 1: 791–803.

80. Hollander H, Vaaland JL (1968) A reliable staining method for semi-thin sections in experimental neurfanatomy. Brain Res 10: 120–126.

81. Chauhan BC, Levatte TL, Garnier KL, Tremblay F, Pang IH, et al. (2006) Semiquantitative optic nerve grading scheme for determining axonal loss in experimental optic neuropathy. Invest Ophthalmol Vis Sci 47: 634–640.

# 14

# Cystatin A, a Potential Common Link for Mutant Myocilin Causative Glaucoma

**K. David Kennedy, S. A. AnithaChristy, LaKisha K. Buie, Teresa Borrás***

Department of Ophthalmology, University of North Carolina School of Medicine, Chapel Hill, North Carolina, United States of America

## Abstract

Myocilin (MYOC) is a 504 aa secreted glycoprotein induced by stress factors in the trabecular meshwork tissue of the eye, where it was discovered. Mutations in *MYOC* are linked to glaucoma. The glaucoma phenotype of each of the different *MYOC* mutation varies, but all of them cause elevated intraocular pressure (IOP). In cells, forty percent of wild-type MYOC is cleaved by calpain II, a cysteine protease. This proteolytic process is inhibited by MYOC mutants. In this study, we investigated the molecular mechanisms by which MYOC mutants cause glaucoma. We constructed adenoviral vectors with variants Q368X, R342K, D380N, K423E, and overexpressed them in human trabecular meshwork cells. We analyzed expression profiles with Affymetrix U133Plus2 GeneChips using wild-type and null viruses as controls. Analysis of trabecular meshwork relevant mechanisms showed that the unfolded protein response (UPR) was the most affected. Search for individual candidate genes revealed that genes that have been historically connected to trabecular meshwork physiology and pathology were altered by the *MYOC* mutants. Some of those had known *MYOC* associations (*MMP1, PDIA4, CALR, SFPR1*) while others did not (*EDN1, MGP, IGF1, TAC1*). Some, were top-changed in only one mutant (*LOXL1, CYP1B1, FBN1*), others followed a mutant group pattern. Some of the genes were new (*RAB39B, STC1, CXCL12, CSTA*). In particular, one selected gene, the cysteine protease inhibitor cystatin A (*CSTA*), was commonly induced by all mutants and not by the wild-type. Subsequent functional analysis of the selected gene showed that CSTA was able to reduce wild-type MYOC cleavage in primary trabecular meshwork cells while an inactive mutated CSTA was not. These findings provide a new molecular understanding of the mechanisms of MYOC-causative glaucoma and reveal CSTA, a serum biomarker for cancer, as a potential biomarker and drug for the treatment of MYOC-induced glaucoma.

**Editor:** Reiner Albert Veitia, Institut Jacques Monod, France

**Funding:** This work was supported by National Institutes of Health (USA) grants EY11906 (TB), EY13126 (TB), EY015873 (RHHA), and by a Research to Prevent Blindness unrestricted grant to the UNC Department of Ophthalmology. The funders had no role in study design, data collection and analysis, decision to publish, or preparation of the manuscript.

**Competing Interests:** The authors have declared that no competing interests exist.

* E-mail: tborras@med.unc.edu

## Introduction

The secreted glycoprotein, myocilin (MYOC), was identified in human trabecular meshwork (HTM) cells after prolonged exposure to dexamethasone (DEX) (*Trabecular Meshwork Inducible protein, TIGR*) [1]. It was independently discovered in the ciliary body [2] and in the normal retina [3]. The gene was later found to be expressed in non-ocular tissues, especially in heart and skeletal muscle [4]. However, MYOC retained special properties in the trabecular meshwork and its induction by DEX is specific to this tissue [5]. Soon after its discovery, mutations in the *MYOC* gene were found to be linked to 3–4% of primary open-angle glaucoma (POAG) [6] and to a large percent (10–30%) to juvenile open-angle glaucoma (JOAG), an early-onset and more severe form of the disease [7].

The glaucomas are a group of optic neuropathies caused by the degeneration and death of the retinal ganglion cells. In glaucoma, there is a progressive visual field loss and if left untreated, it leads to irreversible blindness. It is estimated that by 2020 there will be 79.6 million cases of glaucoma worldwide, with a high proportion of women and Asians [8]. POAG is the most common form of the disease, which in most cases, is triggered by an elevated intraocular pressure (IOP). In turn, elevated IOP is the result of an increased resistance of the trabecular meshwork tissue to the aqueous humor outflow.

To date, more than 70 *MYOC* mutations have been associated with glaucoma (http://myocilin.com/) [9]. Each of the mutations results in a slightly different phenotype, it is more prevalent in a given race and some have been speculated to be affected by environmental epigenetic factors (reviewed in [9]). Nevertheless, in every case, mutations in *MYOC* are associated with elevated IOP, ranging from mild to severe (http://myocilin.com/). Because of the relevance of this association, the MYOC protein has been extensively studied.

Myocilin is a 504 amino acid protein with a molecular weight of 55–57 kDa [10,11]. The gene maps to 1q23–q24 [6] and contains three exons, which pretty much define three protein folding domains [4,10]. The N-domain (aa 1 to 202) contains a signal peptide cleavage, a leucine zipper-like motif and is similar to the heavy chain of myosin [4,10]. The C-terminal domain (aa 244 to 505), separated by a central linker (aa 203 to 205), is 40% homologous to olfactomedin, a major component of the extracellular matrix (ECM) of the olfactory neuroepithelium. The original finding that *MYOC* mutants mapped to the olfactomedin domain has held, and today, over 90% percent of pathogenic mutations are known to occur in that third exon of the protein (http://myocilin.com/).

Although considerable progress has been made, many questions regarding the function of wild-type MYOC and the molecular correlations of the different mutant variants to disease severity remain. Myocilin is processed and shed inside vesicles [12,13]. In contrast to the wild-type, recombinant mutants in the olfactomedin domain, whether generic, glaucoma-associated, stop or missense, are unable to exit the cell in all cell types tried [5,12,14,15]. Our earlier work also showed that mutant MYOC proteins lacking the olfactomedin domain are misfolded, form insoluble aggregates and accumulate in the endoplasmic reticulum (ER) [11]. Further, presence of increasing amounts of the recombinant mutant induces a fraction of the soluble, wild-type MYOC to move to the insoluble fraction and hamper its secretion [11]. Glaucoma-associated mutants are likewise insoluble [16] and hetero-oligomers with the wild-type are sequestered in the ER [17], leading to ER stress, activation of the unfolded protein response (UPR) and potential cytotoxicity [18,19]. This data, supported by clinical findings on the absence of POAG in homozygous patients for certain MYOC mutants [20] led to the conclusion that MYOC-linked glaucoma was due to a gain of function.

In addition to glucocorticoids, *MYOC* expression is induced by a number of stress factors. Mechanical stretch, TGF-β, oxidative stress, heat shock and elevated IOP all induce *MYOC* in cells and tissues (review in [21,22]. In addition, expression of *MYOC* mutants sensitizes cells to oxidative stress [23]. Myocilin interacts with several intracellular and extracellular matrix proteins (review in [24]). Recently it was shown to interact with components of the WNT signaling pathway [25], which was independently found to be associated to regulation of IOP [22,26].

In the ER, MYOC undergoes an intracellular endoproteolytic cleavage in the central linker domain [27,28]. This processing occurs in ~40% of the wild-type protein and yields a 35 kDa fragment which is co-secreted with the full-length [28]. Myocilin mutants inhibit the proteolytic processing and the extent of inhibition has been correlated with the severity of the glaucoma phenotypes [28]. In addition, this proteolytic process modulates the molecular interactions of myocilin and reduces the formation of myocilin homoaggregates [29]. The enzyme responsible for this cleavage has been identified as Calpain II [30], a calcium-dependent cysteine protease present in most mammalian tissues.

All these findings put together reveal the potential involvement of many different genes in the functions leading to the *MYOC*-linked glaucoma. Previously, we reported a first microarray analysis using wild-type *MYOC* and high density oligonucleotide Affymetrix U133A GeneChips [31]. To now identify molecular differences among the effects of the causative glaucoma *MYOC* mutants, in this study we conducted an expression analysis on the transcriptome of primary human trabecular meshwork cells overexpressing *MYOC* mutants, and performed the analysis using the upgraded Affymetrix U133 Plus 2.0 GeneChips. We selected four representative mutants, based on different clinical outcomes, populations and/or relevance of the mutated codon. The Q368X variant is the most common (29% of the diseased causing variants) and results in a mild phenotype (http://myocilin.com/). Mutations R342K and D380N comprise 0.8% of the causing variants each, and are very severe, with a mean maximum IOP of 54 and 39 mmHg [32]. Both mutations have been reported only in one population, that of Ghana in West Africa. However while there is only one variant utilizing amino acid Arg342, the amino acid Asp380, highly conserved in all vertebrates, has produced four disease causing variants (D380N, D380H, D380A, D380G) [9], a

recurrence known to occur very rarely in genetics. These four variants appear in different populations and in particular, the His and Ala changes result in intermediate glaucoma phenotypes and biochemical protein effects [15,28,33]. The last mutation, K423E, was selected because it occurs in two unrelated Caucasian populations [20,34], has a severe clinical outcome and exhibits the interesting feature that homozygous patients do not manifest the disease [20]. A similar analysis recently published utilized transgenic flies and analyzed changes in the transcriptome of 2–3 day old insects' whole heads [19].

Cystatin A (CSTA) is a member of the cystatin superfamily of proteins, some of which are active cysteine protease inhibitors, such as cystatin A (review in [35]). Within the cystatin superfamily, CSTA is characterized as a stefin [36]. Proteins of the stefin family, lack carbohydrates and disulfide bonds and have a molecular weight ~11 kDa. This single chain protein forms tight complexes and inhibits the activity of papain-type proteases, cathepsin B, H and L [36], and presumably other intracellular cysteine protease inhibitors. The short N-terminal region of CSTA, and in particular the evolutionary conserved Gly-4 residue has been shown to play a key role in the binding of the CSTA inhibitor to the target proteases, papain, cathepsin B and L [37]. Mutations of Gly-4 to aminoacids with longer side chains like arginine were also shown to be more deleterious for the binding that mutations to alanine or serine which have small side chains [37]. Cystatin A is present in various tissues (epidermis, polymorphonuclear granulocytes, liver and spleen) and has also been found in extracellular fluids [35]. A loss of function mutation for CSTA was recently linked to two families of Middle Eastern origin exhibiting exfoliative ichthyosis, a scaly skin disease [38]. Cystatin A is a known myoepithelial cell marker and its downregulation plays a role in carcinogenesis, from breast to brain tumors [35]. It is believed that CSTA regulates cellular proliferation, tumor growth and metastasis. Cystatin A expression is a negative prognostic marker in breast tumors of lymph node negative patients [35]. Recently, levels of CSTA in serum, together with manganese superoxide dismutase and MMP2, were shown to be reliable biomarkers for the detection of nasopharyngeal carcinomas patients [39].

In the present study, we searched for genes and mechanisms affected by overexpression of four myocilin mutants in primary human trabecular meshwork cells. Using microarray profiles, we found that the myocilin mutants altered a high number of genes which had been previously associated with trabecular meshwork physiological and glaucomatous conditions. Some genes were shared by all mutants while some were mutant-specific. The extracellular matrix gene ontology (GO) category was the most enriched and most significant. Of the four most common mechanisms, genes in the UPR list were changed the most. More important, this study uncovered cystatin A, a cysteine protein inhibitor induced by all mutants, which reduced the processing of wild-type myocilin in vitro. These findings provide a molecular insight into mechanisms that trigger MYOC-glaucoma and raise the possibility of using silencing or inhibition of *CSTA* as a potential treatment of the MYOC-mutant development of glaucoma.

## Materials and Methods

### Generation of Adenoviruses Carrying Wild-type and MYOC Glaucoma-associated Mutants

Plasmids carrying point mutations corresponding to four human *MYOC* mutations genetically linked to glaucoma were generated by site-directed mutagenesis using as a template clone pMC2 [11] and the QuickChange mutagenesis kit (Stratagene, La Jolla, CAL) [19]. The plasmids contained the MYOC mutations Q368X, R342K, D380N, and K423E (Figure1). All mutant clones were re-amplified with 5'-*KpnI*-3'-*BamHI* ended primers to remove the *PmeI* site (*MYOC* nucleotides (nt) 4–1566) (all *MYOC* nt numbering is from access number AF001620) and subcloned into pCR2.1 (Invitrogen, Carlsbad, CA) for confirmation of sequence and presence of the mutations (clones pGL6, pGL9, pAC10, pAC14). *KpnI-NotI* restricted mutant cDNA fragments (1,596 nucleotides) were gel purified and inserted into pShuttle-CMV (generously donated by B. Vogelstein [40] for the generation of the recombinant adenoviral plasmid vectors (pGL7, pGL10, pAC11, pAC15). For the wild-type, the pKM1 plasmid (see below) was digested with *KpnI-NotI* and the isolated fragment inserted into the same pShuttle-CMV vector to yield pAC18 (total insert 1,601 bp containing 46 bp 5' and 33 bp 3'plasmid sequences flanking the 1,522 *MYOC* wild-type coding region).

The shuttle vectors were then linearized with *PmeI* and electroporated into BJ5183-Ad1 cells for homologous recombination with an adenovirus backbone plasmid using the AdEasy Adenoviral Vector System (Stratagene) following manufacturer's recommendations. The resultant Ad plasmid vectors (pGL8, pGL11, pAC12, pAC16, pAC19) were linearized with *PacI* and calcium phosphate-transfected (Clontech, Mountain View, CA) into early passages QBI-Human Embryonic Kidney (HEK) 293A cells (Qbiogene, Montreal, Quebec, Canada) for the production of the adenoviral recombinants (Adh.Q368X, Adh.R342K, Adh.D380N, Adh.K423E and Adh.MYOCWT). These viruses therefore carry each of the four *MYOC* mutants driven by the same CMV promoter. High titer stocks were obtained by propagation in the same QBI-HEK 293A cells and purification by double binding CsCl density centrifugation as described [41]. A control virus carrying the same promoter and no transgene (Ad5.CMV-Null) was purchased from Qbiogene (Montreal, Canada) and grown and purified in our laboratory. For Adh.Q368X, the virus particle number was determined by measurement of its optical density at 260 nm using the formula 1 $\mu$g of DNA = 2.2 X $10^{10}$ particles. For the remaining recombinants, physical particles were titered as viral genomes (vg)/ml as described [41] using a *MYOC* fluorescent TaqMan primers/probe Hs00165345_m1 (Applied Biosystems, ABI, Foster City, CA) and the *MYOC* plasmid pAC12 for the generation of the standard curve. Viral infectivity (infectious units [IFU]/ml) was measured with a rapid titer kit (AdenoX; Clontech) also as described [41]. Viral lots used in these studies had concentrations between 2 X $10^{11}$ and 1 X $10^{12}$ vg/ml with infectivity values between 2 X $10^9$ and 5 X$10^{10}$ IFU/ml A second set of viral stocks were grown at the University of North Carolina Vector Core facility. All viral stocks used in the experiments were checked for the overexpression of *MYOC* mRNA by TaqMan PCR (probe Hs00165345_m1) and MYOC protein by western blot (goat anti-human polyclonal, Santa Cruz Biotechnology #21243, Santa Cruz, CA)).

## Primary Culture of Human Trabecular Meshwork Cells

Primary human trabecular meshwork (HTM) HTM-72 and HTM-137 cell lines were generated respectively from the trabecular meshworks dissected from residual cornea rims of 29 and 39 years old donors (North Carolina Eye Bank) after surgical corneal transplants at the University of North Carolina Eye Clinic. The tissue was cut into small pieces, carefully attached to the

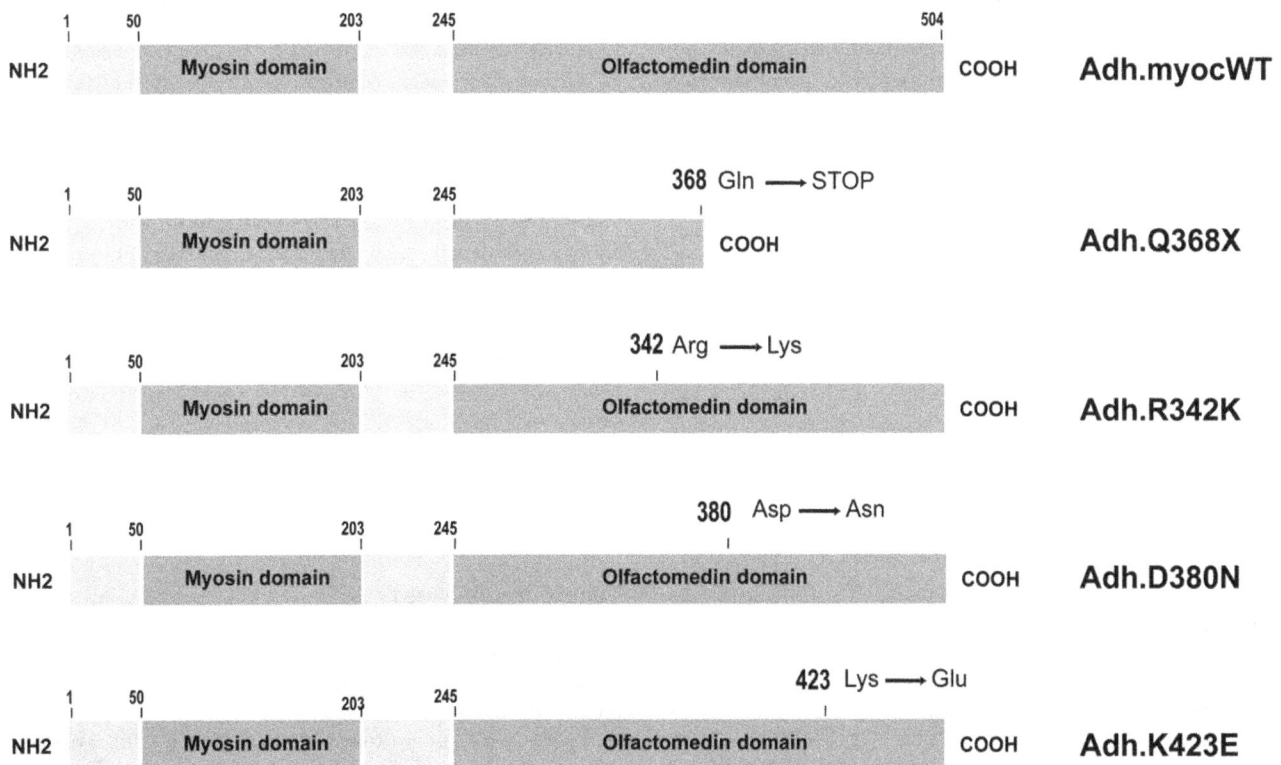

**Figure 1. Schematic representation of MYOC wild-type and mutant proteins used for the adenoviral constructions.** Myocilin protein contains a signal peptide cleavage (aa 1–50) and three folding domains. An N-terminal myosin domain (aa 50–203), a linker region (aa 203–245), and C-terminal olfactomedin domain (aa 245–504). All four selected mutants have mutations in the C-terminal olfaction domain. The Q368X mutation produces a truncated protein.

bottom of the 2% gelatin-coated 35 mm dish, and covered slipped with a drop of MEM Richter's Modification medium (IMEM, HyClone, Thermo Fisher Scientific, Waltham, MA) supplemented with 20% heat-inactivated fetal bovine serum (FBS, GIBCO catalog # 16140-071), 50 μg/ml gentamicin (Invitrogen). Cells from these specimens were not treated with enzymes and were allowed to grow from the explant for a period of 4 weeks changing the media every other day; upon confluency, cells were harvested and stored in liquid nitrogen. When reconstituted, these primary non-transformed cells are grown in complete medium consisting of IMEM, heat inactivated 10% FBS, gentamicin and subsist for seven to eight passages. In this study all cells were used at passage 4. These outflow pathway cultures comprise all cell types involved in maintaining resistance to flow. That includes cells from the three distinct regions of the trabecular meshwork plus cells lining the Schlemm's canal. Because most of the cells in these cultures come from the trabecular meshwork, they are commonly referred to as "trabecular meshwork cells".

## Delivery of Recombinant Adenoviruses to Primary Human Trabecular Meshwork Cells

Human trabecular meshwork primary cells at passage 4, seeded on either 3 cm or 10 cm dishes, were grown to between 65–90% confluency, washed twice with PBS and exposed to the recombinant adenoviruses (Adh.Q368X, Adh.R342K, Adh.D380N, Adh.K423E, Adh.MYOCWT and Ad5.CMV-Null) in 1 ml or 3 ml serum-free medium respectively. Multiplicity of infections (moi) ranged from $1.6 \times 10^3$–$1.6 \times 10^4$ vg/cell and were randomly distributed among the replicas. After exposure to the virus for 90 min, complete media was added and incubation continued for 48 h or 72 h. Mutant-Null infections were always performed in the same day, but interspersed replicas expand over two years. Although FBS lot number was not recorded in each experiment, the same supplier, same catalog number of heat inactivated FBS was used in all experiments.

## RNA Extraction, Reverse Transcription and TaqMan-PCR Assays

Human trabecular meshwork cells cells were scraped from tissue culture dishes with guanidine thiocyanate buffer (RLT, Qiagen, Valencia, CA). Total RNA was extracted by loading the solution onto a QIA Shredder™ column (Qiagen) and continued by the use of the RNeasy Mini kit with on-column RNase-free DNAse digestion according to manufacturer's recommendations (Qiagen). Purified RNA was eluted in 30 μl RNase-free water and the concentration measured with a NanoDrop ND-100 spectrophotometer (Thermo Fisher Scientific). Total RNA recoveries averaged 65.4±3.6 μg and 11.9±1.1 μg per 10 and 3 cm culture dishes respectively. RNA quality was assessed by measuring the size distribution on an Agilent Bioanalyzer (Agilent Technologies, Santa Clara, CA).

Reverse transcription (RT) reactions were conducted with 1 μg HTM cells RNA in a 20 μl total volume of proprietary RT buffer with RNAse inhibitor (High Capacity cDNA kit) (ABI) following manufacturer's recommendations (25°C 10 min, 37°C 2 h, 85°C 5 min, then 4°C). Fluorescently labeled TaqMan probe/primers sets for human MYOC, CSTA, CXCL2, IGF1, MMP1, MMP3, MMP12, SFRP1, STC1, SNCA, RAB39B, THBD and 18S RNA were purchased from the ABI TaqMan Gene Expression Assays (ABI). The human probes used were: *MYOC* (Hs00165345_m1), *CSTA* (Hs00193257_m1), *CXCL2* (Hs00235956_m1), IGF1 (Hs00153126_m1), *MMP1* (Hs00233958_m1), *MMP3* (Hs00968305_m1), *MMP12* (Hs00899662_m1), *SFRP1*

(Hs00610060_m1), *STC1* (Hs00174970_m1), SNCA (Hs01103383_m1), *RAB39B* (Hs00293395_m1) and *THBD* (Hs000264920_s1). All but one probe corresponded to sequences from different exons. The 18S RNA probe corresponded to sequences surrounding position nucleotide 609 (Hs99999901_s1). Reactions were performed in triplicate 20 μl aliquots using TaqMan Universal PCR Master mix No AmpErase UNG, run on an Applied Biosystems 7500 Real-Time PCR System, and analyzed by 7500 System SDS v.2.0.4 software (ABI). Relative Quantification (RQ) values between treated and untreated samples were calculated by the formula $2^{-\Delta\Delta C_T}$ where $C_T$ is the cycle at threshold, $\Delta C_T$ is $C_T$ of the assayed gene minus $C_T$ of the endogenous control (18S), and $\Delta\Delta C_T$ is the $\Delta C_T$ of the normalized assayed gene in the treated sample minus the $\Delta C_T$ of the same gene in the untreated one (calibrator). Because of the high abundance of the 18S rRNA used as the endogenous control and in order to get a linear amplification, RT reactions from treated and untreated samples were diluted $10^4$ times prior to their hybridization to the 18S TaqMan probe. Statistical analysis was performed by the Student's *t-test*.

## RNA Microarrays Hybridization

The RNAs from cells infected with *MYOC* mutants viral recombinants were prepared for hybridization to Human Genome U133 Plus 2.0 (n = 17) GeneChips (Affymetrix, Santa Clara, CA) at the University of North Carolina Functional Genomics Core Facility. These oligonucleotide microarrays contain 54,678 probe sets representing approximately 39,500 well-characterized human genes. The level of transcription of each gene represented on these chips is measured using the 11 nucleotide sequences which comprise each probe set. For the hybridization, total RNA (~0.7 μg) was reverse transcribed into cDNA using a cDNA kit from Life Technologies with a T7-(dT)$_{24}$ primer. Biotinylated cRNA was then generated from the cDNA reaction using the BioArray High Yield RNA Transcript Kit. The cRNA was then fragmented in fragmentation buffer (5X fragmentation buffer: 200 mM Tris-acetate, pH 8.1, 500 mM KOAc, 150 mM MgOAc) at 94°C for 35 min before the chip hybridization. 15 μg of fragmented cRNA was then added to a hybridization cocktail (0.05 μg/μl fragmented cRNA, 50 pM control oligonucleotide B2, *BioB*, *BioC*, *BioD*, and *cre* hybridization controls, 0.1 mg/ml herring sperm DNA, 0.5 mg/ml acetylated BSA, 100 mM MES, 1M [Na$^+$], 20 mM EDTA, 0.01% Tween 20). 10 μg of cRNA was used for hybridization. Arrays were hybridized for 16 h at 45°C in the GeneChip Hybridization Oven 640. The arrays were washed and stained with R-phycoerythrin streptavidin in the GeneChip Fluidics Station 450. After this, arrays were scanned with the GeneChip Scanner 3000 7G Plus. Sample quality was assessed by examination of 3' to 5' intensity ratios of certain genes.

## GeneSpring Analyses

Row data CEL files from Affymetrix were imported into GeneSpring GX Expression Analysis software, version GS10 (Agilent Technologies). For analysis of expression changes between the *MYOC* mutants, *MYOC* wild-type and null infected samples, their files were pre-processed through the Robust Multichip Average (RMA) and replicas from each of the mutant, wild-type or control chips were grouped using the grouping feature of the program. An interpretation was created which identified the treated versus the control selecting average over replicates in each of the two conditions. To eliminate genes expressed at lower levels in at least one out of the conditions compared, normalized data were filtered by expression level using the signal intensity raw data at a lower cutoff value of 50.

To identify top-changers, data were subsequently filtered on Fold Change (FC) to select genes that exhibited at least a 1.5-fold increase or decrease in the MYOC infected cells. Variance of the samples was obtained by the unpaired *t*-test. Lists with genes altered FC ≥ 1.5 were generated in GS10 and exported to the hard drive. These original gene lists contain many annotations with no Entrez number, repeated annotations with the same Entrez gene, a few annotations recognizing more than one Entrez number (almost identical genes, often pseudogenes) as well as genes encoding hypothetical proteins and undefined open reading frames genes. Using standard excel sorting applications, we used a rational approach to clean and filter FC 1.5-fold gene lists for each of the redundant and the undefined genes parameters (see results below). Heat maps of the full range FC of the mutants on categories of genes from a given function (calcification, elastin collagen crosslinking, WNT signaling pathway, stress and UPR response and molecular signature of glaucoma) were created in GS v7.3. The custom made gene-function lists contained one Affymetrix ID per gene. In the case that one of the genes from the list was represented by more than one Affymetrix ID in the chip, we chose the ID which was more altered by the Q368X mutation. Overlapping Venn diagrams were created in GS10 with re-imported gene lists containing Entrez numbers (IDs with no Entrez removed). Gene ontologies of the overlapping gene list altered in all-mutants were created in GS v7.3. They were obtained from the GO SLIMS lists available in the GS7 software, which contain subsets of the terms in the whole GO.

## Microarray Data Submission

All microarray data is MIAME compliant and the raw data has been deposited in the ArrayExpress MIAME compliant database. The accession numbers of each of the five experiments along with login information are as follows:

Experiment name: MYOC.Q368XvsNull
ArrayExpress accession: **E-MEXP-3427.**
Username: Reviewer_E-MEXP-3427
Password: ebr8fswC

Experiment name: MYOC.R342KvsNull
ArrayExpress accession: **E-MEXP-3435.**
Username: Reviewer_E-MEXP-3435
Password: nzsut632

Experiment name: MYOC.D380NvsNull
ArrayExpress accession: **E-MEXP-3434.**
Username: Reviewer_E-MEXP-3434
Password: uuvvpXH4

Experiment name: MYOC.K423EvsNull
ArrayExpress accession: **E-MEXP-3439**
Username: Reviewer_E-MEXP-3439
Password: Ljwhbanh

Experiment name: MYOC.WTvsNull
ArrayExpress accession: **E-MEXP-3440**
Username: Reviewer_E-MEXP-3440
Password: kdXjkn3s

## Plasmids and Transfections

A human *MYOC* full coding recombinant expression vector was generated by amplifying pMC2 with primers 5'CACCTGCAAT-GAGGTTCTTCTGTG3' (forward) and 5'TTTTCA-CATCTTGGAGAGCTTGAT3' using Platinum Taq DNA

Polymerase (Invitrogen) and cloning of the gel purified insert into pCDNA3.1D V5-His-TOPO (Invitrogen). The new plasmid, pKM1, contains 1522 bp (from -4ATG to TGA+3) of wild-type *MYOC* cDNA (19–1540 nt). A *MYOC*-V5 fused clone was generated by amplifying pKM1 with the same forward primer and a 5'TTTCATCTTGGAGAGCTTGATGTC3' (reverse) which skips the stop codon (19–1534 nt) using high fidelity Advantage HD Polymerase Mix (Clontech). The gel purified fragment was incubated with pCDNA3.1D V5-His-TOPO to yield plasmid pMG29. A pCDNA3.1D V5-His-TOPO empty (CMV promoter, no transgene) was obtained during the sequence screening of above cloning procedures (pEmpty). All plasmids were transformed in TOP10 cells (Invitrogen) and confirmed by sequence. A TrueORFGold clone of human *CSTA* (stefin A) was obtained from Origene (Rockville, MD, cat.# RC203115). The pCSTA plasmid contains the full coding *CSTA* cDNA (nt 130–424 accession # NM_005213) fused to Myc-DDK tags. A TrueORF-Gold clone of human mutant *CSTA* (*CSTAm*) was designed and custom ordered to Origene. The *CSTAm* was obtained by site-directed mutagenesis of the codon GGA at nucleotide 10–12 of the ORF, coding for Glycine, to AGG coding for Arginine [37]. Change of the evolutionary conserved Gly-4 residue has been shown to decrease affinity of the binding of the CSTA inhibitor to Cathepsin B [37]. Plasmid DNAs were isolated either using either a Midi-Prep plasmid kit (QIAGEN) or a PowerPrep™ HP Plasmid Purification kit (Origene), which results in lower toxicity after the nucleofector transfection (unpublished).

Transfection of HEK293 cells was performed by the standard calcium phosphate method precipitating 7 µg of DNA (pMG29:pCSTA or pEmpty 1:2.5) in 120 mM calcium phosphate (Clontech) per 3 cm dish, 40% confluent cells. After overnight exposure, cells were quickly washed with 1 mM EGTA/PBS, and incubated in IMEM 2% FBS for an additional 48 h. A change of medium was done 24 h before harvesting. Transfection of primary HTM cells was performed using nucleofector technology (Amaxa Lonza, Basel, Switzerland), their basic kit for Primary Mammalian Endothelial Cells and the protocol previously described [42]. Briefly, cells were split 24 h before transfection, trypsinized, counted, and centrifuged at 100 g for 10 min. Cell pellets were resuspended in the proprietary mammalian endothelial solution at a concentration of 4 X $10^5$ cells/100 µl. Plasmid DNA encoding the V5-fused MYOC protein (pMG29) was mixed with that of plasmids encoding either the DDK-fused *CSTA* (pCSTA) or an empty transgene (pEmpty) and added to the cells at a total of 3 µg (pMG29:pCSTA or pEmpty 1:2). Cells-DNA solution was electroporated on the nucleofector apparatus (Amaxa Lonza) using program T-23 and allowed to recover for 15 min in pre-warmed serum-containing media inside the $CO_2$ incubator. Following the recovery period, cells were gently transferred to warm medium-containing 3 cm dishes. After 24 h, media was changed with IMEM 10% serum followed by replacement with serum-free media 8 h later. Cells were then maintained for an additional 24 h (48 h post transfection) before being harvested for the extraction of proteins.

## Western-Blots and Antibodies

Proteins extracted from transfected HEK293 and HTM primary cells were assayed for levels of the different forms of the MYOC protein. Cultured media was collected and saved. Adhered cells were washed 2X with cold PBS and scraped from the dish with 100 µl of modified RIPA buffer containing 1X protease inhibitor cocktail (Roche Applied Science, Indianapolis, IN). Aliquots of 4 µl from either the cell lysates or the media were mixed (1:2 vol) with Laemmli buffer (Bio-Rad, Hercules, CA) containing 5% β-mercaptoethanol and loaded onto 4–15% SDS-PAGE Tris-HCl polyacrylamide gels (Bio-Rad). After running, gels were electro-transferred to PVDF membranes (Bio-Rad), blocked with 5% nonfat dry milk (Bio-Rad) in PBS-0.2% Tween 20 (Sigma-Aldrich, Saint Louis, MO) for 2–5 h and incubated at 4°C for 3 h to overnight with anti-V5 mouse monoclonal antibody (Invitrogen) (1:400). Primary antibody reaction was followed by incubation with anti-mouse IgG secondary antibodies conjugated to horseradish peroxidase (1:2000; Pierce Biotechnology, Rockford, IL) for 1 h at room temperature. Immunoreactive bands were visualized by chemiluminescence ECL Plus western blotting detection system (GE Healthcare Biosciences, Piscataway, NJ) and membranes were exposed to X-ray film (BioMax MR; Kodak, Rochester, NY). For controls, blots were re-probed with a monoclonal anti β-actin (synthetic peptide) (Sigma) (1:5000) and a monoclonal anti-DDK (synthetic peptide) (1:200) (Origene) for 1 h at room temperature and overnight at 4°C, followed by anti-mouse IgG secondary antibodies conjugated to horseradish peroxidase (1:5000; Pierce Biotechnology). Full length and processed MYOC bands were captured using a Chemi System equipped with a GelCam 310 camera, PCI digitizing image acquisition board, EpiChemi II Darkroom with transilluminator and VisonWorksLS image acquisition software v.7.0.1 (UVP, Upland, CA). Densitometry of each band was performed with the provided software to obtain mean intensity values (average of intensities of all pixels of band region, minus average intensity of the background pixels). Default background is equal to the sum total of the perimeter around each band region, three pixels wide. The percentage of the processed band in each treatment was calculated by dividing its mean density by the sum of the mean density of the process plus unprocessed bands.

## Results

### Adenoviral Vectors Carrying four MYOC Mutants Linked to Glaucoma

The adenoviral vectors were constructed as indicated in methods and the *MYOC* mutant proteins encoded by their inserted cassettes are shown in Figure 1. Prior to the generation of RNA to hybridize to the Affymetrix chips, the mutants vectors were tested on HTM cells for the overexpression of *MYOC* RNA and proteins using TaqMan PCR and WB as described above. Upon normalization to 18S, the levels of MYOC RNA on cells infected with each of the mutants over the levels of MYOC RNA on cells infected with Ad.Null increased significantly for all mutants. Infection with Adh.Q368X produced the truncated form of the protein while Adh.R342K, Adh.D380N and Adh.K423E produced the same size protein as the wild-type. Although the TaqMan mRNA levels produced by Adh.K423E mutant were similar to those of the other mutants, the levels of its produced protein were the lowest, indicating either a higher susceptibility to degradation of this MYOC mutant protein, or a lower recognition by the antibody due to faulty folding.

### Number of Genes Altered in HTM Cells Overexpressing each of the Four MYOC Mutants

To gain a first insight into the extent of changes occurring in the transcriptome of HTM cells overexpressing *MYOC* mutants we counted the number of genes altered between the mutants and controls cells (cells infected with Ad5.CMV-Null viruses). To further understand the differences caused by the mutants and the wild-type, we re-analyzed the comparisons using the chips of the *MYOC* mutants versus those of the *MYOC* wild-type. To override the potential differences between primary cell lines derived from different individuals, all overexpression experiments were conducted in the same cell line at the same passage (HTM-72, passage 4).

All comparisons were done using non-redundant lists of overexpressed genes. For this, the gene lists generated in Gene Spring were cleaned according to the following criteria. Affymetrix IDs that did not have an Entrez number were removed. In the few cases where one Affymetrix probe set ID number recognized more than one gene (usually almost identical genes or pseudogenes), one of them was selected. In the cases of redundant Entrez numbers, that is, when there were several Affymetrix IDs for the same Entrez number, we selected the ID that had been most altered.

Using replicas for each of the mutants and for the controls (Adh.MYOC n = 10, 2 per construct; Ad.CMV-Null n = 7) and selecting the methodology and filters outlined above, we generated lists of 1.5-fold altered genes. Out of the 54,678 spots in the array, the total number of non-redundant genes altered ≥1.5X was higher in the wild-type than in each of the mutants (Figure 2A). Overexpression of the wild-type induced the change of 4,337 genes while that of the Q368X mutation, which was the second highest, altered 2,603 genes. While the number of genes altered in the D380N (2,237) and K423E (2,283) mutations were pretty similar to those changed by the stop mutation, the mutation R342K induced only 803 changes in the HTM transcriptome (Figure 2A). From the total number of altered genes, the number of up- and downregulated seemed to be similar in wild-type and mutants with approximately one-half of the total altered in each category. The highest difference was observed in the R342K mutant, which had a higher number of downregulated genes (274 genes up- and 529 genes downregulated) (Figure 2A).

When comparing the number of genes altered in the mutants with those altered in the wild-type, we found that the stop mutation Q386X had the highest difference with a total of 6,716 (3,342 up and 3,374 down) (Figure 2B). Overall, looking at this parameter, it appeared that the mutants fell into two groups with considerably different patterns. The mutations Q368X and R342K had similar gene number changes and were much higher than those of D380N and K423E which in turn were similar to each other (1,411 and 1,384). Together this result on the absolute number of altered genes indicates that different *MYOC* mutants can alter the HTM transcriptome to a different extent and could therefore have a different severity outcome on the function of the tissue.

### Selected Top-changers Trabecular Meshwork Relevant (TMR) Genes from MYOC Mutants Induced Lists

The 100 top-changers (50 upregulated and 50 downregulated) (p≤0.05) from each of the mutants compared to Ad5.CMV-Null are submitted as supporting material (Tables S1, S2, S3, and S4). To generate these lists we started with the non-redundant lists obtained above and rationally eliminated those ID numbers with annotations for LOC hypothetical proteins, FAM (family w/ sequence similarity), noncoding RNAs and pseudogenes. Myocilin was the most upregulated gene in all lists except in that of the K423E mutant, serving as a control of the overexpression. Levels of overexpressed *MYOC* were identical after infections with Q368X and R342K, and about half after D380N, though still at the top of the list (Tables S1, S2, S3, S4, S5, and S6). TaqMan PCR confirmed that the K423E mutant was highly overexpressing *MYOC*, so its absence from the top gene in the array list was interpreted as a low efficiency of this mutant's cDNA to hybridize to the *MYOC* Affymetrix gene chip spot.

To further get an insight into the extent of how many of those *MYOC* mutant-induced genes were encoding trabecular meshwork

**A.**

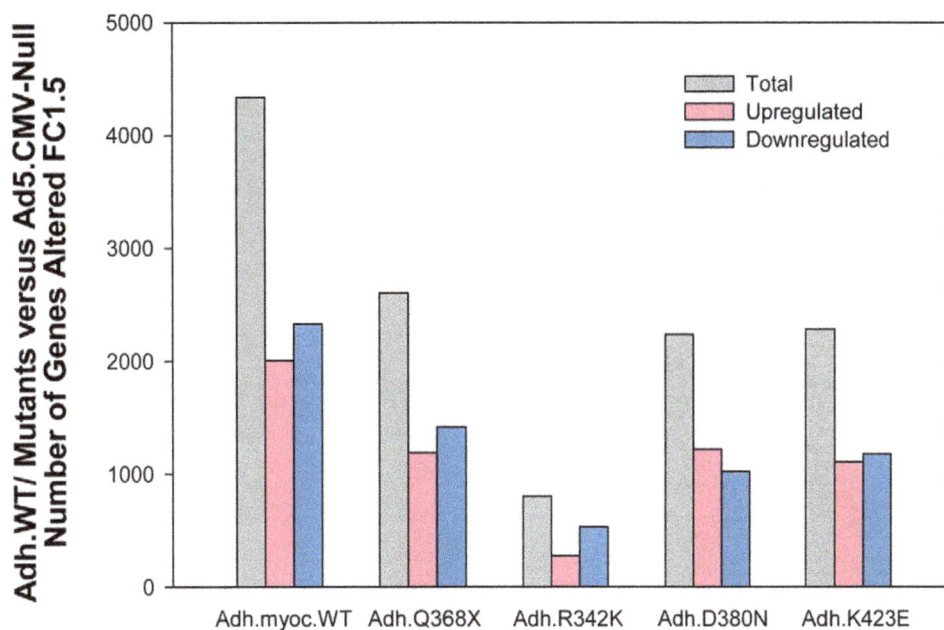

**B.**

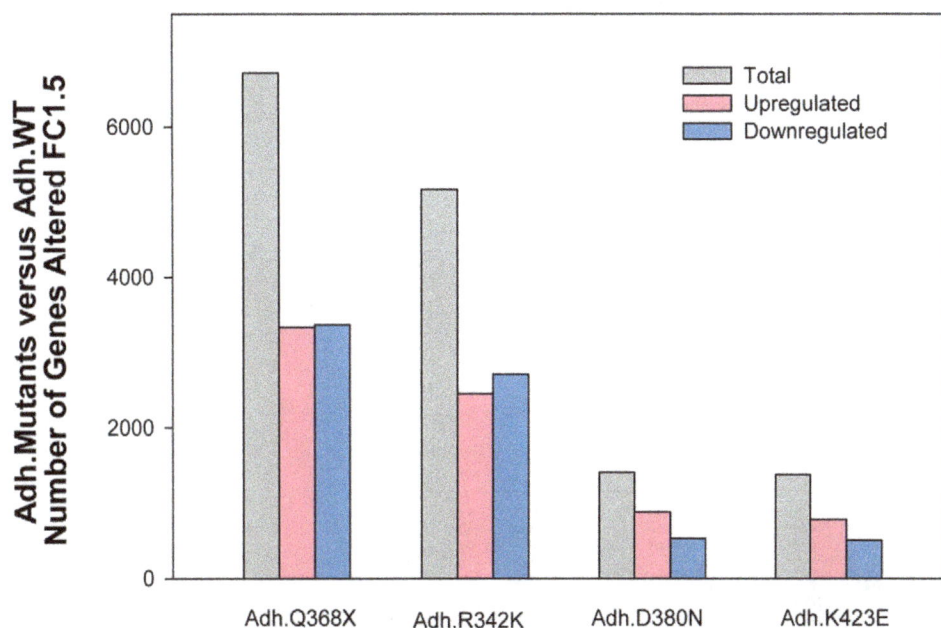

**Figure 2. Wild-type *MYOC* and different *MYOC* mutants alter different gene numbers on the trabecular meshwork transcriptome.** Adenoviral vectors carrying either wild type, four *MYOC* mutations cassettes or no transgene (Ad5.CMV-Null) were infected on primary human trabecular meshwork cell line HTM-72 to overexpress MYOC proteins. The expression of genes in the wild-type or mutant-treated cells was obtained using Affymetrix GeneChips (n = 17). GeneSpring 10 and Excel software were used to generate non-redundant gene lists with cutoff fold-change values of ≥ and ≤ 1.5. A: number of genes altered in cells treated with the wild-type or each of the mutants compared with the number altered in cells treated with the empty virus (Adh.WT/Mutants versus Ad5.CMV-Null). B: number of genes altered in cells treated with the each of the mutants compared with the number altered in cells treated with the wild type virus (Adh.Mutants versus Adh.WT).

**A. Rationally selected 20 TMR upregulated genes in the MYOC mutants**

### Adh.Q368X vs Ad.Null

| Gene Name | Symbol | FC | Entrez ID |
|---|---|---|---|
| Tachykinin 1 (Substance P) | TAC1 | 43.2 | 6863 |
| Lysosomal-associated membrane 3 | LAMP3 | 28.5 | 27074 |
| Spexin | C12orf39 | 12.0 | 80763 |
| Ras-related protein 39B | RAB39B | 10.2 | 116442 |
| Cadherin 15 ( M-cadherin) | CDH15 | 9.7 | 1013 |
| Heat shock 70KDa protein 5 | HSPA5 | 5.9 | 3309 |
| Protein disulfide isomerase A4 | PDIA4 | 4.6 | 9601 |
| Interleukin 1 receptor-like 1 | IL1RL1 | 4.1 | 9173 |
| Cystatin A (Stefin A) | CSTA | 3.4 | 1475 |
| Stanniocalcin 2 | STC2 | 2.4 | 8614 |
| Apoptosis regulator Bcl2 | BCL2 | 2.3 | 596 |
| Calreticulin | CALR | 2.3 | 811 |
| Talin 2 | TLN2 | 2.2 | 83660 |
| Nerve growth factor | NGF | 2.1 | 4803 |
| Extracellular matrix protein 2 | ECM2 | 2.1 | 1842 |
| Calnexin | CANX | 1.9 | 821 |
| Matrix metallopeptidase 1 | MMP1 | 1.9 | 4312 |
| Dentin sialoprotein | DSPP | 1.6 | 1834 |
| Fibrillin 2 | FBN2 | 1.6 | 2201 |
| Neuregulin 1 | NRG1 | 1.5 | 3084 |

### Adh.R342K vs Ad.Null

| Gene Name | Symbol | FC | Entrez ID |
|---|---|---|---|
| Tachykinin 1 (Substance P) | TAC1 | 13.4 | 6863 |
| Spexin | C12orf39 | 6.1 | 80763 |
| Lysosomal-associated membrane 3 | LAMP3 | 4.6 | 27074 |
| Heat shock 70KDa protein 5 | HSPA5 | 3.3 | 3309 |
| Ras-related protein 39B | RAB39B | 3.2 | 116442 |
| Cystatin A (stefin A) | CSTA | 3.2 | 1475 |
| Cadherin 15 ( M-cadherin) | CDH15 | 2.7 | 1013 |
| Osteoglycin | OGN | 2.2 | 4969 |
| Protein disulfide isomerase A4 | PDIA4 | 2.1 | 9601 |
| Extracellular matrix protein 2 | ECM2 | 2.1 | 1842 |
| Lysyl oxidase | LOX | 1.9 | 4015 |
| Apoptosis regulator Bcl2 | BCL2 | 1.8 | 596 |
| Osteomodulin | OMD | 1.8 | 4958 |
| Prostacyclin I2 synthase | PTGIS | 1.7 | 5740 |
| Nerve growth factor | NGF | 1.7 | 4803 |
| Intercellular adhesion molecule 1 | ICAM1 | 1.7 | 3383 |
| Interleukin 1 receptor-like 1 | IL1RL1 | 1.6 | 9173 |
| Calnexin | CANX | 1.6 | 821 |
| Caldesmon 1 | CALD1 | 1.6 | 800 |
| Stanniocalcin 2 | STC2 | 1.5 | 8614 |

### Adh.D380N vs Ad.Null

| Gene Name | Symbol | FC | Entrez ID |
|---|---|---|---|
| Aldo-keto reductase 1 | AKR1C1 | 3.8 | 1645 |
| Angiopoietin-like 2 | ANGPTL2 | 3.7 | 23452 |
| Aldehyde dehydrogenase 5 A1 | ALDH5A1 | 3.5 | 7915 |
| Chemokine (C-X-C motif) ligand 12 | CXCL12 | 3.3 | 6387 |
| Growth arrest-specific 1 | GAS1 | 2.5 | 2619 |
| Synuclein alpha | SNCA | 2.5 | 6622 |
| Eukaryotic elongation factor 1 A1 | EEF1A1 | 2.3 | 1915 |
| Podoplanin | PDPN | 2.3 | 10630 |
| Cathepsin O | CTSO | 2.2 | 1519 |
| Prostacyclin I2 synthase | PTGIS | 2.1 | 5740 |
| Ras-related protein 39B | RAB39B | 2.1 | 116442 |
| Extracellular matrix protein 2 | ECM2 | 1.9 | 1842 |
| Lysosomal-associated membrane 2 | LAMP2 | 1.9 | 3920 |
| Fibronectin 1 | FN1 | 1.8 | 2335 |
| Osteoglycin | OGN | 1.7 | 4969 |
| Pigment epithelium-derived factor | PEDF | 1.7 | 5176 |
| Angiopoietin-like 7 | ANGPTL7 | 1.7 | 10218 |
| Cathepsin F | CTSF | 1.7 | 8722 |
| Insulin-like growth factor 1 | IGF1 | 1.5 | 3479 |
| Cystatin A (stefin A) | CSTA | 1.5 | 1475 |

### Adh.K423E vs Ad.Null

| Gene Name | Symbol | FC | Entrez ID |
|---|---|---|---|
| Insulin-like growth factor 1 | IGF1 | 3.9 | 3479 |
| Podoplanin | PDPN | 3.8 | 10630 |
| Selenoprotein P1 | SEPP1 | 3.0 | 6414 |
| Angiopoietin-like 2 | ANGPTL2 | 2.9 | 23452 |
| Chemokine (C-X-C motif) ligand 12 | CXCL12 | 2.5 | 6387 |
| Fibronectin 1 | FN1 | 2.4 | 2335 |
| Ras-related protein 39B | RAB39B | 2.3 | 116442 |
| Matrix Gla protein | MGP | 2.1 | 4256 |
| Synuclein alpha | SNCA | 2.1 | 6622 |
| Prostaglandin F receptor | PTGFR | 2.0 | 5737 |
| Caldesmon 1 | CALD1 | 2.0 | 800 |
| Aldo-keto reductase 1 | AKR1C1 | 2.0 | 1645 |
| Cystatin A (stefin A) | CSTA | 1.8 | 1475 |
| Cathepsin O | CTSO | 1.7 | 1519 |
| Bone morphogenetic protein 2 | BMP2 | 1.7 | 650 |
| Stanniocalcin 2 | STC2 | 1.7 | 8614 |
| Fibrillin 1 | FBN1 | 1.7 | 2200 |
| Extracellular matrix protein 2 | ECM2 | 1.6 | 1842 |
| Lysosomal-associated membrane 3 | LAMP3 | 1.6 | 27074 |
| Eukaryotic elongation factor 1 A1 | EEF1A1 | 1.5 | 1915 |

**B.**

**Rationally selected 20 TMR downregulated genes in the MYOC mutants**

### Adh.Q368X vs Ad.Null

| Gene Name | Symbol | FC | Entrez ID |
|---|---|---|---|
| Stanniocalcin 1 | STC1 | -5.4 | 6781 |
| Sphingosine-1-phosphate receptor 3 | S1PR3 | -4.1 | 1903 |
| Insulin-like growth factor binding protein 5 | IGFBP5 | -3.6 | 3488 |
| Chemokine (C-X-C motif) ligand 12 | CXCL12 | -3.0 | 6387 |
| Microtubule-assoc protein 2 | MAP2 | -2.8 | 4133 |
| Parathyroid hormone-like hormone | PTHLH | -2.8 | 5744 |
| Secreted frizzled-related protein 1 | SFRP1 | -2.5 | 6422 |
| Cytochrome P450, 26B | CYP26B1 | -2.5 | 56603 |
| Thrombospondin 2 | THBS2 | -2.5 | 7058 |
| Thrombomodulin | THBD | -2.2 | 7056 |
| Podoplanin | PDPN | -2.1 | 10630 |
| Insulin-like growth factor 1 | IGF1 | -2.1 | 3479 |
| Synuclein alpha | SNCA | -2.1 | 6622 |
| Lysyl oxidase-like 1 | LOXL1 | -2.0 | 4016 |
| Matrix Gla protein | MGP | -2.0 | 4256 |
| Osteoglycin | OGN | -1.9 | 4969 |
| Endothelin 1 | EDN1 | -1.9 | 1906 |
| Interleukin 8 | IL8 | -1.8 | 3576 |
| Angiopoietin 2 | ANGPT2 | -1.8 | 285 |
| Biglycan | BGN | -1.8 | 633 |

### Adh.R342K vs Ad.Null

| Gene Name | Symbol | FC | Entrez ID |
|---|---|---|---|
| Matrix metallopeptidase 1 | MMP1 | -4.5 | 4312 |
| Microtubule-assoc protein 2 | MAP2 | -2.8 | 4133 |
| Parathyroid hormone-like hormone | PTHLH | -2.4 | 5744 |
| Sphingosine-1-phosphate receptor 3 | S1PR3 | -2.4 | 1903 |
| Matrix metallopeptidase 12 | MMP12 | -2.1 | 4321 |
| Secreted frizzled-related protein 1 | SFRP1 | -1.9 | 6422 |
| Chemokine (C-X-C motif) ligand 12 | CXCL12 | -1.9 | 6387 |
| Cytochrome P450, 26B | CYP26B1 | -1.8 | 56603 |
| Stanniocalcin 1 | STC1 | -1.8 | 6781 |
| Thrombomodulin | THBD | -1.8 | 7056 |
| Periostin, osteoblast specific factor | POSTN | -1.7 | 10631 |
| Angiopoietin 2 | ANGPT2 | -1.7 | 285 |
| Dickkopf homolog 1 | DKK1 | -1.7 | 22943 |
| Procollagen C-endopeptidase enhancer 2 | PCOLCE2 | -1.7 | 26577 |
| Insulin-like growth factor 1 | IGF1 | -1.6 | 3479 |
| Follistatin | FST | -1.6 | 10468 |
| Endothelin 1 | EDN1 | -1.6 | 1906 |
| Carbonic anhydrase II | CA2 | -1.5 | 760 |
| Tenascin C | TNC | -1.5 | 3371 |
| Statherin | STATH | -1.5 | 6779 |

### Adh.D380N vs Ad.Null

| Gene Name | Symbol | FC | Entrez ID |
|---|---|---|---|
| Matrix metallopeptidase 1 | MMP1 | -5.5 | 4312 |
| Matrix metallopeptidase 12 | MMP12 | -5.3 | 4321 |
| Tenascin C | TNC | -3.9 | 3371 |
| Versican | VCAN | -3.7 | 1462 |
| Parathyroid hormone-like hormone | PTHLH | -3.3 | 5744 |
| Dickkopf homolog 1 | DKK1 | -3.2 | 22943 |
| Claudin 1 | CLDN1 | -3.1 | 9076 |
| Matrix metallopeptidase 3 | MMP3 | -3.0 | 4314 |
| Stanniocalcin 1 | STC1 | -2.5 | 6781 |
| Endothelin 1 | EDN1 | -2.5 | 1906 |
| Interleukin 8 | IL8 | -2.3 | 3576 |
| Angiopoietin 2 | ANGPT2 | -2.0 | 285 |
| Thrombomodulin | THBD | -2.0 | 7056 |
| Periostin, osteoblast specific factor | POSTN | -1.9 | 10631 |
| Carbonic anhydrase II | CA2 | -1.9 | 760 |
| Microtubule-assoc protein 2 | MAP2 | -1.8 | 4133 |
| Interleukin 6 | IL6 | -1.8 | 3569 |
| Neuregulin 1 | NRG1 | -1.6 | 3084 |
| Osteomodulin | OMD | -1.6 | 4958 |
| Secretogranin II | SCG2 | -1.6 | 7857 |

### Adh.K423E vs Ad.Null

| Gene Name | Symbol | FC | Entrez ID |
|---|---|---|---|
| Matrix metallopeptidase 12 | MMP12 | -4.0 | 4321 |
| Lysyl oxidase-like 2 | LOXL2 | -3.0 | 4017 |
| Matrix metallopeptidase 3 | MMP3 | -2.8 | 4314 |
| Lysyl oxidase | LOX | -2.8 | 4015 |
| Cytochrome P450, 1B1 | CYP1B1 | -2.7 | 1545 |
| Calmodulin 1 | CALM1 | -2.7 | 801 |
| Heat shock protein 90 | HSP90AB | -2.5 | 3326 |
| Claudin 1 | CLDN1 | -2.4 | 9076 |
| Interleukin 8 | IL8 | -2.2 | 3576 |
| Zyxin | ZYX | -2.0 | 7791 |
| Presenilin 1 | PSEN1 | -2.0 | 5663 |
| Biglycan | BGN | -1.9 | 633 |
| Endothelin 1 | EDN1 | -1.8 | 1906 |
| Calreticulin | CALR | -1.8 | 811 |
| Calnexin | CANX | -1.8 | 821 |
| Stanniocalcin 1 | STC1 | -1.7 | 6781 |
| Insulin-like growth factor binding protein 5 | IGFBP5 | -1.7 | 3488 |
| Neuregulin 1 | NRG1 | -1.6 | 3084 |
| Angiopoietin 2 | ANGPT2 | -1.5 | 285 |
| Secreted frizzled-related protein 1 | SFRP1 | -1.5 | 6422 |

**Figure 3. *MYOC* mutants' top-changers contained numerous human trabecular meshwork relevant genes.** Adenoviral vectors carrying four *MYOC* mutations cassettes and no transgene (Ad5.CMV-Null) were infected on primary human trabecular meshwork cell line HTM-72 to overexpress MYOC mutant proteins. The expression of genes in the mutant-treated cells was compared with that of the cells treated with the empty virus, using Affymetrix GeneChips (n = 15). Non-redundant gene lists from the cutoff FC value of ≥ and ≤ 1.5 of each mutant were screened for trabecular meshwork relevant (TMR) genes. Each selected TMR gene was manually cross-checked to identify its expression in the other three mutants. A: twenty selected upregulated TMR genes in Q368X, R342K, D380N and K423E. B: twenty selected downregulated genes in Q368X, R342K, D380N and K423E.

functions, and to investigate whether there was sharing of genes among the four mutants, we screened each of the FC 1.5 lists for TMR. For this analysis, we separated the up- and downregulated genes of each mutant list, sort them by FC and, without taking into account the microarray p-values, scrolled down to rationally select 20 genes from each direction with TM and/or glaucoma-related functions (TMR) (total 160 genes). Then, we performed a manual cross-check and identified whether each of the selected genes in each mutant was present in the other three (Figure 3A and 3B).

Overall, we had a total of 75 unique TMR genes altered in any of four *MYOC* mutants, many of which had previously been reported as responders to glaucomatous insults in independent studies. Eight genes were altered in all the mutants. *Ras-related protein 39B (RAB39B), Cystatin A (CSTA)* and *Extracellular matrix protein 2 (ECM2)* were upregulated, while *Endothelin 1 (EDN1), Angiopoietin 2 (ANGPT2)* and *Stanniocalcin 1 (STC1)* were downregulated. *Chemokine (C-X-C) ligand 12 (CXCL12) and Insulin-like growth factor 1 (IGF1, Somatomedin C)* showed different regulation depending on the mutants.

The upregulated TMR genes induced by the Q368X mutant appeared to be more similar to those induced by R342K and different from those induced by D380N and K423E. Thus, including the all-common genes, 14 out of the 20 TMRs (70%) in Q368X were shared by R342K while only 6 and 7 in each of these were shared by either D380N and/or K432E respectively. Interestingly, upregulated D380N and K423E lists shared a higher similarity between themselves (12 out of 20, 60%).

The dowregulated TMR genes induced by the Q368X, were however very similar in the four mutants. Thirteen out of 20 downregulated TMR in Q368X were altered in R342K and all genes but one, *Lysyl oxidase-like 1 (LOXL1)*, were altered in D380N and K423E. *LOXL1*, a gene recently linked to pseudoexfoliation glaucoma [43] was altered only by the Q368X mutation.

Among the altered genes shared by Q368X and R342K (mutant set #1) and not by D380N and K423E (mutant set #2), were *Tachykinin 1 (TAC1), Protein disulfide isomerase A4 (PDIA4), Cadherin 15 (CDH15), Apoptosis regulator BCL2 (BCL2)* and *CYP26B1*. The *TAC1* gene, encoding the precursor of neuropeptide substance P, was previously identified as a mechanosensitive gene in the human trabecular meshwork intact tissue [22,44]. Protein disulfide isomerase A4, which plays a key role in protein folding, had been found to be altered by TGFβ2, DEX and by elevated IOP in the trabecular meshwork tissue during the homeostatic response period [44–46].

Among the genes altered by set #2 and not by set #1 mutants we found Aldo-ketoreductase 1 (AKR1C1), Angiopoietin-like 2 (ANGPTL2), Fibronectin 1(FN1), Matrix metallopeptidase 3 (MMP3) and α-Synuclein (SNCA), which affect various functions, such steroid metabolism, inflammatory signaling and ECM organization. The synucleins are proteins highly expressed in the brain and are involved in presynaptic signaling and membrane trafficking.

Two of the all-common genes (*IGF1* and *CXCL12*) support the notion that mutant's set #1 had similar effects on the trabecular

meshwork transcriptome, which were different from those of set #2. Expression of *IGF1* and *CXCL12* was down in set #1 and up in set #2. Insulin growth factor 1 was classified as an individual responder to elevated IOP in human perfused organ cultures and pressure [22] while *CXCL12* is a member of the same chemokine family as CXCL2, a general responder to elevated IOP. Another case where *MYOC* mutants had opposite effects on a given gene was that of *Podoplanin (PDPN)*, a lymphatic marker regulated by elevated IOP. Podoplanin is upregulated by D380N and K423E while is downregulated by Q368X.

There were only a few TMR genes that were altered by just one mutant. These were: *Lysyl oxidase-like 1 (LOXL1)* (downregulated by Q368X), *Procollagen C-endopeptidase enhancer 2 (PCOLCE2)* (downregulated by R342K), *Pigment epithelium-derived factor (PEDF)* (downreguled by D380N), *Lysyl oxidase-like 2 (LOXL2)* and *Cytochrome P450 1B1 (CYP1B1)* (downregulated by K423E), *and Bone morphogenetic protein 2 (BMP2)* and *Fibrillin 1 (FBN1)* (upregulated by K423E). Curiously, three of these genes have been genetically linked to glaucoma [43,47,48], suggesting an additional physiological link of the mutants with glaucoma at the molecular level.

Another trabecular meshwork gene previously known to be altered under other insults (IOP and DEX) was *Thrombomodulin (THBD)* [45]. Thrombomodulin is a vascular endothelial cell receptor that binds to thrombin and is involved in the inhibition of blood clotting. It has been speculated that *THBD* plays a role in maintaining the fluidity of the aqueous humor [45]. In this study, *THBD* was downregulated in all but the K423 mutant, suggesting a potential detrimental effect caused by the *MYOC* mutants. The same occurred with insult-altered metallopeptidases *Matrix metallopeptidase 3 (MMP3) (Stromelysin* 1) [49] and *Matrix metallopeptidase 12 (MMP12) (Macrophage elastase)* [22] which were shown downregulated here by the *MYOC* mutants suggesting that they would contribute to a decrease outflow.

Although many of the rationally selected TMR genes had significant microarray FC values, some of them had not. Thus, a representative sample of ten genes with no significant microarray p-values in at least one mutant were analyzed in triplicate by the more rigorous TaqMan PCR assay in a different primary cell line. HTM-137 and HTM-134 lines were infected with Adh.Q368X, Adh.R342K, Adh.D380N, Adh.K423E plus the control Ad.Null viruses, their RNA extracted at 48 h post-infection and reversed transcribed. Results are included in Table S5. Although not in every case the absolute TaqMan FC alteration value was similar to that of the microarray data (different individual, different culture and different viral stock), only four of the forty TaqMan assays performed showed a p-value higher than 0.05. Of the four (MMP1 and SFRP1 in Adh.Q368X and MMP12 and SFRP1 in Adh.K423E), two of them had a p<0.05 in the microarrays (Table S5). The remaining of the genes exhibited highly significant p-values in all mutants (Table S5).

Altogether these results indicate that overexpression of *MYOC* mutants share many elicited changes with other known glaucomatous insults. Further, they indicate that distinct *MYOC* mutants could have specific effects on the trabecular meshwork cells transcriptome.

## Pattern of Expression of Trabecular Meshwork Relevant Functions (TMR.F) Gene Lists in the Four MYOC Mutants

Next we investigated the overall expression pattern of set of genes known to be associated with selected TMR.F. In other words, we wanted to know whether genes involved in calcification mechanisms [50], collagen-elastin cross-linking functions [51], the WNT signaling pathway [22,25,26] and stress response had been affected by overexpression of *MYOC* mutants. We custom made comprehensive gene lists of the four mechanisms each containing 20–21 genes, and ran heat maps against the complete FC lists of each of the *MYOC* mutants (Figure 4). Each row of the map represents the response of a single gene to the overexpression of each of the four *MYOC* mutants, expressed in FC of the *MYOC* mutant- versus Ad5.CMV-Null infected cells. Each column represents the set of genes selected per category. The range of the FCs of the genes in the calcification, collagen-elastin and WNT maps by all mutants was between +2.1- and −3.3-fold. The range of FC of the stress and UPR genes was much larger, between +8.5 and −2.0-fold. Altered *MYOC* mutant genes which did not pass the minimal expression criteria (absent signals) have no color and appear as gray-cells. Overall, most of the genes of in each of the four functional categories were up or down regulated by at least one of the *MYOC* mutants and only a few were not affected in any mutant (represented by yellow colors). The trend of the similarities of the mutants in set #1 distinct from those in set #2 can be also seen here, mostly on genes with highest or lowest changes.

**Calcification genes.** The mutation Q368X downregulated most of the genes in the calcification category, including *Matrix Gla* (*MGP*), an inhibitor of calcification and one of the ten most abundant genes in the trabecular meshwork [52,53]. Concurrently, Q368X upregulated *BMP2*, an inducer of calcification and bone formation which loses its activity upon binding to the inhibitor *MGP* [54]. These two changes together would suggest that the Q368X mutant is prone to induce calcification in the HTM cells which in turn would provoke hardening of the tissue and reduce outflow facility. In contrast, the same *MGP* gene was upregulated in the set #2 mutants, where *BMP2* was moderately reduced, indicating a different degree of involvement of this pathway by different *MYOC* mutants. The *Connective Tissue Growth Factor* (*CTGF*) gene, which has been extensively studied for its relevance in ECM deposition in trabecular meshwork function [55] was the less altered in all mutants, and *Collagen type 1 alpha 1* (*COL1A1*), an important structural component of the trabecular meshwork ECM, was downregulated in the four mutants assayed. Genes like *Osteomodulin* (*OMD*) and *Osteoglycin* (*OGN*, also known as *Mimecan*), members of the SLPRs family of proteoglycans were markedly upregulated only by mutant R342K and appeared downregulated by Q368X. These two genes are markers of osteoblast differentiation [56], and respond to mechanical stress [44,46]; *OGN* was found upregulated in tissues from POAG patients [57]. Another gene, *Periostin* (*POSTN*, also known as *Osteoblast- specific factor2*), secreted by osteoblasts, was highly upregulated only in K423E. Periostin was previously shown to be upregulated by the glaucomatous insults of mechanical strain and TGFβ2 [58,59]. Lastly, *Transglutaminase2* (*TGM2*), which catalyzes the cross-linking of numerous ECM proteins, whose presence in vascular smooth muscle cells (VSMC) is key to mineralize their matrix and which is present in the aqueous humor of glaucomatous patients [60] was very much downregulated in Q368X (Figure 4 upper left panel).

**Collagen-Elastin Crosslinking.** The most upregulated genes in this TMR.F category were *Fibrillin 2* (*FBN2*) and to a lesser extent *Lysyl oxidase* (*LOX*). They were induced with different intensities in mutant's set #1 Q368X and R342K. Lysyl oxidase is an enzyme involved in post-translational modifications of collagen and elastin and in the formation of intra/intermolecular cross-links, and *FBN2* is involved elastic fiber assembly. Lysyl oxidase-like 1, which is linked to Pseudoexfoliation (PEX) glaucoma, and which is heavily bound to the PEX material of PEX patients was very downregulated in Q368X, while other two PEX relevant components [51], *FBN1 and Fibulin 5* (*FBLN5*), were slightly altered in all four mutants. The mutation D380N most dowregulated *Versican* (*VCAN*), another PEX component and mechanical strain regulated gene [44], and two metalloproteinases/inhibitors, *ADAM metallopeptidase 20* (*ADAM20*) and *Tissue inhibitor of metalloproteinases 3* (*TIMP3*), which are involved in maintaining the balance of the ECM and therefore affecting the elastin network. Overall it seemed that the effect of the four *MYOC* mutants had subtle effects on genes involved in the formation of the elastin network and that such light effect was mostly that of downregulation (Figure 4 right panel).

**WNT signaling.** Genes involved in this pathway were downregulated preferentially by mutant's set #1. Mutant Q368X most downregulated *Secreted frizzled-related protein 1* (*SFPR-1*), an IOP responder gene [22] which is present in glaucomatous trabecular meshwork cells and causes elevated pressure [26]. The most differently regulated gene between set #1 and set #2 was *Transcription factor 4* (*TCF4*), which interacts with β-catenin and mediates transcription of WNT targeted genes. The upregulation of *TCF4* in D380N and K423E could be an indication that these two *MYOC* mutants would utilize more the WNT pathway to induce transcription than the other two. In contrast, *Dickkopf-1* (*DKK-1*), an antagonist that prevents activation the WNT pathway, was downregulated by all mutants, especially by D380N. Two of the genes of this pathway, the intronless transmembrane receptor *Frizzled family receptor 10* (*FZD10*), and the WNT protein inhibitor *WNT inhibitory factor 1* (*WIF1*), were not expressed in these set of trabecular meshwork cells (Figure 4, lower left panel).

**Stress and Unfolded Protein Response (UPR).** Because *MYOC* mutants are known to accumulate in the ER and thus affect the UPR [11,18,19,23], we next examined the expression of twenty genes encoding the most common stress proteins (Figure 4, lower right panel). We found that expression of genes in the stress category was considerably affected by the *MYOC* mutants. Furthermore, expression of these genes was clearly different in set #1 and #2 mutants. The mutant having a major effect on this TMR.F was the stop mutation Q368X. In this mutant, the expression of all but two of the selected most commonly associated proteins were markedly altered. Among them the canonical UPR proteins *Bone-inducing protein* (*BIP*), *DAN-damage-inducible transcript 3* (*CHOP*) and *Calreticulin* (*CALR*) were markedly upregulated, as well as chaperones *Der1-like protein 3* (*DERL3*) and heat shock proteins *HSP90B1, DNAJB9 and DJC6*. Interestingly, *CALR*, an ER Ca$^+$ binding protein that binds to the glucocorticoid receptor, together with *Stress-induced-phosphoprotein 1* (*STIP1*) was one of the most down regulated protein in the set #2 mutants. Another protein in which the direction of expression was clearly reversed in both sets was *SNCA*, an important component of the amyloid plaques in Alzheimer patients. *SNCA* was the most UPR upregulated transcript in D380N and K423E and the most downregulated in Q368X and R342K. Except for the *NADH dehydrogenase (ubiquinone) 1 alpha subcomplex, assembly factor 1* (*NDUFAF1*), the UPR proteins altered in transgenic flies carrying these mutants [19] are also

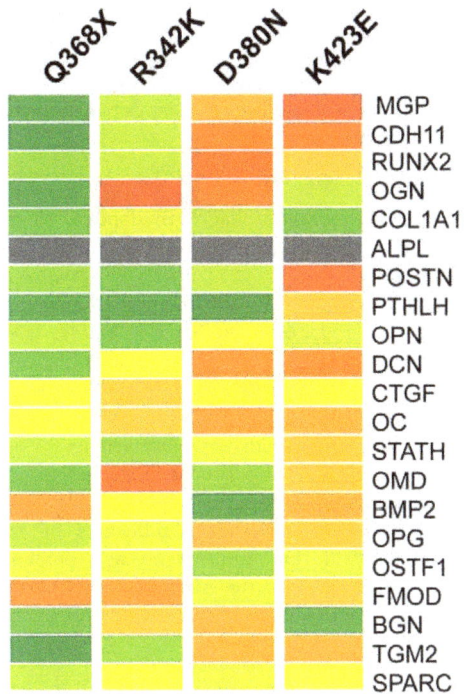

**Calcification genes**

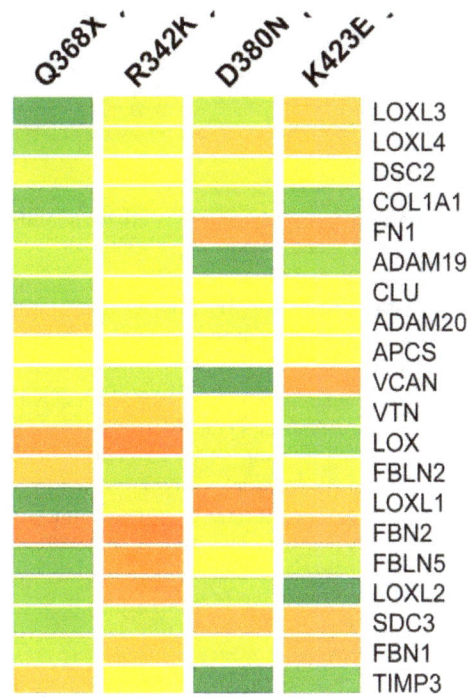

**Collagen-Elastin crosslinking genes**

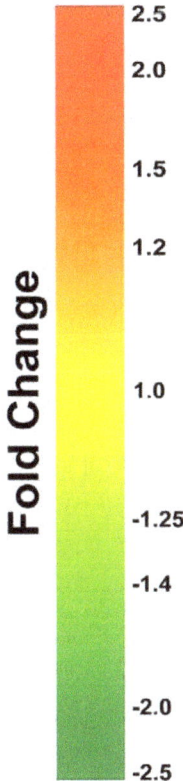

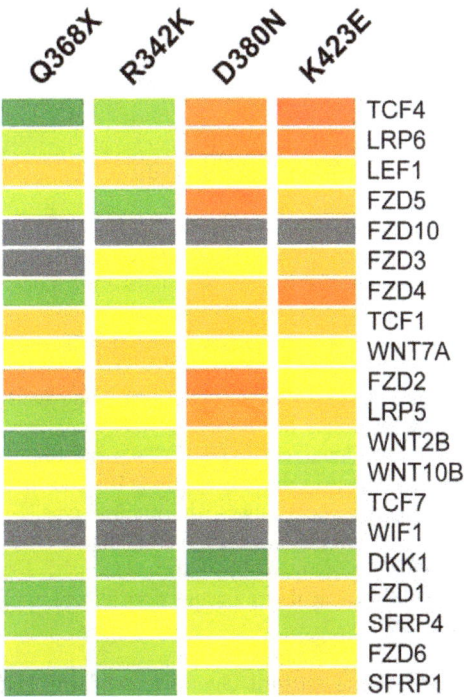

**WNT signaling pathway genes**

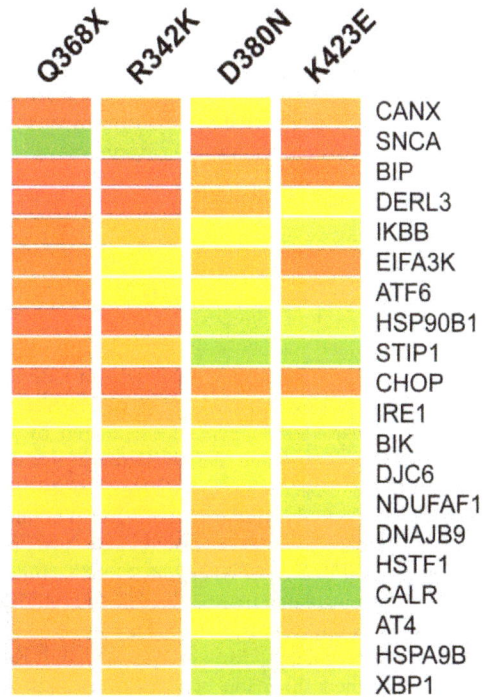

**Stress and Unfolded Protein Response genes**

**Figure 4. _MYOC_ mutants induced changes on genes of trabecular meshwork relevant functions, especially on the UPR.** Heat maps of set of genes representing four relevant trabecular meshwork functions. The four categories gene lists were costumed generated by literature review. Each row represents the fold change (Adeno.MYOC mutant over Adeno.Null) for a single gene in each of the four mutants. Each column represents the fold changes for all genes of the category in one _MYOC_ mutant. The fold change for each gene is visually represented by a color, which is given by the scale bar in the center of the figure. Heat maps were generated with genes lists containing the full range of fold changes. Gray cells indicate that the expression of the giving gene was below the signal intensity cutoff value and was considered absent.

altered in the human trabecular meshwork tissue, validating the fly system as a good genetic model of glaucoma.

## Pattern of Expression of the Physiological Trabecular Meshwork Biomarkers Gene List in the Overexpressed Four _MYOC_ Mutants

We next were interested to determine the ability of the _MYOC_ mutants to alter a set of genes potentially associated with glaucoma and or glaucomatous insult. The 50 gene list is based on a previously published potential molecular signature of glaucoma genes [45]. It is also based on a more recent list of physiological biomarkers of glaucoma built on a revision of trabecular meshwork gene expression studies from us and other investigators (Table S6). The results of the heat map showing the expression of the 50 genes in all the mutants are shown in Figure 5. All genes except _Endothelial adhesion molecule 1_ (_ELAM1_) were present in all the mutants, indicating that _ELAM1_ did not pass the filter set up for analysis of expression in the HTM-72 cell line. Because expression of this gene has been detected in whole trabecular meshwork tissues [22], its absence here indicates a marked downregulation of the gene when the cells are set up in culture.

Although some of the genes were expressed in set #1 differently than in set #2, the overall patterns of the different sets was not as marked as seen in the other gene lists categories. It is interesting to observe that 78% of the genes from this independent gene list were shown to be altered more ≥1.5X in at least one of the four _MYOC_ mutants (Tables S1, S2, S3, S4, and Figure 3A and Figure 3B), an indication of the physiological causative role of _MYOC_ in glaucoma. Very few genes were altered in the same direction in all four mutants. Two of the three downregulated genes, _EDN1_ and _MMP12_, had been mentioned above. The third one, _Parathyroid hormone-like hormone_ (_PTHLH_), is a protein that regulates vascular calcification [61] and that has previously been shown to be induced by DEX in the trabecular meshwork [62]. Only the gene encoding _Prostaglandin D2 synthase_ (_PTGDS_), an enzyme that catalyzes the conversion of PGH2 to PGD2, was lightly upregulated in the four mutants.

Overall, a similar number of genes were up- and downregulated in mutants Q368X, D380N and K423E while R342K showed a lower number of downregulated genes. However, alteration of specific genes varied. The genes most altered by Q368X were _TAC1_, _CDH15_, _PDIA4_ and _HSP90B1_ (upregulated 43X, 9.7X, 4.6X and 3.3X respectively), and _PTHLH_, _SFRP1_ and _Thrombospondin2_ (_THBS2_) (all downregulated −2.5X). The mutant R342K shared the four most upregulated and two of the most downregulated (_PTHLH_, _SFRP1_) with Q368X. Interestingly, the gene most downregulated by R342K, _MMP1_ (−4.5X), was shared with the D380N and K423E mutants but not with Q368X, where _MMP1_ was upregulated. Mutants D380N and K423E shared _PDPN_ among their three top upregulated and the metallopeptidases _MMP3_ and _MMP12_ among the top downregulated. Another interesting difference among the effect of the four mutants on the transcriptome was the total lack of expression of _TAC1_ (precursor of the substance P neuropeptide) in D380N and K423E, while it was the most induced gene in Q368X and R342K. Mutant Q368X was the only one to exhibit genes with unique responses,

that is, with changes in expression that were opposite to the changes incurred by the other three (_MMP1_, _MMP3_ and _Prostacyclin synthase, PTGIS_).

Of the four genes induced by the highest number of glaucomatous insults, _Angiopoietin-like 7_ (_ANGPTL7_), _PDIA4_, _Superoxide dismutase 1_ (_SOD1_) and _Tropomysin 4_ (_TPM4_) (Table S6), only _PDIA4_ (upregulated in Q368X and R342K), and _TPM4_ (downregulated in K423E) were markedly altered in some of the mutants. _PDIA4_ is an ER protein with isomerase activity on S-S bonds, and _TPM4_ is actin binding protein involved in the contractile system of the cell.

Altogether, these different and common influences on the transcriptome triggered by the four mutants reveal a potential molecular reason as to why each of the _MYOC_ mutants have a distinct clinical outcome and affect a particular group of the population.

## Genes Altered in All Mutants

In addition to finding genes by which each of the mutants may exert their damage, we were interested in searching for a common altered gene whose mechanism of action could potentially be applied to all _MYOC_-causing glaucomas. For this we compared the 1.5X altered genes from wild-type (Adh.MYOCWT) and Adh.Mutants using the Venn map feature of the GS10 program. Because this feature uses the Affymetrix ID numbers for the comparisons, for this analysis we used 1.5-fold redundant gene lists (all spots for a given Entrez number included). Fold change ≥1.5 lists of each of the wild-type and mutants versus the null virus were created as indicated in methods, exported to the hard drive, and cleaned of IDs that did not have an Entrez number.

To first get an insight on the extent of sharing changes between the wild-type and the mutants, re-imported all Entrez lists were Venn mapped comparing each of the mutants to the wild-type (Figure 6A). This comparison showed that the number of altered genes in each mutant that did not overlap with those altered in the wild-type varied. The stop mutation Q368X contained the highest number of non-overlapping genes, both in absolute numbers and in percentage (2,247; 64%) (Figure 6A). The mutation R342K, whose absolute number of altered genes is the lowest of the mutants studied (Figure 2), contained 542 non overlapping genes, which amounts to a still high percentage of the total (56%) (Figure 6A). The other two mutants (set #2), D380N and K423E had a lower number of non-overlapping genes (24% and 22% respectively), sharing more of the changes with the wild-type.

To study the number of genes which were simultaneously altered in all mutants, we Venn mapped their FC ≥1.5 lists (Figure 6B). We found that a total of 73 genes were altered in all four mutants (Figure 6B).

## Enriched Functions of the Mutant Overlapping Gene List

To investigate functions potentially involved in a common causative action of the four mutants studied, we searched for the GO enriched functions in the 73 mutant overlapping gene list. We analyzed the three GO SLIMS major functional categories of Biological Processes, Cellular Components and Molecular Functions, and sorted them by percent of genes in each of their

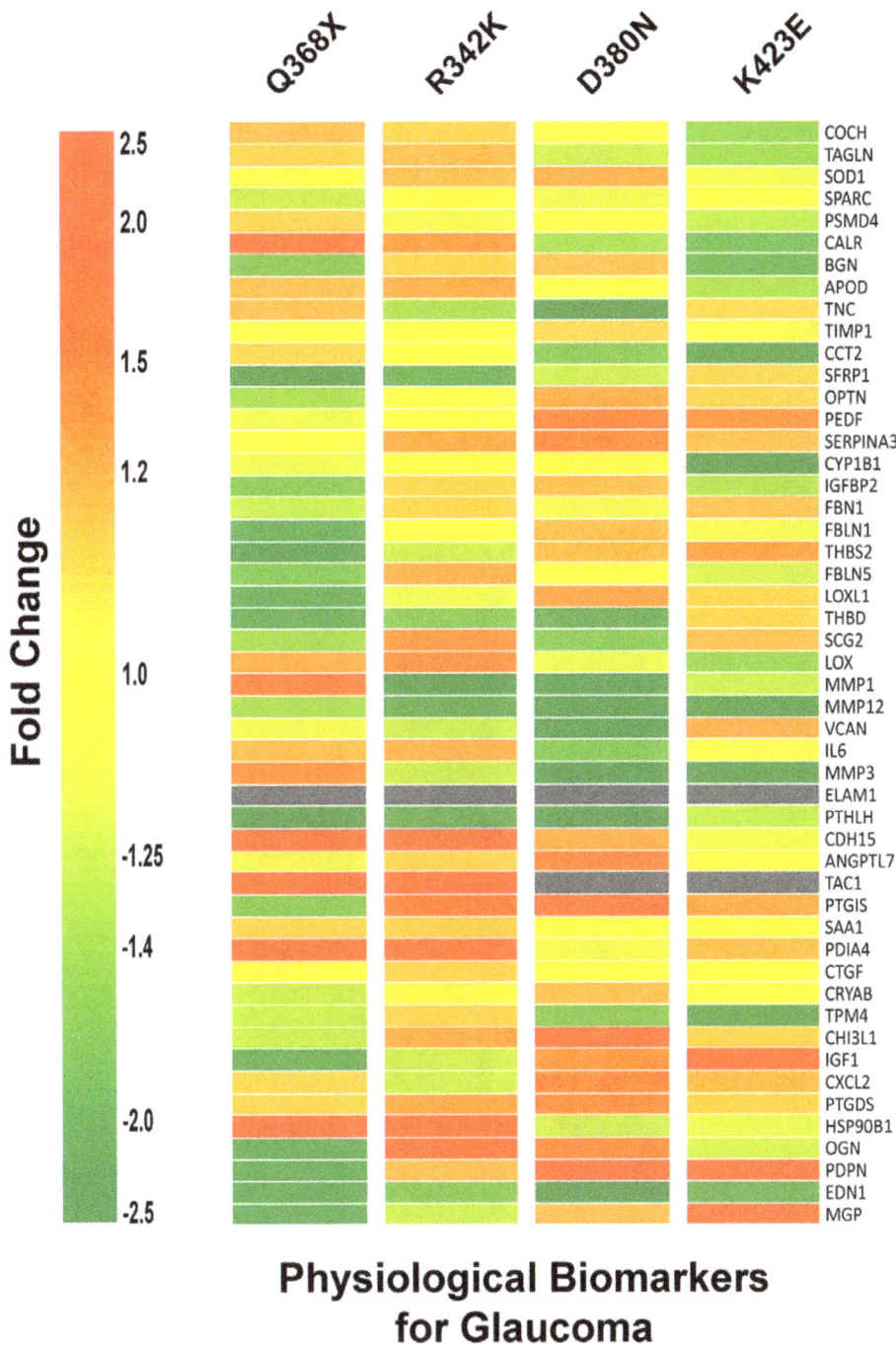

**Figure 5. *MYOC* mutants altered most physiological biomarkers of glaucoma.** Heat maps of a gene list containing 50 potential biomarkers for the human trabecular meshwork (Table S6). The biomarker gene list was generated by a comprehensive review of trabecular meshwork expression studies as indicated in the result section. Each row represents the fold change (Adeno.MYOC mutant over Adeno.Null) for a single gene in each of the four mutants. Each column represents the fold changes for all biomarkers in one *MYOC* mutant. The fold change for each gene is visually represented by a color, which is given by the scale bar at left. Heat maps were generated with genes lists containing the full range of fold changes. Gray cells indicate that the expression of the giving gene was below the cutoff of signal intensity value and was considered absent.

subcategories which were statistically significant (P≤0.05). The diagram of the top seven subcategories from each main group is shown in Figure 7 top. In Biological Processes, cell cycle (GO:7049) contained the highest percent of genes number (23.1%, P≤0.0003,) and DNA replication (GO:6260) was the most significant (P≤0.000009, 13.5% genes). In Cellular Components, the extracellular region subcategory (GO:5576) was both the one with highest percentage of genes and most significant (25.9%, P≤0.0001). In the Molecular Function category, the subcategory with more genes was that of receptor binding (GO:5102) (15.8%, P≤0.0009) while the one most significant was the ATPase inhibitor activity (GO:42030) (P≤0.00008, 3.5% genes) (Figure 7 top).

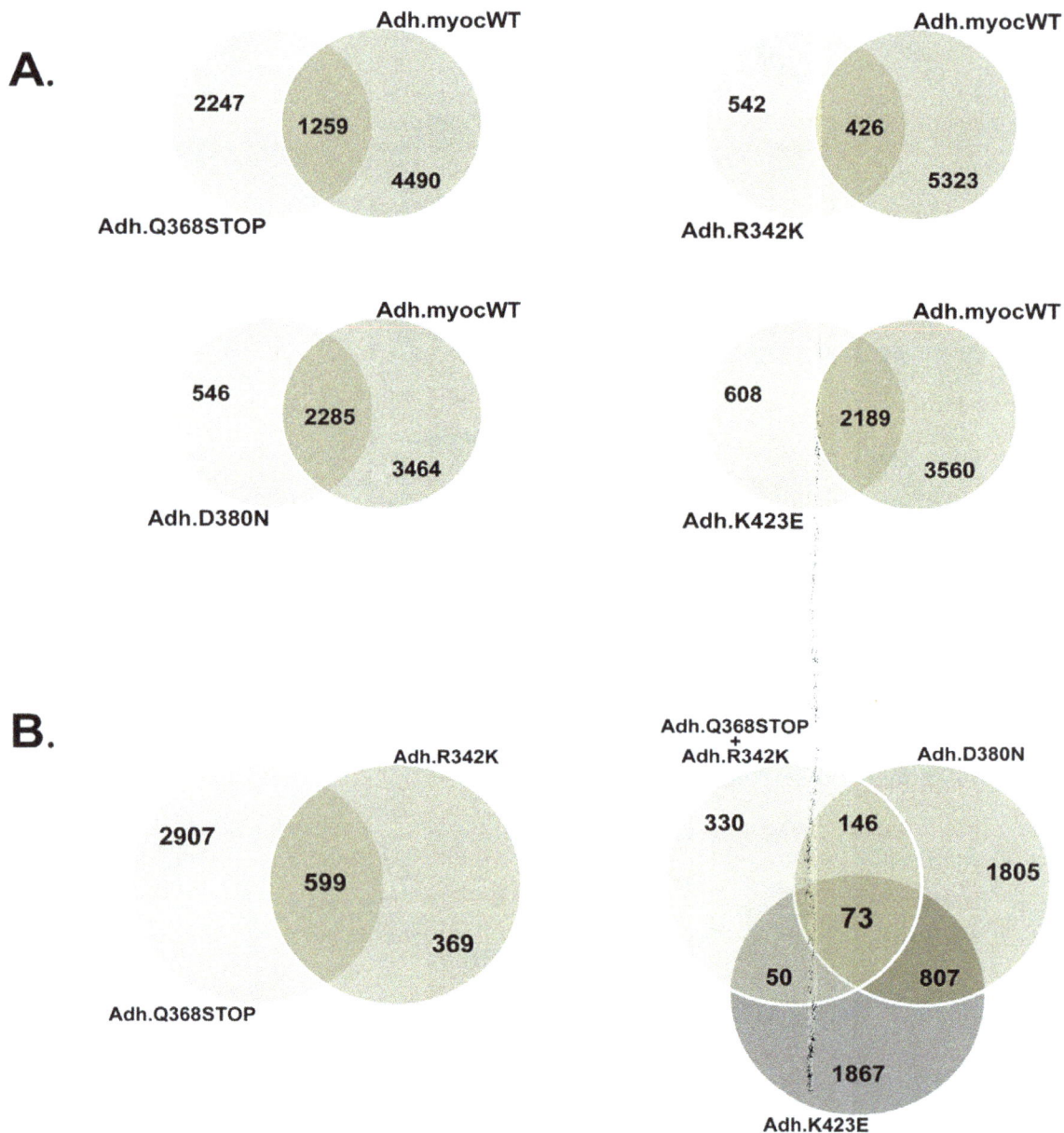

**Figure 6.** *MYOC* **mutants shared different gene percentages with** *MYOC* **wild-type, and shared 73 genes among themselves.** Venn diagrams of genes differentially altered 1.5-fold in response to overexpression of *MYOC* wild-type and *MYOC*-mutants. Each circle represents one condition. Intersections indicate numbers of genes that are shared between the different conditions. A) genes shared of each of the mutants with the wild-type. B) genes shared by all mutants.

Genes selected from each of the lists of the subcategories are shown in Figure 7 lower panel. As expected, some of these genes coincide with those selected above through other selection means, ratifying the relevance of their potential involvement in the association of *MYOC* mutants with glaucoma. Among the genes, we observed the signaling cytokine *CXCL12*, the vasoconstrictor *EDN1*, the extracellular matrix constituent *ECM2*, the cysteine protease *CSTA*, the calcium homeostasis proteins *STC1*, *STC2* and the growth factors *IGF1* and *FGF1*. It is likely that a different extent combination of the functions encoded by these genes is what it would cause the *MYOC* mutants to trigger the development of the disease.

## Genes Altered in All Mutants and not in the Wild-type. Identification of Cystatin A

Next we were interested to investigate whether the genes altered in all mutants were also altered in the wild-type. To determine how many of the 73 genes in the mutants' overlapping list were mutant-specific, we performed a Venn map comparing the shared mutant list with that of the 5,749 genes altered by the wild-type. Looking for non-overlapping genes, we found that only 10 out of the 73 genes were altered specifically in all mutants and were not shared with the altered genes of the wild-type (Figure 8).

Analysis of the functions of the 10 specific genes revealed the presence of a cysteine protease inhibitor, *CSTA* (alias *Stefin A*), which showed a no change 1.0-fold in the wild-type and an increase of 3.4-, 3.2-, 1.5- and 1.9-fold in Q368X, R342K, D380N

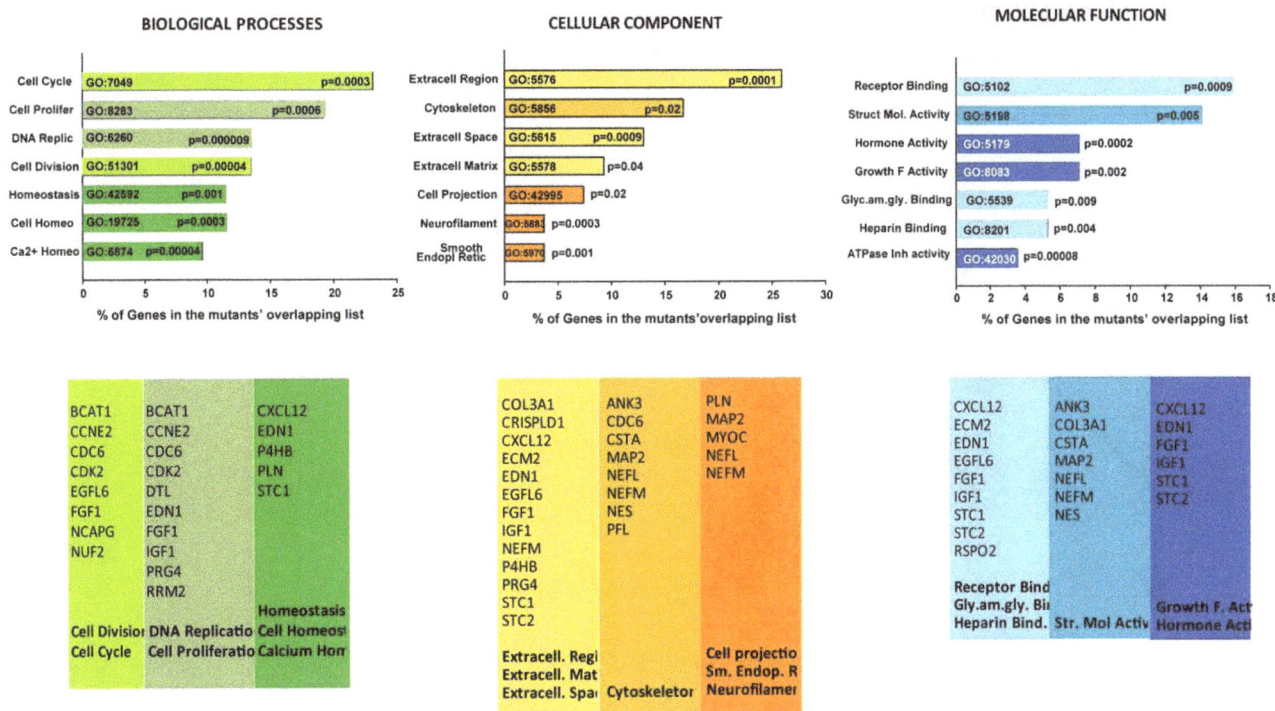

**Figure 7. Gene ontology. The ECM category (GO:5576) contained the highest percent and significance of MYOC-induced genes.** *Top:* enriched GO categories of the 73 gene list shared by all mutants (from Figure 6) sorted by *P* values. *Bottom:* genes selected from the categories shown on top (color coded).

and K423E respectively. The induction of CSTA in all cells overexpressing the MYOC mutants was validated by TaqMan PCR in a different HTM primary cell line (HTM-137) and using new viral stocks. Cells were infected with each of the four mutants, Ad5.CMV-Null and Adh.MYOCWT as indicated in methods. RNA was extracted 48 h post-infection and its cDNA assayed for expression of *CSTA*, using *MYOC* as a positive control and 18S as the endogenous calibrator. Results were expressed in FC values of each of the genes in the treated (MYOCs) over negative control (Ad5.CMV.Null), and normalized to their own 18S. In cells infected with Q368X, R342K, D380N and K423E, *CSTA* was induced 4.6-fold (P = 0.012), 3.7-fold (P = .001), 6.45-fold (p = 0.015), and 5.7-fold (P = 0.002) respectively. In cells infected with Adh.MYOCWT, rather than a no change as it occurred in the chip, *CSTA* was reduced −3.0-fold (P = 0.0001), a result most likely due to the highest sensitivity to the TaqMan assay. The overexpression of *MYOC* in each of the dishes (mutants and wild-type infected) was used as a positive control and ranged from 891 to 7,131 FC over that in Ad5.CMV-Null.

## Functional Assay of Cystatin A. Involvement in Wild-type Myocilin Processing

In order to investigate whether overexpression of the selected *CSTA* gene would affect the processing of the wild-type *MYOC* protein we generated tagged recombinant plasmids, containing both genes (Figure 9A). Plasmid pMG29 contains 1513 nt of wild-type *MYOC* fused to the V5 tag in a pCDNA3.1D V5-His-TOPO background. Plasmid pCSTA contains the full coding *CSTA* cDNA (Origene) fused to the DDK and MYC elements. Plasmid pCSTAm derives from pCSTA but contains a mutation at nucleotide 139 (G to A) that converts N-terminal Gly-4 residue to an Arginine and inactivates the binding of the inhibitor to the

cathepsin B protease [37]. Plasmid pEmpty does not contain any transgene cDNA (see methods) and was used as a control. pMG29 was co-transfected with either pCSTA or pEmpty in HEK293 and primary HTM-137 cells in a ratio of 1:2 (Figures. 9B and 9C). Extracted intracellular and secreted proteins were run in PAGE gels, blotted and cross-reacted with an antibody against the V5 tag fused to MYOC. Blots were then re-probed with beta-actin for equal loading control and with anti-DDK antibody to confirm the presence of CSTA. The 35 K processed C-terminal appeared as a doublet. In both cell lines, the processing of the wild-type was reduced in the presence of the CSTA protein.

In the HEK293 cells secreted fraction, densitometry of the wild-type and processed C-terminal fragments showed a mean density of the processed MYOC bands to be a 48.6% of the total secreted MYOC in the cells transfected with pEmpty and 36.4% in the cells transfected with pCSTA (a percent reduction of 25.1%). The difference was more marked in the intracellular fraction where the processed MYOC was 49.8% of the total in the control and 12.5% in the cells transfected with *CSTA* (a percent reduction of 74.9%).

In the primary HTM cells secreted fraction, densitometry of the wild-type and processed C-terminal fragments bands showed the mean density of the processed MYOC to be 33.0% of the total secreted MYOC in the cells transfected with pEmpty controls and 17.2% in the cells transfected with pCSTA (a percent reduction of 47.9%). The difference was more marked in the intracellular fraction where the processed MYOC was 36.5% of the total in the control and 6.6% in the cells transfected with *CSTA* (percent reduction of 89.1%). Protein extracts were run in duplicate gels and transfections were repeated on the HEK293 to confirm the findings. Confirmation of the processing effect of CSTA in wild-type MYOC was achieved by the transfection and overexpression of HTM-137 cells with pCSTAm, a plasmid where the activity of

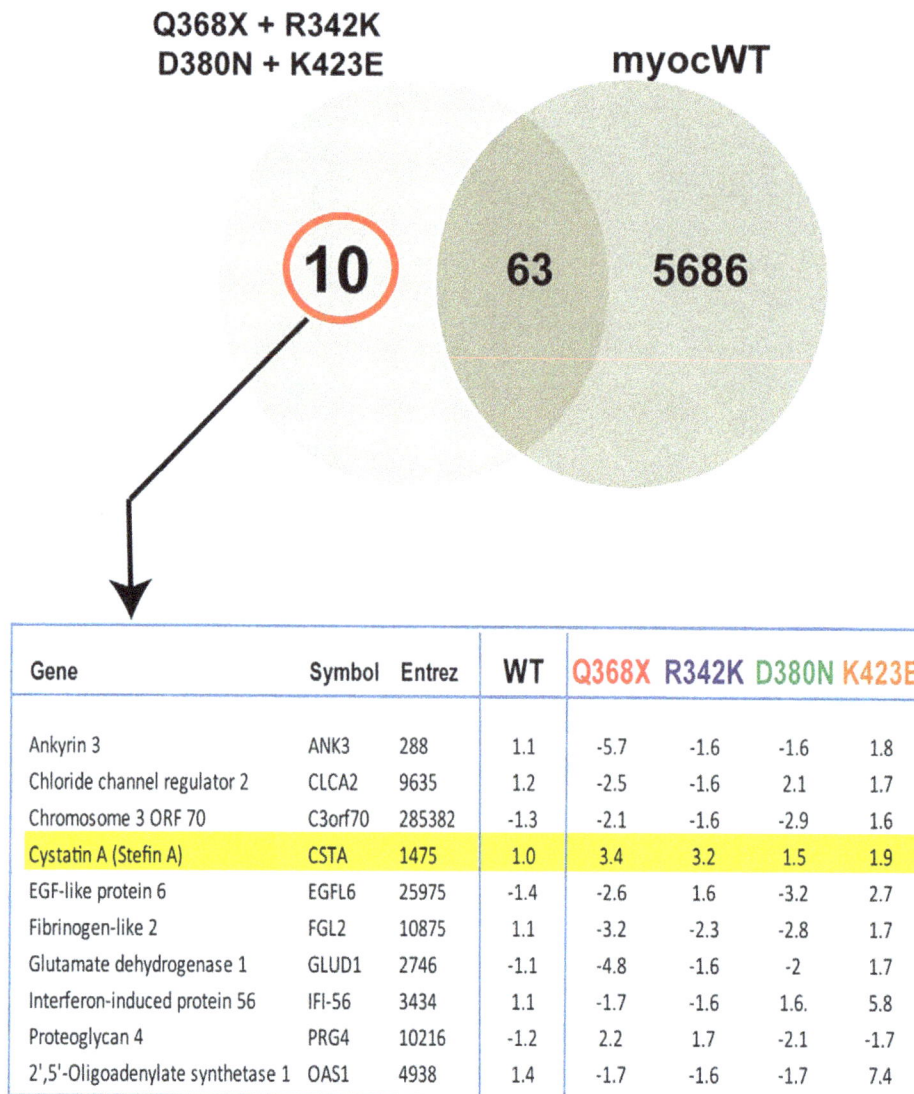

**Figure 8. Cystatin A is induced in all *MYOC* mutants and not in *MYOC* wild-type.** *Top*: Venn diagram comparing genes altered 1.5-fold in all *MYOC* mutants (left circle) with those altered in the *MYOC* wild-type (right circle) (from Figure 6). Intersection indicates numbers of altered genes which are shared between all the mutants and those altered in the wild-type. Number of genes specifically altered by the mutants is outside the intersection and circled in red. *Bottom*: list of specific genes highlighting Cystatin A and its altered fold change values in each condition.

the CSTA protein is destroyed by the mutation of the conserved residue Gly-4 to Arg [37] (Figure 9D). In the secreted fraction, densitometry readings of the mutant experiments showed the processed MYOC in cells transfected with pEmpty and pCSTAm to be 23.6% and 37.1% respectively of the total secreted, while in cells transfected with pCSTA was 10.5% (percent reductions of 55.5 and 71.7% respectively). In the intracellular fraction, the processed MYOC was 17.2% and 20.4% of the total MYOC in cells transfected with pEmpty and pCSTAm and 9.5% in cells transfected with pCSTA (percent reductions of 44.8% and 53.4% respectively).

These results indicate that the increased levels of the protease inhibitor CSTA, but not those of the inactivated CSTA, are able to inhibit the processing of MYOC. In both cell types the inhibition occurred in both fractions and the reduction seems to be higher in the non-transformed trabecular meshwork specific cells than in the transformed embryonic kidney HEK293 line. Therefore the previously reported protein processing reduction

observed in the MYOC mutants [28] might be due to overexpression of *CSTA*. The finding could lead to a common treatment of the inhibition of *CSTA* to ameliorate the development of the disease caused by *MYOC* mutants.

## Discussion

Our goal in this study was to gain insight into the molecular mechanisms linking *MYOC* mutants to the development of glaucoma. Even if the *MYOC* gene is expressed in several non-ocular tissues, *MYOC* mutants are associated to only one disease, glaucoma. Because myocilin is induced by a variety of stress factors (from oxidative stress to mechanical strain), it is very likely that the disease caused by the *MYOC* mutants would be aggravated by their induced overexpression under stress conditions. To date, a few studies have addressed the effect of overexpressing some *MYOC* mutants in ocular and non-ocular cells [15,18,23,28]. However, except for one study in fruit flies [19], most of them

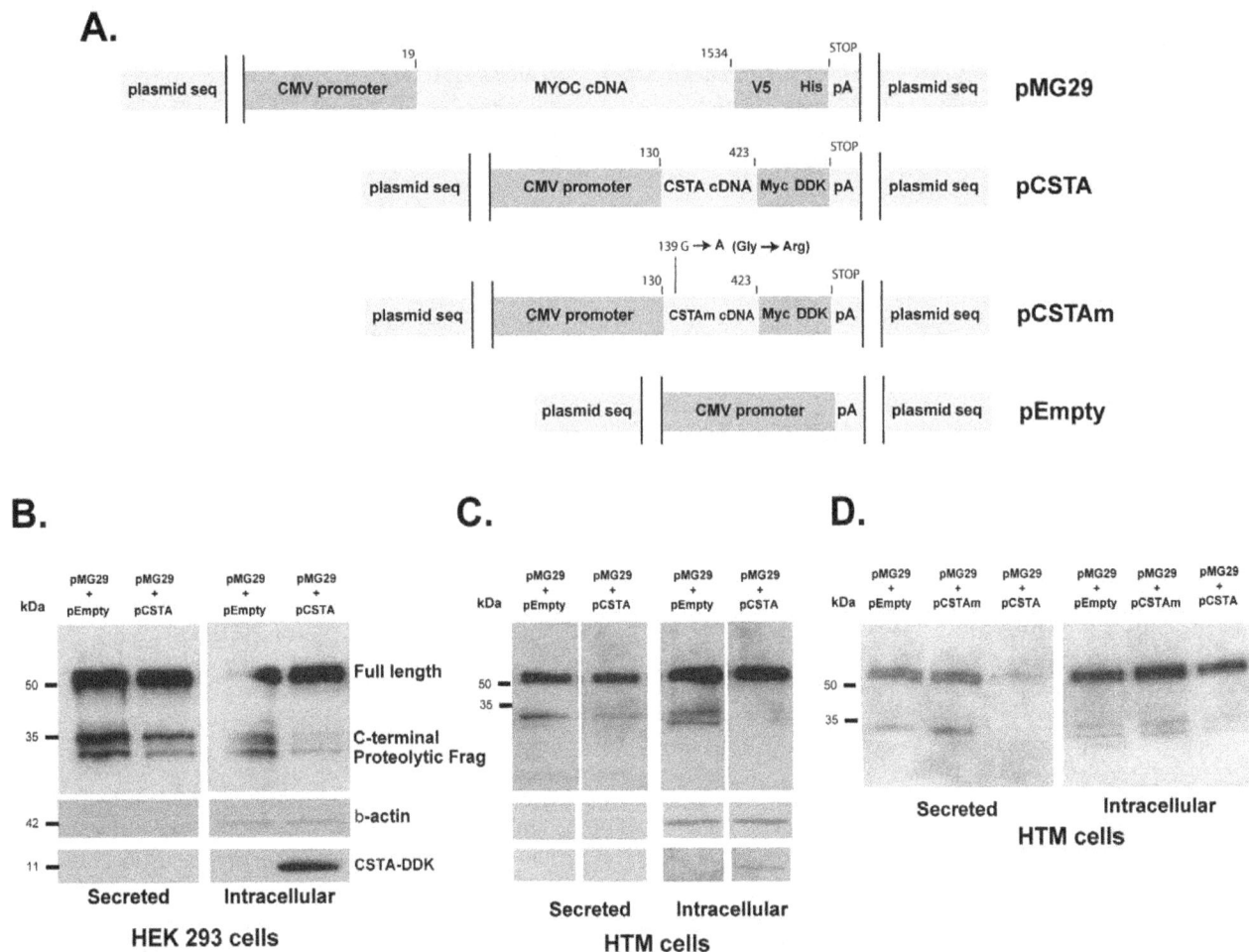

**Figure 9. Cystatin A inhibits the processing of MYOC wild-type in cultured cells.** Recombinant expression plasmids containing tag-fused full coding wild-type *MYOC* (pMG29), *CSTA,* and controls plasmids, inactive mutated *CSTA (CSTAm)* and pEmpty, were generated as indicated in Methods. pMG29 was co-transfected with either pCSTA, pCSTAm or pEmpty (1:2) and harvested at 48 h post-transfection. Equivalent volumes of cell extracts and of their supernatants were loaded onto 4–15% SDS-PAGE gels, transferred to PVDF membranes and analyzed by immunoblotting. Different MYOC protein forms (full length and processed) were detected with an anti-V5 mouse monoclonal followed by an anti-mouse horseradish peroxidase antibodies. Blots were re-probed with β-actin and DDK antibodies for loading and identification controls. Percent of the MYOC processed band was calculated by densitometry. A) schematic representation of the expression cassettes of the recombinant plasmids. B, C and D: Representative western blots with extracts from transfected cells. B) extracts from HEK293 co-transfected by calcium phosphate. C and D) extracts from primary HTM-137 cells co-transfected by nucleofector electroporation.

focused on the effect of the mutants in a few cellular mechanisms. Because *MYOC* mutants cause high tension glaucoma in humans, and because an elevated IOP phenotype is the result of a dysfunctional trabecular meshwork, here we studied the effect of overexpressing them in primary non-transformed, human trabecular meshwork cells. With the intent of uncovering new mechanisms, our approach entailed the examination of global changes induced by the mutants in the entire transcriptome of the cell.

## Genes, known and New

When we examined the most altered genes induced by all four mutants, we observed a high number of genes which had been previously identified as functionally relevant for the trabecular meshwork at either physiological or glaucomatous stress conditions. Among those genes are *EDN1, MGP, IGF1, CALR, PDIA4, PCLOCE2, MMP1, MMP3, SFRP1, FN1, PDPN, OGN, OSF2,* THBS2, *THBD,* LOX, LOX-L1, *TAC1, Secretogranin II (SCG2)* and *SNCA.* Some of these had already been reported to be associated

with *MYOC* mutants (e.g. *MMP1, CALR,* and *PDI)* or wild-type (SFRP1, *FN1)* in other studies [18,19,41] [25,63], and validates the finding. However, the association of most of them with *MYOC* mutants was unknown.

As is not uncommon in this type of studies, some of the found genes appeared to serve a counteracting purpose while others appeared to be directly related to the detrimental effect. For example, *END1* was on the top downregulated list in all four mutants. Endothelin protein is processed to secrete a potent vasoconstrictor peptide with a well-established connection to glaucoma [64]. Endothelin can lower IOP by contracting the ciliary muscle, but conversely, an antagonist of its receptor can also lower IOP in glaucomatous monkeys [64]. The endogenous *EDN1* downregulation by myocilin mutants seen here is curious. It could be interpreted as either a signal for contributing to the high IOP phenotype of the mutants or to a counteracting effect.

A gene that could enlighten the correlation between the mutants and elevated IOP is *MMP1.* In this study all mutants but one (Q368X) downregulated *MMP1,* while the wild-type upregulated its expression. Matrix metallopeptidase 1 breaks down collagen type 1, an important component of the ECM of the outflow tissue. Increased levels of *MMP1* have been extensively associated with increasing outflow facility and lowering of IOP [41,65]. Therefore, the *MMP1* downregulation observed here could be seen as a contribution to the build-up of an ECM excess, increase of aqueous humor resistance and consequent elevated IOP produced by the mutants. The unexpected upregulation of *MMP1* by Q368X (confirmed repeatedly by TaqMan PCR) could then be explained as one of the molecular reasons as to why this mutation causes a milder outcome of the disease. Curiously, we had previously reported an interesting feedback loop regulation of expression between the *MMP1/MYOC* genes [31,41,66], where overexpression of wild-type *MYOC* induced the expression of *MMP1* [31] while overexpression of *MMP1* reduced that of wild-type *MYOC* [41,66]. It is possible that a homeostatic balance between these two proteins would be disrupted by the presence of the mutated protein form.

Another potentially relevant gene found in these studies was *PDIA4*. In an earlier report overexpressing Q368X in trabecular meshwork cells, Kee and co-workers [18] had observed increased PDI levels in the treated cells. In this study *PDIA4* expression was induced by both the Q368X and R342K mutants, but not by D380N and K423E. This enzyme which catalyzes the formation and breakage of disulfide bonds is a key component of the protein folding mechanism. Myocilin folding and complex formation is relevant for its function and has been known to be mediated by the formation of covalent disulfide bonds involving its five cysteine residues [67]. Although the fifth residue 433Cys is not present in the Q368X stop mutation, the induction of the PDI is bound to affect the stability of the proteins and even perhaps affect the secretion of other proteins [68]. In our early work, *PDIA4* was induced in response to elevated pressure [45,46]. It is known that mechanical strain causes deformation of proteins, triggering them to unfold and subsequently refold [69]. Protein disulfide isomerase induction could thus be a mediator of this effect and represent a cellular defense response against the altered protein, as it also occurs in Creutzfeld-Jacob disease [70]. Why *PDIA4* it is only induced by two of the mutants is not yet clear and might be a sign of the different avenues through which each mutant contributes to the disease.

Some of the genes altered by these mutants were new. These include among others RAB39B, *STC1*, *CDH15*, *CXCL12*, *CSTA*, *ECM2* and *Lysosomal-associated membrane protein 3* (*LAMP3*), a gene which is expressed in lymphoid organs and dendritic cells. Some of these genes were commonly altered in all mutants while others where changed only in one or two of them. Their encoded functions could play a role on the mutant's linkage to the disease. Thus, *RAB39B*, upregulated in all mutants, is a small GTPase binding protein described as being specific to neurons and involved in vesicular trafficking [71]. This mechanism, which includes the ability to secrete the protein, has been shown to play a key role in myocilin function [12,13] and was suggested to be disrupted by *MYOC* mutants [11]. It would be possible that upregulation of RAB39B could have a role on the trafficking and non-secretion of the MYOC mutants.

Another new gene, *STC1*, was in contrast downregulated in all mutants. Stanniocalcin regulates calcium and phosphate transport in the kidney and has been postulated to prevent hypercalcemia [72]. The downregulation of *STC1* could be an indication that the *MYOC* mutants are favoring a trend towards calcification of the trabecular meshwork.

Few of the genes encoding proteins reported to interact with Myocilin made the 1.5X FC cutoff. Two of them did. Secreted

frizzled protein 1, [25] which was downregulated in mutants Q368X and R342K, and *FN1* [63], that was upregulated in D380N and K423E. The *SNCA* gene which was also upregulated in D380N and K423E is from the same family as the *MYOC* binding protein γ-synuclein, but in contrast, showed no co-localization and thus, not binding [73]. α-Synuclein, is a protein abundant in neurons and involved in Parkinson and other neurodegenerative disorders and in here could play the role of a pathological chaperone, as it has been described in other systems [74]. α-Synuclein peptides are a major component of amyloid plaques in the brains of patients with Alzheimer's disease [75], which has been speculated to have some common mechanistic features with Glaucoma [76].

## Differences between Mutants

Overall, there were many similarities between Q368X and R342K (which we termed set #1). Those similarities were distinct from the changes induced by the other two mutants D380N and K423E (set #2). This was an unexpected finding, since there are not described phenotypic similarities shared between the mutants of the same group, or described phenotypic differences between the two groups. At the moment we can postulate that, in addition to IOP, there may yet be undefined glaucoma biomarkers in the altered genes pool which could differently influence the development of the disease in sets #1 and #2.

A look at the genes representing trabecular meshwork relevant functions and physiological markers of glaucoma by the use of heat maps (Figures 4 and 5) revealed that most of genes in those lists are affected by overexpression of *MYOC* mutants. The trend of similarities between the two sets of mutants is clearly seen in the genes involved in calcification, WNT signaling and stress, while it is less obvious in those genes encoding collagen-elastin cross-linking and in the biomarkers' list. The intensity of the changes was considerably greater in the stress and UPR function group, especially for the Q368X mutation. This mutation clearly downregulated genes that could induce elevated IOP, such *TGM2* and *SFRP1* [26,60] while inducing others that have a role in protein folding, such as *CALR* and *Calnexin* (*CANX*). This combined regulation could be beneficial and contribute to the milder outcome of the disease in the Q368X mutant. In contrast, the lower induction of the same genes (*CALR* and *CANX*) by R342K, together with the upregulation of the calcification genes *OGN* and *OMD* (heat map Figure 4) could provide this mutant (otherwise similar to the stop mutation) with the difference needed to induce an elevated pressure.

Although each of the *MYOC* mutants exhibited individual characteristics which are most likely instrumental in triggering different disease severities, there was a need to search for a common thread. In a Venn map comparison with wild-type we observed that the four *MYOC* mutants exhibited a different percentage of non-shared altered genes. Set #1 mutants had a larger non-shared percentage than set #2. This could be an indication that set #1 would be further away from the proposed protective mechanism of the wild-type than set #2 or, that these mutants require a higher number of changes to cause the disease. When comparing the four mutants against themselves, we found only 73 altered common genes. And from the 73, only 10 were not altered in the wild-type.

## Cystatin A as a Potential Common Link

One of the genes found elevated in all mutants and not elevated in the wild-type was *CSTA*, which encodes for the cysteine protease inhibitor cystatin A. This gene is present in most tissues, its expression is associated with tumor growth and it is a serum biomarker for screening cancer patients. The upregulation of the *CSTA* mRNA by the *MYOC* mutants is intriguing. Because the protein involved in the processing of myocilin, calpain II, is a cysteine protease, and because myocilin cleavage is inhibited by MYOC mutants, one could reasonably infer that *CSTA* plays a role in the inhibition of the process. Whether the elevation of cystatin A seen here can result also in the inhibition of calpain is not yet known. Cystatin A is known to inhibit papain and cathepsins, not calpains. However, a recent study investigating induced cell death in monocytes and macrophages has shown that calpain activation occurred downstream of cathepsin B (a CSTA substrate) [77]. They concluded that cathepsin B activated calpain [77]. Such finding would implicate that increased levels of cystatin A would, by inactivating cathepsin B, result in the inactivation of calpain. In our functional assay, overexpression of cystatin A reduced the processing of wild-type myocilin while overexpression of an inactive CSTA did not. This effect could then have been achieved by either a downstream inactivation of calpain through the inactivation of cathepsin B, or by a direct cleavage of myocilin by cathepsin B.

It is important to point out that *MYOC*-causative glaucoma occurs only in heterozygous individuals, and that *MYOC* forms wild-type/mutant hetero-oligomers which lead to the formation of insoluble aggregates (gain of function) [12,17]. It would be logical to assume that myocilin processing, affected by the expression of the mutants, plays a fundamental role in the formation of the hetero-aggregates. The fact that hetero-aggregation could also modulate the extracellular environment [15] provides an additional support for the relevance of faulty hetero-aggregates in the development of glaucoma.

Finally, although several mechanisms are bound to be involved in the association of *MYOC* mutants to glaucoma, it looks that activation of cysteine protease inhibitors could be a common, general one. It would be interesting to investigate whether the application of an inhibitor to *CSTA*, such as its siRNA, could restore the normal *MYOC* processing and affect the outcome of the disease. Our results showing that overexpression of an inactive CSTA reverted the decrease processing would support this possibility. It would also be of interest to determine whether a screening of CSTA levels in the serum could be applied to glaucoma as it is presently occurring in cancer [39].

## Conclusions

Our study on the transcripts altered by overexpression of *MYOC* mutants in glaucoma-relevant primary human cells provides key insights on the potential mechanisms leading to the development of *MYOC*-linked glaucoma. We uncovered that each mutant's phenotype could result from its unique effect on the transcriptome. We learned that a number of important genes which have been historically associated with physiological and pathological mechanisms of the human trabecular meshwork are altered by the expression of these MYOC mutants. On overall mechanisms, we identified that, genes of the UPR pathway were the most affected. On individual gene analyses, we confirmed the involvement of previously MYOC-associated genes (e.g. *MMP1, PDIA4, CALR, SFPR1*) and revealed the relevance of some new ones (e.g. *STC1, RAB39B, CXCL12*). Most importantly, we discovered a mutant-specific induced gene, *CSTA*. This inhibitor of cysteine proteases was functional, and inhibited MYOC protein processing in cultured cells. We believe these findings do significantly impact our understanding of *MYOC*-caused glaucoma and could provide the basis for the potential development of a broad-spectrum therapy for the mutant disease.

## Supporting Information

**Table S1   Q368STOP. The 100 most altered genes.** a) 50 upregulated; b) 50 downregulated

**Table S2   R342K. The 100 most altered genes.** a) 50 upregulated; b) 50 downregulated

**Table S3   D380N. The 100 most altered genes.** a) 50 upregulated; b) 50 downregulated

**Table S4   K423E. The 100 most altered genes** a) 50 upregulated; b) 50 downregulated

**Table S5   Taqman FC and p-values of selected relevant genes.** Comparison to microarray FC

**Table S6   Physiological Biomarkers List for Glaucoma (Trabecular Meshwork).**

## Acknowledgments

The authors thank Drs. M.A. Carbone and R.R.H. Anholt for providing the myocilin mutant plasmids. They also thank members of the laboratory, Dr. M.G. Spiga for generating the fusion myocilin clone, M.H. Smith and R. Elliott for generation of the gene tables and Dr. J. Carabaña for critical reading of the manuscript.

## Author Contributions

Conceived and designed the experiments: TB KDK SAA. Performed the experiments: KDK SAA LKKB. Analyzed the data: TB KDK SAA. Contributed reagents/materials/analysis tools: KDK SAA LKKB. Wrote the paper: TB KDK.

## References

1. Polansky JR, Kurtz RM, Fauss DJ, Kim RY, Bloom E (1991) *In vitro* correlates of glucocorticoid effects on intraocular pressure. In: Krieglstein GK, ed. Glaucoma Update IV. Berlin, Heilderberg: Springer-Verlag. pp 20–29.

2. Escribano J, Ortego J, Coca-Prados M (1995) Isolation and characterization of cell-specific cDNA clones from a subtractive library of the ocular ciliary body of a single normal human donor: transcription and synthesis of plasma proteins. J Biochem 118: 921–931.

3. Kubota R, Noda S, Wang Y, Minoshima S, Asakawa S, et al. (1997) A novel myosin-like protein (myocilin) expressed in the connecting cilium of the photoreceptor: molecular cloning, tissue expression, and chromosomal mapping. Genomics 41: 360–369.

4. Ortego J, Escribano J, Coca-Prados M (1997) Cloning and characterization of subtracted cDNAs from a human ciliary body library encoding TIGR, a protein involved in juvenile open angle glaucoma with homology to myosin and olfactomedin. FEBS Lett 413: 349–353.

5. Lo WR, Rowlette LL, Caballero M, Yang P, Hernandez MR, et al. (2003) Tissue differential microarray analysis of dexamethasone induction reveals potential mechanisms of steroid glaucoma. Invest Ophthalmol Vis Sci 44: 473–485.

6. Stone EM, Fingert JH, Alward WL, Nguyen TD, Polansky JR, et al. (1997) Identification of a gene that causes primary open angle glaucoma. Science 275: 668–670.

7. Shimizu S, Lichter PR, Johnson AT, Zhou Z, Higashi M, et al. (2000) Age-dependent prevalence of mutations at the GLC1A locus in primary open-angle glaucoma. Am J Ophthalmol 130: 165–177.

8. Quigley HA, Broman AT (2006) The number of people with glaucoma worldwide in 2010 and 2020. Br J Ophthalmol 90: 262–267.

9. Gong G, Kosoko-Lasaki O, Haynatzki GR, Wilson MR (2004) Genetic dissection of myocilin glaucoma. Hum Mol Genet 13 Spec No 1: R91–102.

10. Nguyen TD, Chen P, Huang WD, Chen H, Johnson D, et al. (1998) Gene structure and properties of TIGR, an olfactomedin-related glycoprotein cloned from glucocorticoid-induced trabecular meshwork cells. J Biol Chem 273: 6341–6350.

11. Caballero M, Borrás T (2001) Inefficient processing of an olfactomedin-deficient myocilin mutant: potential physiological relevance to glaucoma. Biochem Biophys Res Commun 282: 662–670.

12. Caballero M, Rowlette LL, Borrás T (2000) Altered secretion of a TIGR/MYOC mutant lacking the olfactomedin domain. Biochim Biophys Acta 1502: 447–460.

13. Perkumas KM, Hoffman EA, McKay BS, Allingham RR, Stamer WD (2007) Myocilin-associated exosomes in human ocular samples. Exp Eye Res 84: 209–212.

14. Jacobson N, Andrews M, Shepard AR, Nishimura D, Searby C, et al. (2001) Non-secretion of mutant proteins of the glaucoma gene myocilin in cultured trabecular meshwork cells and in aqueous humor. Hum Mol Genet 10: 117–125.

15. Aroca-Aguilar JD, Sanchez-Sanchez F, Martinez-Redondo F, Coca-Prados M, Escribano J (2008) Heterozygous expression of myocilin glaucoma mutants increases secretion of the mutant forms and reduces extracellular processed myocilin. Mol Vis 14: 2097–2108.

16. Zhou Z, Vollrath D (1999) A cellular assay distinguishes normal and mutant TIGR/myocilin protein. Hum Mol Genet 8: 2221–2228.

17. Gobeil S, Rodrigue MA, Moisan S, Nguyen TD, Polansky JR, et al. (2004) Intracellular sequestration of hetero-oligomers formed by wild-type and glaucoma-causing myocilin mutants. Invest Ophthalmol Vis Sci 45: 3560–3567.

18. Joe MK, Sohn S, Hur W, Moon Y, Choi YR, et al. (2003) Accumulation of mutant myocilins in ER leads to ER stress and potential cytotoxicity in human trabecular meshwork cells. Biochem Biophys Res Commun 312: 592–600.

19. Carbone MA, Ayroles JF, Yamamoto A, Morozova TV, West SA, et al. (2009) Overexpression of myocilin in the Drosophila eye activates the unfolded protein response: implications for glaucoma. PLoS One 4: e4216.

20. Morissette J, Clepet C, Moisan S, Dubois S, Winstall E, et al. (1998) Homozygotes carrying an autosomal dominant TIGR mutation do not manifest glaucoma. Nat Genet 19: 319–321.

21. Tamm ER (2002) Myocilin and glaucoma: facts and ideas. Prog Retin Eye Res 21: 395–428.

22. Comes N, Borrás T (2009) Individual molecular response to elevated intraocular pressure in perfused postmortem human eyes. Physiol Genomics 38: 205–225.

23. Joe MK, Tomarev SI (2010) Expression of myocilin mutants sensitizes cells to oxidative stress-induced apoptosis: implication for glaucoma pathogenesis. Am J Pathol 176: 2880–2890.

24. Menaa F, Braghini CA, Vasconcellos JP, Menaa B, Costa VP, et al. (2011) Keeping an eye on myocilin: a complex molecule associated with primary open-angle glaucoma susceptibility. Molecules 16: 5402–5421.

25. Kwon HS, Lee HS, Ji Y, Rubin JS, Tomarev SI (2009) Myocilin is a modulator of Wnt signaling. Mol Cell Biol 29: 2139–2154.

26. Wang WH, McNatt LG, Pang IH, Millar JC, Hellberg PE, et al. (2008) Increased expression of the WNT antagonist sFRP-1 in glaucoma elevates intraocular pressure. J Clin Invest 118: 1056–1064.

27. Goldwich A, Ethier CR, Chan DW, Tamm ER (2003) Perfusion with the olfactomedin domain of myocilin does not affect outflow facility. Invest Ophthalmol Vis Sci 44: 1953–1961.

28. Aroca-Aguilar JD, Sanchez-Sanchez F, Ghosh S, Coca-Prados M, Escribano J (2005) Myocilin mutations causing glaucoma inhibit the intracellular endoproteolytic cleavage of myocilin between amino acids Arg226 and Ile227. J Biol Chem 280: 21043–21051.

29. Aroca-Aguilar JD, Martinez-Redondo F, Sanchez-Sanchez F, Coca-Prados M, Escribano J (2010) Functional role of proteolytic processing of recombinant myocilin in self-aggregation. Invest Ophthalmol Vis Sci 51: 72–78.

30. Sanchez-Sanchez F, Martinez-Redondo F, Aroca-Aguilar JD, Coca-Prados M, Escribano J (2007) Characterization of the intracellular proteolytic cleavage of myocilin and identification of calpain II as a myocilin-processing protease. J Biol Chem 282: 27810–27824.

31. Borrás T, Bryant PA, Chisolm SS (2006) First look at the effect of overexpression of TIGR/MYOC on the transcriptome of the human trabecular meshwork. Exp Eye Res 82: 1002–1010.

32. Challa P, Herndon LW, Hauser MA, Broomer BW, Pericak-Vance MA, et al. (2002) Prevalence of myocilin mutations in adults with primary open-angle glaucoma in Ghana, West Africa. J Glaucoma 11: 416–420.

33. Wirtz MK, Samples JR, Choi D, Gaudette ND (2007) Clinical features associated with an Asp380His Myocilin mutation in a US family with primary open-angle glaucoma. Am J Ophthalmol 144: 75–80.

34. Bruttini M, Longo I, Frezzotti P, Ciappetta R, Randazzo A, et al. (2003) Mutations in the myocilin gene in families with primary open-angle glaucoma and juvenile open-angle glaucoma. Arch Ophthalmol 121: 1034–1038.

35. Rivenbark AG, Coleman WB (2009) Epigenetic regulation of cystatins in cancer. Front Biosci 14: 453–462.

36. Martin JR, Craven CJ, Jerala R, Kroon-Zitko L, Zerovnik E, et al. (1995) The three-dimensional solution structure of human stefin A. J Mol Biol 246: 331–343.

37. Estrada S, Nycander M, Hill NJ, Craven CJ, Waltho JP, et al. (1998) The role of Gly-4 of human cystatin A (stefin A) in the binding of target proteinases. Characterization by kinetic and equilibrium methods of the interactions of

cystatin A Gly-4 mutants with papain, cathepsin B, and cathepsin L. Biochemistry 37: 7551–7560.

38. Blaydon DC, Nitoiu D, Eckl KM, Cabral RM, Bland P, et al. (2011) Mutations in CSTA, encoding Cystatin A, underlie exfoliative ichthyosis and reveal a role for this protease inhibitor in cell-cell adhesion. Am J Hum Genet 89: 564–571.

39. Chang KP, Wu CC, Chen HC, Chen SJ, Peng PH, et al. (2010) Identification of candidate nasopharyngeal carcinoma serum biomarkers by cancer cell secretome and tissue transcriptome analysis: potential usage of cystatin A for predicting nodal stage and poor prognosis. Proteomics 10: 2644–2660.

40. He TC, Zhou S, da Costa LT, Yu J, Kinzler KW, et al. (1998) A simplified system for generating recombinant adenoviruses. Proc Natl Acad Sci U S A 95: 2509–2514.

41. Spiga MG, Borrás T (2010) Development of a gene therapy virus with a glucocorticoid-inducible MMP1 for the treatment of steroid glaucoma. Invest Ophthalmol Vis Sci 51: 3029–3041.

42. Comes N, Buie LK, Borrás T (2011) Evidence for a role of angiopoietin-like 7 (ANGPTL7) in extracellular matrix formation of the human trabecular meshwork: implications for glaucoma. Genes Cells 16: 243–259.

43. Thorleifsson G, Magnusson KP, Sulem P, Walters GB, Gudbjartsson DF, et al. (2007) Common sequence variants in the LOXL1 gene confer susceptibility to exfoliation glaucoma. Science 317: 1397–1400.

44. Borrás T (2008) Mechanosensitive genes in the trabecular meshwork at homeostasis: elevated intraocular pressure and stretch. In: Tombran-Tink J, Barnstable CJ, Shields MB, eds. Mechanisms of the Glaucomas: Disease Processes and Therapeutic Modalities. New York: Humana Press, Inc. pp 329–362.

45. Borrás T (2008) What is Functional Genomics teaching us about intraocular pressure regulation and glaucoma? In: Civan MM, ed. The Eye's Aqueous Humor, Second Edition. San Diego: Elsevier. pp 323–377.

46. Vittitow J, Borrás T (2004) Genes expressed in the human trabecular meshwork during pressure-induced homeostatic response. J Cell Physiol 201: 126–137.

47. Xu H, Acott TS, Wirtz MK (2000) Identification and expression of a novel type I procollagen C-proteinase enhancer protein gene from the glaucoma candidate region on 3q21-q24. Genomics 66: 264–273.

48. Stoilov I, Akarsu AN, Sarfarazi M (1997) Identification of three different truncating mutations in cytochrome P4501B1 (CYP1B1) as the principal cause of primary congenital glaucoma (Buphthalmos) in families linked to the GLC3A locus on chromosome 2p21. Hum Mol Genet 6: 641–647.

49. Gonzalez P, Epstein DL, Borrás T (2000) Genes upregulated in the human trabecular meshwork in response to elevated intraocular pressure. Invest Ophthalmol Vis Sci 41: 352–361.

50. Borrás T, Comes N (2009) Evidence for a calcification process in the trabecular meshwork. Exp Eye Res 88: 738–746.

51. Schlötzer-Schrehardt U (2009) Molecular pathology of pseudoexfoliation syndrome/glaucoma–new insights from LOXL1 gene associations. Exp Eye Res 88: 776–785.

52. Gonzalez P, Epstein DL, Borrás T (2000) Characterization of gene expression in human trabecular meshwork using single-pass sequencing of 1060 clones. Invest Ophthalmol Vis Sci 41: 3678–3693.

53. Tomarev SI, Wistow G, Raymond V, Dubois S, Malyukova I (2003) Gene expression profile of the human trabecular meshwork: NEIBank sequence tag analysis. Invest Ophthalmol Vis Sci 44: 2588–2596.

54. Xue W, Wallin R, Olmsted-Davis EA, Borrás T (2006) Matrix GLA protein function in human trabecular meshwork cells: inhibition of BMP2-induced calcification process. Invest Ophthalmol Vis Sci 47: 997–1007.

55. Junglas B, Yu AH, Welge-Lussen U, Tamm ER, Fuchshofer R (2009) Connective tissue growth factor induces extracellular matrix deposition in human trabecular meshwork cells. Exp Eye Res 88: 1065–1075.

56. Balint E, Lapointe D, Drissi H, van der Meijden C, Young DW, et al. (2003) Phenotype discovery by gene expression profiling: mapping of biological processes linked to BMP-2-mediated osteoblast differentiation. J Cell Biochem 89: 401–426.

57. Diskin S, Kumar J, Cao Z, Schuman JS, Gilmartin T, et al. (2006) Detection of differentially expressed glycogenes in trabecular meshwork of eyes with primary open-angle glaucoma. Invest Ophthalmol Vis Sci 47: 1491–1499.

58. Vittal V, Rose A, Gregory KE, Kelley MJ, Acott TS (2005) Changes in gene expression by trabecular meshwork cells in response to mechanical stretching. Invest Ophthalmol Vis Sci 46: 2857–2868.

59. Zhao X, Ramsey KE, Stephan DA, Russell P (2004) Gene and protein expression changes in human trabecular meshwork cells treated with transforming growth factor-beta. Invest Ophthalmol Vis Sci 45: 4023–4034.

60. Tovar-Vidales T, Roque R, Clark AF, Wordinger RJ (2008) Tissue transglutaminase expression and activity in normal and glaucomatous human trabecular meshwork cells and tissues. Invest Ophthalmol Vis Sci 49: 622–628.

61. Jono S, Nishizawa Y, Shioi A, Morii H (1997) Parathyroid hormone-related peptide as a local regulator of vascular calcification. Its inhibitory action on in vitro calcification by bovine vascular smooth muscle cells. Arterioscler Thromb Vasc Biol 17: 1135–1142.

62. Rozsa FW, Reed DM, Scott KM, Pawar H, Moroi SE, et al. (2006) Gene expression profile of human trabecular meshwork cells in response to long-term dexamethasone exposure. Mol Vis 12: 125–141.

63. Filla MS, Liu X, Nguyen TD, Polansky JR, Brandt CR, et al. (2002) In vitro localization of TIGR/MYOC in trabecular meshwork extracellular matrix and binding to fibronectin. Invest Ophthalmol Vis Sci 43: 151–161.

64. Yorio T, Krishnamoorthy R, Prasanna G (2002) Endothelin: is it a contributor to glaucoma pathophysiology? J Glaucoma 11: 259–270.

65. Bradley JM, Vranka J, Colvis CM, Conger DM, Alexander JP, et al. (1998) Effect of matrix metalloproteinases activity on outflow in perfused human organ culture. Invest Ophthalmol Vis Sci 39: 2649–2658.

66. Buie L, Spiga M, Kennedy K, Fowler W, Borrás T (2010) Overexpression of MMP1 by an Adenoviral Vector (Ad) Hampers Myocilin (MYOC) Expression. Invest Ophthalmol Vis Sci ARVO: # 3222.

67. Fautsch MP, Vrabel AM, Peterson SL, Johnson DH (2004) In vitro and in vivo characterization of disulfide bond use in myocilin complex formation. Mol Vis 10: 417–425.

68. Mukaiyama H, Tohda H, Takegawa K (2010) Overexpression of protein disulfide isomerases enhances secretion of recombinant human transferrin in Schizosaccharomyces pombe. Appl Microbiol Biotechnol 86: 1135–1143.

69. Kleiner A, Shakhnovich E (2007) The mechanical unfolding of ubiquitin through all-atom Monte Carlo simulation with a Go-type potential. Biophys J 92: 2054–2061.

70. Yoo BC, Krapfenbauer K, Cairns N, Belay G, Bajo M, et al. (2002) Overexpressed protein disulfide isomerase in brains of patients with sporadic Creutzfeldt-Jakob disease. Neurosci Lett 334: 196–200.

71. Giannandrea M, Bianchi V, Mignogna ML, Sirri A, Carrabino S, et al. (2010) Mutations in the small GTPase gene RAB39B are responsible for X-linked mental retardation associated with autism, epilepsy, and macrocephaly. Am J Hum Genet 86: 185–195.

72. Zeiger W, Ito D, Swetlik C, Oh-Hora M, Villereal ML, et al. (2011) Stanniocalcin 2 Is a Negative Modulator of Store-Operated Calcium Entry. Mol Cell Biol 31: 3710–3722.

73. Surgucheva I, Park BC, Yue BY, Tomarev S, Surguchov A (2005) Interaction of myocilin with gamma-synuclein affects its secretion and aggregation. Cell Mol Neurobiol 25: 1009–1033.

74. Giasson BI, Forman MS, Higuchi M, Golbe LI, Graves CL, et al. (2003) Initiation and synergistic fibrillization of tau and alpha-synuclein. Science 300: 636–640.

75. Eller M, Williams DR (2011) alpha-Synuclein in Parkinson disease and other neurodegenerative disorders. Clin Chem Lab Med 49: 403–408.

76. McKinnon SJ (2003) Glaucoma: ocular Alzheimer's disease? Front Biosci 8: s1140–s1156.

77. Hentze H, Lin XY, Choi MS, Porter AG (2003) Critical role for cathepsin B in mediating caspase-1-dependent interleukin-18 maturation and caspase-1-independent necrosis triggered by the microbial toxin nigericin. Cell Death Differ 10: 956–968.

# 15

# A New Safety Concern for Glaucoma Treatment Demonstrated by Mass Spectrometry Imaging of Benzalkonium Chloride Distribution in the Eye, an Experimental Study in Rabbits

Françoise Brignole-Baudouin[1,2,3,4,9]*, Nicolas Desbenoit[1,2,3,5], Gregory Hamm[8], Hong Liang[1,2,3,4], Jean-Pierre Both[6], Alain Brunelle[5], Isabelle Fournier[7], Vincent Guerineau[5], Raphael Legouffe[8], Jonathan Stauber[8], David Touboul[5], Maxence Wisztorski[7], Michel Salzet[7], Olivier Laprevote[9], Christophe Baudouin[1,2,3,4,10,11]

1 INSERM, U968, Paris, France, 2 UPMC Univ Paris 06, UMR_S 968, Institut de la Vision, Paris, France, 3 CNRS, UMR_7210, Paris, France, 4 Centre Hospitalier National d'Ophtalmologie des Quinze-Vingts, INSERM-DHOS CIC 503, Paris, France, 5 Centre de recherche de Gif, Institut de Chimie des Substances Naturelles, CNRS, Gif-sur-Yvette, France, 6 Laboratoire d'Intégration des Systèmes et des Technologies, CEA-LIST, Gif-sur-Yvette, France, 7 Laboratoire de Spectrométrie de Masse Biologique, Fondamentale et Appliquée, EA 4550, Université Lille Nord de France – Université Lille 1, Villeneuve d'Ascq, France, 8 Imabiotech Campus Cité Scientifique, Villeneuve d'Ascq, France, 9 Chimie Toxicologie Analytique et Cellulaire, EA 4463, Faculté des Sciences Pharmaceutiques et Biologiques, Université Paris Descartes, Paris, France, 10 Université Versailles Saint-Quentin-en-Yvelines, Versailles, France, 11 Assistance Publique - Hôpitaux de Paris Hôpital Ambroise Paré, Service d'Ophtalmologie, Boulogne-Billancourt, France

## Abstract

We investigated in a rabbit model, the eye distribution of topically instilled benzalkonium (BAK) chloride a commonly used preservative in eye drops using mass spectrometry imaging. Three groups of three New Zealand rabbits each were used: a control one without instillation, one receiving 0.01%BAK twice a day for 5 months and one with 0.2%BAK one drop a day for 1 month. After sacrifice, eyes were embedded and frozen in tragacanth gum. Serial cryosections were alternately deposited on glass slides for histological (hematoxylin-eosin staining) and immunohistological controls (CD45, RLA-DR and vimentin for inflammatory cell infiltration as well as vimentin for Müller glial cell activation) and ITO or stainless steel plates for MSI experiments using Matrix-assisted laser desorption ionization time-of-flight. The MSI results were confirmed by a round-robin study on several adjacent sections conducted in two different laboratories using different sample preparation methods, mass spectrometers and data analysis softwares. BAK was shown to penetrate healthy eyes even after a short duration and was not only detected on the ocular surface structures, but also in deeper tissues, especially in sensitive areas involved in glaucoma pathophysiology, such as the trabecular meshwork and the optic nerve areas, as confirmed by images with histological stainings. CD45-, RLA-DR- and vimentin-positive cells increased in treated eyes. Vimentin was found only in the inner layer of retina in normal eyes and increased in all retinal layers in treated eyes, confirming an activation response to a cell stress. This ocular toxicological study confirms the presence of BAK preservative in ocular surface structures as well as in deeper structures involved in glaucoma disease. The inflammatory cell infiltration and Müller glial cell activation confirmed the deleterious effect of BAK. Although these results were obtained in animals, they highlight the importance of the safety-first principle for the treatment of glaucoma patients.

**Editor:** Bang V. Bui, Univeristy of Melbourne, Australia

**Funding:** This study was supported by the Agence Nationale de la Recherche (grant ANR-09-PIRI-0012 MASDA-EYE). The funders had no role in study design, data collection and analysis, decision to publish, or preparation of the manuscript.

**Competing Interests:** The authors acknowledge the fact that three authors are employed by Imabiotech Campus Cité Scientifique, a company specializing in mass spectrometry. These authors made independent analyses that confirmed the results obtained by the other members of the consortium in different laboratories.

* E-mail: francoise.brignole@inserm.fr

## Introduction

Glaucoma is a severe optic neuropathy leading to blindness without treatment and affecting more than 70 million people worldwide. This insidious disease is the main cause of irreversible blindness and is associated with increased intraocular pressure due to a resistance in the trabecular meshwork outflow pathway of aqueous humor [1]. Once diagnosed, treatment must be taken throughout life to prevent or halt retinal ganglion cell loss and visual deterioration. Consequently, patients have to be treated for the rest of their life with intraocular pressure (IOP)-lowering multi-dose eye drops (1). Most of these eye drops contain a preservative: the most commonly used is benzalkonium chloride (BAK), a quaternary ammonium salt composed of a mixture of benzodo-decinium $C_{21}H_{38}N^+$ (BAK $C_{12}$) and myristalkonium $C_{23}H_{42}N^+$

(BAK $C_{14}$) chlorides. BAK is a cationic surfactant and tensioactive compound, acting as a detergent for the lipid layer of the tear film as well as for the lipids of cell plasma membranes. It is reputed to increase bioavailability or penetration of active compounds and can be used as a penetration enhancer [2,3]. At a concentration ranging from 0.004 to 0.2% in eye drops, this preservative is required by pharmacopeia guidelines to prevent the multidose eye drop containers from bacterial and fungi contamination [4,5]. Although it has the advantage of inducing fewer allergic-type side effects and of being relatively well tolerated, it has been reported to induce ocular surface disorders combining irritation, inflammation and cell death processes, especially in long-term treatment [6]. There is a growing body of evidence that BAK induces apoptosis, oxidative stress and inflammation on the ocular surface epithelia, unlike antiglaucoma active compounds that have been demonstrated to be safe for epithelial cells [6]. While the deleterious effects of BAK could be negligible for a short-term treatment, they need to be considered for long-term or repeated treatment such as in chronic open-angle glaucoma. In this case, patients are most often treated for the rest of their life, often with several BAK-containing eye drops, since about 40% of patients require multiple therapies to control their IOP and prevent further optic nerve damage [7]. The ocular surface structures, tear film, cornea, conjunctiva as well as the eyelids are the tissues most apparently involved in treatment tolerance. BAK-containing antiglaucoma eye drops have been reported to cause disruption of the blood–aqueous barrier inducing cystoid macular edema following cataract surgery [8].

Little is known about BAK penetration and distribution in the eye. A study reported its presence in the conjunctiva after a single drop of BAK up to 7 days after instillation [9]. In an in vivo study, Chou et al. found abnormal electroretinograms (ERG) with a reduction in the a- and b-wave amplitudes in rabbits receiving subconjunctival injections of beta-blockers associated with BAK, showing a pathway for BAK to reach the eye's posterior segment [10]. Recently, Garrett and colleagues found BAK in the outer periphery of a human donor eye using a mass spectrometry imaging (MSI) technique [11]. In fact, the use of MSI to study tissue distribution is continuously growing. In contrast to the autoradiography technique classically used for tissue distribution analysis of a radio-labeled compound, MSI by matrix-assisted laser desorption/ionization (MALDI) is a powerful label-free technique that can identify a compound as well as its metabolites by detecting specific peaks in their mass spectra with a histologic resolution of about 50 μm [12,13,14,15]. It has already been used for pharmacokinetics studies of drug distribution in the eye [16]. Actually, in the particular case of glaucoma treatment, it is crucial to ensure the absence of adverse effects, not only for the ocular surface tissues to promote tolerance and compliance, but also for deeper ocular tissues such as the trabecular meshwork, lens, retina or optic nerve to preserve visual function. Our objective was therefore to investigate BAK penetration using MSI in a rabbit model. This enabled us to see whether was able to reach sensitive ocular areas involved in glaucoma physiopathology that could compromise treatment efficacy and threaten visual function over the long term.

## Materials and Methods

### Chemicals

HPLC-grade acetonitrile and water were purchased from BioSolve (Valkenswaard, Netherlands) or Sigma-Aldrich (Saint-Quentin Fallavier, France). Alpha-cyano-4-hydroxycinnamic acid (CHCA), trifluoroacetic acid (TFA), hematoxylin, eosin, ethanol and benzalkonium chlorides (BAK) were purchased from Sigma-Aldrich (Saint-Quentin Fallavier, France). The chemical structures of benzalkonium homologs BAK $C_{12}$ and BAK $C_{14}$ (2:1) used in this study are presented in figure 1.

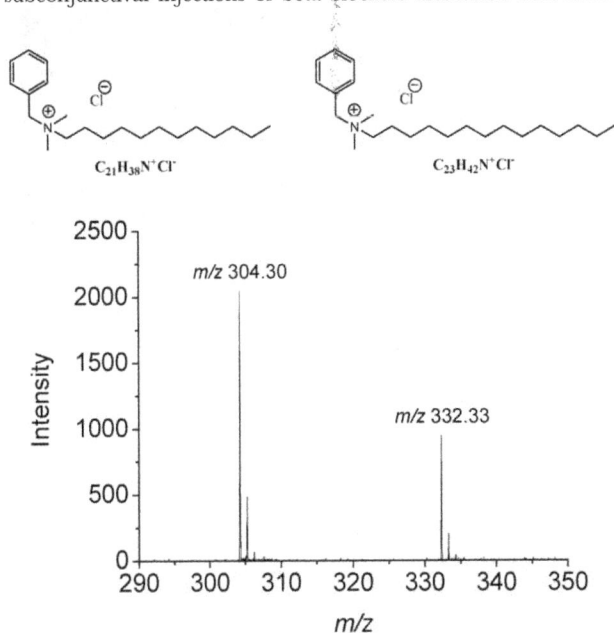

**Figure 1. Chemical structures and MALDI-TOF spectra.** Chemical structure and MALDI-TOF spectrum of benzalkonium homologs used in this study, BAK $C_{12}$ and BAK $C_{14}$, are presented with their respective MALDI-TOF spectrum in positive ion mode. The BAK solution instilled in the rabbit eyes contained two thirds of BAK $C_{12}$ (m/z 304.30) and one third of BAK $C_{14}$ (m/z 332.33).

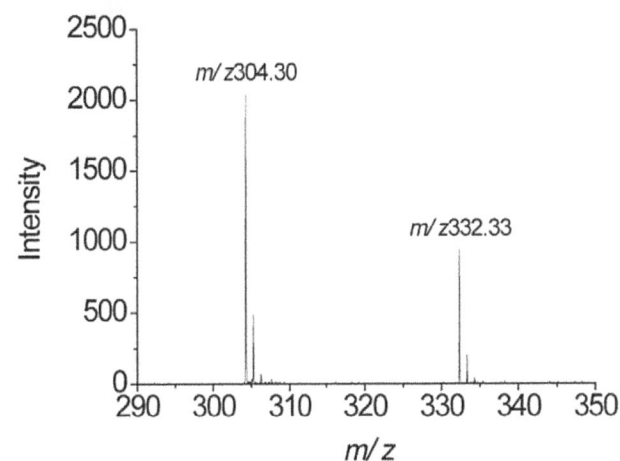

**Figure 2. MALDI-TOF imaging of whole eye section of a control rabbit.** MALDI-TOF imaging shows the absence of benzalkonium chloride (BAK) in the control eye. (a) Histology image of an adjacent cryosection stained with hematoxylin-eosin (HE) showing three areas of interest: cornea (area 1), nasal iridocorneal angle (area 2) and near the optic nerve (area 3). (b, c) Overlays between HE and MALDI-TOF images of BAK $C_{12}$ and $C_{14}$ eye distributions at m/z 304.32 and 332.36, respectively. Intensities of the ions are represented in colour, based on the intensity scale provided (from black to white). Field of view 18× 6 mm. (d, e, f) MALDI-TOF mass spectra extracted from areas 1, 2 and 3, respectively confirming the absence of BAK $C_{12}$ and $C_{14}$.

## Animals

All rabbits used in this study (n = 3 in each group) were white New Zealand albino rabbits weighing 2–2.5 kg and were purchased from Cegav, St Mars-d'Egrenne, France. They were housed individually in stainless-steel wire-bottom cages in environmentally controlled rooms with a 12-h light/12-h dark cycle, a 30–70% humidity range and a22–24°C temperature range. They were allowed to drink tap water and to eat *ad libitum*.

## Ethics Statement

This study was conducted in accordance with the Association for Research in Vision and Ophthalmology (ARVO) statement for the Use of Animals in Ophthalmic and Vision research and was approved by the local ethics committee for animal experimentation at the Faculty of Pharmaceutical and Biological Sciences, Sorbonne Paris Cité University.

## Study Design

New Zealand albino rabbits were instilled with BAK solutions in PBS containing 65.7% $C_{12}$ and 30.7% $C_{14}$ homologs; a MALDI mass spectrum is shown in Figure 1. Two different toxicity models were used in this study. The first one, called the Low Chronic model (LCm) was intended to simulate chronic use with a low BAK concentration for a long time, *i.e.*, instillation of one drop of 0.01% BAK concentration, the most commonly used concentration in eye drops, twice a day for 5 months. The second model, called the High Sub-Chronic model (HSCm) was used to mimic a subchronic use at a high concentration for a shorter time with a 0.2% BAK concentration once daily for 1 month. This latter model was selected in order to maximize the toxic effect and to be able to see the eye penetration pathways. Non-instilled rabbits were used as controls.

## Sample Processing

After sacrifice, the eyes were quickly enucleated and embedded in tragacanth gum (Alfa Aesar, Schiltigheim, France) and frozen at −80°C. Serial cryosections (14 μm thick) were cut at −30°C with a CM3050-S cryostat (Leica Microsystems SA, Nanterre, France) and deposited on stainless steel plates for MALDI MSI experiments. Before MSI analyses, the samples were dried in a vacuum, at a pressure of a few hectopascals for 15 min, with no further treatment. Optical images were recorded with an Olympus BX51 microscope (Olympus, Rungis, France) equipped with ×1.25 to ×50 lenses and a Color View I camera, monitored by Cell[B] software (Soft Imaging System, GmbH, Münster, Germany). Cryosections of rabbit eyes adjacent to sections dedicated to MSI were stained with hematoxylin-eosin (HE) and analyzed using a DM5000 optic microscope (Leica Microsystems SA, Nanterre, France) in order to align the MS images with histology patterns.

## MALDI Mass Mpectrometry Imaging

MALDI mass spectrometry images were acquired in two different laboratories, which are named in the following text ImaBiotech and CNRS-ICSN, respectively.

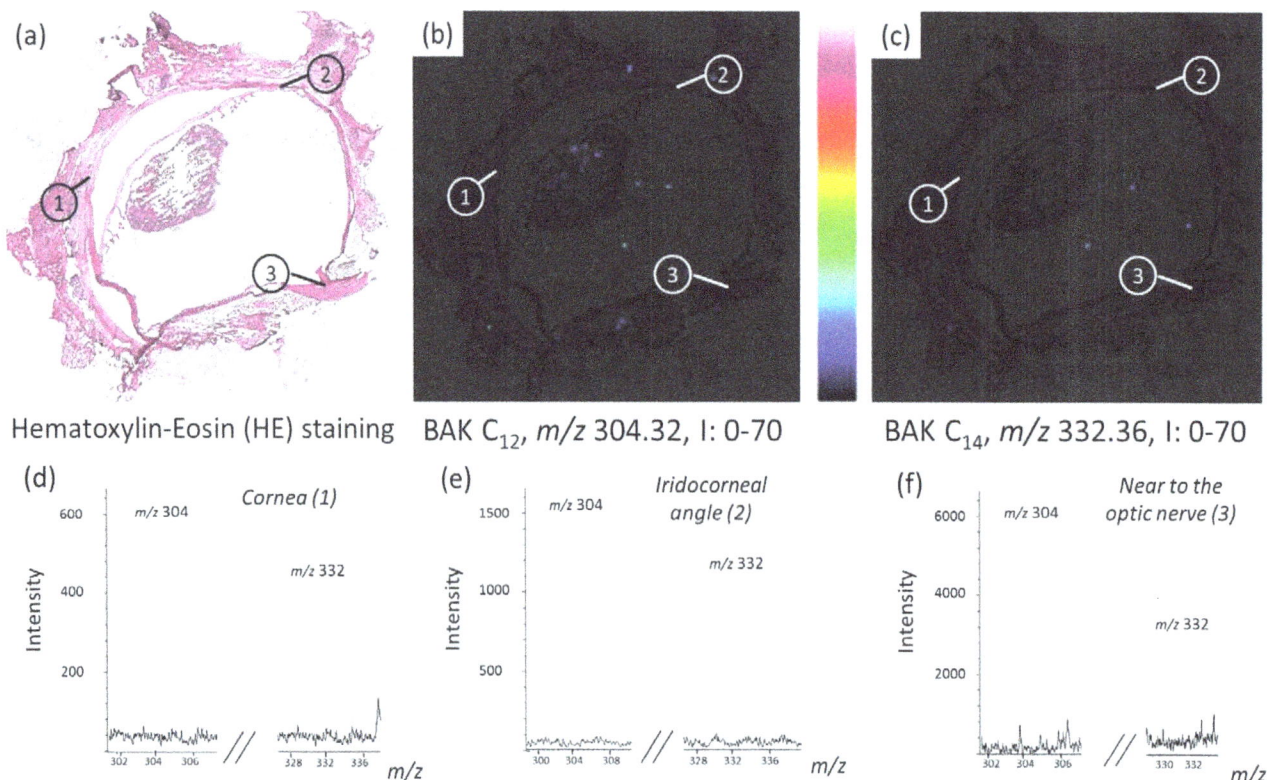

**Figure 3. MALDI-TOF imaging of whole eye section of a rabbit instilled twice a day with one drop of 0.01% benzalkonium chloride (BAK) for 5 months.** MALDI-TOF imaging shows the BAK distribution in a BAK-treated eye. (a) Histology image of an adjacent cryosection stained with hematoxylin-eosin (HE) showing three areas of interest: cornea (area 1), nasal iridocorneal angle (area 2) and optic nerve area (area 3). (b, c) Overlays between HE staining and MALDI-TOF ion images of BAK $C_{12}$ and $C_{14}$ distributions in whole eye section at *m/z* 304.30 and 332.33, respectively. (d, e) MALDI-TOF ion images of BAK $C_{12}$ and $C_{14}$ distributions at *m/z* 304.30 and 332.33, respectively. Intensities of the ions are represented in colour, based on the intensity scale provided (from black to white). Field of view 16×15 mm. (f, g, h) MALDI-TOF mass spectra extracted from areas 1, 2 and 3, respectively, showing BAK $C_{12}$ and $C_{14}$ ion peaks.

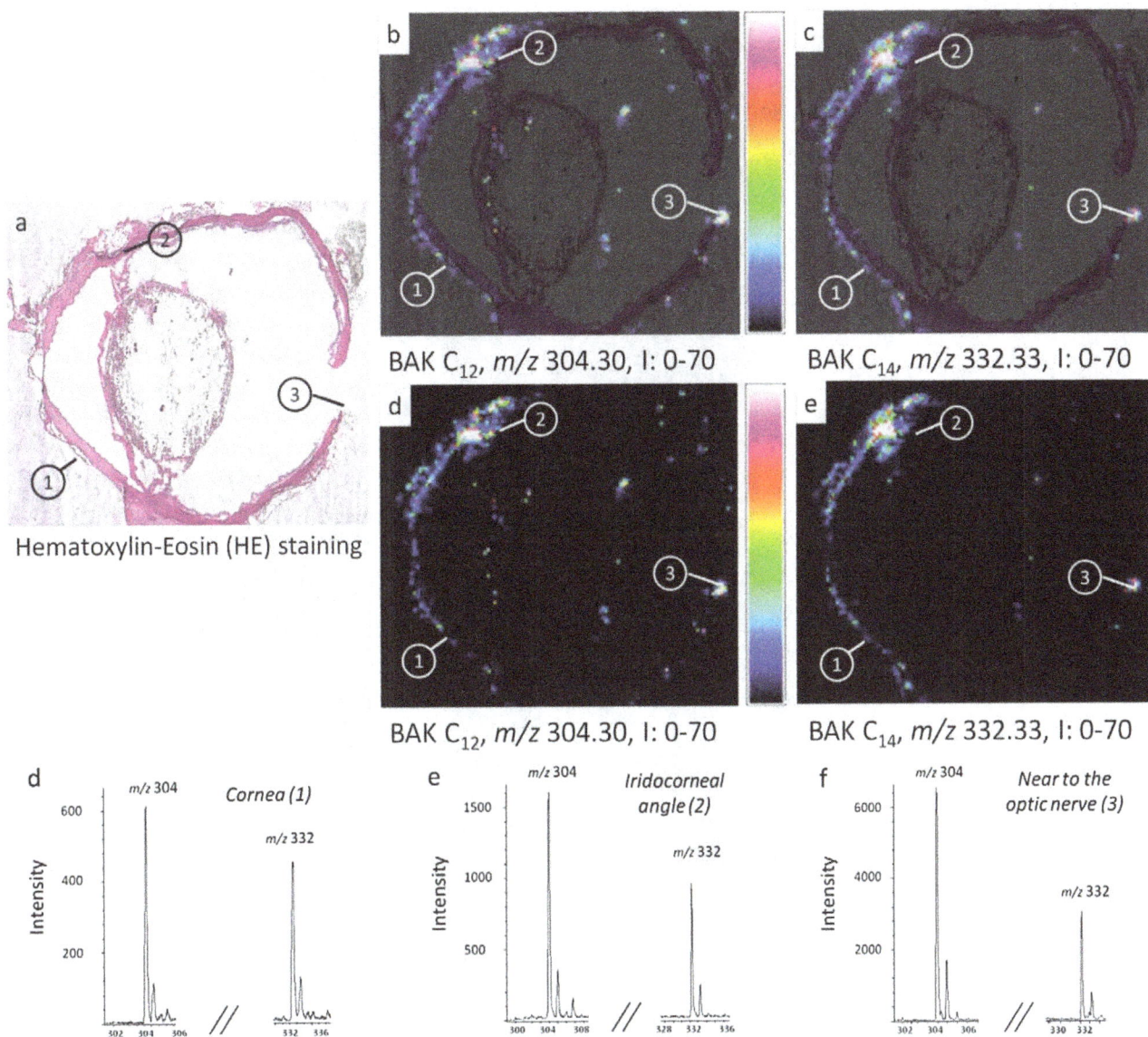

Figure 4. Round-robin experiment using the AutoFlex speed LRF MALDI-TOF mass spectrometer (ImaBiotech). MALDI-TOF imaging generated by the AutoFlex speed LRF MALDI-TOF mass spectrometer (ImaBiotech) shows the BAK distribution in whole eye section of a rabbit instilled once a day with one drop of 0.2% benzalkonium chloride (BAK) for 1 month. (a) Histology image of an adjacent cryosection stained with hematoxylin-eosin (HE) showing three areas of interest: cornea (area 1), nasal iridocorneal angle (area 2) and optic nerve area (area 3). (b, c) Overlays between HE staining and MALDI-TOF ion images of BAK $C_{12}$ and $C_{14}$ distributions in whole eye section at $m/z$ 304.30 and 332.33, respectively. (d, e) MALDI-TOF ion images of BAK $C_{12}$ and $C_{14}$ distributions in whole eye section at $m/z$ 304.30 and $m/z$ 332.33, respectively. Intensities of the ions are represented in colour, based on the intensity scale provided (from black to white). Field of view 8×10 mm. (f, g, h) MALDI-TOF mass spectra extracted from areas 1, 2 and 3, respectively, showing BAK $C_{12}$ and $C_{14}$ ion peaks.

**MALDI mass spectrometry imaging (ImaBiotech).** Optical images of each stained section were acquired using an HP scan (Hewlett-Packard, Palo Alto, CA, USA). CHCA at 10 mg/mL in acetonitrile/water/trifluoroacetic acid (ACN/H$_2$O/TFA, 60/40/0.1, V/V/V) was used as the matrix solution. The matrix solution was sprayed onto the eye sections using the SunCollect automatic sprayer (SunChrom, Friedrichsdorf, Germany). Each layer was sprayed at a 20-µL/min flow rate, and 15 layers were overlaid to achieve a homogeneous matrix coating. MS images were acquired with an AutoFlex speed LRF MALDI-TOF mass spectrometer (Bruker Daltonics, Bremen, Germany) equipped with a Smart beam II laser used at a repetition rate of 1000 Hz. All instrumental parameters were optimized before the imaging experiment on standard samples of BAK $C_{12}$ and $C_{14}$ at $m/z$ 304.30 and $m/z$ 332.33, respectively. Positive ion mass spectra were acquired within the 100- to 1000-$m/z$ range. The mass spectrometer was operated in the reflectron mode and the mass spectrum obtained for each image position corresponds to the averaged mass spectra of 700 consecutive laser shots at the same location. Two image raster steps were selected: (1) 150 µm for MS imaging of eye sections from the control rabbit (Figure 2) and from a rabbit treated for 5 months with 0.01% BAK solution (Figures 3 and 4) and (2) 80 µm for the rabbit treated 1 month with 0.2% BAK solution (Figure 5). Flex Control 3.0 and Flex Imaging 2.1 software packages (Bruker Daltonics, Bremen, Germany) were used to control the mass spectrometer, set imaging

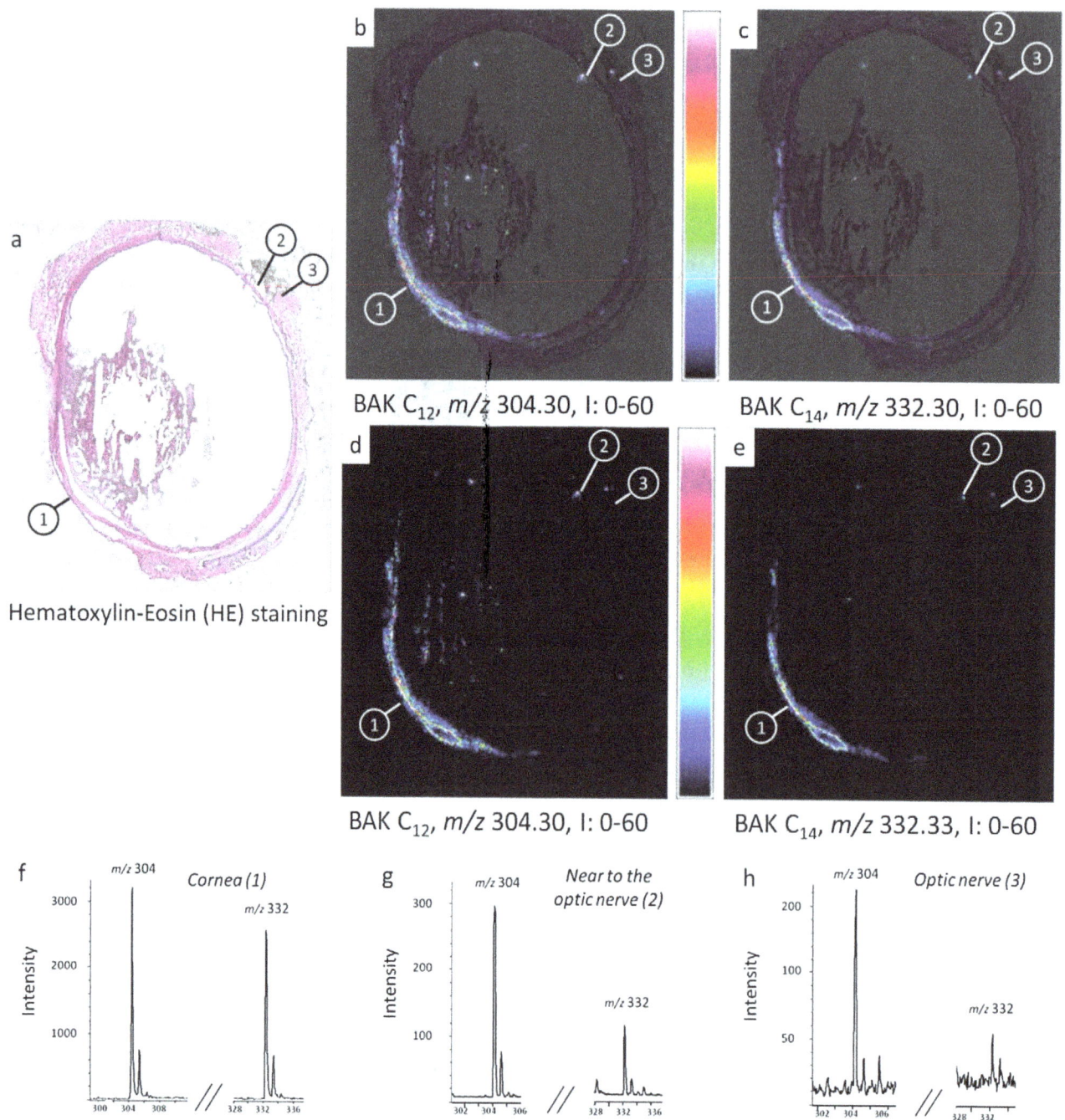

Hematoxylin-Eosin (HE) staining

BAK C$_{12}$, *m/z* 304.30, I: 0-60

BAK C$_{14}$, *m/z* 332.30, I: 0-60

BAK C$_{12}$, *m/z* 304.30, I: 0-60

BAK C$_{14}$, *m/z* 332.33, I: 0-60

**Figure 5. Round-robin experiment using the 4800 MALDI-TOF/TOF mass spectrometer (ICSN-CNRS).** MALDI-TOF imaging generated by the 4800 MALDI-TOF/TOF mass spectrometer (ICSN-CNRS) shows the BAK distribution in whole eye section of a rabbit instilled once a day with one drop of 0.2% benzalkonium chloride (BAK) for 1 month. (a) Histology image of an adjacent cryosection stained with hematoxylin-eosin (HE) showing three areas of interest: cornea (area 1), near to optic nerve area (area 2) and optic nerve (area 3). (b, c) Overlays between HE staining and MALDI-TOF ion images of BAK C$_{12}$ and C$_{14}$ distributions in whole eye section at *m/z* 304.32 and *m/z* 332.36, respectively. (d, e) MALDI-TOF ion images of BAK C$_{12}$ and C$_{14}$ distributions in whole eye section at *m/z* 304.30 and *m/z* 332.33, respectively, with intensity scale from 0 to 714. Intensities of the ions are represented in color, based on the intensity scale provided (from black to red). Field of view 18×23 mm. (f, g, h) MALDI-TOF mass spectra extracted from areas 1, 2 and 3, respectively, showing BAK C$_{12}$ and C$_{14}$ ion peaks.

parameters and visualize imaging data. After MALDI image acquisition, the matrix was washed off the sections in 100% methanol and conventional hematoxylin-eosin (HE) staining was performed.

**MALDI mass spectrometry imaging (ICSN, CNRS).** CHCA matrix solution at 10 mg/mL concentrations

in acetonitrile/water/trifluoroacetic acid (ACN/H$_2$O/TFA, 60/40/0.1, V/V/V) was prepared for positive ion mode analysis. Rabbit eye sections were homogeneously covered by matrix using a TM-Sprayer (HTX-Imaging, Carrboro, NC, USA). In this system, the nozzle/air spray system is heated to 120°C and coupled to an isocratic pump, which provides a constant flow rate of

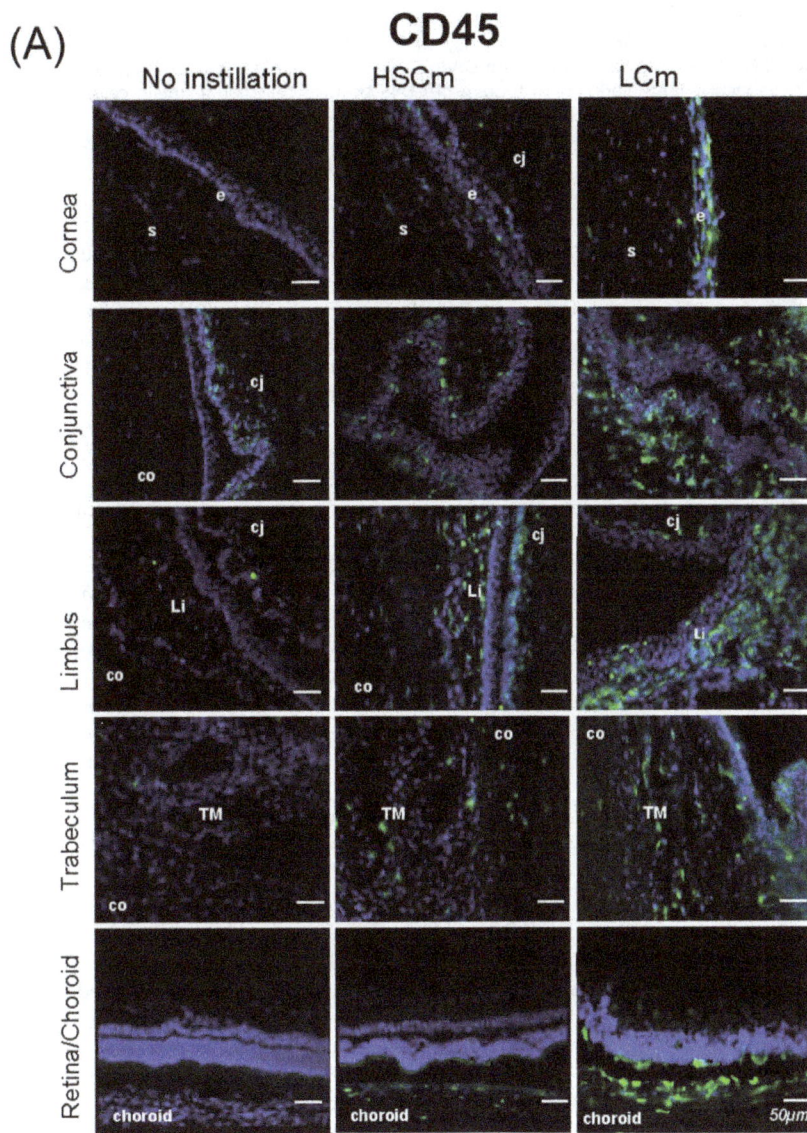

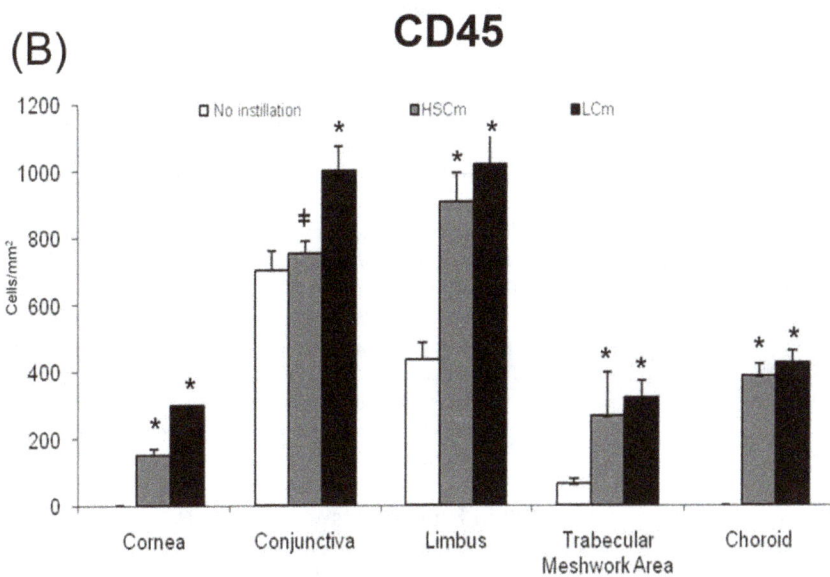

**Figure 6. CD45-positive cell infiltration. (A)** Immunofluorescence staining of leucocytes with CD45 (in green) in rabbit eye cryosections in normal noninstilled rabbit eyes compared with rabbit eye instilled with BAK 0.01% twice a day for 5 months (Low Chronic model, LCm) and 0.2% once a day for 1 month (High Sub-Chronic model, HSCm). Nuclei are stained in blue with DAPI. Scale bar, 50 mm. Cj: conjunctiva; Co: cornea; Li: limbus; s: corneal stroma; e: superficial epithelium; TM: trabecular meshwork. **(B)** Histogram of CD45 positive cells count (mean cells/mm$^2$±SD) *$P<0.001$ compared with the normal eye; I $P<0.0001$ HsCm versus LCm.

240 μL/min of matrix solution. The MALDI target plate is anchored on an x–y axis stage, and matrix coating is achieved by moving the sample plate under the fixed nozzle/air system at a linear velocity of 120 cm/min. Data were acquired with a 4800 MALDI TOF/TOF mass spectrometer (AB SCIEX, Les Ulis, France) equipped with a 200-Hz tripled-frequency Nd/YAG pulsed laser (355 nm) and an electrostatic mirror, providing a routine mass resolution of about 15,000 in MS mode. The data were acquired in the positive reflectron ion mode at an accelerating potential of 20 kV and a delayed extraction of450 ns (80%). Internal mass calibration was achieved using known ions present at the sample surface such as $m/z$ 379.09 (protonated CHCA dimer) or 877.73 (triacylglycerol, [TG (54:7) + H]$^+$). The number of laser shots per pixel was set to 120. The distance between two adjacent pixels was set to 80 μm, which roughly corresponds to the laser spot diameter and which thus defines the lateral resolution. This leads to acquisition times of several hours, depending on the surface size analyzed. The images were recorded using 4000 Series Imaging software (www.maldi-msi.org, M. Stoeckli, Novartis Pharma, Basel, Switzerland), processed using Tissue View software (AB Sciex, Les Ulis, France), and are presented in Figure 5.

## Immunohistological Study in Cryosections and Positive Cell Counts

Whole rabbit eye cryosections were fixed in 4% PFA for 15 mn at 4°C, washed in PBS with 1% BSA, permeabilized with 0.01%-diluted Triton X100® (Sigma Chemical Company, St Louis, MO, USA) for 5 min and incubated for 2 h at 4°C with mouse immunoglobulins directed against rabbit pan-leukocyte antigen CD45 (1:50; CBL1412, Cymbus Biotechnology, Chandlers Ford, UK), rabbit MHC Class II Leukocyte Antigen RLA-DR (1:100; RDR34, Beckman coulter, Miami, FL, USA) and vimentin (V9; 1/50, Dako, Glostrup, Denmark)in order to detect inflammatory cell infiltration: leukocytes, antigen-presenting cells and Müller cell activation, respectively. Normal mouse IgG (Beckman Coulter, Miami, FL, USA) were used as negative controls of fluorescence. Regarding vimentin, it is normally expressed by epithelial cells, keratocytes and fibroblasts but is highly expressed by mesenchymal infiltrating cells [17], mainly immune cells, and was used here to confirm the inflammatory infiltration and also to investigate the level of Müller glial cell activation [18]. Sections were then incubated with the secondary antibody (Alexa Fluor®488 anti-mouse immunoglobulin, 1:500) for 1 h. After three washes in PBS, they were incubated in DAPI for 3 min (Sigma-Aldrich) to stain the nuclei. Slides were then mounted in an antifade medium (Vectashield; Vector Laboratories). Images were digitized using an epifluorescence microscope DM5000 (Leica, Wetzlar, Germany). Immunopositive cells were counted on cryosections from three rabbits using a 100×100-μm reticule in the cornea, conjunctiva, limbus, trabecular meshwork area and retina.

## Statistical Analysis

The results are expressed as means ± standard errors (SE). The groups for analysis were compared using factorial analysis of variance (ANOVA) followed by the Fisher method (GraphPad Software, La Jolla, CA, USA).

## Results

### Identification of BAK C$_{12}$/C$_{14}$ Homolog Mass Spectra

A MALDI mass spectrum of BAK solution was first recorded as a reference sample. Two intense ion signals at $m/z$ 304.30 (BAK C$_{12}$) and $m/z$ 332.32 (BAK C$_{14}$) were detected with a relative ratio of 2 to 1 corresponding to the relative concentration in the solution (Figure 1). Then sections of non-instilled normal rabbit eyes were analyzed according to the two MSI protocols (Figure 2). No signal corresponding to BAK C$_{12}$ or C$_{14}$was detected in the ion images or in the extracted mass spectra of the cornea (area 1), nasal iridocorneal angle (area 2) and near the optic nerve (area 3). This experiment clearly indicated that the control sample was not contaminated by BAK and that no natural product in the eye could interfere with BAK signals. For all following MSI experiments, we used complete MS images with corresponding adjacent HE-stained histology images (a in all figures) and we constructed overlays (b, c in all figures) of HE staining and BAK ion images (d, e in all figures) in order to visualize the anatomical structures of the eye. We particularly focused on three areas of interest: (1) the ocular surface with cornea and conjunctiva as the first ocular defense, (2) the iridocorneal angle and (3) the optic nerve area, the two ocular structures involved in glaucoma. Parts of the mass spectra are presented showing the peaks of BAK C$_{12}$ and C$_{14}$.

In instilled rabbit eyes–with one drop twice a day for 5 months of 0.01% BAK (LCm; Figure 3) or with one drop a day for 1 month of 0.2% BAK (HsCm; Figure 4) – BAK was detected in the cornea, the conjunctiva and the limbus, as expected with a topically applied compound. Furthermore, concerning the Low Chronic Model (LCm), similar results have been obtained between the 4800 MALDI-TOF/TOF and the AutoFlex speed LRF MALDI-TOF mass spectrometers. Interestingly, the presence of BAK was also found in deeper structures such as the sclera, near the trabecular meshwork, the filter primarily impaired in glaucoma and increasing intraocular pressure, and finally the optic nerve and its surrounding area, the structure that anti-glaucoma treatments specifically aim at protecting. Some hot spots were also observed in the lens showing BAK penetration *via* a transcorneal/aqueous humor pathway (Figure 4). Hot colored spots were also seen surrounding the eyeball, this peripheral localization suggesting that the conjunctival/scleral route could be another BAK penetration pathway to reach the retina. Moreover, a series of images were acquired from adjacent sections of an animal to assess the repeatability of the results. Supplementary figures of the MS images of whole eyes are given to show such consistency (Figures S1 A, B). More than a dozen of full eye images were performed on the three groups that received the different treatments. Other images were taken by focusing only on very specific areas of the eye (cornea, iridocorneal angle, retina, optic nerve region) and were repeatedly verified, in order to assess the consistency of the results.

### Round-Robin Experiments

A round-robin study on two adjacent sections was set up by two laboratories involved in the study (ImaBiotech and ICSN, CNRS) using different sample preparation methods, mass spectrometers

# RLA-DR

(A)

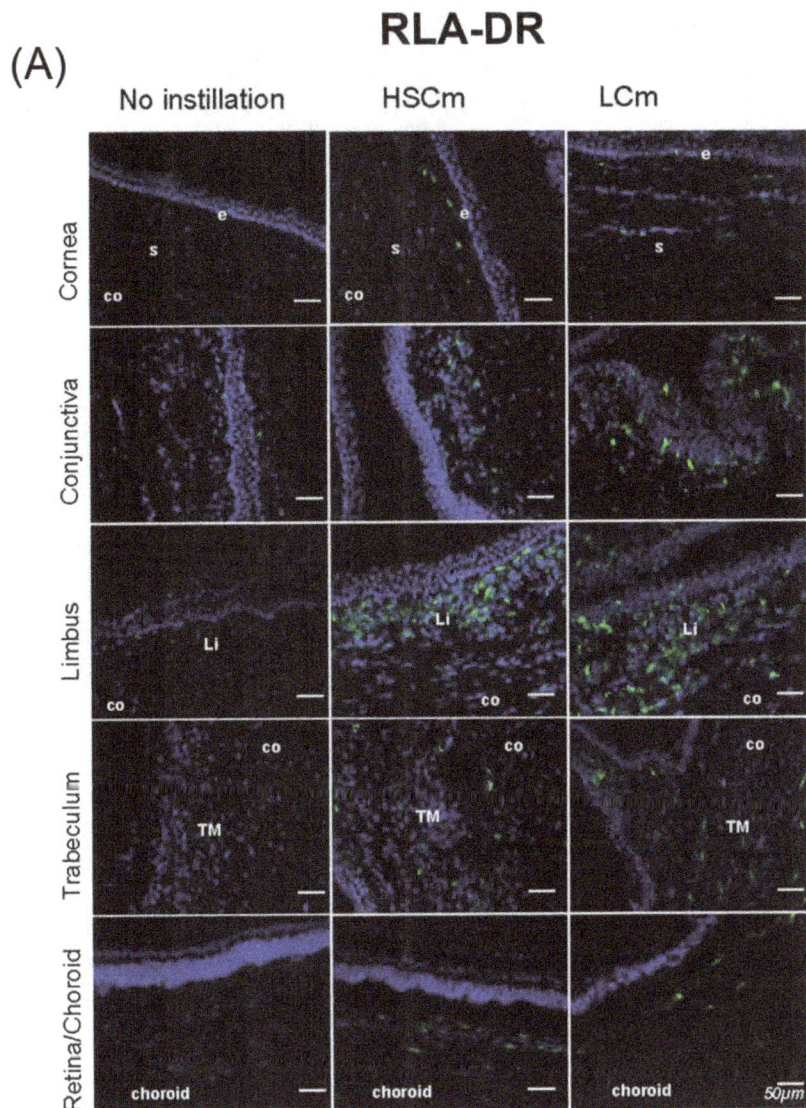

(B)

# RLA-DR

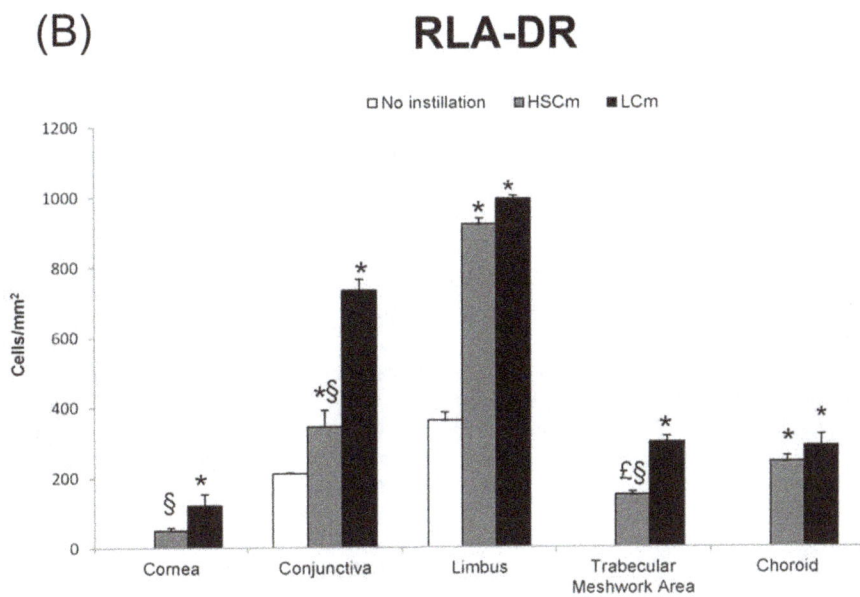

**Figure 7. RLA-DR-positive cell infiltration.** (A) Immunofluorescence staining of antigen presenting cells expressing RLA-DR (in green) in rabbit eye cryosections in normal non instilled rabbit eyes compared with rabbit eye instilled with BAK 0.01% twice a day for 5 months (Low Chronic model, LCm) and 0.2% once a day for 1 month (High SubChronic model, HSCm). Nuclei in blue are stained with DAPI. Scale bar, 50 mm. Cj: conjunctiva; Co: cornea; Li: limbus; s: corneal stroma; e: superficial epithelium; TM: trabecular meshwork. (B) Histogram of RLA-DR positive cells count (mean cells/$mm^2 \pm$SD) *$P<0.001$ compared with the normal eye or £ $P<0.001$ compared with the normal eye; § $P<0.01$ HsCm versus LCm.

and data analysis software, as described above, in order to test the robustness of the entire MSI method independently of the instrumentation. A set of four adjacent eye sections was prepared. The MALDI matrix was deposited by the Sun Collect sprayer for two sections and by the TM-Sprayer for two additional sections. Then two sections prepared using each method were analyzed by each spectrometer, i.e., the 4800 MALDI TOF/TOF and the AutoFlex, respectively. Finally, the dedicated software was subsequently used for data analysis. Two of the images are shown in Figures 4 and 5. The results were very similar: BAK localizations were the same with the two methods, which demonstrated the robustness of MSI. These results were also validated for both toxicological models differing in the time and the concentrations used and showed similar results (Figures 2–5). Intensities in the spectra could not be compared between the two round-robin experiments (Figures 4 and 5). The intensities could nevertheless be directly compared between different areas of the same ion image. These comparisons could be made only if we could assume that the environment had no effect on BAK desorption/ionization, indicating that the same amount of BAK in different areas of the eye induced the same intensities in the spectra. Figure 4 shows that the intensity of BAK was higher in the optic nerve than in the iridocorneal angle and in the cornea, for the rabbit eye instilled twice a day with one drop of 0.01% BAK for 5 months (a factor of ~10). An opposite variation was observed for the rabbit eye instilled once a day with one drop of 0.2% BAK for 1 month, in which BAK was more concentrated in the cornea than in the optic nerve (greater than tenfold concentration; Figures 4 and 5). Small relative variations between intensities of BAK $C_{12}$ and BAK $C_{14}$, compared to the spectrum shown in Figure 1, were observed, especially in the cornea (Figures 3f and 4f), possibly indicating a different penetration of BAK in cornea depending on the length of the chain.

## Immunohistological Study in Cryosections and Positive Cell Counts

In normal non instilled eyes, CD45, RLA-DR and vimentin positive cells were not found in the cornea, and the retina/choroid, only few CD45 positive cells could be observed in the trabecular meshwork area (Figures 6, 7, 8). Conversely, positive cells are normally found in the conjunctiva and the limbus.

In the eyes instilled with BAK, immunohistological examinations clearly showed globally higher expressions of the markers tested in the LCm than in the HsCm, except for the retina/choroid area, suggesting that time had a greater effect than the BAK concentration (Figures 6, 7, 8). As RLA-DR-positive cells represent a cell subpopulation of the whole CD45-positive cell population, CD45- and RLA-DR-positive cell populations increased in the same manner but with a lower density for the RLA-DR population (Figures 6 and 7).

No positive cells could be found in the normal cornea, while CD45 and RLA-DR increased in the HsCmodel ($p<0.001$ versus control for CD45, non statistically significant increase for RLA-DR) and many positive cells were observed in the LCm ($p<0.001$ versus control; Figures 6B and 7B).

In the normal conjunctiva, CD45-positive cells were observed as expected, the conjunctiva containing lymphocytes as well as

dendritic cells. These CD45-positive cells, however, increased in the two toxicological models with a tremendous increase in the LCm ($p<0.0001$ versus control and HsCm) but the difference between HsCm and control was not statistically significant (Figure 6B). The number of RLA-DR positive cells increased in the two models ($p<0.0001$ versus control) with greater values in LCm than in HsCm ($p<0.01$, figure 7B).

In the limbus, we observed an important increase in CD45 and RLA-DR positive cells ($p<0.0001$ versus control) without any difference between the two models. The same patterns were found for CD45 in the trabecular meshwork area with the same statistically significant difference with the normal rabbit control ($p<0.0001$). The number of RLA-DR positive cells increased in this area in the two models, with higher values in LCm ($p<0.001$ between HsCm and control and $p<0.01$ between LCm and HsCm).

In addition, the number of CD45 and RLA-DR positive cells was increased in the inner part of the choroid and the retinal pigment epithelium. The numeration of the cells in these areas did not differ between the two models but confirmed an increase in the two models when compared with the control ($p<0.001$).

In the corneal stroma, some vimentin positive cells were observed in the HSCm and many cells were found in the LCm ($p<0.0001$ versus control for LCm). This increase was higher for LCm than for HSCm, ($p>0.0001$) as shown on the graph (Figure 8B). We observed an increase in the number of cells expressing high levels of vimentin in the conjunctiva (Figure 8; $p<0.0001$ versus control for LCm and $p<0.001$ for HsCm with no difference between them. Numerous cells expressing high levels of vimentin were observed in the trabecular meshwork in LCm and only few positive cells in the HSCm (without difference when compared to control; $p<0.0001$ between the two models). In the limbus, positive cells increased gradually from the HSCm to the LCm. In the retina, anti-vimentin labeling extended within Müller cells from the ganglion cell layer to the outer limiting membrane with expression increasing in a time-dependent manner, reflecting an activation state of the Müller glial cells.

## Discussion

As it is relatively difficult to obtain fresh human eyes from glaucoma donors treated with BAK-containing eye drops, we undertook a toxicological study using two different conditions in New Zealand rabbits, classically considered animals of choice for toxicological studies [19]. The first model was based on the instillation of the 0.01% BAK solution, which is the concentration commonly used in eye drops, twice a day for 5 months and the other model was based on the instillation of one drop of 0.2% BAK solution once daily for 1 month. We chose this toxicological approach in order to simulate the long-term antiglaucoma treatment as much as possible according to Haber's rule suggesting that the exposure concentration (c) multiplied by the exposure duration (t) corresponds to a constant (k) in terms of biological effect [20]. By combining the advantages of mass spectrometry (MS) and microscopy in a single experiment, the emerging MSI technology offers an extraordinarily powerful tool to understand the molecular complexity of any tissue [21]. Among the various techniques aiming to map the surface of the sample, MSI is the

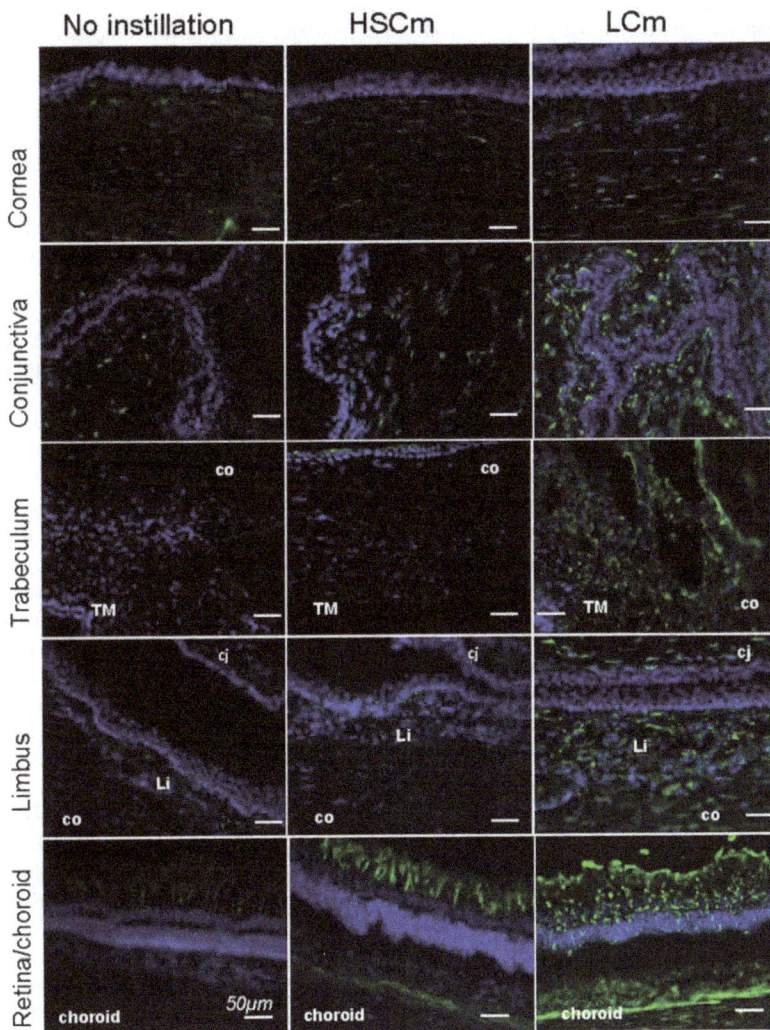

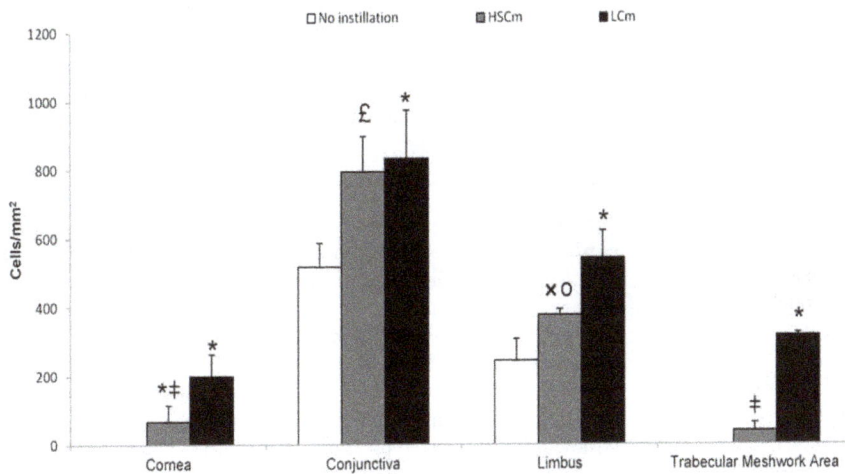

**Figure 8. Vimentin-positive cell infiltration.** (A) Immunofluorescence stainings of vimentin (in green) in rabbit eye cryosections in normal non instilled rabbit eyes compared with rabbit eye instilled with BAK 0.01% twice a day for 5 months (Low Chronic model, LCm) and 0.2% once a day for 1 month (High SubChronic model, HSCm). Nuclei in blue are stained with DAPI. Scale bar, 50 mm. Cj: conjunctiva; Co: cornea; Li: limbus; s: corneal stroma; e: superficial epithelium; TM: trabecular meshwork. (B) Histogram of vimentin positive cells count (mean cells/mm$^2\pm$SD) *$P<0.001$ compared with the normal eye or £ $P<0.001$ or × $P<0.005$ compared with the normal eye; I $P<0.0001$ or ○ $P<0.0001$ HsCm versus LCm.

only analytical method capable of providing, in a single run, the spatial distribution of a wide range of molecules over the surface of a biological sample, in the present study the surface of non-fixed rabbit eye cryosections. Compared to traditional biochemical techniques based on antibodies, which are often limited by the specificity of the applied labels and the number of compounds that can be studied simultaneously, or on radiolabeling, which is difficult to carry out on living animals, MSI retrieves the molecular content of samples without requiring a priori knowledge of the target compounds [22]. Therefore, to characterize the spatial distribution of BAK, we used the matrix-assisted laser desorption/ionization MSI technique coupled to time-of-flight mass spectrometry (MALDI-TOF MS). Even if this method requires the deposition of an organic compound, called matrix, on top of the eye section to improve ionization, it is now well established that this ionization source offers excellent sensitivity, which is needed when examining the distribution of exogenous compounds in a tissue section. The robustness of this technique was also demonstrated by a round robin organized between two laboratories involved in the study using similar preparations but with different instrumentations. They resulted in similar observations regarding BAK detection in particular histological structures, such as the iridocorneal angle or the optic nerve area. Eventually, we evaluated the repeatability of MS imaging on more than thirty MS images from several animals, carried out in two separate laboratories, all leading to the same conclusion about the distribution of BAK and its accumulation in some histological areas of the rabbit eyes after instillation. Beyond inter-laboratory reproducibility, these results nicely demonstrate the consistency of the measurements. BAK was thus detected in ocular surface structures, cornea and conjunctiva, but also in the trabecular meshwork and optic nerve areas. Interestingly, we demonstrated that even relatively short exposure in a healthy eye might not prevent BAK from deeply entering the eye. Immunohistochemistry was indeed consistent with MSI findings, as we repeatedly found retinal changes in BAK treated eyes. This is in favor of the presence of BAK molecules that could stimulate inflammatory cell infiltration. Indeed, in the areas where BAK was observed, we showed the presence of CD45- and RLA-DR-positive cells as well as vimentin-positive cells. CD45, a pan-leukocyte marker, was used to detect any leukocyte infiltrating the tissue. HLA-DR is a MHC class II antigen expressed on antigen-presenting cells, monocytes/macrophages, B-lymphocytes and dendritic cells, and was used to confirm the presence of immune cells. Moreover, the intermediate filament vimentin, which is normally expressed in retina at the end feet of Müller cell processes, was found expressed throughout the Müller cells and up to the outer limiting membrane, as is classically observed in altered retina [18].

The immunological analyses found a greater toxic effect in the 5-month application model than in the 1-month model, suggesting that the duration of the application time has a greater impact than the BAK concentration used. This is an important finding to consider in appreciating glaucoma treatments. However, clinical studies in glaucoma patients using conjunctival impression cytology have shown that the inflammatory markers increased with the number of therapies used. Cornea and conjunctiva/sclera are the main drug absorption pathways. Drug physiochemical

properties, lipophilicity, molecular size, and ionic state greatly influence absorption [23]. In addition, penetration of BAK may be enhanced in patients treated with multiple therapies and in those with an impaired ocular surface, mainly as a consequence of BAK toxicity to surface epithelia. As BAK can be detected in deep eye tissues, especially in the vicinity of the trabecular meshwork, it could be hypothesized that preserved topical antiglaucoma drugs can induce adverse effects: it may at the same time decrease IOP but cause further toxicity to this structure, resulting in an increase of aqueous outflow resistance and therefore increasing IOP. In a very recent paper, related to a clinical trial, BAK was shown to induce anterior chamber inflammation in previously untreated patients with ocular hypertension using a laser flare/cellmeter, confirming the BAK penetration inside deep ocular structures [24]. This combination of a positive IOP-lowering effect and the deleterious effects of BAK in the long run could result in apparent progressive loss of efficiency of IOP-lowering compounds. This progressive failure of treatment efficacy actually corresponds to widely observed situations in clinical practice. Indeed, nearly 40% of patients require additional eye drops in the years after diagnosis as the initial therapy fails to control pressure [7]. Additionally, as the aim of antiglaucoma drugs is to decrease IOP and consequently to protect the optic nerve, the potential presence and most likely toxicity of BAK along the optic nerve raises major sight-threatening issues. Prostaglandin F2 alpha analogs are currently the first-line treatment for reducing IOP in glaucoma patients. In a rabbit model as well as in humans, these molecules have been reported to increase optic nerve head blood flow in an IOP-reduction-independent manner, suggesting that they may reach the retina to increase blood flow [25,26]. Moreover, Miyake proposed the term 'pseudophakic preservative maculopathy' for cystoid macular edema caused by antiglaucoma eyedrops, explaining that the preservative increases synthesis of prostaglandins and other inflammatory mediators and intensifies postoperative inflammation [8]. BAK could therefore cause a side effect that would be indistinguishable from the disease outcome, as the treatment would be both protective and, to a lesser but significant extent, deleterious. Such findings could account for the glaucomatous patients whose disease progresses despite good IOP control [27,28]. Further studies with humans, whenever possible, would confirm such findings. However, we conclude that preservative-free compounds should become the first choice therapy for patients suffering from glaucoma and any other disease requiring chronic drug administration in their eyes.

## Supporting Information

**Figure S1 Repeated ion images of whole eye section of rabbit eye.** (A) Rabbit eye instilled twice a day with one drop of 0.01% benzalkonium chloride (BAK) for 1 and 5 months (Low Chronic model, LCm): two images (separated by a dotted red line) for each model (separated by a red line) showing the BAK distribution using MALDI-TOF mass spectrometry imaging: (Lines 1 and 2) MALDI-TOF ion images of BAK $C_{12}$ and BAK $C_{14}$ distributions in whole eye section, respectively; (Line 3) Histology images of cryosections stained with hematoxylin-eosin and unstained contrast phase optical views for each model. (B) Rabbit eye instilled once a day with one drop of 0.2% benzalkonium chloride (BAK) for 1 month (High Sub-Chronic model, HSCm): three images (separated by a dotted red line) showing BAK distribution using MALDI-TOF mass spectrometry imaging. (Lines 1 and 2) MALDI-TOF ion images of BAK $C_{12}$ and BAK $C_{14}$ distributions in whole eye section, respectively; (Line 3) Histology images of cryosections stained with hematoxylin-eosin (right and left) and unstained contrast phase optical views (middle).

## Acknowledgments

The authors wish to thank Mrs. Razika Nanache for her technical assistance in immunohistochemical analysis.

## Author Contributions

Conceived and designed the experiments: OL CB FBB AB JPB JS. Performed the experiments: FBB ND GH HL JPB AB IF MS VG RL DT MW. Analyzed the data: FBB ND GH HL JPB AB IF MS VG RL DT MW OL CB. Contributed reagents/materials/analysis tools: FBB ND GH HL AB IF MS DT MW. Wrote the paper: FBB ND AB CB GH.

## References

1. Quigley HA (2011) Glaucoma. Lancet 377: 1367–1377.
2. Okabe K, Kimura H, Okabe J, Kato A, Shimizu H, et al. (2005) Effect of benzalkonium chloride on transscleral drug delivery. Invest Ophthalmol Vis Sci 46: 703–8.
3. Chetoni P, Burgalassi S, Monti D, Saettone MF (2003) Ocular toxicity of some corneal penetration enhancers evaluated by electrophysiology measurements on isolated rabbit corneas. Toxicol In Vitro 17: 497–504.
4. The United State Pharmacopoeia 24th rev (2000) The National Formulary 19th ed. Rockville, MD: the United States Pharmacopeial Convention, Inc.
5. European Pharmacopoeia 7th ed (2010) Council of Europe, Strasbourg.
6. Baudouin C, Labbé A, Liang H, Brignole-Baudouin F (2010) Preservatives in eyedrops: The good, the bad and the ugly. Prog Retin Eye Res 29: 312–334.
7. Kass MA, Heuer DK, Higginbotham EJ, Johnson CA, Keltner JL, et al. (2002) The Ocular Hypertension Treatment Study: a randomized trial determines that topical ocular hypotensive medication delays or prevents the onset of primary open-angle glaucoma. Arch Ophthalmol 120: 701–713.
8. Miyake K, Ibaraki N, Goto Y, Oogiya S, Ishigaki J, et al. (2003) ESCRS Binkhorst lecture 2002: pseudophakic preservative maculopathy. J Cataract Refract Surg 29: 1800–1810.
9. Champeau E, Edelhauser H (1986) Effect of ophthalmic preservatives on the ocular surface: conjunctival and corneal uptake and distribution of benzalkonium chloride and chlorhexidinedigluconate. In: Holly, F. (Ed.), The preocular tear film. Dry Eye Institute, Inc, Lubbock, TX 292–302.
10. Chou A, Hori S, Takase M (1985) Ocular toxicity of beta-blockers and benzalkonium chloride in pigmented rabbits: electrophysiological and morphological studies. Jpn J Ophthalmol 29: 13–23.
11. Garrett TJ, Menger RF, Dawson WW, Yost RA (2011) Lipid analysis of flat-mounted eye tissue by imaging mass spectrometry with identification of contaminants in preservation. Anal Bioanal Chem 401: 103–113.
12. Kafka AP, Kleffmann T, Rades T, McDowell A (2011) The application of MALDI TOF MS in biopharmaceutical research. Int J Pharm 417: 70–82.
13. Balluff B, Schöne C, Höfler H, Walch A (2011) MALDI imaging mass spectrometry for direct tissue analysis: technological advancements and recent applications. Histochem Cell Biol 136: 227–44.
14. Pól J, Strohalm M, Havlíček V, Volný M (2010) Molecular mass spectrometry imaging in biomedical and life science research. Histochem Cell Biol 134: 423–443.
15. Touboul D, Laprévote O, Brunelle A (2011) Micrometric molecular histology of lipids by mass spectrometry imaging. Curr Opin Chem Biol 15: 725–32.
16. Yamada Y, Hidefumi K, Shion H, Oshikata M, Haramaki Y (2011) Distribution of chloroquine in ocular tissue of pigmented rat using matrix-assisted laser desorption/ionization imaging quadrupole time-of-flight tandem mass spectrometry. Rapid Commun Mass Spectrom 25: 1600–1608.
17. Sappino AP, Schurch W, Gabbiani G (1990) Biology of disease: Differentiation repertoire of fibroblastic cells: Expression of cytoskeletal proteins as marker of phenotypic modulations. Lab Invest 63: 144–161.
18. Lewis GP, Fisher SK (2003) Up-regulation of glial fibrillary acidic protein in response to retinal injury: its potential role in glial remodeling and a comparison to vimentin expression. Int Rev Cytol 230: 263–90.
19. Short BG (2008) Safety evaluation of ocular drug delivery formulations: techniques and practical considerations. Toxicol Pathol 36: 49–62.
20. Shustermann D, Matovinovic E, Salmon A (2006) Does Haber's Law Apply to Human Sensory Irritation? Inhal Toxicol 18: 457–471.
21. Stoeckli M, Chaurand P, Hallahan DE, Caprioli RM (2001) Imaging mass spectrometry: a new technology for the analysis of protein expression in mammalian tissues. Nat Med 7: 493–496.
22. Benabdellah F, Seyer A, Quinton L, Touboul D, Brunelle A, et al. (2010) Mass spectrometry imaging of rat brain sections: nanomolar sensitivity with MALDI versus nanometer resolution by TOF-SIMS. Anal Bioanal Chem 396: 151–162.
23. Ichhpujani P, Katz LJ, Hollo G, Schields CL, Schields JA, et al. (2011) Comparison of human ocular distribution of bimatoprost and latanoprost. J Ocul Pharmacol Ther 28: 134–45.
24. Stevens AM, Kestelyn PA, De Bacquer D, Kestelyn PG (2012) Benzalkonium chloride induces anterior chamber inflammation in previously untreated patients with ocular hypertension as measured by flare meter: a randomized clinical trial. Acta Ophthalmol 90: e221–e224.
25. Yamagishi R, Aihara M, Araie M (2011) Neuroprotective effects of prostaglandin analogues on retinal ganglion cell death independent of intraocular pressure reduction. Exp Eye Res 93: 265–70.
26. Akaishi T, Kurashima H, Odani-Kawabata N, Ishida N, Nakamura M (2010) Effects of repeated administrations of tafluprost, latanoprost, and travoprost on optic nerve head blood flow in conscious normal rabbits. J Ocul Pharmacol Ther 26: 181–186.
27. Brubaker RF (1996) Delayed functional loss in glaucoma: LII Edward Jackson Memorial Lecture. Am J Ophthalmol 121: 473–483.
28. Tezel G, Siegmund KD, Trinkaus K, Wax MB, Kass MA, et al. (2001) Clinical factors associated with progression of glaucomatous optic disc damage in treated patients. Arch Ophthalmol 119: 813–818.

# 16

# Early Ahmed Glaucoma Valve Implantation after Penetrating Keratoplasty Leads to Better Outcomes in an Asian Population with Preexisting Glaucoma

**Ming-Cheng Tai[1,2], Yi-Hao Chen[1,2], Jen-Hao Cheng[1], Chang-Min Liang[1,2], Jiann-Torng Chen[1,2], Ching-Long Chen[1,2], Da-Wen Lu[1,2]***

**1** Department of Ophthalmology, Tri-Service General Hospital, National Defense Medical Center, Taipei, Taiwan, **2** Graduate Institute of Medical Science, National Defense Medical Center, Taipei, Taiwan

## Abstract

***Background:*** To evaluate the efficacy of Ahmed Glaucoma Valve (AGV) surgery and the optimal interval between penetrating keratoplasty (PKP) and AGV implantation in a population of Asian patients with preexisting glaucoma who underwent PKP.

***Methodology/Principal Findings:*** In total, 45 eyes of 45 patients were included in this retrospective chart review. The final intraocular pressures (IOPs), graft survival rate, and changes in visual acuity were assessed to evaluate the outcomes of AGV implantations in eyes in which AGV implantation occurred within 1 month of post-PKP IOP elevation (Group 1) and in eyes in which AGV implantation took place more than 1 month after the post-PKP IOP evaluation (Group 2). Factors that were associated with graft failure were analyzed, and the overall patterns of complications were reviewed. By their final follow-up visits, 58% of the patients had been successfully treated for glaucoma. After the operation, there were no statistically significant differences between the groups with respect to graft survival (p = 0.98), but significant differences for IOP control (p = 0.049) and the maintenance of visual acuity (VA) (p<0.05) were observed. One year after surgery, the success rates of IOP control in Group 1 and Group 2 were 80% and 46.7%, respectively, and these rates fell to 70% and 37.3%, respectively, by 2 years. Factors that were associated with a high risk of AGV failure were a diagnosis of preexisting angle-closure glaucoma, a history of previous PKP, and a preoperative IOP that was >21 mm Hg. The most common surgical complication, aside from graft failure, was hyphema.

***Conclusions/Significance:*** Early AGV implantation results in a higher probability of AGV survival and a better VA outcome without increasing the risk of corneal graft failure as a result of post-PKP glaucoma drainage tube implantation.

**Editor:** James T. Rosenbaum, Oregon Health & Science University, United States of America

**Funding:** This study is supported, in part, by grants from the Tri-Service General Hospital (TSGHC100-008-006-6-S03 and TSGH-C100-086). No additional external funding received for this study. The funders had no role in study design, data collection and analysis, decision to publish, or preparation of the manuscript.

**Competing Interests:** The authors have declared that no competing interests exist.

* E-mail: p310849@ms23.hinet.net

## Introduction

The presence of glaucoma following a penetrating keratoplasty (PKP) procedure is the second most common cause of corneal graft failure [1]. Some patients who have corneal pathology that requires PKP have preexisting glaucoma; Reinhard et al [2] estimated that the 3-year graft survival rate in these patients is approximately 71%, as opposed to an 89% survival rate in patients with no history of glaucoma. The implantation of glaucoma drainage devices (GDDs) has therefore played an important role in the surgical treatment of glaucoma in patients who have undergone PKPs [3]. Several reports have shown that using GDDs as a method of treating glaucoma, as is the case with Ahmed valve (AGV) implantation, is an effective method of controlling intraocular pressure (IOP) in glaucoma patients. In a number of studies, 50–80% of the patients experienced post-operative corneal graft rejections that affected their visual acuities (VAs) [4–6]. At

present, there is no consensus regarding the amount of time between PKP and AGV implantation that is optimal for controlling IOP, improving graft survival, and preserving VA in patients with preexisting glaucoma. Moreover, there have been no studies that compare the surgical outcomes of patients who received AGV implantations at various intervals after undergoing PKPs.

The purpose of the present study was to evaluate the procedure of using AGV implantation to control preexisting glaucoma following PKP in patients from an Asian population. This study compares the IOP, corneal graft, and visual acuity outcomes of post-PKP patients who received AGV implantation either within 1 month of post-PKP IOP elevation or more than 1 month after IOP elevation. The outcome measures were monitored for as long as 2 years after PKP. In addition, the factors that were associated with AGV failure in these patients, and the overall complications that they experienced were also analyzed. Finally, we found that earlier AGV implantation following post-PKP IOP elevation in patients with preexisting glaucoma and who underwent PKPs improved the probability of tube survival and preserved VA without increasing the likelihood of corneal graft failure.

## Methods

### Objectives

AGV implantation is a suitable treatment method for various types of glaucoma, including the treatment of glaucoma that is associated with undergoing a PKP procedure. For the most part, the present study aimed to evaluate whether more aggressive glaucoma treatment (early AGV implantation) was of greater benefit to patients with preexisting glaucoma who had undergone PKP. The study also placed a minor focus on evaluating the risk of AGV failure in these patients.

### Participants

We reviewed the medical records of patients with preexisting glaucoma and significant corneal disease that required PKP who were subsequently treated with AGV implantation at the Department of Ophthalmology of the Tri-Service General Hospital, Taipei, Taiwan, between January 2000 and December 2010. In total, 73 cases were reviewed, and 28 cases were excluded because the medical records were incomplete. A total of 45 eyes of 45 patients were included. All of the AGV implantation surgeries were performed by the corresponding author, and no other GDDs were used during the study period. Prospective patients who were not able to attend follow-up visits during an extended postoperative period were also excluded.

The patients were divided into 2 groups: Group 1 included patients in whom AGV implantation was performed within 1 month of determining the presence of persistent IOP elevation (measured IOP of $\geq 21$ mm Hg at three successive visits), and Group 2 included patients in whom AGV implantation was performed more than 1 month after a persistent IOP elevation was established. Our hospital is a tertiary referral center, so most of the patients who were recruited for participation in our study were referred from other hospitals. To ensure corneal graft survival, we performed surgical interventions as soon as was possible. The criteria that were used in grouping these patients were therefore based on the information contained in the referral documents that we received when the patient was referred to our hospital.

### Description of Procedures

Pre- and postoperative patient demographics and clinical characteristics, including their ages, genders, IOP measurements (using a Goldmann applanation tonometer), corneal diagnoses, types of preexisting glaucoma and use of antiglaucoma medications, were documented and subjected to statistical analysis.

A similar surgical technique was used to perform AGV implantation in all patients. Under peribulbar anesthesia, we created a fornix-based conjunctival flap in the superotemporal quadrant between 2 adjacent recti muscles. After creating a 3×3 mm triangular scleral flap, the AGV (model S2 with a 185 mm$^2$ polypropylene plate; New World Medical, Rancho Cucamonga, CA, USA) was irrigated with balanced saline solution (BSS; Alcon, Fort Worth, TX, USA) to prime the valve mechanism. The polypropylene body of the implant was placed 8 mm posterior to the corneoscleral limbus and was sutured to the sclera with an 8–0 prolene suture (Ethicon Inc., Somerville, NJ, USA). The tube of the AGV implant was then trimmed so that the bevel of it faced the corneal endothelial surface and was subsequently inserted into the anterior chamber through a needle track that had been made with a 23-gauge needle. A scleral patch graft from a human donor was placed on the tube so that the anterior edge was adjacent to the limbus and was then sutured to the sclera with an 8–0 prolene suture. After the implant and graft had been inserted, 0.5 cc of a viscoelastic solution (Healon GV®; Advanced Medical Optics, Santa Ana, CA, USA) was injected into the anterior chamber to avoid early hypotony. Finally, the conjunctiva was sutured to the limbus, and the eye received a subconjunctival injection of steroids and antibiotics. No adjunctive metabolites were used.

After the operation, topical eye drops containing 0.3% ofloxacin (Tarvid, Santen, Osaka, Japan) and 1% prednisolone acetate (EconoPred Plus, Alcon, Texas, USA) were prescribed, and their use was tapered slowly over a period of 4–8 weeks. Antiglaucoma medication prescriptions were adjusted on the basis of both the IOP and the clinical status of the eye that had received the implant. Patients were examined at a specific series of postoperative intervals (1 day, 1 week, and 1 month after surgery) and every 3 months thereafter for a total follow-up period of 2 years. Slit-lamp examinations were performed, and VA, IOP, and any surgical complications were assessed at each follow-up visit.

The outcome variable that we used to measure the success of AGV survival was postoperative IOP control after AGV implantation. Complete success was defined as having a final IOP that was <21 mm Hg, >6 mm Hg, and accompanied by a pressure reduction of at least 20% relative to pre-surgery levels in the absence of any loss of light perception, the need for any additional antiglaucoma medication, or AGV implant removal. Partial success was defined as a final IOP that was <21 mm Hg, >6 mm Hg, and accompanied by a pressure reduction of at least 20% relative to pre-surgery levels in conjunction with a need for additional antiglaucoma medication. Patients with IOPs that were $\geq 21$ mm Hg or that were $\leq 6$ mm Hg were given treatment that attempted to lower or raise their IOPs, respectively, and they were re-examined within several days to a week. Because these patients required more frequent postoperative examinations than patients in whom the AGV implant had been partially or completely successful, the results of their additional examinations were averaged to generate statistics for a single time frame. Neither success nor failure was defined until at least 2 consecutive examinations after the 3- to 6-month time frame had taken place. Success and failure of graft clarity survival were defined as follows: success was defined as the corneal graft remaining clear, and failure was determined by the presence of corneal graft decomposition. Additional outcome parameters included changes in visual acuity, operative complications, and postoperative complications.

### Ethics

The study followed the principles that were established in the Declaration of Helsinki and was approved by the Institutional Review Board of the hospital.

### Statistical methods

The Mann-Whitney $U$ test and Fisher's exact test were used to compare non-parametric continuous and categorical variables, respectively, within the groups. Differences between the preoperative IOPs and the IOPs that were measured at each follow-up examination were analyzed using Wilcoxon signed-rank tests. Means were used to describe non-parametric data, and categorical data were represented by numbers and percentages. Kaplan-Meier life-table analysis was used to calculate IOP and graft survival curves. The following factors that may have influenced the rates of AGV failure were assessed in a logistic regression model:

age, gender, diagnosis of glaucoma, total number of antiglaucoma medications, lens status, total number of previous PKPs, and postoperative IOP. All statistical assessments were two-tailed, and a P-value of P≤0.05 was considered statistically significant. Statistical analyses were performed using version 15.0 of the SPSS statistical software package (SPSS Inc., Chicago, IL, USA).

## Results

Demographic and preoperative characteristics of Groups 1 and 2 are listed in Table 1. Data that were collected include the ages, genders, preoperative IOPs, mean numbers of PKPs, types of preexisting glaucoma and corneal disease diagnoses. The most common type of glaucoma that was diagnosed in both groups was chronic angle-closure glaucoma (55% and 60% of patients in Groups 1 and 2, respectively). The major corneal disorder in both groups was pseudophakic bullous keratopathy (60% and 52% in Groups 1 and 2, respectively). The average follow-up period for patients in Group 1 and Group 2 was 22.4 months (SD, 11.3) and 17.8 months (SD, 12.0), respectively. The average time between PKP and AGV implantation was 74.5 days (SD, 40.5) in the Group 1 patients and 111.4 days (SD, 43.4) in the Group 2 patients ($P<0.05$).

Figure 1 shows the IOP data that were obtained during the preoperative examination and postoperative follow-up periods in patients from Groups 1 and 2. The mean preoperative IOP of Group 1 patients was 27.8 mm Hg (SD, 7.3), and the mean preoperative IOP of the Group 2 patients was 29.0 mm Hg (SD, 10.9). After the operation, the mean IOPs of both groups decreased significantly at postoperative day 1, month 1, month 3, month 6, month 9, year 1, year 2, and year 3 ($P<0.05$). The mean IOP at the final follow-up examination had also decreased significantly in both groups; it reached a final value of 14.9 mm Hg (SD, 4.4) in group 1 ($P<0.001$) and a final value of 15.0 mm Hg (SD, 4.1) in Group 2 ($P<0.001$).

The rate of completely successful Ahmed valve implantation was 40.0% (18/45), and the partial success rate of AGV implantation was 17.8% (8/45) in all patients at the last visit.

The Kaplan-Meier life-table analysis for AGV survival in the 2 groups is shown in Figure 2. The overall cumulative probability of success was 58.9% at 1 year after implantation and was 49.4% at 2 years after implantation. The probabilities of success in Group 1 and Group 2 were 80% and 46.7% at 1 year and 70% and 37.3% at 2 years, respectively. There was a statistically significant difference between the two groups with respect to final success rate of IOP reduction (log-rank test = 0.049).

The overall cumulative probabilities of corneal graft success were 74.0% and 52.2% at 1 and 2 years postoperatively, respectively (Figure 3). These probabilities were 73.8% and 73.6% at 1 year and 53.7% and 50.5% at 2 years in the Group 1 and Group 2 patients, respectively. There was no statistically significant difference between the two groups with respect to final rate of corneal graft survival (log-rank test = 0.98).

Figure 4 shows a comparison of the final changes in the visual acuities of the two groups. There was a significant difference in the final VAs of the "worsened" (p = 0.04, Fisher's exact test) and "improved" (p = 0.02) subgroups. However, there were no differences between either of these groups and the subgroup that experienced "no change." In Group 1, 8 patients (40%) showed no change in VA, 4 patients (20%) showed a decline in VA, and 8 patients (40%) showed an improvement in VA. Similarly, 10 patients in Group 2 (40%) had no change in VA, 8 patients (32%) showed a decline in VA, and 7 patients (28%) showed an improvement in VA.

The average number of antiglaucoma medications that patients were using prior to AGV implantations was 2.3 (SD, 1.3) in Group 1 and 1.9 (SD, 0.9) in Group 2, and the difference between the numbers of medications taken by each group was significant ($P<0.05$). After undergoing various operations, the mean number of medications was 1.0 (SD, 1.1) in the Group 1 patients and 1.3 (SD, 1.2) in the Group 2 patients; the difference between the two groups was not significant.

As shown in Table 2, age, gender, diagnosis, lens status, number of previous PKPs and pre-operative IOP were analyzed as potential risk factors for AGV implantation failure. The Cox proportional hazards model indicated that the hazard ratio of

**Table 1.** Preoperative characteristics of study patients in both groups.

|  | Group 1 | Group 2 | P-value |
|---|---|---|---|
| Patients (Number) | 20 | 25 | 0.063 |
| Age (Mean) | 62.8 | 59.5 | 0.77 |
| Female, No. (%) | 11 (55%) | 15 (60%) | 0.38 |
| Preoperative IOP (mmHg), mean (SD) | 30.3 (5.28) | 27 (6.25) | 0.057 |
| Duration between PK and persistent IOP elevation (days), mean (SD) | 56.3 (39.9) | 58.0 (42.3) | 0.93 |
| Preoperative antiglaucoma medications, mean (SD) | 2.3 (1.3) | 1.9 (0.9) | 0.03[a] |
| Type of preexisting glaucoma diagnosis, No. (%) |  |  | 0.43 |
| Primary open angle | 4 (20) | 5 (20) |  |
| Chronic angle closure | 11 (55) | 15 (60) |  |
| Secondary (trauma, uveitis) | 3 (15) | 4 (16) |  |
| Other | 3 (15) | 1 (4) |  |
| Type of corneal diagnosis, No. (%) |  |  | 0.58 |
| Pseudophakic bullous keratopathy | 12 (60) | 13 (52) |  |
| Failed PK | 5 (25) | 7 (28) |  |
| Other | 3 (15) | 5 (20) |  |

Abbreviations: IOP = intraocular pressure; SD = standard deviation; [a]Denotes statistical significance.

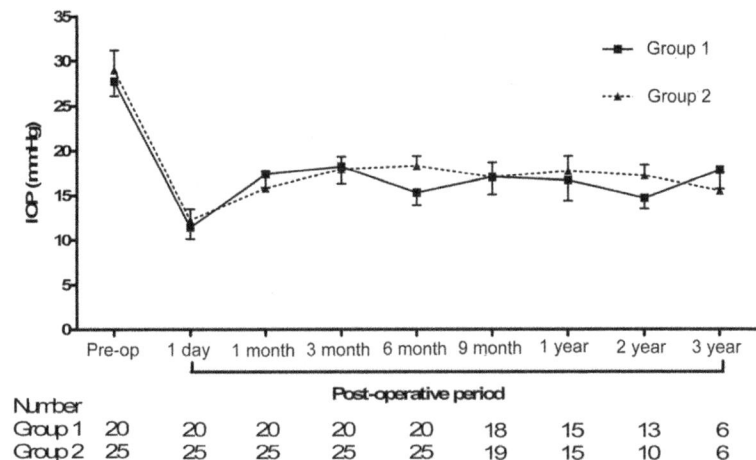

**Figure 1. Pre- and postoperative intraocular pressures following Ahmed glaucoma valve implantation surgery in Group 1 and Group 2 over time.** A marked decrease in the median IOP relative to the baseline IOP was noted during each postoperative period.

AGV implant failure was significantly increased by having a diagnosis of preexisting glaucoma, the number of previous PKPs, and the pre-operative IOP after the AGV. The chronic angle-closure glaucoma patients appeared to be predisposed to higher rates of failure compared with other patients (OR, 3.55; 95% CI, 1.05–5.79; $P = 0.034$). In addition, having two or three previous PKPs was associated with an elevated risk of failure (ORs, 1.63 and 1.92, respectively; 95% CIs, 1.39–1.93 and 1.78–2.28, respectively; $P = 0.042$) as was an individual's preoperative IOP (OR, 3.01; 95% CI; 2.50–5.20; $P = 0.02$).

The postoperative complications that occurred in patients in both groups are summarized in Table 3. The most frequent complications (in order of decreasing frequency) were as follows: corneal graft failure or rejection, hyphema, and the presence shallow anterior chamber.

## Discussion

Ahmed glaucoma valve implantation often enables the successful control of refractory glaucoma in cases in which other surgical modalities are ineffective [7–12]. This undoubtedly poses a chal-

lenge to the surgical management of patients with preexisting glaucoma who have undergone PKPs. It has also been shown that pre-existing glaucoma is a risk factor for graft failure [13]. Although various types of GDDs have been effective in IOP control, many patients who received GDD implants have shown poor corneal graft outcomes with graft failure rates that ranged from 10 to 51% [3,14–18]. Several studies have investigated the effect of the relative sequence of PK and GDD on graft survival. Rapuano et al [19] found evidence of a tendency toward decreased graft survival when a GDD was implanted after a patient had undergone PK. However, Coleman et al [6] found that there was no difference in outcomes when an AGV was implanted concurrently with or after a PK. Kwon et al [10] reported that eyes in which a GDD had been implanted prior to PK have a higher risk for graft failure than eyes in which GDDs were implanted concurrently with or after PKs. They also considered the fact that these patients tend to have severe glaucoma, which in turn could affect graft survival. In the case series that we reviewed in the present study, the total corneal graft survival rate was 52.2% at 2 years postoperatively, which is similar to the survival rate that

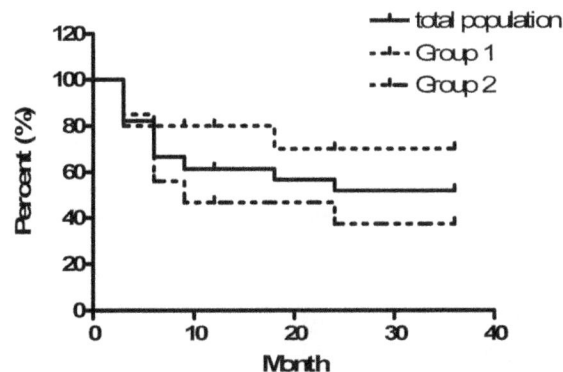

**Figure 2. Kaplan-Meier life-table analysis showing the cumulative probabilities of IOP control at 1 year and 2 years post-PKP in Group 1, Group 2, and the entire sample population following Ahmed glaucoma valve implantation either with or without the use of antiglaucoma medications.** (Log-Rank test = 0.049).

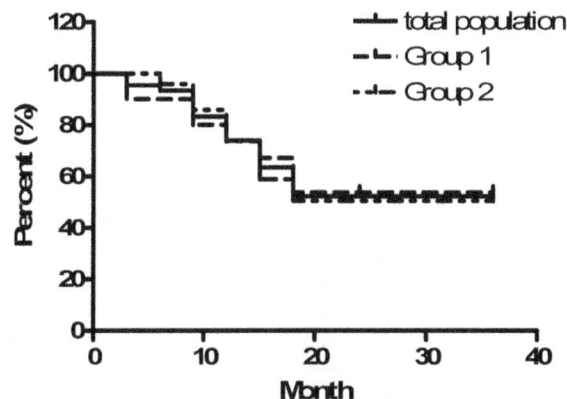

**Figure 3. Kaplan-Meier life-table analysis showing the cumulative probabilities of graft survival at 1 year and 2 years post-PKP in Group 1, Group 2, and the entire sample population following Ahmed glaucoma valve implantation either with or without the use of antiglaucoma medications.** (Log-Rank test = 0.98).

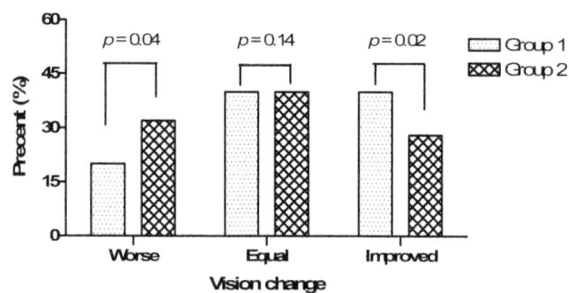

**Figure 4. Visual acuity status at the final follow-up visit in Groups 1 and 2.**

has been reported in previous studies. Moreover, there was no statistically significant difference in the graft survival rates of the two groups. However, the success rate for controlling glaucoma was significantly higher among Group 1 patients compared with the success rate among Group 2 patients. These results demonstrate that early surgery can effectively improve the success rate in controlling glaucoma without inducing an increased risk of graft failure. In addition, several other mechanisms have been associated with a potentially higher risk of graft failure, such as excessive surgical time, multiple procedures, excessive postoperative inflammation, or early tube endothelial touch [10,14]. Fortunately, these factors did not play especially strong roles in the clinical histories and outcomes of our patients. We performed anterior chamber injections of 0.5 cc of a viscoelastic solution (Healon GV®; Advanced Medical Optics, Santa Ana, CA, USA) and used AGV tubes of relatively short lengths to avoid complications such as early shallow anterior chamber and early tube endothelial touch after the suture in our patients.

Goldberg's study found that 71% of patients with pre-existing glaucoma developed increased IOPs early in the postoperative course following PKP [20]. In the present case series, AGV implantation succeeded in controlling glaucoma in 80% and 71% of patients at 1 and 2 years, respectively. Alvarenga et al [14] reported that eyes in which Ahmed valves were implanted had glaucoma control success rates of 74% and 63.1% at 1 and 2 years, respectively, which are higher than the success rates in our patients. This finding may be a result of the time at which the AGV was implanted. In our study, an aggressive therapeutic protocol in which an AGV was implanted within 1 month of the establishment of elevated IOP (Group 1) showed survival rates of AGV implantation that were similar to those of previous reports, whereas a less intensive treatment protocol in which AGV implantation occurred more than 1 month after an elevated IOP was established (Group 2) yielded an opposite result. Furthermore, the inclusion of eyes with different types of preexisting glaucoma may play a role in this issue. Our study differs from other studies that have been mentioned in that the majority of patients who were included in it had chronic angle-closure glaucoma. In general, AGV implantation has been thought to be relatively effective with respect to controlling glaucoma in different types of patients [21,22], and neither glaucoma nor corneal diagnosis has been shown to influence the success of long-term glaucoma control with GDDs. However, our experience has shown the success rate of AGV implantation may be influenced by the type of glaucoma; for example, we have found evidence of poor outcomes of AGV implantation in controlling neovascular glaucoma [22]. Furthermore, our Cox regression analysis also showed that the patients with preexisting angle-closure glaucoma had an increased risk of AGV failure compared with other patients. Thus, we believe that

**Table 2.** Logistic regression analysis of risk factors for AGV failure at 2 years.

|  | Hazard Ratio | 95% CI | P-value |
|---|---|---|---|
| Age (years) |  |  | 0.054 |
| <60 | 1.00 | – |  |
| ≥60 | 1.03 | (1.00, 1.05) |  |
| Gender |  |  | 0.494 |
| Male | 1.00 | – |  |
| Female | 1.08 | (0.55, 3.44) |  |
| Diagnosis (glaucoma type) |  |  | 0.034[a] |
| Primary open angle | 1.00 | – |  |
| Chronic angle closure | 3.55 | (1.05, 5.79) |  |
| Secondary (trauma, uveitis) | 2.44 | (0.84, 4.41) |  |
| Lens status |  |  | 0.064 |
| Pseudophakia | 1.00 | – |  |
| Aphakia | 1.17 | (0.77, 5.16) |  |
| Phakia | 1.08 | (0.73, 4.98) |  |
| Previous PKs |  |  | 0.041[a] |
| One | 1.00 | – |  |
| Two | 1.63 | (1.39, 1.93) |  |
| Three | 1.92 | (1.78, 2.28) |  |
| Postoperative IOP |  |  | 0.02[a] |
| <21 | 1.00 | – |  |
| ≥21 | 3.01 | (2.5, 5.2) |  |

Abbreviations: CI = confidence interval; IOP = intraocular pressure; PK = penetrating keratoplasty; [a]Denotes statistical significance.

the clinical characteristics of patients with different types of glaucoma may differ and could result in diverse outcomes.

Escalation of glaucoma therapy often immediately follows PKP in patients with a preexisting glaucoma condition [23] in which the rapid onset of IOP control could diminish the severity of optic nerve damage. In our study, a short latency between PKP and AGV implantation is related to the improved success rate of AGV implantation and to the preservation of VA. An increased duration of elevated IOP prior to Ahmed valve implantation may lead to greater inflammation that could cause further damage to the trabecular cells [24]. Therefore, earlier AGV implantation may

**Table 3.** Postoperative complications in the 2 study groups.

|  | Group 1 (No., %) | Group 2 (No., %) |
|---|---|---|
| Shallow anterior chamber | 2, 10 | 3, 12 |
| Corneal graft failure or rejection | 8, 40 | 8, 32 |
| Serous choroidal detachment | 1, 5 | 0, 0 |
| Encapsulated bleb | 1, 5 | 1, 4 |
| Tube malposition | 1, 5 | 1, 4 |
| Diplopia | 0, 0 | 1, 4 |
| Hypotony | 2, 10 | 2, 8 |
| Fibrinous iridocyclitis | 0, 0 | 1, 4 |
| Hyphema | 3, 15 | 3, 12 |

preserve the residual functioning of trabecular meshwork by lessening the degree of trabecular cell death. In addition, we also found that patients who underwent AGV implantation shortly after PKP generally had better VA outcomes than patients for whom the interval between PKP and AGV implantation was longer. Although the visual field data to support this result were not available, we speculate that this result might be due to the lessening of optic damage that resulted from early IOP control.

The Cox regression analysis that we conducted showed that the type of glaucoma with which a patient had been diagnosed, the number of previous PKPs, and the duration of IOP elevation prior to AGV implantation were all associated with an increased risk of AGV failure. The majority of our patients had chronic angle-closure glaucoma, which was associated with a higher risk of AGV failure. No previous study has found evidence of an increased rate of AGV failure in angle-closure glaucoma. We suggest that this increase may result from having a narrow angle space that is occupied by a tube. The presence of the tube may easily cause anterior chamber inflammation due to friction against the angle walls. Moreover, inflammation in the anterior chamber may decrease the AGV success rate, which is the case in uveitic glaucoma [25]. Multiple previous PKPs can lead to an increased tendency to develop anterior chamber synechiae and corneal neovascularization [26], which may also result in a high risk of AGV failure. Preoperative IOP elevation may reflect a refractory disease status in which the disease cannot readily be controlled by drugs or by laser therapy. Thus, the elevated risk of AGV failure that has been observed in these patients was reasonable.

In our study, the most common early postoperative complication was hyphema, followed by a shallow anterior chamber. The incidence of hyphema following AGV implantation has been reported to occur in approximately 2%–20% of patients, and it typically resolves without surgical intervention [17,21,27,28]. The incidence of a shallow anterior chamber following the implantation of an Ahmed valve has been reported to be 0–15% [17,21,27,28]. Differences between these reports and our findings might be explained by the clinical statuses of our patients and by the particular variation in the surgical technique that we used in which a viscoelastic solution was injected immediately following valve implantation to prevent early hypotony or choroidal effusions. Fortunately, this condition typically resolves spontaneously without additional surgery. No serious complications that involved VA losses or blindness occurred among our patients.

There are several limitations to our study. The retrospective design with variable follow-up intervals may result in certain patient selection biases, and the inclusion of patients with various glaucoma diagnoses resulted in a relatively small sample size. However, it is difficult to conduct a prospective and randomized trial because of ethical concerns and because the amount of time that elapses between PKP and AGV implantation cannot be masked. Moreover, the continual availability of new drugs makes it impossible to control for type of ocular medications. The VAs of some patients might be influenced by both corneal pathology and preexisting glaucoma, which in turn may also result in certain biases in the assessment of VA. Antiglaucoma drug use was more prominent among patients in group 1, which may reflect a generally greater severity of glaucoma in this group. The elevated severity of glaucoma may have proceeded to interfere with the success rate of AGV implantation. Another possible reason for some of the observed inter-group differences is that the patients in group 1 were referred by an aggressive corneal specialist who may have attempted to use an intensive protocol for controlling IOP that involved the use of multiple antiglaucoma drugs. In contrast, better IOP control should be more easily achieved in patients with less severe diagnoses, and our results showed that IOP control was more successful in the group with more severe glaucoma. In other words, patients who were categorized as belonging to Group 1 were primarily treated during the latter half of the 10-year study period, which means that a change in surgical practice and decision making may have occurred. A change in surgical practice would suggest that the observed improvement in the IOPs of Group 1 patients was actually due to earlier intervention more than to the possibility of a patient selection bias.

In conclusion, AGV implantation appears to be a viable option for controlling IOP in patients with preexisting glaucoma after penetrating keratoplasty (PKP). In addition, we found that early AGV implantation results in a higher rate of AGV implant survival and a better VA outcome compared with delayed AGV implantation without increasing the risk of graft failure. There is also a low incidence of severe postoperative complications with the notable exception of graft decomposition. However, graft failure remains a challenge in such patients.

## Author Contributions

Conceived and designed the experiments: M-CT Y-HC D-WL. Performed the experiments: J-HC C-LC D-WL. Analyzed the data: C-ML J-TC. Contributed reagents/materials/analysis tools: M-CT Y-HC J-HC D-WL. Wrote the paper: Y-HC J-HC.

## References

1. Muenzler WS, Harms WK (1981) Visual prognosis in aphakic bullous keratopathy treated by penetrating keratoplasty: a retrospective study of 73 cases. Ophthalmic Surg 12: 210–212.
2. Reinhard T, Kallmann C, Cepin A, Godehardt E, Sundmacher R (1997) The influence of glaucoma history on graft survival after penetrating keratoplasty. Graefes Arch Clin Exp Ophthalmol 235: 553–557.
3. Ayyala RS (2000) Penetrating keratoplasty and glaucoma. Surv Ophthalmol 45: 91–105.
4. Al-Torbak AA (2004) Outcome of combined Ahmed glaucoma valve implant and penetrating keratoplasty in refractory congenital glaucoma with corneal opacity. Cornea 23: 554–559.
5. Kwon YH, Taylor JM, Hong S, Honkanen RA, Zimmerman MB, et al. (2001) Long-term results of eyes with penetrating keratoplasty and glaucoma drainage tube implant. Ophthalmology 108: 272–278.
6. Coleman AL, Mondino BJ, Wilson MR, Casey R (1997) Clinical experience with the Ahmed Glaucoma Valve implant in eyes with prior or concurrent penetrating keratoplasties. Am J Ophthalmol 123: 54–61.
7. Kook MS, Yoon J, Kim J, Lee MS (2000) Clinical results of Ahmed glaucoma valve implantation in refractory glaucoma with adjunctive mitomycin C. Ophthalmic Surg Lasers 31: 100–106.
8. Lai JS, Poon AS, Chua JK, Tham CC, Leung AT, et al. (2000) Efficacy and safety of the Ahmed glaucoma valve implant in Chinese eyes with complicated glaucoma. Br J Ophthalmol 84: 718–721.
9. Taglia DP, Perkins TW, Gangnon R, Heatley GA, Kaufman PL (2002) Comparison of the Ahmed Glaucoma Valve, the Krupin Eye Valve with Disk, and the double-plate Molteno implant. J Glaucoma 11: 347–353.
10. Das JC, Chaudhuri Z, Sharma P, Bhomaj S (2005) The Ahmed Glaucoma Valve in refractory glaucoma: experiences in Indian eyes. Eye (Lond) 19: 183–190.
11. Al-Aswad LA, Netland PA, Bellows AR, Ajdelsztajn T, Wadhwani RA, et al. (2006) Clinical experience with the double-plate Ahmed glaucoma valve. Am J Ophthalmol 141: 390–391.
12. Brasil MV, Rockwood EJ, Smith SD (2007) Comparison of silicone and polypropylene Ahmed Glaucoma Valve implants. J Glaucoma 16: 36–41.
13. Yamagami S, Suzuki Y, Tsuru T (1996) Risk factors for graft failure in penetrating keratoplasty. Acta Ophthalmol Scand 74: 584–588.
14. Alvarenga LS, Mannis MJ, Brandt JD, Lee WB, Schwab IR, et al. (2004) The long-term results of keratoplasty in eyes with a glaucoma drainage device. Am J Ophthalmol 138: 200–205.
15. McDonnell PJ, Robin JB, Schanzlin DJ, Minckler D, Baerveldt G, et al. (1988) Molteno implant for control of glaucoma in eyes after penetrating keratoplasty. Ophthalmology 95: 364–369.

16. Al-Torbak A (2003) Graft survival and glaucoma outcome after simultaneous penetrating keratoplasty and ahmed glaucoma valve implant. Cornea 22: 194–197.

17. Topouzis F, Coleman AL, Choplin N, Bethlem MM, Hill R, et al. (1999) Follow-up of the original cohort with the Ahmed glaucoma valve implant. Am J Ophthalmol 128: 198–204.

18. Sherwood MB, Smith MF, Driebe WT Jr., Stern GA, Beneke JA, et al. (1993) Drainage tube implants in the treatment of glaucoma following penetrating keratoplasty. Ophthalmic Surg 24: 185–189.

19. Rapuano CJ, Schmidt CM, Cohen EJ, Rajpal RK, Raber IM, et al. (1995) Results of alloplastic tube shunt procedures before, during, or after penetrating keratoplasty. Cornea 14: 26–32.

20. Goldberg DB, Schanzlin DJ, Brown SI (1981) Incidence of increased intraocular pressure after keratoplasty. Am J Ophthalmol 92: 372–377.

21. Wilson MR, Mendis U, Paliwal A, Haynatzka V (2003) Long-term follow-up of primary glaucoma surgery with Ahmed glaucoma valve implant versus trabeculectomy. Am J Ophthalmol 136: 464–470.

22. Tai MC, Cheng JH, Chen JT, Liang CM, Lu DW (2010) Intermediate outcomes of Ahmed glaucoma valve surgery in Asian patients with intractable glaucoma. Eye (Lond) 24: 547–552.

23. Doyle JW, Smith MF (1994) Glaucoma after penetrating keratoplasty. Semin Ophthalmol 9: 254–257.

24. Babizhayev MA, Yegorov YE (2011) Senescent phenotype of trabecular meshwork cells displays biomarkers in primary open-angle glaucoma. Curr Mol Med 11: 528–552.

25. Yalvac IS, Eksioglu U, Satana B, Duman S (2007) Long-term results of Ahmed glaucoma valve and Molteno implant in neovascular glaucoma. Eye (Lond) 21: 65–70.

26. Sit M, Weisbrod DJ, Naor J, Slomovic AR (2001) Corneal graft outcome study. Cornea 20: 129–133.

27. Ishida K, Netland PA, Costa VP, Shiroma L, Khan B, et al. (2006) Comparison of polypropylene and silicone Ahmed Glaucoma Valves. Ophthalmology 113: 1320–1326.

28. Ayyala RS, Zurakowski D, Smith JA, Monshizadeh R, Netland PA, et al. (1998) A clinical study of the Ahmed glaucoma valve implant in advanced glaucoma. Ophthalmology 105: 1968–1976.

# 17

# Altered Spontaneous Brain Activity in Primary Open Angle Glaucoma: A Resting-State Functional Magnetic Resonance Imaging Study

Yinwei Song[1,9], Ketao Mu[2,9], Junming Wang[1,9], Fuchun Lin[3]*, Zhiqi Chen[1], Xiaoqin Yan[1], Yonghong Hao[2], Wenzhen Zhu[2]*, Hong Zhang[1]*

1 Department of Ophthalmology, Tongji Hospital, Tongji Medical College, Huazhong University of Science and Technology, Wuhan, China, 2 Department of Radiology, Tongji Hospital, Tongji Medical College, Huazhong University of Science and Technology, Wuhan, China, 3 Wuhan Center for Magnetic Resonance, State Key Laboratory of Magnetic Resonance and Atomic and Molecular Physics, Wuhan Institute of Physics and Mathematics, Chinese Academy of Sciences, Wuhan, China

## Abstract

*Background:* Previous studies demonstrated that primary open angle glaucoma (POAG) is associated with abnormal brain structure; however, little is known about the changes in the local synchronization of spontaneous activity. The main objective of this study was to investigate spontaneous brain activity in patients with POAG using regional homogeneity (ReHo) analysis based on resting state functional magnetic resonance imaging (rs-fMRI).

*Methodology/Principal Findings:* Thirty-nine POAG patients and forty-one age- and gender- matched healthy controls were finally included in the study. ReHo values were used to evaluate spontaneous brain activity and whole brain voxel-wise analysis of ReHo was carried out to detect differences by region in spontaneous brain activity between groups. Compared to controls, POAG patients showed increased ReHo in the right dorsal anterior cingulated cortex, the bilateral medial frontal gyrus and the right cerebellar anterior lobe, and decreased ReHo in the bilateral calcarine, bilateral precuneus gyrus, bilateral pre/postcentral gyrus, left inferior parietal lobule and left cerebellum posterior lobe. A multiple linear regression analysis was performed to explore the relationships between clinical measures and ReHo by region showed significant group differences in the POAG group. Negative correlations were found between age and the ReHo values of the superior frontal gyrus ($r = -0.323$, $p = 0.045$), left calcarine ($r = -0.357$, $p = 0.026$) and inferior parietal lobule ($r = -0.362$, $p = 0.024$). A negative correlation was found between the ReHo values of the left precuneus and the cumulative mean defect ($r = -0.400$, $p = 0.012$).

*Conclusions:* POAG was associated with abnormal brain spontaneous activity in some brain regions and such changed regional activity may be associated with clinical parameters. Spontaneous brain activity may play a role in POAG initiation and progression.

**Editor:** Sanjoy Bhattacharya, Bascom Palmer Eye Institute, University of Miami School of Medicine;, United States of America

**Funding:** This study was supported by National Natural Science Foundation(Grants No 81170842 and 81171308) of China, and National Program of the Ministry of Science and Technology of China during the "12th Five-year Plan" (Grants No 2011BAI08B10). The funders had no role in study design, data collection and analysis, decision to publish, or preparation of the manuscript.

**Competing Interests:** The authors have declared that no competing interests exist.

\* E-mail: fclin@wipm.ac.cn (FL); zhuwenzhen@hotmail.com (WZ); dr_zhanghong@126.com (HZ)

⑨ These authors contributed equally to this work.

## Introduction

Primary open angle glaucoma (POAG), a neurodegenerative optic disease, is the leading cause of irreversible blindness in the world. Clinical features include optic nerve rim loss, retinal nerve fiber damage and visual field defect. The risk of glaucomatous optic neuropathy increases with multiple risk factors, including elevated intraocular pressure (IOP), age greater than 60 years, a family history of glaucoma and African race. However, a fundamental understanding of the pathology and mechanism of POAG is important because, thus far, no comprehensive theory has been developed to explain all clinical presentations. Previous studies agree with that not only does POAG injure the optic nerve but cross-synaptic degeneration also extends into the lateral geniculate body, as well as to the tertiary neuron in the visual cortex [1–7].

Recently, advanced magnetic resonance imaging (MRI) technology permits visualization of minor changes in the whole brain in vivo. We applied both techniques of proton density sequence and gray matter sequence to measure the height and volume of the lateral geniculate nucleus in POAG. Both sequences revealed that the maximum height and volume of the lateral geniculate nucleus in POAG patients were significantly reduced compared with healthy volunteers and correlated with cumulative clinical glaucoma stage [8,9]. The diffusion tensor imaging technique can detect myelin and axonal damage, which represent nerve fiber remodeling. Previous studies have shown that the diffusion tensor imaging parameters of fractional anisotropy, mean diffusivity and radial diffusivity are altered in the optic nerve, chiasm and optic radiations of glaucoma patients [10–13]. Voxel-based morphometry (VBM) studies have shown that neural degeneration extends to the primary visual cortex, as well as to other related cortical areas [11,14–19]. Furthermore, some studies have focused on whole brain changes within and beyond the visual pathway in glaucoma [14,19]. However, all of the above-mentioned techniques only show neuronal morphological changes in POAG, and there is a lack of direct evidence of changes in brain function. Resting-state functional magnetic resonance imaging (rs-fMRI) can show both spontaneous brain activity and the endogenous/ background neurophysiological processes of the human brain. Blood oxygenation level-dependent (BOLD) technique, an imaging technique that detect changes in the concentration of oxygenated and deoxygenated hemoglobin, reflecting neuronal activity. Regional homogeneity (ReHo) analysis based on BOLD is widely used to detect the function of various brain areas. Taking into account the previous studies and the most current MRI techniques, we used BOLD technique to quantify the spontaneous change in neuronal activity in patients with POAG and in matched controls in the resting state.

## Materials and Methods

### Subjects

From October 2010 to January 2013, 42 patients with POAG who were admitted to the Ophthalmology Department at Tongji Hospital, Medical College, Huazhong University of Science and Technology and who met the following criteria were prospectively included: (1) one or both eyes with glaucomatous-type optic disc cupping, or patients with thinning of the inferior and/or superior rim with a cup/disc ratio (CDR) asymmetry >0.2; (2) normal anterior chamber with an open angle in both eyes; (3) matched glaucomatous visual field defects; and (4) right-handedness. The control group was comprised of age- and gender-matched healthy subjects. Exclusion criteria were secondary glaucoma and any other ocular or neurological disorder that could affect the optic visual pathway. Subjects unable to undergo MRI scanning due to metal implantation or those with a history of cigarette consumption, claustrophobia or other psychological disorders were excluded.

Forty-two POAG patients (33 males and 9 females) met the inclusion criteria: a total of 39 formed the POAG group (two patients had head movement >3 mm, and one patient had incomplete data). Of the 42 age- and gender-matched controls selected, 41 formed the control group (one had incomplete data).

The cumulative clinical measurement, such as mean defect (MD), retinal nerve fiber layer thickness (RNFLT), cup to disc ratio (CDR) and intraocular pressure (IOP) was calculated as the sum of the measurements of both eyes in each individual.

Table 1 shows the demographic information and clinical measures for POAG patients and healthy controls. POAG patients were matched with the controls in age (p = 1.00) and gender (p = 0.86) distribution. There were significant differences in the best-corrected visual acuity (p<0.0001), CDR (p<0.0001), MD and RNFLT (p<0.0001) of the bilateral eyes, and the IOP of the left eye (p<0.027), while a trend difference in the IOP of the right eye (p<0.095) was seen between groups.

The study followed the tenets of the Declaration of Helsinki and was approved by the Ethics Committee of the Tongji Hospital, Medical College, Huazhong University of Science and Technology Institute, Wuhan, P.R. China. Written informed consent was obtained from subjects after the purposes of the research study

**Table 1.** Demographic and ocular characteristics (mean ± standard deviation) in patients with primary open-angle glaucoma (POAG) and control group.

| Issues | Groups | | P |
| --- | --- | --- | --- |
| | **POAG** | **Normal Control** | |
| Male/Female | 32/7 | 33/8 | |
| Age (years) | 34.82±9.90 | 34.83±9.65 | 0.997 |
| Best-corrected VA-Right | 0.80±0.42 | 1.12±0.10 | <0.001 |
| Best-corrected VA-Left | 0.78±0.43 | 1.14±0.11 | <0.001 |
| Refraction (D)-Right | −2.74±2.87 | −1.85±2.09 | 0.116 |
| Refraction (D)-Left | −2.55±2.79 | −1.78±1.97 | 0.156 |
| IOP-Right | 17.08±8.71 | 14.34±2.30 | 0.056 |
| IOP-Left | 17.33±6.47 | 14.44±2.38 | 0.011 |
| CDR-Right | 0.81±0.17 | 0.30±0.05 | <0.001 |
| CDR-Left | 0.77±0.23 | 0.31±0.06 | <0.001 |
| MD-Right | −16.09±9.76 | −1.35±0.93 | <0.001 |
| MD-Left | −13.64±13.94 | −1.53±0.99 | <0.001 |
| RNFLT-Right | 58.22±21.59 | 111.28±8.29 | <0.001 |
| RNFLT-Left | 66.62±26.16 | 111.27±8.29 | <0.001 |

VA visual acuity; D diopters; IOP intraocular pressure; CDR cup/disc ratio; MD mean defect; RNFLT retinal nerve fiber thickness.

were explained. The individuals in this manuscript gave written informed consent to publish these case details.

### Data Acquisition

All subjects were examined by a 3 T magnetic resonance scanner (Signa HDxt, GE Healthcare, Milwaukee, WI) with an 8-channel phased-array head coil. The rs-fMRI data were acquired with the following parameters: repetition time = 2,000 ms; echo time = 30 ms; flip angle = 90°; acquisition matrix = 64×64; field of view = 240×240 mm2; slice thickness = 3 mm with a 1 mm gap. Each brain volume comprised 33 axial slices and each run contained 240 volumes. During the rs-fMRI data acquisition, subjects were instructed to keep their eyes closed, relax their minds but not fall asleep, and remain as motionless as possible.

### Data Processing

Data processing was carried out using SPM8 (http://www.fil. ion.ucl.ac.uk/spm). For each subject, the first 10 volumes were discarded to allow for magnetization equilibration. The remaining volumes were corrected for the acquisition time and realigned to correct for head motion. Subjects with maximum displacement in any direction of more than 3.0 mm or head rotation of more than 3.0°were excluded from this study. Subjects with incomplete data were also excluded. As a result, data of three POAG patients and one control subject were excluded and a total of 80 subjects (39 POAG patients and 41 controls) were analyzed. The realigned images were then spatially normalized to the Montreal Neurological Institute space and resampled to 3 mm isotropic voxels. Finally, the linear trend of the time series was removed and bandpass filtering (0.01–0.08 Hz) was performed to reduce the effects of physiological noise.

ReHo was used to evaluate spontaneous brain activity in POAG patients. ReHo analysis was carried out using the Resting-State fMRI Data Analysis Toolkit (http://restfmri.net/forum/REST). ReHo was defined as the Kendall's coefficient of concordance (KCC) of the time series of a given voxel with its nearest 26 neighboring voxels. Each individual ReHo map was generated by a voxel-wise manner [20]. Finally, the ReHo maps were smoothed by 6 mm full width at half maximum (FWHM) Gaussian kernel.

## Statistical Analysis

A voxel-wise two-sample t-test with age and gender as covariates was performed to detect group differences in ReHo across the whole brain between POAG patients and healthy controls. The statistical map was set at a combined threshold of $p<0.005$ for each voxel with a minimum cluster size of 26 voxels ($702 \text{ mm}^3$), resulting in a corrected threshold of $p_{alpha}<0.05$ as determined by Monte Carlo simulation (AlphaSim with the following parameters: single voxel $p = 0.005$, FWHM = 6 mm, cluster connection radius $r = 5$ mm, with the Automated Anatomical Labelling template as a mask).

Additionally, although the groups were well matched for age and gender, brain function is still highly dependent on age, a fact that must be taken into account as a confounding variable in any analysis involving brain function. An analysis of stepwise multiple linear regression analysis (ANCOVA) with age, gender, cumulative IOP, cumulative MD, cumulative CDR and cumulative RNFLT as covariates was performed to assess the relationships between clinical variables and spontaneous brain activity in the affected regions showing changed ReHo values in POAG patients. A p value of less than 0.05 was considered statistically significant. Statistical analyses were performed by using the Statistical Product and Service Solutions Statistics, Version 20.0 for Windows (IBM SPSS Statistics-win64).

## Results

The within-group ReHo maps for the healthy controls and POAG patients were shown in Figure 1. For both the two groups, extensive grey matter regions showed significant larger-than-global-mean ReHo values. Those regions include sensorimotor areas, visual areas, auditory areas, prefrontal cortex, temporal cortex, parietal cortex, insula, cerebellum, striatum, thalamus and the default mode network.

Compared with healthy controls, POAG patients had significantly increased ReHo values in the brain regions of the right dorsal anterior cingulated cortex, the bilateral medial frontal gyrus and the right cerebellar anterior lobe (Figure 2 red and Table 2). Brain areas with significant decreased ReHo values in POAG were located in the bilateral calcarine, bilateral precuneus, bilateral precentral/postcentral gyrus, left inferior parietal lobule and left cerebellar posterior lobe (Figure 2 blue and Table 2).

Negative correlations were found between age and the ReHo values of the superior frontal gyrus ($r = -0.323$, $p = 0.04$), left inferior parietal lobule($r = -0.362$, $p = 0.024$) and left calcarine ($r = -0.357$, $p = 0.026$) in the POAG group but not in the control group.

In the POAG group, the ReHo values of the left precuneus were negatively correlated with the cumulative MD ($r = -0.400$, $p = 0.012$) (Figure 3).

## Discussion

Glaucoma is well understood at the level of the retina and optic nerve, but remains poorly understood at the level of the whole brain. Various mechanisms such as endoplasmic reticulum stress, dendrite disruption and astrogliosis activation are involved in the plasticity of the neural system, resulting in functional deficits and reorganization of the whole brain network. Many previous MRI studies have shown altered brain structure in POAG patients; however, little has been published regarding where or how spontaneous underlying brain activity differs between POAG patients and healthy subjects. Rs-fMRI technology enables observation of the functional alterations in POAG patients. ReHo, a voxel-wise method of rs-fMRI analysis, was used in the current study to provide rapid mapping of regional activity across the whole brain [20].

Our result is consistent with previous studies which show both morphological atropy and functional deterioration in the visual cortex of POAG patients [19,21,22]. However, our study differs Chen's study in important ways. The previous study found increased gray matter volume in the bilateral middle temporal gyrus and precuneus, and decreased gray matter volume in the superior and inferior frontal gyrus [19]. In our study, on the other hand, neuroactivity was significantly increased in the medial and

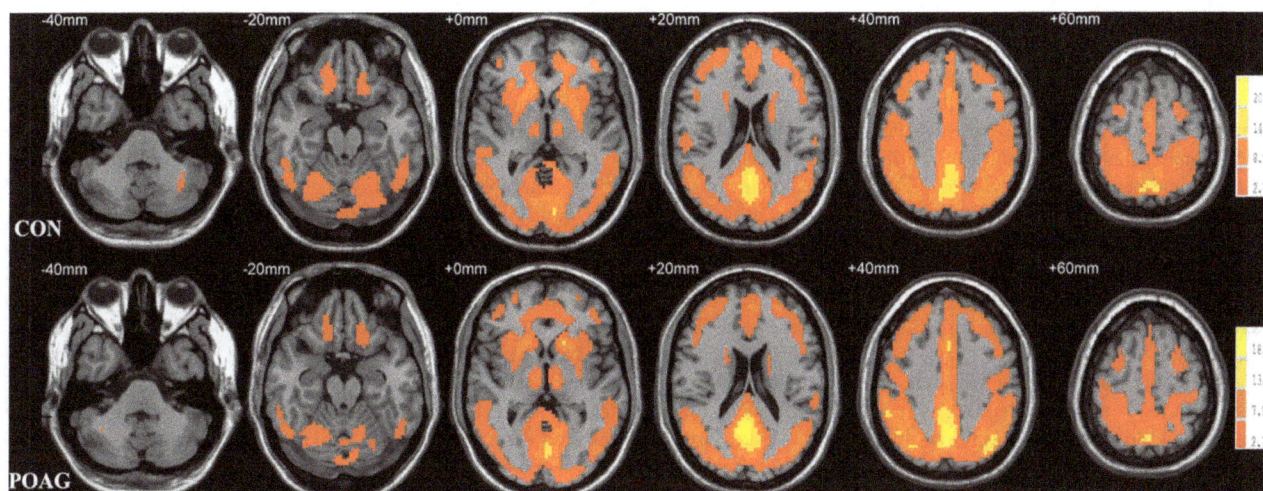

**Figure 1. Results from one-sample t-test on ReHo maps for healthy subjects (CON, upper) and POAG patients (lower).** Threshold was set to p<0.05 with AlphaSim correction.

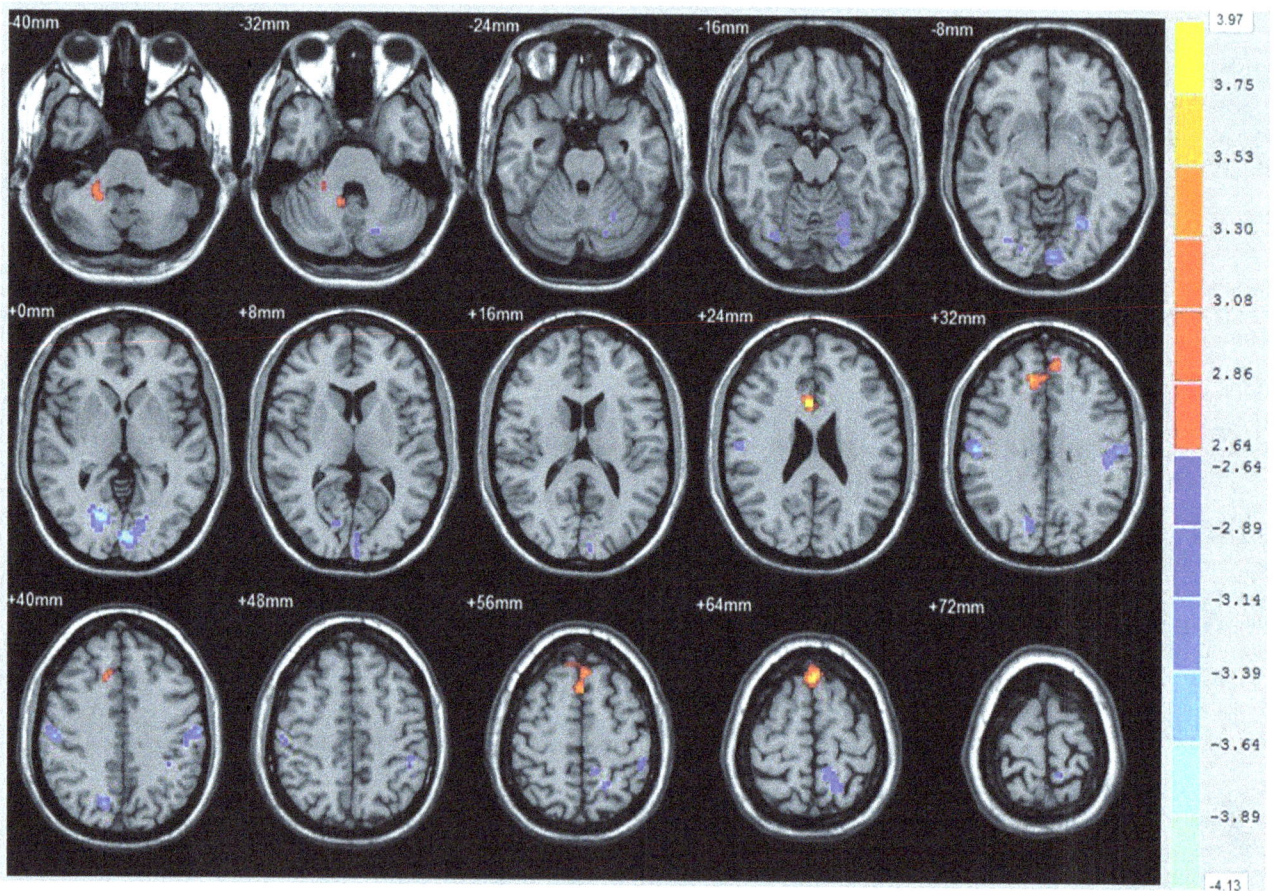

**Figure 2. Significant differences of spontaneous brain activity between the POAG group and normal control group (p<0.05 with AlphaSim correction).** The right dorsal anterior cingulate, bilateral medial superior frontal gyrus, bilateral medial frontal gyrus and right cerebellum anterior lobe showed increased spontaneous brain activity in POAG group (red). The bilateral calcarine, right lingual gyrus, bilateral precuneus gyrus, left cerebellum posterior lobe, left inferior parietal lobule, bilateral precentral and postcentral gyrus showed decreased spontaneous brain activity in POAG group (blue).

medial superior frontal gyrus, but not in the middle temporal gyrus. The differences may stem from the fact that that our study included patients with POAG of any stage from 0–5, including bilateral asymmetric optic nerve damage, but Chen's study included only symmetric terminal stage patients. Another reason may be the different scan sequences and analytical methods used. VBM is a semi-automated technique that detects morphological changes at the whole-brain level, but rs-fMRI uses the BOLD technique to, reflect neuronal activity and changes in functional connections at the whole-brain level. Although in most situations the functional changes agree with the morphological changes, the results are sometimes inconsistent. Therefore, using a combination of both techniques may provide greater insight into the pathological mechanisms of POAG.

In the current study, spontaneous neuronal activity was decreased in the primary visual cortex (BA17) and the secondary visual cortex (BA 18 and 19), caused by apoptosis of retinal ganglion cells. Morphological research indicates that the visual cortex gradually atrophies as POAG progresses [1]. Recently, Duncan revealed decreased cerebral blood flow in the visual cortex of those with POAG [22], suggesting that regional metabolism and blood flow contribute to the phenomenon. Visual information is known to be transmitted through the dorsal and ventral pathways. The former involves the parietal gyrus and responds to spatial information and motional orientation; the latter

pathway extends into the temporal lobe and responds to color and shapes [23]. Previous studies found that the occipital cortex predominantly, but also the temporal-parietal regions constitute an intrinsic connectivity network for visual processing [24,25]. In a recent investigation using rs-fMRI, Dai et al. reported that in POAG patients, voxel-wise analysis showed decreased functional connectivity decreased between the primary visual cortex and the right inferior temporal, left fusiform, left middle occipital, right superior occipital, left postcentral, right precentral gyri and the anterior lobe of the left cerebellum [26]. Obviously, the most affected area of functional connectivity was located in the ventral pathway in Dai's study; the dorsal pathway changed little. However, clinical features indicate injury to both visual pathways [27]. This contradiction arises from the method by which functional connectivity is measured. Since connectivity represents a correlation of two spatially distinct regions, it is modulated by cerebral blood flow from both regions [28]. Our measuring method has the advantage of clarifying the spontaneous brain activity and cerebral blood flow of each independent region. We detected decreased regional activity in the precuneus and inferior part of the parietal lobe, but no change in regional activity in the temporal lobe. The precuneus is located in the superior region and connects with visual areas in the cuneus and with the primary visual cortex. Functional imaging studies have found that the precuneus and the inferior parietal lobe play an important role in a

**Table 2.** Brain regions with significant differences in ReHo between control and POAG group (P(corrected)<0.05, P(uncorrected)< 0.005 and cluster voxels>26).

| Brain areas | Hemisphere | BA | MNI coordinates (cluster maxima, mm) | | | Peak T values | Cluster size (voxels) |
|---|---|---|---|---|---|---|---|
| | | | X | Y | Z | | |
| **POAG<CON** | | | | | | | |
| Dorsal Cingulate Cortex | Right | 33 | 6 | 18 | 24 | 3.97 | 47 |
| Medial Superior Frontal Gyrus | Bilateral | | 0 | 27 | 63 | 3.71 | 90 |
| Medial Frontal Gyrus | Bilateral | 9 | 12 | 36 | 33 | 3.45 | 64 |
| Cerebellum Anterior Lobe | Right | | 24 | −42 | −36 | 3.09 | 31 |
| **POAG<CON** | | | | | | | |
| Calcarine | Left | 17 | −3 | −90 | 0 | 4.13 | 132 |
| Calcarine/Lingual Gyrus | Right | 18 | 15 | −75 | 0 | 4.13 | 97 |
| Precentral/Postcentral Gyrus | Left | 4 | −60 | −18 | 36 | 3.78 | 57 |
| Precentral/Postcentral Gyrus | Right | 3 | 57 | −18 | 33 | 3.75 | 68 |
| Occipital/Cerebellum Posterior Lobe | Left | | −27 | −63 | −9 | 3.58 | 87 |
| Precuneus | Left | | −12 | −45 | 69 | 3.55 | 55 |
| Precuneus | Right | | 15 | −72 | 39 | 3.51 | 39 |
| Inferior Parietal Lobule | Left | | −45 | −39 | 48 | 3.14 | 27 |

BA Brodmann area; MNI: Montreal Neurological Institute;
ReHo: regional homogeneity; POAG: primary open-angle glaucoma;

wide spectrum of highly integrated tasks, such as visuospatial imagery, episodic memory retrieval, self-reflection, and aspects of consciousness [29–31]. Therefore, decreased regional activity in the precuneus and the inferior parietal lobe could reflect impaired visual function in the POAG group. The potential mechanism for the decrease in spontaneous activity in the precentral/postcentral gyrus is unknown, but a previous study indicated that the precentral/postcentral gyrus is associated with primary visual areas in the resting state [32]. Although little is known on the mechanism of the decreased activity in the observed above

regions, but the neurons accept similar stimulate may have similar structures, and this could partly explain why decreased activity is occurring in some but not the whole brain [33].

The regions of hyperactivity in the current study include the right anterior cingulate cortex (ACC) and the bilateral medial frontal gyrus. The dorsal region of the ACC is the cognitive subdivision of the ACC. It is connected with the prefrontal cortex, the parietal cortex, the motor system and the frontal eye fields, and modulates the frontal eye field, visual attention particularly during the tracking of visible targets [34]; it is also involved in the

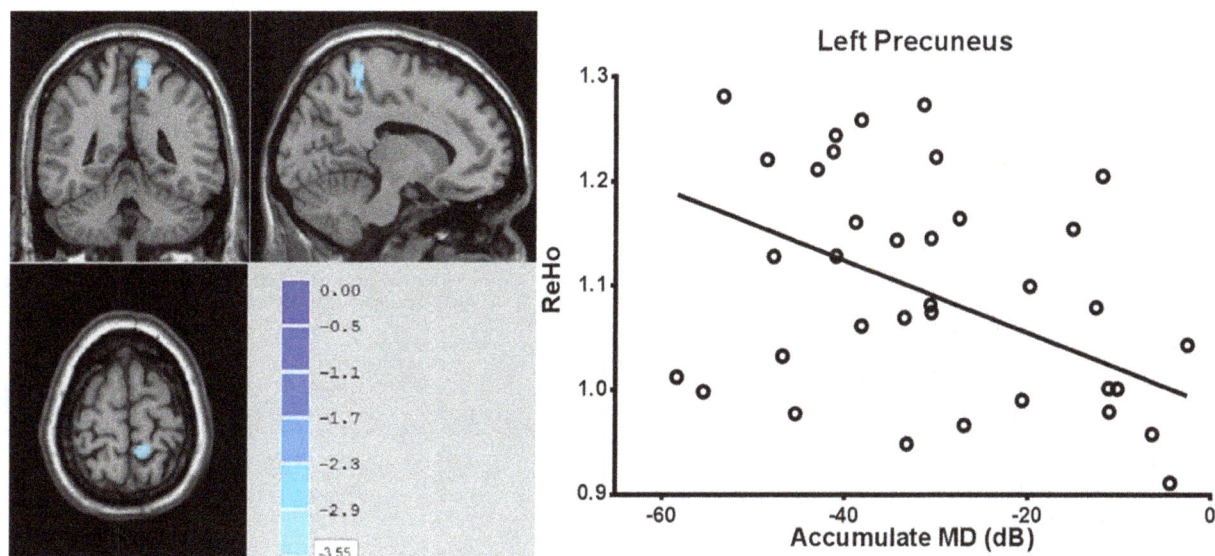

Figure 3. ReHo values of the left precuneus showed negative correlation with cumulative MD values in POAG group (r = −0.400, p = 0.012).

categorical recognition of visual objects [35]. Clinically, when the right dorsal ACC is invaded by a mass, such as a tumor, visual function deficits occur; once the tumor is removed, visual attention and visual memory improves [36]. The frontal lobe helps in the optic localization, coordinating multiple retinal fields and determining the fixation point. It processes the coordination of spatial information beyond the categorical processing [37], and transmits the visual information to the oculomotor complex [38]. The frontal lobe also processes language tasks [39]. Increased neuronal activity in the superior and medial frontal gyrus is due to cerebral plastic change, including neurodegeneration and structural reconstruction. In the current study, we also found that regional activity was increased in the left cerebellar posterior lobe, but decreased in the right cerebellar anterior lobe. This results partly confirms the notion that different cerebellar subregions play different roles in different intrinsic connectivity networks [40].

In the POAG group but not the control group, age was negatively correlate with the ReHo values of the superior frontal gyrus, the left inferior parietal lobule and the left calcarine. The results of our study suggests that POAG may aggravate the degeneration of central nerve system that occurs with age, and furthermore, that changes in distant neuronal populations may aggravate of existing central nervous system disease [41].

Interestingly, a negative correlation was also found between the ReHo values of the left precuneus and the cumulative MD in POAG group$(r = -0.400, p = 0.012)$. A previous study reported that the precuneus plays a role in peripheral vision [42]. It is difficult to determine why there is a negative correlation between the spontaneous activity in this region and cumulative MD, because this region had decreased activity. However, a very recent study indicated that, early in POAG, the brain goes through a temporary compensated stage in which most brain structures become larger, before they develop structural atrophy [43]. This brain change is a result of the defense mechanism of suppressing neuronal activity at the early stage of the disease, accompanied by a compensatory mechanism of increasing neuronal activity and increasing dendritic arborization and axonal tracts [44].

Some limitations in our research should be mentioned. Firstly, the number of subjects included in the study was relatively small for obtaining subgroup differences within the POAG group. However, this emerging tool showed statistically significant differences between the POAG group and the control group. The underlying mechanism of these intriguing results, once elucidated, promises to provide further insight into the neurobiology and functional consequences of POAG. Secondly, an unresolved issue is the number of independent clusters needed to neither overestimate the regional activity nor over-split the main networks [45]. Thirdly, the current research is just a first step toward understanding the abnormal condition in the resting state in POAG patients, which may play an important role in neuronal functional reconstruction and POAG development. The next step is to determine the different connections of the resting state networks. Fourth, although some previous researches indicated that some areas were rhythm-related and IOP-related, we found no correlation between IOP and spontaneous brain activity. The most important reason may be most subjects were received IOP-lowing therapy, so that there was no significant difference in IOP between two groups. And it is still unclear why some area differences are unilateral.

In conclusion, rs-fMRI reveals, abnormal regional spontaneous activity involved in brain changes associated with POAG. Our study, showing a negative correlation between the spontaneous activity of the precuneus and clinical severity, enhances our understanding of the retinotopy in the brain. Future studies are needed to determine the complete structural and functional changes that occur from the early to the end stage of POAG.

## Author Contributions

Conceived and designed the experiments: YS ZC HZ. Performed the experiments: KM YH WZ FL YS XY. Analyzed the data: YS FL. Contributed reagents/materials/analysis tools: YS JW HZ WZ KM FL. Wrote the paper: YS HZ.

## References

1. Gupta N, Ang LC, Noel de Tilly L, Bidaisee L, Yucel YH (2006) Human glaucoma and neural degeneration in intracranial optic nerve, lateral geniculate nucleus, and visual cortex. Br J Ophthalmol 90: 674–678.
2. Yucel YH, Zhang Q, Weinreb RN, Kaufman PL, Gupta N (2001) Atrophy of relay neurons in magno- and parvocellular layers in the lateral geniculate nucleus in experimental glaucoma. Invest Ophthalmol Vis Sci 42: 3216–3222.
3. Gupta N, Ly T, Zhang Q, Kaufman PL, Weinreb RN, et al. (2007) Chronic ocular hypertension induces dendrite pathology in the lateral geniculate nucleus of the brain. Exp Eye Res 84: 176–184.
4. Abouzeid H, Youssef MA, ElShakankiri N, Hauser P, Munier FL, et al. (2009) PAX6 aniridia and interhemispheric brain anomalies. Mol Vis 15: 2074–2083.
5. Ito Y, Shimazawa M, Chen YN, Tsuruma K, Yamashima T, et al. (2009) Morphological changes in the visual pathway induced by experimental glaucoma in Japanese monkeys. Exp Eye Res 89: 246–255.
6. Ito Y, Shimazawa M, Inokuchi Y, Yamanaka H, Tsuruma K, et al. (2011) Involvement of endoplasmic reticulum stress on neuronal cell death in the lateral geniculate nucleus in the monkey glaucoma model. Eur J Neurosci 33: 843–855.
7. Dai Y, Sun X, Yu X, Guo W, Yu D (2012) Astrocytic responses in the lateral geniculate nucleus of monkeys with experimental glaucoma. Vet Ophthalmol 15: 23–30.
8. Dai H, Mu KT, Qi JP, Wang CY, Zhu WZ, et al. (2011) Assessment of lateral geniculate nucleus atrophy with 3T MR imaging and correlation with clinical stage of glaucoma. AJNR Am J Neuroradiol 32: 1347–1353.
9. Chen Z, Wang J, Lin F, Dai H, Mu K, et al. (2013) Correlation between lateral geniculate nucleus atrophy and damage to the optic disc in glaucoma. J Neuroradiol 40: 281–287.
10. Chen Z, Lin F, Wang J, Li Z, Dai H, et al. (2013) Diffusion tensor magnetic resonance imaging reveals visual pathway damage that correlates with clinical severity in glaucoma. Clin Experiment Ophthalmol 41: 43–49.
11. Dai H, Yin D, Hu C, Morelli JN, Hu S, et al. (2013) Whole-brain voxel-based analysis of diffusion tensor MRI parameters in patients with primary open angle glaucoma and correlation with clinical glaucoma stage. Neuroradiology 55: 233–243.
12. Nucci C, Mancino R, Martucci A, Bolacchi F, Manenti G, et al. (2012) 3-T Diffusion tensor imaging of the optic nerve in subjects with glaucoma: correlation with GDx-VCC, HRT-III and Stratus optical coherence tomography findings. Br J Ophthalmol 96: 976–980.
13. Nucci C, Martucci A, Cesareo M, Mancino R, Russo R, et al. (2013) Brain involvement in glaucoma: advanced neuroimaging for understanding and monitoring a new target for therapy. Curr Opin Pharmacol 13: 128–133.
14. Zikou AK, Kitsos G, Tzarouchi LC, Astrakas L, Alexiou GA, et al. (2012) Voxel-based morphometry and diffusion tensor imaging of the optic pathway in primary open-angle glaucoma: a preliminary study. AJNR Am J Neuroradiol 33: 128–134.
15. Boucard CC, Hernowo AT, Maguire RP, Jansonius NM, Roerdink JB, et al. (2009) Changes in cortical grey matter density associated with long-standing retinal visual field defects. Brain 132: 1898–1906.
16. Hernowo AT, Boucard CC, Jansonius NM, Hooymans JM, Cornelissen FW (2011) Automated morphometry of the visual pathway in primary open-angle glaucoma. Invest Ophthalmol Vis Sci 52: 2758–2766.
17. Duncan RO, Sample PA, Weinreb RN, Bowd C, Zangwill LM (2007) Retinotopic organization of primary visual cortex in glaucoma: a method for comparing cortical function with damage to the optic disk. Invest Ophthalmol Vis Sci 48: 733–744.
18. Duncan RO, Sample PA, Weinreb RN, Bowd C, Zangwill LM (2007) Retinotopic organization of primary visual cortex in glaucoma: Comparing fMRI measurements of cortical function with visual field loss. Prog Retin Eye Res 26: 38–56.
19. Chen WW, Wang N, Cai S, Fang Z, Yu M, et al. (2013) Structural brain abnormalities in patients with primary open-angle glaucoma: a study with 3T MR imaging. Invest Ophthalmol Vis Sci 54: 545–554.
20. Zang Y, Jiang T, Lu Y, He Y, Tian L (2004) Regional homogeneity approach to fMRI data analysis. Neuroimage 22: 394–400.

21. Qing G, Zhang S, Wang B, Wang N (2010) Functional MRI signal changes in primary visual cortex corresponding to the central normal visual field of patients with primary open-angle glaucoma. Invest Ophthalmol Vis Sci 51: 4627–4634.

22. Duncan RO, Sample PA, Bowd C, Weinreb RN, Zangwill LM (2012) Arterial spin labeling fMRI measurements of decreased blood flow in primary visual cortex correlates with decreased visual function in human glaucoma. Vision Res 60: 51–60.

23. Stiers P, Peeters R, Lagae L, Van Hecke P, Sunaert S (2006) Mapping multiple visual areas in the human brain with a short fMRI sequence. Neuroimage 29: 74–89.

24. Damoiseaux JS, Rombouts SA, Barkhof F, Scheltens P, Stam CJ, et al. (2006) Consistent resting-state networks across healthy subjects. Proc Natl Acad Sci U S A 103: 13848–13853.

25. De Luca M, Beckmann CF, De Stefano N, Matthews PM, Smith SM (2006) fMRI resting state networks define distinct modes of long-distance interactions in the human brain. Neuroimage 29: 1359–1367.

26. Dai H, Morelli JN, Ai F, Yin D, Hu C, et al. (2013) Resting-state functional MRI: functional connectivity analysis of the visual cortex in primary open-angle glaucoma patients. Hum Brain Mapp 34: 2455–2463.

27. Rauscher FG, Chisholm CM, Edgar DF, Barbur JL (2013) Assessment of novel binocular colour, motion and contrast tests in glaucoma. Cell Tissue Res 353: 297–310.

28. Li Z, Zhu Y, Childress AR, Detre JA, Wang Z (2012) Relations between BOLD fMRI-derived resting brain activity and cerebral blood flow. PLoS One 7: e44556.

29. Cavanna AE, Trimble MR (2006) The precuneus: a review of its functional anatomy and behavioural correlates. Brain 129: 564–583.

30. Steinmetz MA, Constantinidis C (1995) Neurophysiological evidence for a role of posterior parietal cortex in redirecting visual attention. Cereb Cortex 5: 448–456.

31. Urner M, Sarri M, Grahn J, Manly T, Rees G, et al. (2013) The role of prestimulus activity in visual extinction. Neuropsychologia 51: 1630–1637.

32. Wang K, Jiang T, Yu C, Tian L, Li J, et al. (2008) Spontaneous activity associated with primary visual cortex: a resting-state FMRI study. Cereb Cortex 18: 697–704.

33. Ghiso JA, Doudevski I, Ritch R, Rostagno AA (2013) Alzheimer's disease and glaucoma: mechanistic similarities and differences. J Glaucoma 22 Suppl 5: S36–38.

34. Ding J, Powell D, Jiang Y (2009) Dissociable frontal controls during visible and memory-guided eye-tracking of moving targets. Hum Brain Mapp 30: 3541–3552.

35. Schettino A, Loeys T, Delplanque S, Pourtois G (2011) Brain dynamics of upstream perceptual processes leading to visual object recognition: a high density ERP topographic mapping study. Neuroimage 55: 1227–1241.

36. Shinoura N, Yamada R, Tabei Y, Shiode T, Itoi C, et al. (2013) The right dorsal anterior cingulate cortex may play a role in anxiety disorder and visual function. Neurol Res 35: 65–70.

37. Mazzarella E, Ramsey R, Conson M, Hamilton A (2013) Brain systems for visual perspective taking and action perception. Soc Neurosci 8: 248–267.

38. Leichnetz GR, Gonzalo-Ruiz A (1987) Collateralization of frontal eye field (medial precentral/anterior cingulate) neurons projecting to the paraoculomotor region, superior colliculus, and medial pontine reticular formation in the rat: a fluorescent double-labeling study. Exp Brain Res 68: 355–364.

39. Kamada K, Sawamura Y, Takeuchi F, Kuriki S, Kawai K, et al. (2007) Expressive and receptive language areas determined by a non-invasive reliable method using functional magnetic resonance imaging and magnetoencephalography. Neurosurgery 60: 296–305; discussion 305–296.

40. Sang L, Qin W, Liu Y, Han W, Zhang Y, et al. (2012) Resting-state functional connectivity of the vermal and hemispheric subregions of the cerebellum with both the cerebral cortical networks and subcortical structures. Neuroimage 61: 1213–1225.

41. Ramulu P (2009) Glaucoma and disability: which tasks are affected, and at what stage of disease? Curr Opin Ophthalmol 20: 92–98.

42. Simon O, Mangin JF, Cohen L, Le Bihan D, Dehaene S (2002) Topographical layout of hand, eye, calculation, and language-related areas in the human parietal lobe. Neuron 33: 475–487.

43. Williams AL, Lackey J, Wizov SS, Chia TM, Gatla S, et al. (2013) Evidence for widespread structural brain changes in glaucoma: a preliminary voxel-based MRI study. Invest Ophthalmol Vis Sci. 54: 5880–7.

44. Johansen-Berg H (2007) Structural plasticity: rewiring the brain. Curr Biol 17: R141–144.

45. Auer DP (2008) Spontaneous low-frequency blood oxygenation level-dependent fluctuations and functional connectivity analysis of the 'resting' brain. Magn Reson Imaging 26: 1055–1064.

# 18

# Subfoveal Choroidal Thickness and Glaucoma: The Beijing Eye Study 2011

Ya Xing Wang[1], Liang Xu[1], Lei Shao[1], Ya Qin Zhang[1], Hua Yang[1], Jin Da Wang[1], Jost B. Jonas[1,2¶], Wen Bin Wei[3*¶]

1 Beijing Institute of Ophthalmology, Beijing Tongren Hospital, Capital Medical University, Beijing, China, 2 Department of Ophthalmology, Medical Faculty Mannheim of the Ruprecht-Karls-University, Heidelberg, Germany, 3 Beijing Tongren Eye Center, Beijing Tongren Hospital, Capital Medical University, Beijing, China

## Abstract

*Purpose:* To examine subfoveal choroidal thickness (SFCT) in eyes with glaucoma, using enhanced depth imaging spectral domain optical coherence tomography.

*Methods:* The population-based Beijing Eye Study 2011 included 3468 individuals with a mean age of $64.6\pm9.8$ years (range: 50–93 years). A detailed ophthalmic examination was performed including spectral-domain optical coherence tomography (SD-OCT) with enhanced depth imaging for measurement of SFCT, and assessment of fundus photographs for presence of glaucoma. In addition, the group of patients with chronic angle-closure glaucoma (ACG) from the Beijing Eye Study (n = 37) was merged with a group of patients with chronic ACG from the Tongren hospital (n = 52).

*Results:* Assessments of SFCT and glaucoma were available for 3232 (93.2%) subjects. After adjusting for age, axial length, gender, anterior chamber and lens thickness, SFCT was not significantly associated with presence of glaucoma ($P = 0.08$; regression coefficient B:$-15.7$). As a corollary, in logistic regression analysis with adjustment for age, axial length and intraocular pressure, presence of glaucoma was not significantly associated with SFCT ($P = 0.20$). If only open-angle glaucoma was considered, multivariate analysis revealed no significant association between SFCT and presence of open-angle glaucoma ($P = 0.44$). As a corollary, in logistic regression analysis, open-angle glaucoma was not significantly associated with SFCT ($P = 0.91$). In a similar manner if only ACG was taken into account, SFCT was not significantly associated with the presence of ACG ($P = 0.27$) in multivariate analysis. As a corollary in binary regression analysis, presence of ACG was not significantly associated with SFCT ($P = 0.27$).

*Conclusions:* In multivariate analysis with adjustment for age, axial length, gender, anterior chamber and lens thickness, neither OAG nor ACG was associated with an abnormal SFCT.

**Editor:** Paul Baird, Centre for Eye Research Australia, Australia

**Funding:** This work was supported by the State Natural Sciences Fund (81041018) and the Natural Sciences Fund of Beijing Government (7092021, 7112031). The funders had no role in study design, data collection and analysis, decision to publish, or preparation of the manuscript.

**Competing Interests:** JBJ was or has been a member of advisory boards for the following companies: Allergan Inc., Merck Sharp & Dohme Co., Inc., Alimera Co., Boehringer Ingelheim Co. The authors state that these advisory board activities did not have anything to do with the present study.

* Email: wenbing_wei@yahoo.com.cn

¶ These authors share the last authorship.

## Introduction

Glaucomatous optic neuropathy is characterized by the loss of retinal ganglion cell axons, leading to marked morphological changes in the optic nerve head and the inner retinal layers [1]. Additional glaucoma-related changes in the deep retinal layers and the choroid were suggested by few histomorphometric studies and by some recent clinical studies, while other investigations contradicted the notion of glaucomatous changes at the level of the photoreceptors, retinal pigment epithelium and choroid [2–11]. Investigations focused on patients with acute angle-closure glaucoma suggested that eyes with angle-closure glaucoma have an abnormally thick choroid. It has been discussed, that this choroidal abnormality may be involved in the pathogenesis of angle-closure glaucoma [12,13]. Other studies did not find differences in subfoveal choroidal thickness (SFCT) between eyes with open-angle glaucoma and control eyes or assessed the choroidal thickness in the parapapillary or perifoveal region [14–26]. Since the previous studies were hospital-based investigations with the potential risk of a bias due to the referral of patients or since these studies measured the ocular dimensions in fixed eyes with postmortal swelling and fixation induced shrinkage, it remains unclear whether patients with open-angle glaucoma and patients with angle-closure glaucoma show abnormalities in choroidal thickness. Knowledge about the choroidal thickness in glaucoma would help in the discussion whether glaucoma is additionally associated with changes in the deep retinal layers and the choroid. It may also be of interest for the diagnosis of glaucoma, since deep retinal changes show a different pattern in the psychophysical examinations such as perimetry and color vision testing, and since glaucoma related changes in the deep retinal layers and in the choroid could be visualized and analyzed by optical coherence tomography (OCT). We therefore planned and prospectively performed this study to measure the choroidal thickness in patients with glaucoma and non-glaucomatous subjects in a population-based setting. We defined glaucoma by the appearance of the optic nerve head and graduated the amount of glaucomatous optic nerve damage by the thickness of the retinal nerve fiber layer.

## Methods

### Ethics Statement

The Medical Ethics Committee of the Beijing Tongren Hospital approved the study protocol of the Beijing Eye Study and the protocol for including the additional patients examined in the Beijing Tongren hospital and all participants gave informed written consent, according to the Declaration of Helsinki.

The Beijing Eye Study 2011 is a population-based cross-sectional study in Northern China [27,28]. It was carried out in 5 communities in the urban district of Haidian in the North of Central Beijing and in 3 communities in the village area of Yufa of the Daxing District south of Beijing. The only eligibility criterion for inclusion into the study was an age of 50+ years. In 2011, the 8 communities had a total population of 4403 individuals aged 50 years or older. In total, 3468 individuals (1963 (56.6%) women) participated in the eye examination, corresponding to an overall response rate of 78.8%. The study was divided into a rural part (1633 (47.1%) subjects; 943 (57.7%) women) and an urban part (1835 (52.9%) subjects; 1020 (55.6%) women). The mean age was 64.6±9.8 years (median, 64 years; range, 50–93 years). All study participants underwent an interview with standardized questions on their family status, level of education, physical activity, and known major systemic diseases. The ophthalmic examination included measurement of presenting visual acuity, uncorrected visual acuity, and best corrected visual acuity, tonometry, slit lamp examination of the anterior and posterior segment of the eye, biometry for measurement of the anterior corneal curvature, central corneal thickness, anterior chamber depth, lens thickness and axial length, and digital photography of the cornea, lens, macula and optic disc (fundus camera Type CR6-45NM; Canon Inc, Tokyo, Japan). The retinal nerve fiber thickness was measured by spectral domain OCT (Spectralis, Heidelberg Engineering Co., Heidelberg, Germany).

SFCT was measured using spectral domain optical coherence tomography (SD-OCT; Spectralis, Wavelength: 870 nm; Heidelberg Engineering Co., Heidelberg, Germany) with enhanced depth imaging (EDI-OCT) modality after pupil dilation [28,29]. Seven sections, each comprising 100 averaged scans, were obtained in an angle of 5°–30° rectangle centered onto the fovea. The horizontal section running through the center of the fovea was selected for further analysis. Subfoveal choroidal thickness was defined as the vertical distance from the hyperreflective line of the Bruch's membrane to the hyperreflective line of the inner surface of the sclera. The measurements were performed using the Heidelberg Eye Explorer software (version 5.3.3.0; Heidelberg Engineering Co., Heidelberg, Germany). Only the right eye of each study participant was measured. The images were taken by one technician (CXC) and the images were assessed by two ophthalmologists (LS, KFD). The reproducibility of the technique was previously examined and revealed a high reproducibility (Bland-Altman plot with 1.9% (61/3233) points outside the 95% limits of agreement; intra-class coefficient: 1.00; mean coefficient of variation: 0.85%±1.48%) [30].

Examining the digital photographs of the optic disc and macula, glaucoma was defined by a glaucomatous appearance of the optic disc. The optic nerve head was glaucomatous (1) if the inferior-superior-nasal-temporal (ISNT)-rule of the neuroretinal rim shape was not fulfilled in early glaucoma and in eyes with a normally shaped optic disc (it included a notch in the neuroretinal rim in the temporal inferior region and/or the temporal superior region); or (2) if the neuroretinal rim was too small in relation to the size of the optic disc. For all situations, the retinal nerve fiber layer had to show a localized and/or diffuse loss. The assessment of the optic disc photographs was carried in a masked manner without knowledge of intraocular pressure. Each photograph of a glaucomatous optic disc was independently adjudicated by three senior graders (LX, YXW, JBJ). The whole glaucoma group was differentiated into subjects with open-angle glaucoma and with primary angle closure glaucoma. Open-angle glaucoma was characterized by an open anterior chamber angle, in addition to a normal depth of the anterior chamber as assessed by slit lamp biomicroscopy. In angle-closure glaucoma, the anterior chamber angle was occluded or occludable. Using the definition by Foster and colleagues, the anterior chamber angle was defined as occludable, if ≥270° of the posterior trabecular meshwork could not be seen upon gonioscopy [31]. In addition, other features for angle-closure glaucoma were iris whirling and glaukomflecken in the anterior subcapsular lens region, in combination with a narrow anterior chamber angle.

For a subgroup of study participants, optical coherence tomography (iTVue SD-OCT; Optovue, Inc. Fremont, CA, U.S.A.) of the optic nerve head was performed and the vertical cup/disc diameter ratio among other optic disc parameters was measured. For this subgroup, we additionally assessed the presence of glaucoma using criteria of the International Society of Geographic and Epidemiological Ophthalmology ISGEO [31].

Statistical analysis was performed using a commercially available statistical software package (SPSS for Windows, version 20.0, IBM-SPSS, Chicago, IL). In a first step, we examined the mean values (presented as mean ± standard deviation) of SFCT. In a second step, we compared the SFCT between the study groups. In a third step, we performed a multivariate linear regression analysis, with SFCT as dependent parameter and those parameters as independent parameters which had previously been shown to be associated with SFCT.[28] Odds ratios (OR) and 95% confidence intervals (CI) were presented. All $P$-values were 2-sided and were considered statistically significant when the values were less than 0.05.

## Results

Out of the 3468 participants, measurements of the SFCT and assessments for glaucoma were available for 3232 (93.2%) subjects (1817 (56.2%) women). The mean age was 64.3±9.6 years (median: 63 years; range: 50 to 93 years), mean refractive error (spherical equivalent) was −0.18±1.98 diopters (median: 0.25 diopters; range: −20.0 to +7.00 diopters), and mean axial length was 23.24±1.11 mm (median: 23.13 mm; range: 18.96–30.88 mm). The group of subjects without measurements of the SFCT and without assessment of glaucoma as compared with the group of subjects with both examinations was significantly ($P<$ 0.001) older (69.5±10.9 years versus 64.3±9.6 years) and was more myopic (−1.57±4.47 diopters versus −0.18±1.98 diopters; $P=0.002$) and did not vary significantly in gender ($P=0.09$).

Glaucomatous optic neuropathy was detected in 128 (4.0%) patients. The glaucoma group could be further subdivided into subjects with open-angle glaucoma (n = 90 (2.8%)), primary angle-closure glaucoma (n = 37 (1.1%) and secondary angle-closure glaucoma (n = 1 (0.03%)). The glaucoma group as a whole and differentiated into the open-angle glaucoma group and the primary angle-closure glaucoma group as compared with the control group was significantly ($P<0.001$) older (Table 1). Axial length was significantly longer in the total glaucoma group ($P = 0.01$) and in the open-angle glaucoma group ($P = 0.001$) than in the control group, while the angle-closure glaucoma and the control group did not differ significantly ($P = 0.09$) in axial length (Table 1). Mean retinal nerve fiber layer thickness was significantly thinner in the glaucoma group than in the non-glaucomatous group ($101.5 \pm 11.6$ µm versus $85.5 \pm 17.1$ µm; $P<0.001$).

In univariate analysis, mean SFCT was significantly ($P<0.001$) thinner in the total glaucoma group as a whole ($201 \pm 102$ µm (median: 188 µm; range: 9 µm to 537 µm)), and separated into the open-angle glaucoma group ($210 \pm 105$ µm (median: 210 µm; range: 9 µm to 537 µm)), and into the angle-closure glaucoma group ($184 \pm 94$ µm (median: 155 µm; range: 49 µm to 399 µm)) than in the control group ($256 \pm 107$ µm (median: 252 µm; range: 8 µm to 854 µm)) (Table 1).

Since SFCT has been shown to be associated with younger age, shorter axial length, male gender, deeper anterior chamber, thicker lens and presence of diabetes mellitus in the study population of the Beijing Eye Study [28,32], we performed a multivariate analysis with SFCT as dependent variable and age, axial length, gender, anterior chamber depth, lens thickness, presence of diabetes mellitus and presence of glaucoma as independent variables. It revealed that SFCT was significantly associated with younger age ($P<0.001$), shorter axial length ($P<0.001$), male gender ($P<0.001$), deeper anterior chamber ($P<0.001$), larger lens thickness ($P<0.001$) and presence of diabetes mellitus ($P = 0.01$), while the presence of glaucoma ($P = 0.07$) was not significantly associated (Table 2). Analysis of collinearity revealed that the variance inflation factors were <1.90 for all parameters included into the analysis. The variance inflation factor for the presence of glaucoma was 1.02. If intraocular pressure was added to the list of independent parameters, neither glaucoma ($P = 0.09$) nor intraocular pressure ($P = 0.94$) were significantly associated with SFCT. If a logistic regression analysis was performed with the presence of glaucoma as dependent variable, and age, axial length, intraocular pressure (factors which in a previous study were significantly associated with the prevalence of glaucoma) and SFCT as independent variables [27], presence of glaucoma was significantly associated with older age ($P<0.001$; regression coefficient B: 0.07; OR: 1.07 (95%CI: 1.05, 1.09) and higher intraocular pressure ($P = 0.004$; B: 0.13; OR: 1.14 (95%CI: 1.07, 1.21), while axial length ($P = 0.08$; B: 0.15; OR: 1.16 (95%CI: 0.99, 1.36) and SFCT ($P = 0.20$; B: −0.001; OR: 1.00 (95%CI: 1.00, 1.00) were not significantly associated with glaucoma.

Within the total glaucoma group, retinal nerve fiber layer thickness was significantly ($P = 0.003$) associated with SFCT in univariate analysis. If age was added to the list of independent parameters, only age was correlated with SFCT ($P<0.001$; correlation coefficient: −0.46), while SFCT was not related with retinal nerve fiber layer thickness ($P = 0.65$). A similar result was obtained, if additionally axial length was added to the multivariate analysis. If the association was adjusted for age, axial length, gender, anterior chamber depth and lens thickness, the relationship between SFCT and retinal nerve fiber layer thickness again was not statistically significant ($P = 0.62$). If the whole glaucoma group was split up into the open-angle glaucoma subgroup and the angle-glaucoma subgroup, the SFCT was not significantly related with retinal nerve fiber layer thickness, neither in the open-angle

**Table 1.** Demographic parameters, ocular parameters and subfoveal choroidal thickness (mean ± standard deviation) in groups of patients with different types of glaucoma and the remaining control group in the Beijing Eye Study 2011.

| | Total Glaucoma Group | Open-Angle Glaucoma | Angle Closure | Control Group | P-Value (1) | P-Value (2) | P-Value (3) |
|---|---|---|---|---|---|---|---|
| n | 128 | 90 | 37 | 3104 | | | |
| Age | 70.9±9.8 | 70.0±10.1 | 72.9±8.8 | 63.9±9.5 | <0.001 | <0.001 | <0.001 |
| Refractive Error | −0.50±2.24 | −0.67±2.41 | −0.13±2.14 | −0.16±1.96 | 0.11 | 0.053 | 0.91 |
| Axial Length | 23.5±1.3 | 23.8±1.4 | 23.0±0.8 | 23.2±1.1 | 0.01 | 0.001 | 0.09 |
| SFCT | 201.4±02.4 | 210.1±104.7 | 184.2±93,6 | 255.9±107.0 | <0.001 | <0.001 | <0.001 |

P-Value (1): Statistical significance of the difference between the total glaucoma group and the control group.
P-Value (2): Statistical significance of the difference between the open-angle glaucoma group and the control group.
P-Value (3): Statistical significance of the difference between the angle-closure glaucoma group and the control group.
One glaucoma patient had secondary angle-closure glaucoma.

**Table 2.** Associations (multivariate analysis) between subfoveal choroidal thickness, general parameters and glaucoma in the Beijing Eye Study 2011.

| Parameter | P-Value | Standardized Coefficient Beta | Regression Coefficient B | 95% Confidence Intervals for B |
|---|---|---|---|---|
| Age (Years) | <0.001 | −0.41 | −4.63 | −5.02, −4.24 |
| Axial Length (mm) | <0.001 | −0.38 | −36.8 | −40.4, −33.1 |
| Gender (Men/Women) | <0.001 | −0.15 | −32.7 | −39.6, −25.8 |
| Anterior Chamber Depth (mm) | <0.001 | −0.08 | 26.4 | 13.5, 39.4 |
| Lens Thickness (mm) | <0.001 | 0.08 | 25.0 | 13.0, 37.0 |
| Diabetes Mellitus | 0.01 | 0.04 | 11.7 | 2.43, 21.0 |
| Glaucoma | 0.07 | −0.03 | −16.7 | −34.8,1.32 |

glaucoma subgroup ($P = 0.69$) nor in the angle-glaucoma subgroup ($P = 0.85$).

Optical coherence tomography of the optic disc was performed on 1587 (49.1% from the study population) subjects with a mean age of 66.1±9.9 years and a mean axial length of 23.39±1.12 mm. Out of these 1587 subjects, 42 subjects had a vertical cup/disc ratio of 0.91 (i.e. 97.5 percentile) or larger, 29 subjects had history of glaucoma treatment, and 59 subjects had an inferior or superior rim area less than the 97.5% percentile. Altogether (including the overlapping cases), 97 (6.1%) subjects fulfilled at least one of the criteria. Using this glaucoma definition and re-calculating the multivariable analysis revealed that SFCT was significantly associated with younger age ($P < 0.001$), shorter axial length ($P < 0.001$), and male gender ($P < 0.001$). It was not significantly associated with anterior chamber ($P = 0.08$), lens thickness ($P = 0.11$) presence of diabetes mellitus ($P = 0.86$) nor presence of glaucoma ($P = 0.42$).

If only the group of patients with open-angle glaucoma was considered, SFCT was significantly associated with younger age ($P < 0.001$), shorter axial length ($P < 0.001$), male gender ($P < 0.001$), deeper anterior chamber ($P < 0.001$), larger lens thickness ($P < 0.001$) and presence of diabetes mellitus ($P = 0.01$), while the presence of open-angle glaucoma ($P = 0.41$) was not significantly associated (Table 3). If intraocular pressure was added to the list of independent parameters, neither open-angle glaucoma ($P = 0.40$) nor intraocular pressure ($P = 0.99$) were significantly associated with SFCT. If a logistic regression analysis was performed with the presence of open-angle glaucoma as dependent variable, and age, axial length and intraocular pressure and SFCT as independent variables, presence of open-angle glaucoma was significantly associated with older age ($P < 0.001$; regression coefficient B: 0.07; OR: 1.07 (95%CI: 1.04, 1.09), higher intraocular pressure ($P = 0.004$; B: 0.12; OR: 1.13 (95%CI: 1.05, 1.21) and longer axial length ($P = 0.001$; B: 0.30; OR: 1.35 (95%CI: 1.13, 1.61), while SFCT ($P = 0.91$) was not significantly associated with open-angle glaucoma. Within the group with open-angle glaucoma, 7 (8%) eyes had undergone anti-glaucomatous filtering surgery one or more years prior to inclusion into the study. The subgroup with glaucoma surgery and the subgroup without glaucoma surgery did not vary significantly in SFCT (262±96 μm versus 206±105 μm; $P = 0.18$) or in age (71.9±10.3 years versus 70.1±10.1 years; $P = 0.81$), while axial length was significantly shorter in the surgical subgroup (22.5±1.1 mm versus 23.9±1.4 mm; $P = 0.01$). After adjusting for axial length, SFCT was again not significantly associated with previous glaucoma surgery.

If only the group of patients with primary angle-closure glaucoma was considered, thicker SFCT was significantly associated with younger age ($P < 0.001$), shorter axial length ($P < 0.001$), male gender ($P < 0.001$), deeper anterior chamber ($P < 0.001$), larger lens thickness ($P < 0.001$), presence of diabetes mellitus ($P = 0.01$), and the absence of angle-closure glaucoma ($P = 0.044$) (Table 4). If intraocular pressure was added to the list of independent parameters, neither angle-closure glaucoma ($P = 0.07$) nor intraocular pressure ($P = 0.97$) were significantly associated with SFCT. If a logistic regression analysis was performed with the presence of angle-closure glaucoma as dependent variable, and age, axial length and intraocular pressure, and SFCT as independent variables, presence of angle-closure glaucoma was significantly associated with older age ($P < 0.001$; regression coefficient B: 0.08; OR: 1.08 (95%CI: 1.04, 1.13), higher intraocular pressure ($P = 0.004$; B: 0.15; OR: 1.16 (95%CI: 1.05, 1.29), shorter axial length ($P = 0.048$; B: −0.34; OR: 0.71 (95%CI: 0.50, 1.00), and thinner SFCT ($P = 0.04$; B: −0.01; OR: 0.995 (95%CI: 0.991, 1.00). Within the group with angle-closure glaucoma, 8 (22%) eyes had undergone anti-glaucomatous filtering surgery one or more years prior to inclusion into the study. The subgroup with glaucoma surgery and the subgroup without glaucoma surgery did not vary significantly in SFCT (185±98 μm versus 184±94 μm; $P = 0.98$) or in age (71.9±10.3 years versus 73.2±8.4 years; $P = 0.74$) or in axial length 22.6±0.9 mm versus 23.1±0.7 mm; $P = 0.12$).

Since the number of individuals with primary angle-closure glaucoma was relatively small (n = 37), we added a second group of patients (n = 52) with chronic primary angle-closure glaucoma who had been diagnosed and treated in the Beijing Tongren hospital. There had been no known glaucoma attack in at least two months preceding the examination. As the participants of the Beijing Eye Study, the patients with chronic angle-closure glaucoma from the Tongren hospital had undergone an ophthalmological examination including spectral-domain OCT with enhanced depth imaging to visualize and measure the SFCT. Mean age was 62.3±7.2 years (median: 62 years; range: 44–76 years). If this hospital-based group of patients with angle-closure glaucoma was merged with the population-based group of patients with angle-closure glaucoma, SFCT was significantly thinner in the chronic angle-closure glaucoma group than in the non-glaucomatous group (222±90 μm versus 256±107 μm; $P < 0.001$). In multivariate analysis, with SFCT as a dependent variable and refractive error, age and presence of chronic angle-closure glaucoma as independent variables, thinner SFCT was significantly associated with the older age ($P < 0.001$; beta: −0.43; B: −4.84 (95%CI: −5.18, −4.50)) and myopic refractive error ($P < 0.001$; beta: 0.29; B: 16.2 (95%CI: 14.5, 17.8)) while it was not significantly associated with the presence of chronic angle-closure glaucoma

**Table 3.** Associations (multivariate analysis) between subfoveal choroidal thickness, general parameters and open-angle glaucoma in the Beijing Eye Study 2011.

| Parameter | P-Value | Standardized Coefficient Beta | Regression Coefficient B | 95% Confidence Intervals for B |
|---|---|---|---|---|
| Age (Years) | <0.001 | −0.41 | −4.65 | −5.04, −4.26 |
| Axial Length (mm) | <0.001 | −0.38 | −36.9 | −40.5, −33.2 |
| Gender (Men/Women) | <0.001 | −0.15 | −32.8 | −39.7, −25.9 |
| Anterior Chamber Depth (mm) | <0.001 | −0.08 | 25.1 | 12.0, 38.1 |
| Lens Thickness (mm) | <0.001 | 0.08 | 24.7 | 12.7, 36.7 |
| Diabetes Mellitus | 0.01 | 0.04 | 11.6 | 2.34, 20.9 |
| Open-Angle Glaucoma | 0.41 | −0.01 | −9.1 | −30.5, 12.4 |

($P = 0.27$; beta: −0.02; B: −13.1 (95%CI: −38.8, 11.0)). In binary regression analysis, presence of chronic angle-closure glaucoma was significantly associated with older age ($P<0.001$; OR: 1.08 (95%CI: 1.05, 1.12)) but not with SFCT ($P = 0.27$; OR: 0.998 (95%CI: 0.005, 1.001)).

To reduce the potential influence of outliers, the analysis was repeated after excluding all subjects with a SFCT measurement outside of the 95% confidence intervals (i.e. smaller than 69 μm or larger than 464 μm). It revealed that SFCT was significantly associated with younger age ($P<0.001$; standardized coefficient beta: −0.40; regression coefficient B: −4.04 (95%CI: −4.39, −3.68), shorter axial length ($P<0.001$; beta: −0.36; B: −32.9 (95%CI: −36.4, −29.4)), male gender ($P<0.001$; beta: −0.14; B: −25.6 (95%CI: −31.9, −19.3)), deeper anterior chamber ($P<0.001$; beta: −0.08; B: 21.4 (95%CI: 9.5, 33.2)) and larger lens thickness ($P<0.001$; beta: 0.08; B: 22.4 (95%CI: 11.6, 33.3)), while presence of diabetes mellitus and presence of glaucoma ($P = 0.08$; beta: −0.03; B: −14.8 (95%CI: −31.4, 1.8)) were not significantly associated. In a similar manner, open-angle glaucoma ($P = 0.36$) nor angle-closure glaucoma ($P = 0.08$) were significantly associated with SFCT.

## Discussion

Since the landmark study by Spaide and colleagues on the development of enhanced depth imaging by optical coherence tomography [29], an increasing number of studies have addressed choroidal thickness in normal eyes, the factors associated with choroidal thickness in normal eyes, and associations of choroidal thickness with various retinal and retino-choroidal disorders [33–35]. These studies have revealed that the mean subfoveal choroidal thickness (SFCT) in normal eyes is approximately

250 μm in a population with a mean age of 65 years [28]; that it shows a huge range between values as low as 8 μm and values as large as 854 μm, that it decreases with age by 4 μm per year of age and with increasing myopia by 15 μm per diopter of myopia; and that it is additionally associated with male gender, a deeper anterior chamber and thicker lens [28]. Clinical studies also showed that patients with central serous chorioretinopathy have a thickened SFCT in the affected eye as well as in the contralateral unaffected eye [33], and that patients with polypoidal vascular choroidopathy have an increased thickness of the subfoveal choroid in association with a dilatation of the large choroidal vessels [34]. In our population-based study on a relatively large study population, we found that neither patients with open-angle glaucoma nor patients with chronic angle-closure glaucoma have an abnormal SFCT in multivariate analysis with adjustment for age, axial length, gender, anterior chamber and lens thickness.

The finding that patients with open-angle glaucoma did not differ in SFCT from normal subjects agrees with previous hospital-based studies. In the study by Mwanza and colleagues, 36 eyes with unilateral advanced glaucoma as compared with the contralateral eyes with no or mild glaucoma were examined [19]. After adjusting for axial length and intraocular pressure, choroidal thickness did not differ significantly between both groups ($P = 0.78$ to 0.99). Visual field mean deviation did not correlate with choroidal thickness measurements. In a similar manner in our study, SFCT was not significantly ($P = 0.65$) related with retinal nerve fiber layer thickness as another surrogate for the amount of optic nerve damage in glaucoma. Maul et al. reported in another study that choroidal thickness did not differ among normal subjects, patients with normal-pressure glaucoma and patients with primary open-angle glaucoma [16]. SFCT was not signifi-

**Table 4.** Associations (multivariate analysis) between subfoveal choroidal thickness, general parameters and angle-closure glaucoma in the Beijing Eye Study 2011.

| Parameter | P-Value | Standardized Coefficient Beta | Regression Coefficient B | 95% Confidence Intervals for B |
|---|---|---|---|---|
| Age (Years) | <0.001 | −0.41 | −4.64 | −5.03, −4.25 |
| Axial Length (mm) | <0.001 | −0.38 | −36.8 | −40.5, −33.2 |
| Gender (Men/Women) | <0.001 | −0.15 | −32.6 | −39.5, −25.8 |
| Anterior Chamber Depth (mm) | <0.001 | −0.08 | 24.8 | 12.8, 36.8 |
| Lens Thickness (mm) | <0.001 | 0.08 | 24.8 | 12.8, 36.8 |
| Diabetes Mellitus | 0.01 | 0.04 | 11.9 | 2.65, 21.2 |
| Angle-Closure Glaucoma | 0.044 | −0.03 | −33.4 | −66.0, −0.89 |

cantly associated with glaucoma damage severity as estimated by visual field mean deviation or nerve fiber layer thickness. In the study by Rhew and coworkers, SFCT was measured in 32 patients with normal-tension glaucoma and compared with 35 normal individuals [25]. The mean SFCT in the normal individual group and the normal-pressure glaucoma patient group were $300.0 \pm 52.7$ and $289.5 \pm 100.4$ µm, with no significant difference between both groups ($P = 0.60$). The peripapillary choroidal thickness in healthy controls and in patients with glaucoma with focal, diffuse and sclerotic glaucomatous optic disc damages were examined by Roberts and colleagues [20]. The authors found that peripapillary choroidal thickness did not differ significantly between glaucoma patients with focal and diffuse optic disc damage as compared to control subjects, while it was approximately 30% lower in patients with sclerotic glaucomatous optic disc damage ($P = 0.001$).

With respect to choroidal thickness in angle-closure glaucoma, Arora and colleagues recently examined 106 patients with open-angle and 79 patients with angle-closure with or without glaucoma and 40 control subjects [12]. Choroidal thickness was significantly greater in the angle-closure glaucoma group than in the open-angle glaucoma group and the normal subjects ($P \leq 0.05$), but there was no significant difference between the open-angle glaucoma group and the normal subjects. After adjusting for age, axial length, intraocular pressure, central corneal thickness, choroidal thickness was significantly greater in the angle-closure glaucoma group than either in the normal or the open-angle glaucoma group ($P = 0.003$ and $P = 0.03$, respectively). Interestingly, the severity of glaucomatous optic nerve damage as measured by cup/disc ratio cup-to-disc ratio or visual field mean deviation was not significantly associated with choroidal thickness. In another investigation, Arora and coworkers found that a significant increase in choroidal thickness and a decrease in anterior chamber depth when a water drinking test was performed in eyes with anterior chamber angle closure as compared to eyes with open anterior chamber angles [13]. While the study by Arora and coworkers agrees with our study in that patients with open-angle glaucoma and normal subjects do not differ significantly in choroidal thickness, both studies disagree on the results for angle-closure: While we found, that eyes with chronic angle-closure glaucoma have a normal SFCT, the choroid was abnormally thick in the subjects with angle-closure in the study by Arora. In another recent study on fellow eyes of 44 patients with unilateral acute primary angle-closure in the contralateral eyes, Zhou and colleagues found that the fellow eyes had a thicker choroid than a group of control eyes after adjusting for age, axial length, and gender [36]. The reasons for the discrepancies between the studies have remained unclear. A potential cause for the discrepancy between the studies could be a difference between acute angle-closure glaucoma and chronic angle-closure glaucoma. Most of the preceding studies showing an association between abnormally thick SFCT and angle-closure glaucoma included patients shortly after an acute angle-closure glaucoma attack. There may be the possibility that shortly after a high intraocular pressure period such as after an acute glaucoma attack, the choroidal vessels show a reactive dilatation. It could lead to an overestimation of choroidal thickness in these eyes with acute angle-closure glaucoma as compared to eyes with chronic angle-closure glaucoma.

Interestingly, a histomorphometric study on human enucleated eyes with absolute secondary angle-closure glaucoma revealed that the choroid was significantly thinner in the glaucoma group than in the control group [2]. In a similar manner, Hayreh and colleagues reported on a positive correlation between the optic nerve head damage and atrophic changes in the temporal peripapillary choroid in monkeys with experimental high-pressure glaucoma [5]. Spraul et al. found that eyes with advanced glaucomatous damage after long standing primary open-angle glaucoma exhibited a decreased density of capillaries of the choriocapillaris and decreased density of large choroidal vessels [7]. In a histologic study by Yin and coworkers, a reduced choroidal thickness was found in enucleated human eyes with primary open-angle glaucoma with a loss of the innermost choroidal vessels [37]. Other studies reported on tissue loss in the deep retinal layers [6,8–10]. These histologic studies were however not corrected for the dependence of choroidal thickness on age and axial length so that it has remained unclear whether and how their results may contribute to the current discussion.

Potential limitations of our study should be mentioned. First, a major concern in any prevalence study is nonparticipation. The Beijing Eye Study 2011 had a reasonable response rate of 78.8%, however, differences between participants and non-participants could have led to a selection artifact. Since the group of subjects without OCT measurements and assessments of the presence of glaucoma as compared to the group of subjects with these measurements was significantly ($P<0.001$) older more myopic ($P = 0.002$), one may argue that the non-participation of a part of the elderly eligible study population may have influenced the results of the investigation. Second, previous studies by Chakraborty and colleagues and others have shown a circadian (diurnal) rhythm of about 20–30 micron change in choroidal thickness measurements by OCT [38]. The participants of our study underwent the OCT examinations at various times of the day. Since these examinations were performed in a randomized manner with respect to when they were performed, it is unlikely that the reported dependence of the choroidal thickness measurement on the time of the day introduced a bias into our study. Third, choroidal thickness was examined only in the right eye of each study participant, so that inter-eye differences and their associations with inter-eye differences of other parameters could not be assessed. Fourth, the definition of glaucoma applied in our study did not follow the recommendations of the International Society of Geographical and Epidemiological Ophthalmology [31]. If however, criteria of the ISGEO were applied for a subgroup of subjects, again the SFCT was not significantly ($P = 0.42$) associated with glaucoma after adjustment for age, axial length, gender, anterior chamber depth, lens thickness and presence of diabetes mellitus. Fifth, some eyes of the study group had undergone anti-glaucomatous filtering surgery. Previous studies have shown that filtering surgery can lead to a change in SFCT, i.e., a thickening. SFCT however was not thicker in the group of eyes with chronic angle-closure glaucoma than in the non-glaucomatous group. Sixth, differences between this study and previous investigations in SFCT and its associations with angle-closure glaucoma may have been due to differences in the ethnic background. The strengths of our study are its design as a population-based investigations and the relatively large number of study participants.

In conclusion, in multivariate analysis with adjustment for age, axial length, gender, anterior chamber and lens thickness, neither open-angle glaucoma nor chronic angle-closure glaucoma was associated with an abnormal SFCT.

## Author Contributions

Conceived and designed the experiments: LX YXW JBJ. Performed the experiments: YXW LX LS YQZ HY JDW JBJ WBW. Analyzed the data: YXW LX LS YQZ HY JDW JBJ WBW. Contributed reagents/materials/analysis tools: LX JBJ. Wrote the paper: YXW LX LS YQZ HY JDW JBJ WBW.

## References

1.  Jonas JB, Budde WM, Panda-Jonas S (1999) Ophthalmoscopic evaluation of the optic nerve head. Surv Ophthalmol 43: 293–320.

2.  Kubota T, Jonas JB, Naumann GO (1993) Decreased choroidal thickness in eyes with secondary angle closure glaucoma. An aetiological factor for deep retinal changes in glaucoma? Br J Ophthalmol 77: 430–432.

3.  Panda S, Jonas JB (1992) Decreased photoreceptor count in human eyes with secondary angle-closure glaucoma. Invest Ophthalmol Vis Sci 33: 2532–2536.

4.  Kendell KR, Quigley HA, Kerrigan LA, Pease ME, Quigley EN (1995) Primary open-angle glaucoma is not associated with photoreceptor loss. Invest Ophthalmol Vis Sci 36: 200–205.

5.  Hayreh SS, Pe'er J, Zimmerman MB (1999) Morphologic changes in chronic high-pressure experimental glaucoma in rhesus monkeys. J Glaucoma 8: 56–71.

6.  Nork TM, Ver Hoeve JN, Poulsen GL, Nickells RW, Davis MD, et al. (2000) Swelling and loss of photoreceptors in chronic human and experimental glaucomas. Arch Ophthalmol 118: 235–245.

7.  Spraul CW, Lang GE, Lang GK, Grossniklaus HE (2002) Morphometric changes of the choriocapillaris and the choroidal vasculature in eyes with advanced glaucomatous changes. Vision Res 42: 923–932.

8.  Kanis MJ, Lemij HG, Berendschot TT, van de Kraats J, van Norren D (2010) Foveal cone photoreceptor involvement in primary open-angle glaucoma. Graefes Arch Clin Exp Ophthalmol 248: 999–1006.

9.  Werner JS, Keltner JL, Zawadzki RJ, Choi SS (2011) Outer retinal abnormalities associated with inner retinal pathology in nonglaucomatous and glaucomatous optic neuropathies. Eye (Lond) 25: 279–289.

10. Choi SS, Zawadzki RJ, Lim MC, Brandt JD, Keltner JL, et al. (2011) Evidence of outer retinal changes in glaucoma patients as revealed by ultrahigh-resolution in vivo retinal imaging. Br J Ophthalmol 95: 131–141.

11. Werner JS, Keltner JL, Zawadzki RJ, Choi SS (2011) Outer retinal abnormalities associated with inner retinal pathology in nonglaucomatous and glaucomatous optic neuropathies. Eye (Lond) 25: 279–289.

12. Arora KS, Jefferys JL, Maul EA, Quigley HA (2012) The choroid is thicker in angle closure than in open angle and control eyes. Invest Ophthalmol Vis Sci 53: 7813–7818.

13. Arora KS, Jefferys JL, Maul EA, Quigley HA (2012) Choroidal thickness change after water drinking is greater in angle closure than in open angle eyes. Invest Ophthalmol Vis Sci 53: 6393–6402.

14. McCourt EA, Cadena BC, Barnett CJ, Ciardella AP, Mandava N, et al. (2010) Measurement of subfoveal choroidal thickness using spectral domain optical coherence tomography. Ophthalmic Surg Lasers Imaging 41 (Suppl.): S28–S33.

15. Mwanza JC, Hochberg JT, Banitt MR, Feuer WJ, Budenz DL (2011) Lack of association between glaucoma and macular choroidal thickness measured with enhanced depth-imaging optical coherence tomography. Invest Ophthalmol Vis Sci 52: 3430–3435.

16. Maul EA, Friedman DS, Chang DS, Boland MV, Ramulu PY, et al. (2011) Choroidal thickness measured by spectral domain optical coherence tomography: factors affecting thickness in glaucoma patients. Ophthalmology 118: 1571–1579.

17. Ehrlich JR, Peterson J, Parlitsis G, Kay KY, Kiss S, et al. (2011) Peripapillary choroidal thickness in glaucoma measured with optical coherence tomography. Exp Eye Res 92: 189–194.

18. Fénolland JR, Giraud JM, Maÿ F, Mouinga A, Seck S, et al. (2011) Evaluation de l'epaisseur choroidienne par tomographie en coherence optique (SD-OCT). Etude preliminaire dans le glaucome a angle ouvert. [Enhanced depth imaging of the choroid in open-angle glaucoma: a preliminary study]. J Fr Ophthalmol 34: 313–317.

19. Mwanza JC, Sayyad FE, Budenz DL (2012) Choroidal thickness in unilateral advanced glaucoma. Invest Ophthalmol Vis Sci 53: 6695–6701.

20. Roberts KF, Artes PH, O'Leary N, Reis AS, Sharpe GP, et al. (2012) Peripapillary choroidal thickness in healthy controls and patients with focal, diffuse, and sclerotic glaucomatous optic disc damage. Arch Ophthalmol 130: 980–986.

21. Hirooka K, Fujiwara A, Shiragami C, Baba T, Shiraga F (2012) Relationship between progression of visual field damage and choroidal thickness in eyes with normal-tension glaucoma. Clin Exp Ophthalmol 40: 576–582.

22. Cennamo G, Finelli M, Iaccarino G, de Crecchio G (2012) Choroidal thickness in open-angle glaucoma measured by spectral-domain scanning laser ophthalmoscopy/optical coherence tomography. Ophthalmologica 228: 47–52.

23. Hirooka K, Tenkumo K, Fujiwara A, Baba T, Sato S, et al. (2012) Evaluation of peripapillary choroidal thickness in patients with normal-tension glaucoma. BMC Ophthalmol 12: 29.

24. Usui S, Ikuno Y, Miki A, Matsushita K, Yasuno Y, et al. (2012) Evaluation of the choroidal thickness using high penetration optical coherence tomography with long wavelength in highly myopic normal-tension glaucoma. Am J Ophthalmol 153: 10.e1–16.e1.

25. Rhew JY, Kim YT, Choi KR (2012) Measurement of subfoveal choroidal thickness in normal-tension glaucoma in Korean patients. J Glaucoma 2012 Jun 4. [Epub ahead of print]

26. Banitt M (2013) The choroid in glaucoma. Curr Opin Ophthalmol 2013 Jan 9. [Epub ahead of print]

27. Wang YX, Xu L, Yang H, Jonas JB (2010) Prevalence of glaucoma in North China. The Beijing Eye Study. Am J Ophthalmol 150: 917–924.

28. Wei WB, Xu L, Jonas JB, Shao L, Du KF, et al. (2013) Subfoveal choriodal thickness: the Beijing Eye Study. Ophthalmology 120: 175–180.

29. Spaide RF, Koizumi H, Pozonni MC (2008) Enhanced depth imaging spectral-domain optical coherence tomography. Am J Ophthalmol 146: 496–500.

30. Shao L, Xu L, Chen CX, Yang LH, Du KF, et al. (2013) Reproducibility of subfoveal choroidal thickness measurements with enhanced depth imaging by spectral-domain optical coherence tomography. Invest Ophthalmol Vis Sci 54: 230–233.

31. Foster PJ, Buhrmann R, Quigley HA, Johnson GJ (2002) The definition and classification of glaucoma in prevalence surveys. Br J Ophthalmol 86: 238–242.

32. Xu J, Xu L, Fang K, Shao L, Chen CX, et al. (2013) Subfoveal choroidal thickness in diabetes and diabetic retinopathy. The Beijing Eye Study 2011. Ophthalmology 2013; In print

33. Kim YT, Kang SW, Bai KH (2011) Choroidal thickness in both eyes of patients with unilaterally active central serous chorioretinopathy. Eye 25: 1635–1640.

34. Chung SE, Kang SW, Lee JH, Kim YT (2011) Choroidal thickness in polypoidal choroidal vasculopathy and exudative age-related macular degeneration. Ophthalmology 118: 840–845.

35. Regatieri CV, Branchini L, Carmody J, Fujimoto JG, Duker JS (2012) Choroidal thickness in patients with diabetic retinopathy analyzed by spectral-domain optical coherence tomography. Retina 32: 563–568.

36. Zhou M, Wang W, Ding X, Huang W, Chen S, et al. (2013) Choroidal thickness in fellow eyes of patients with acute primary angle-closure measured by enhanced depth imaging spectral-domain optical coherence tomography. Invest Ophthalmol Vis Sci 54: 1971–1978.

37. Yin ZQ, Vaegan, Millar TJ, Beaumont P, Sarks S (1997) Widespread choroidal insufficiency in primary open-angle glaucoma. J Glaucoma 6: 23–32.

38. Chakraborty R, Read SA, Collins MJ (2011) Diurnal variations in axial length, choroidal thickness, intraocular pressure, and ocular biometrics. Invest Ophthalmol Vis Sci 52: 5121–5129.

# 19

# The Prevalence of Primary Angle Closure Glaucoma in Adult Asians

**Jin-Wei Cheng**[1]*⁹, **Ying Zong**[2]⁹, **You-Yan Zeng**[3]⁹, **Rui-Li Wei**[1]*

**1** Department of Ophthalmology, Shanghai Changzheng Hospital, Second Military Medical University, Shanghai, China, **2** Department of Health Toxicology, Second Military Medical University, Shanghai, China, **3** School of Nursing, Second Military Medical University, Shanghai, China

## Abstract

*Background:* Primary angle closure glaucoma (PACG) is higher in Asians than Europeans and Africans, with over 80% of PACG worldwide in Asia. Previous estimates of PACG were based largely on early studies, mostly using inappropriate case definitions. Therefore, we did a systematic review and meta-analysis to estimate the prevalence of PACG in adult Asian populations and to quantify its association with age, gender, and region.

*Methods:* All primary reports of population-based studies that reported the prevalence of PACG in adult Asian populations were identified. PACG case definition was compatible with the ISGEO definition. Twenty-nine population-based studies were included. The overall pooled prevalence estimates were calculated using a random effect model, and ethnicity-, age- and gender-specific pooled prevalence estimates were also calculated.

*Results:* The overall pooled prevalence of PACG in those of adult Asians was 0.75% (95% CI, 0.58, 0.96). Ethnicity-specific pooled prevalence estimates were 0.97% (0.22, 4.27) in Middle East group, 0.66% (0.23, 1.86) in South East Asia group, 0.46% (0.32, 0.64) in India group, 1.10% (0.85, 1.44) in China group, and 1.19% (0.35, 3.98) in Japan group, respectively. Age-specific prevalence was 0.21% (0.12, 0.37) for those 40–49 years, 0.54% (0.34, 0.85) for those 50–59 years, 1.26% (0.93, 1.71) for those 60–69 years, and 2.32% (1.74, 3.08) for those 70 years or above. The overall female to male ratio of the PACG prevalence was 1.51:1 (95% CI 1.01, 2.28).

*Conclusions:* PACG affects approximately 0.75% adult Asians, increasing double per decade, and 60% of cases being female. The prevalence rates vary greatly by ethnic region.

**Editor:** Ted S. Acott, Casey Eye Institute, United States of America

**Funding:** This work was supported by Shanghai Rising-Star Program (Grant No. 12QA1404600), Shanghai Municipal Natural Science Foundation (Grant No. 10ZR1439300), and National Natural Science Foundation of China (Grant No. 81000374 and 81170874). The funders had no role in study design, data collection and analysis, decision to publish, or preparation of the manuscript.

**Competing Interests:** The authors have declared that no competing interests exist.

* Email: jinnwave@163.com (JWC); ruiliwei@126.com (RLW)

⁹ These authors contributed equally to this work.

## Introduction

Glaucoma is considered as the leading cause of irreversible blindness worldwide, with Asians accounting for approximately half of the world's glaucoma cases [1]. It also has been accepted that primary angle closure glaucoma (PACG) is higher in Asians than Europeans and Africans, with over 80% of those with PACG in Asia [1,2]. Because PACG appears to cause blindness more frequently than primary open angle glaucoma (POAG), it is an important public health issue.

The current understanding of PACG in Asian populations is based largely on previous studies [1–3]. Early studies using the definitions of glaucoma based on intraocular pressure (IOP) reported that the prevalence of PACG in adults was 0.34% in Japan [4], 1.49% in Mongolia [5], 1.37% in China [6], and 1.18% in India [7], respectively. However, the earlier definitions of glaucoma are no longer accepted [8], and the prevalence rates reported in these earlier studies may not be accurate and comparable [9].

The International Society of Geographical & Epidemiological Ophthalmology (ISGEO) definition has demonstrated the general accepted classification for the diagnosis of glaucoma in population-based prevalence surveys [8]. However, the current understanding of PACG in Asians is based largely on studies using the earlier definitions of glaucoma, but not the ISGEO definition, which increasingly was seen as inadequate for both clinical and research purposes [1,2,9]. Recently, many population-based surveys of glaucoma in Asians using the ISGEO definition have been conducted. Because of the uncertainty surrounding the prevalence of PACG, this systematic review was to summarize the available population-based studies reporting prevalence values in Asians, to estimate an overall prevalence of PACG consistent with the ISGEO definition requiring structural and/or functional evidence of glaucomatous optic neuropathy.

## Materials and Methods

This meta-analysis was performed according to a predetermined protocol, and the methods used conformed to the Meta-analysis of Observational Studies in Epidemiology and the relevant aspects of the PRISMA statement [10,11].

### Search Strategy

We used three methods to identify publications that reported the prevalence of PACG among Asian populations. First, we conducted a systematic search of the PubMed and EMBASE electronic databases from each database's inception date to February 10, 2014. Broad MeSH terms and keywords were used combining terms related to epidemiology (including MeSH search using *exp prevalence**, and *exp epidemiology**, and keyword search using words *prevalence*, *epidemiology*, and *incidence*), terms related to disease (including MeSH search using *exp glaucoma**, and keyword search using words *glaucoma*), and terms related to population (including MeSH search using *exp Asia**, and keyword search using words *Asia*, and *Asian*). Second, we hand-searched the reference lists of the relevant reviews, such as *Rudnicka 2006* [12], *Quigley 2006* [1], *Wong 2006* [2], *Zhou 2007* [3], and *Cheng 2013* [13]. Third, we consulted the reference lists of included articles to find additional studies.

### Study Selection

Published studies were included if they met the following inclusion criteria: (i) population-based, cross-sectional survey studies, with either random or consecutive sampling; (ii) adult Asian populations, customarily aged 40 years and older; (iii) a examination rate of the eligible population sample not less than 50%; (iv) PACG case definitions compatible with the current ISGEO definition based on structural and/or functional evidence of glaucomatous optic neuropathy in the presence of an occludable anterior chamber angle.

To determine study eligibility, three independent researchers screened the titles and abstracts of all search results, and all citations were classified into one of two categories: (i) relevant; (ii) irrelevant. The full articles of relevant citations were retrieved for further review to evaluate whether they met the inclusion criteria or not. Only eligible trials were assessed for methodological quality. Disagreements were resolved by consensus in both phases.

### Data Extraction

The following detailed information was extracted into a customized proforma: (i) study information (study name, publication year, citation, and study type), (ii) basic study data (geographical region, country of survey area, conditions in survey area, data collection year, sample size, and sociodemographic characteristics), (iii) quality-related data and outcome measures data (target population, sampling design, completeness of data/response rate, data collection, prevalence, definition and identification procedures for outcomes). Three reviewers independently carried out the data extraction, and inconsistencies were resolved by discussion with another independent reviewer.

### Risk of Bias Assessment

Two reviewers independently assessed the risk of bias for each included study, using a checklist developed from an existing tool assessing risk of bias in prevalence studies. The tool includes 10 items that assess measurement bias, selection bias, and bias related to the analysis (all rated as either high or low risk) and an overall assessment of risk of bias rated as either low, moderate, or high risk [14,15]. To adapt to the needs of this meta-analysis, we also modified item 9 as "Were the screening process and assessing methods for the parameter of interest appropriate?" [16,17].

Agreement was measured using kappa value as recommended by the Cochrane Handbook for Systematic Reviews of Interventions [18], and disagreement was resolved finally by discussion. Overall agreement between the reviewers was 93% with a kappa value of 0.76, indicating excellent agreement.

### Statistical Analysis

All statistical analyses were performed using Comprehensive Meta-Analysis software version 2.0 (Biostat, Englewood Cliffs, New Jersey) (http://www.meta-analysis.com). The primary outcome for each study was the prevalence proportion, calculated as the ratio of the number of individuals with PACG to the total number of study participants. The $I^2$ statistic was used to determine heterogeneity across studies, which quantify heterogeneity irrespective of the number of studies [19,20]. The estimate and its 95% confidence intervals (CI) of overall proportion was calculated using the random effects model where heterogeneity was found [21], otherwise, the fixed effects model was used [22].

Ethnicity-specific pooled prevalence estimates of PACG were calculated, using a random effect model, which included the dominant ethnic group of five regions in Asia: Middle East, South East Asia, India, China, and Japan [1]. Age- and gender-specific pooled prevalence estimates of PACG were also calculated. A random-effect meta-regression model was built with ethnicity, age, and gender.

In addition, to attempt to control for potential methodologic heterogeneity, a random-effect regression model was also used to evaluate sources of variability in the overall pooled-prevalence estimate, such as urbanicity, the definition of occludable angle and the individual risk-of-bias items.

## Results

### Study Characteristics

**Figure 1** shows the flow chart of the selection process used to identify relevant studies. We reviewed the full text of 117 articles from 1997 studies identified from the literature search, and 88 articles were excluded (**Appendix S1**). Twenty-nine population studies met all the inclusion criteria and were used to calculate the best evidence PACG prevalence estimates in adult Asian populations (**Table 1**) [23–51]. Seven studies (24%) were conducted in China, 5 (17%) in India, 3 (10%) in Singapore, 2 (7%) in Japan, Korea, and Nepal, and 1 (3%) in Bangladesh, Iran, Mongolia, Myanmar, Oman, Qatar, Thailand, and Sri Lanka. Fifteen studies (52%) were undertaken in rural, 6 (21%) in urban, and 8 (28%) in mixed populations. The age ranges of the studied populations were 30 years and over, with the majority of studies (n = 20, 69%) being 40 years and over, and the male portion of the populations ranged from 36% to 64%. Twenty-five studies (86%) used ISGEO definition for the diagnosis of PACG.

### Risk of Bias

Overall, 22 studies (76%) were rated as having a low risk of bias, 7 (24%) were rated as having a moderate risk of bias (**Table 2**). High risk-of-bias ratings were most common for item I (national representativeness/target population), item IV (non-response bias), item VI (case definition), and item VII (study instrument).

### Meta-Analysis

The prevalence of PACG reported in the included studies varied from 0.13% to 2.50% in adult Asian populations (**Figure 2**). The heterogeneity in the prevalence of PACG was

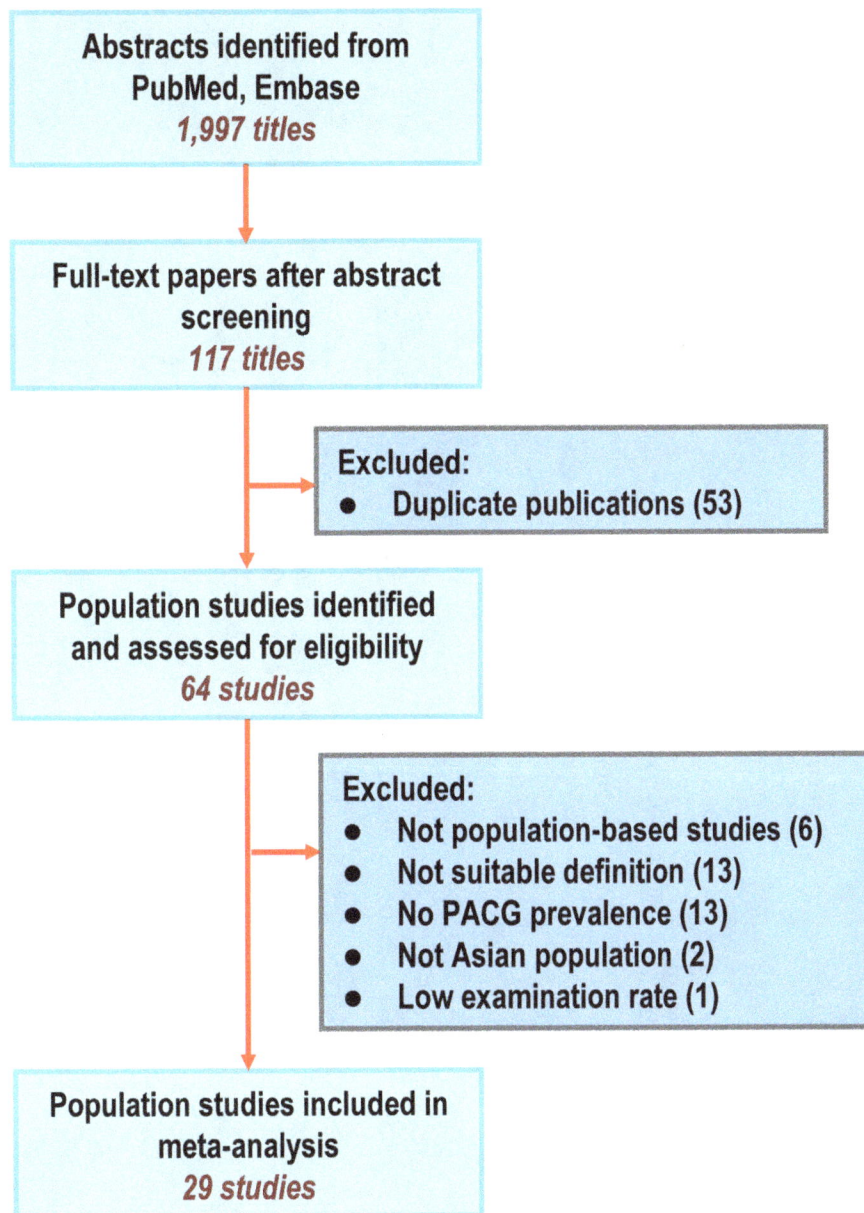

**Figure 1. Flow Diagram of Study Selection.** PACG: primary angle closure glaucoma

statistically significant and substantial in considerable. The overall random-effects estimate of the prevalence of PACG in adult Asian populations was 0.75% (95% CI, 0.58, 0.96).

Ethnicity-specific pooled prevalence estimates of PACG of five Asian regions are shown in Figure 3. The pooled prevalence estimates of PACG were 0.97% (95% CI, 0.22, 4.27) in Middle East group, 0.66% (0.23, 1.86) in South East Asia group, 0.46% (0.32, 0.64) in India group, 1.10% (0.85, 1.44) in China group, and 1.19% (0.35, 3.98) in Japan group, respectively. The meta-regression analyses showed there was a strong association of prevalence with ethnic group ($\beta = 0.27$, $P = 0.009$).

Fifteen studies reported age-specific prevalence of PACG, and twenty-two studies reported gender-specific prevalence. The age-specific prevalence was 0.21% (95% CI, 0.12, 0.37) for those 40–49 years old, 0.54% (0.34, 0.85) for those 50–59 years old, 1.26%

(0.93, 1.71) for those 60–69 years old, and 2.32% (1.74, 3.08) for those 70 years old or above (**Figure 3**). Meta-regression analysis showed a high prevalence rate was strongly associated with an older age of sample ($\beta = 0.74$, $P < 0.0001$). The pooled prevalence was 0.63% (0.49, 0.82) for male and 0.91% (0.68, 1.21) for female (**Figure 3**). Meta-regression analyses showed a strong association between a high prevalence rate and a higher proportion of female gender ($\beta = 0.41$, $P = 0.047$), and the overall female to male ratio of the PACG prevalence was 1.51:1 (95% CI 1.01, 2.28).

The meta-regression analyses showed there was no association of the prevalence rate with urbanicity ($\beta = -0.17$, $P = 0.524$). The prevalence of PACG was also not associated with the definition of occludable angle ($\beta = -0.05$, $P = 0.717$). For risk-of-bias items, the prevalence rate was not associated with a high risk of bias for item

**Table 1.** Population Characteristics of the Studies Reported the Prevalence of Primary Angle Closure Glaucoma in Asians.

| Study | Country | Urbanicity | Examined Year | Response (%) | Age Range (yrs) | N | Sex Ratio (M/F) | Case Definition | Angle Examination | Occludable Angle Definition | Adult PACG n (%) |
|---|---|---|---|---|---|---|---|---|---|---|---|
| Aravind Comprehensive Eye Survey [23] | India | Rural | 1995–1997 | 93.0 | ≥40 | 5150 | 2836/2314 | Angle + (GON ± GVFD) | Gonioscopy | Shaffer grade 0 | 26 (0.50) |
| Mongolia Eye Study [24] | Mongolia | Rural, urban | 1995, 1997 | 95.4 | ≥40 | 1717 | 1007/710 | ISGEO | Gonioscopy | 270° ITM | 28 (1.63) |
| Tanjong Pagar Eye Study [25] | Singapore | Urban | 1997–1998 | 71.8 | 40–79 | 1232 | 557/670 | ISGEO | Gonioscopy | 270° ITM | 14 (1.14) |
| Rom Klao Eye Study [26] | Thailand | Urban | 1999 | 88.7 | ≥50 | 701 | 249/452 | ISGEO | Gonioscopy | 270° ITM | 6 (0.86) |
| Dhaka Eye Study [27] | Bangladesh | Rural | 1997–1998 | 65.9 | ≥35 | 2347 | 1120/1127 | ISGEO | Gonioscopy | 240° ITM | 7 (0.30) |
| Tajimi Study [28] | Japan | Urban | 2000–2001 | 78.1 | ≥40 | 3021 | 1334/1687 | ISGEO | Gonioscopy | 270° ITM | 19 (0.63) |
| Shaanxi Rural Study [29] | China | Rural | 2003 | 81.0 | ≥40 | 2835 | 1246/1587 | Angle+IOP+(GVFD+/−GON) | Gonioscopy | Shaffer grade 0 | 31 (1.09) |
| West Bengal Glaucoma Study [30] | India | Rural | 1998–1999 | 83.1 | ≥50 | 1324 | 611/658 | ISGEO | Gonioscopy | 240° ITM | 3 (0.24) |
| Chennai Glaucoma Study [31] | India | Rural | 2001–2004 | 80.2 | ≥40 | 3850 | 1710/2140 | ISGEO | Gonioscopy | 180° ITM | 34 (0.88) |
| Liwan Eye Study [32] | China | Urban | 2003–2004 | 75.3 | ≥50 | 1405 | 613/792 | ISGEO | Gonioscopy | 270° ITM | 21 (1.53) |
| Meiktila Eye Study [33] | Myanmar | Rural | 2005 | 83.7 | ≥40 | 2076 | 836/1240 | ISGEO | Gonioscopy | 270° ITM | 52 (2.50) |
| Oman Eye Study [34] | Oman | Rural, urban | 2005–2006 | 79.5 | ≥30 | 3324 | 1289/2035 | Angle + (GON ± GVFD) | Gonioscopy | Shaffer grade 2 | 68 (2.05) |
| Singapore Malay Eye Study [35] | Singapore | Urban | 2004–2006 | 78.7 | ≥40 | 3280 | 1576/1704 | ISGEO | Gonioscopy | 180° ITM | 8 (0.24) |
| Kandy Eye Study [36] | Sri Lanka | Rural | 2006–2007 | 79.9 | ≥40 | 1351 | 539/812 | ISGEO | Gonioscopy | 270° ITM | 7 (0.57) |
| Sunsari Eye Study [37] | Nepal | Rural | 2003–2004 | 80.0 | ≥40 | 1600 | 789/811 | Angle+IOP+(GVFD+/−GON) | Gonioscopy | Shaffer grade 0 | 2 (0.13) |
| Andhra Pradesh Eye Disease Study [38] | India | Rural, urban | 1996–2000 | 87.3 | ≥40 | 3724 | 1751/1973 | ISGEO | Gonioscopy | 180° ITM | 35 (0.94) |
| Beijing Eye Study [39] | China | Rural, urban | 2001 | 83.4 | ≥40 | 4315 | 1889/2412 | ISGEO | Gonioscopy | 270° ITM | 44 (1.02) |
| Bin Eye Study [40] | China | Rural | 2000 | 80.0 | ≥40 | 4956 | 2228/2728 | ISGEO | Gonioscopy | 270° ITM | 78 (1.57) |
| Handan Eye Study [41] | China | Rural | 2007 | 90.4 | ≥40 | 5480 | 2557/2923 | ISGEO | Gonioscopy | 180° ITM | 30 (0.55) |

**Table 1.** Cont.

| Study | Country | Urbanicity | Examined Year | Response (%) | Age Range (yrs) | N | Sex Ratio (M/F) | Case Definition | Angle Examination | Occludable Angle Definition | Adult PACG n (%) |
|---|---|---|---|---|---|---|---|---|---|---|---|
| Kailu Eye Study [42] | China | Rural | 2009 | 87.4 | ≥40 | 5158 | 2299/2859 | ISGEO | Gonioscopy | 270° ITM | 90 (1.74) |
| Sangju Eye Study [43] | Korea | Rural | - | 60.0 | ≥50 | 671 | 264/407 | ISGEO | Gonioscopy | 270° ITM | 2 (0.30) |
| Qatar Eye Study [44] | Qatar | Rural, urban | 2009 | 97.7 | ≥40 | 3149 | 2015/1134 | ISGEO | Gonioscopy | 270° ITM | 14 (0.44) |
| Namil Study [45] | Korea | Rural | 2007–2008 | 79.5 | ≥40 | 1426 | 625/801 | ISGEO | Gonioscopy | 270° ITM | 10 (0.70) |
| Bhaktapur Glaucoma Study [46] | Nepal | Rural, urban | 2007–2009 | 83.4 | ≥40 | 3991 | 1819/2172 | ISGEO | Gonioscopy | 270° ITC | 17 (0.43) |
| Kumejima Study [47] | Japan | Rural | 2005–2006 | 81.2 | ≥40 | 3762 | 1833/1929 | ISGEO | Gonioscopy | 270° ITM | 82 (2.18) |
| Yunnan Minority Eye Study [48] | China | Rural | 2010 | 77.8 | ≥50 | 2133 | 769/1364 | ISGEO | Gonioscopy | 270° ITM | 20 (0.94) |
| Central India Eye and Medical Study [49] | India | Rural | 2006–2008 | 80.1 | ≥30 | 4711 | 2191/2520 | ISGEO | Gonioscopy | 270° ITM | 14 (0.30) |
| Singapore Indian Eye Study [50] | Singapore | Urban | 2007–2009 | 75.6 | ≥40 | 3400 | 1706/1694 | ISGEO | Gonioscopy | 180° ITM | 6 (0.18) |
| Yazd Eye Study [51] | Iran | Rural, urban | 2010–2011 | 90.4 | ≥40 | 1990 | 922/1068 | ISGEO | Gonioscopy | 270° ITM | 7 (0.33) |

GON: glaucomatous optic neuropathy; GVFD: glaucomatous visual field defect; IOP: intraocular pressure; ISGEO: International Society of Geographical & Epidemiological Ophthalmology.
ITM: invisible trabecular meshwork; ITC: iridotrabecular contact.
PACG: primary angle closure glaucoma.

**Table 2.** Risk of Bias of the Studies Reported the Prevalence of Primary Angle Closure Glaucoma in Asians.

| Study | I | II | III | IV | V | VI | VII | VIII | IX | X | Overall |
|---|---|---|---|---|---|---|---|---|---|---|---|
| Aravind Comprehensive Eye Survey [23] | High | Low | Low | Low | Low | High | Low | Low | Low | Low | Moderate |
| Mongolia Eye Study [24] | High | Low | Low | Low | Low | Low | Low | Low | Low | Low | Low |
| Tanjong Pagar Eye Study [25] | High | Low | Low | High | Low | Low | Low | Low | Low | Low | Moderate |
| Rom Klao Eye Study [26] | High | Low | Low | Low | Low | Low | Low | Low | Low | Low | Low |
| Dhaka Eye Study [27] | High | Low | Low | High | Low | Low | Low | Low | Low | Low | Moderate |
| Tajimi Study [28] | High | Low | Low | Low | Low | Low | Low | Low | Low | Low | Low |
| Shaanxi Rural Study [29] | High | Low | Low | Low | Low | High | High | Low | Low | Low | Moderate |
| West Bengal Glaucoma Study [30] | High | Low | Low | Low | Low | Low | Low | Low | Low | Low | Low |
| Chennai Glaucoma Study [31] | High | Low | Low | Low | Low | Low | Low | Low | Low | Low | Low |
| Liwan Eye Study [32] | High | Low | Low | Low | Low | Low | Low | Low | Low | Low | Low |
| Meiktila Eye Study [33] | High | Low | Low | Low | Low | Low | Low | Low | Low | Low | Moderate |
| Oman Eye Study [34] | Low | Low | Low | Low | Low | High | Low | Low | Low | Low | Moderate |
| Singapore Malay Eye Study [35] | Low | Low | Low | Low | Low | Low | Low | Low | Low | Low | Low |
| Kandy Eye Study [36] | High | Low | Low | Low | Low | Low | Low | Low | Low | Low | Low |
| Sunsari Eye Study [37] | High | Low | Low | Low | Low | High | Low | Low | Low | Low | Moderate |
| Andhra Pradesh Eye Disease Study [38] | High | Low | Low | Low | Low | Low | Low | Low | Low | Low | Low |
| Beijing Eye Study [39] | High | Low | Low | Low | Low | Low | Low | Low | Low | Low | Low |
| Bin Eye Study [40] | High | Low | Low | Low | Low | Low | Low | Low | Low | Low | Low |
| Handan Eye Study [41] | High | Low | Low | Low | Low | Low | Low | Low | Low | Low | Low |
| Kailu Eye Study [42] | High | Low | Low | Low | Low | Low | Low | Low | Low | Low | Low |
| Sangju Eye Study [43] | High | Low | Low | High | Low | Low | Low | Low | Low | Low | Moderate |
| Qatar Eye Study [44] | Low | Low | Low | Low | Low | Low | Low | Low | Low | Low | Low |
| Namil Study [45] | High | Low | Low | Low | Low | Low | Low | Low | Low | Low | Low |
| Bhaktapur Glaucoma Study [46] | High | Low | Low | Low | Low | Low | Low | Low | Low | Low | Low |
| Kumejima Study [47] | High | Low | Low | Low | Low | Low | Low | Low | Low | Low | Low |
| Yunnan Minority Eye Study [48] | High | Low | Low | Low | Low | Low | Low | Low | Low | Low | Low |
| Central India Eye and Medical Study [49] | High | Low | Low | Low | Low | Low | Low | Low | Low | Low | Low |
| Singapore Indian Eye Study [50] | Low | Low | Low | Low | Low | Low | Low | Low | Low | Low | Low |
| Yazd Eye Study [51] | High | Low | Low | Low | Low | Low | Low | Low | Low | Low | Low |

I    Was the study's target population a close representation of the national population in relation to relevant variables, e.g., age, sex, occupation?

II    Was the sampling frame a true or close representation of the target population?

III    Was some form of random selection used to select the sample, OR, was a census undertaken?

IV    Was the likelihood of non-response bias minimal?

**Table 2.** Cont.

| Study | I | II | III | IV | V | VI | VII | VIII | IX | X | Overall |
|---|---|---|---|---|---|---|---|---|---|---|---|
| V | | | | | | | | | | | |
| VI | | | | | | | | | | | |
| VII | | | | | | | | | | | |
| VIII | | | | | | | | | | | |
| IX | | | | | | | | | | | |
| X | | | | | | | | | | | |

I: Were data collected directly from the subjects (as opposed to a proxy)?
II: Was an acceptable case definition used in the study?
III: Had the study instrument that measured the parameter of interest (e.g., prevalence of PACG) been tested for reliability and validity (if necessary)?
IV: Was the same mode of data collection used for all subjects?
V: Were the screening process and assessing methods for the parameter of interest appropriate?
VI: Were the numerator(s) and denominator(s) for the parameter of interest appropriate?

I ($\beta = 0.48$, $P = 0.217$), item IV ($\beta = -0.40$, $P = 0.391$), item VI ($\beta = 0.06$, $P = 0.882$), and item VII ($\beta = 0.77$, $P = 0.112$).

## Discussion

This comprehensive systematic review was conducted to investigate the prevalence of PACG in Asian, and to understand the reasons of estimate variability. The findings showed that for those of adult Asian populations, 0.75% were estimated to have PACG. This systematic review also quantified the variability in the prevalence of PACG for age, gender and ethnic group. The rate of PACG prevalence increased with age, approximately double per decade. PACG prevalence in women was approximately 1.5 times that in men. There was a strong variability of PACG prevalence rates by ethnic group.

It has been established that the prevalence of glaucoma varies significantly by region [1,9,12,52]. On the basis of the findings from this systematic review, there was also significant ethnic variation in the prevalence of PACG among five Asian regions. The highest prevalence rates of PACG were reported in Japan (1.19%) and China (1.10%), followed by Middle East (0.97%), South East Asia (0.66%), and India (0.46%). A recent systematic review found that the prevalence of PACG in those 40 years or more in European derived populations is 0.4% (95% CI 0.3% to 0.5%) [53]. Therefore, the prevalence of PACG in Asians, especially in East Asians and South East Asians, is higher than those in Europeans. However, the findings should be interpreted with caution, especially for the Japan, Middle East and South East Asia groups, because of the very wide confidence interval of prevalence rates, and the significantly large heterogeneity across included studies.

The pooled prevalence of PACG in five Asian ethnic group from the present review was inconsistent with the results reported in the previous reviews [1,13]. In the previous reviews [1,13], the prevalence of PACG was over-diagnosed in South East Asia, India, and China regions, and under-diagnosed in Middle East and Japan regions. Interpretation of the over- and under-diagnosis of PACG prevalence values is complicated by the inappropriate case definitions used in some studies diagnosing PACG, especially those based only on a narrow anterior chamber angle with raised IOP [13].

An appropriate case definition is the keystone of epidemiological research, and the ISGEO definition has commonly been accepted since it was published [1]. A consensus definition of an "occludable" angle in which the posterior (usually pigmented) trabecular meshwork is seen for less than 90°of angle circumference has come into common usage to indicate the anatomical predisposition to angle closure [1,54,55]. However, the definition of an "occludable" angle excluded around half of all participants who have primary peripheral anterior synechiae (PAS) [54]. Although a slightly more liberal threshold, 180 degrees of iridotrabecular contact (ITC), was used in many population studies, it is still likely to exclude many people who have primary PAS. Therefore, the most widely used epidemiological definition of an "occludable" angle, 180–270 degrees of ITC, is too stringent. The traditional view that primary angle closure becomes a significant possibility in the iridotrabecular angle of 20 degrees probably represents the most inclusive of approaches [54,55]. In addition, gonioscopy using visible light probably under-detects cases where ITC is occurring [55]. Although the results of this present review showed no association between the prevalence of PACG and the definition of occludable angle, in future, the definition of an "occludable angle" used in epidemiological studies of glaucoma still should be reconsidered.

| Study name | Statistics for each study | | | Event rate and 95% CI |
|---|---|---|---|---|
| | Event rate | Lower limit | Upper limit | |
| Aravind Comprehensive Eye Survey | 0.0050 | 0.0034 | 0.0074 | |
| Mongolia Eye Study | 0.0163 | 0.0113 | 0.0235 | |
| Tanjong Pagar Eye Study | 0.0114 | 0.0067 | 0.0191 | |
| Rom Klao Eye Study | 0.0086 | 0.0039 | 0.0189 | |
| Dhaka Eye Study | 0.0030 | 0.0014 | 0.0062 | |
| Tajimi Study | 0.0063 | 0.0040 | 0.0098 | |
| Shaanxi Rural Study | 0.0109 | 0.0077 | 0.0155 | |
| West Bengal Glaucoma Study | 0.0024 | 0.0008 | 0.0073 | |
| Chennai Glaucoma Study | 0.0088 | 0.0063 | 0.0123 | |
| Liwan Eye Study | 0.0153 | 0.0100 | 0.0234 | |
| Meiktila Eye Study | 0.0250 | 0.0191 | 0.0327 | |
| Oman Eye Study | 0.0205 | 0.0162 | 0.0259 | |
| Singapore Malay Eye Study | 0.0024 | 0.0012 | 0.0049 | |
| Kandy Eye Study | 0.0057 | 0.0027 | 0.0119 | |
| Sunsari Eye Study | 0.0013 | 0.0003 | 0.0050 | |
| Andhra Pradesh Eye Disease Study | 0.0094 | 0.0068 | 0.0131 | |
| Beijing Eye Study | 0.0102 | 0.0076 | 0.0137 | |
| Bin Eye Study | 0.0157 | 0.0126 | 0.0196 | |
| Handan Eye Study | 0.0055 | 0.0038 | 0.0078 | |
| Kailu Eye Study | 0.0174 | 0.0142 | 0.0214 | |
| Sangju Eye Study | 0.0030 | 0.0007 | 0.0118 | |
| Qatar Eye Study | 0.0044 | 0.0026 | 0.0075 | |
| Namil Study | 0.0070 | 0.0038 | 0.0130 | |
| Bhaktapur Glaucoma Study | 0.0043 | 0.0026 | 0.0068 | |
| Kumejima Study | 0.0218 | 0.0176 | 0.0270 | |
| Yunnan Minority Eye Study | 0.0094 | 0.0061 | 0.0145 | |
| Central India Eye and Medical Study | 0.0030 | 0.0018 | 0.0050 | |
| Singapore Indian Eye Study | 0.0018 | 0.0008 | 0.0039 | |
| Yazd Eye Study | 0.0033 | 0.0016 | 0.0070 | |
| **Overall** | **0.0075** | **0.0058** | **0.0096** | |

*Test for Heterogeneity: Chi² = 311.760, df = 28 (P < 0.0001); I² = 91.017%*

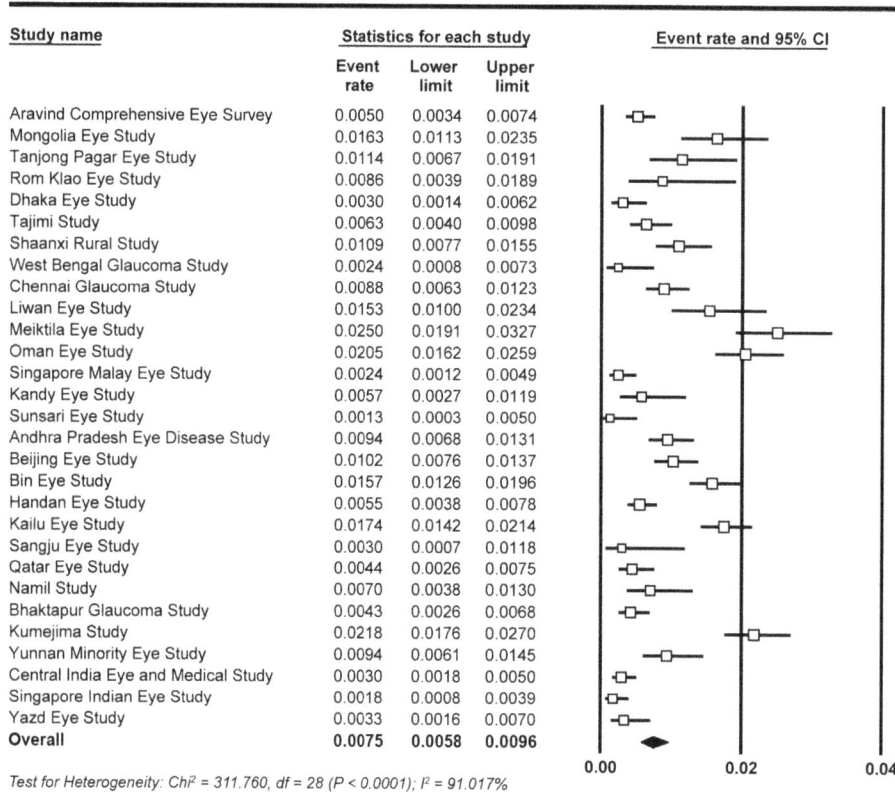

**Figure 2. The forest plot of the prevalence of primary angle closure glaucoma.**

There are several limitations of this systematic review should be discussed. First, similar to most systematic reviews, a potential limitation is the publication bias. We attempted to avoid the potential for publication bias by conducting an extensive search. However, the studies published in languages other than English probably was missed. Second, available studies were from only 14 countries. Thus, more population-based studies should be required to estimates the whole prevalence in Asian populations. Third, the diagnostic criteria for glaucoma and occludable angle also differed among studies. Although no association between the prevalence and case definitions was found, the expanding definition of an 'occludable' angle will allow for better consideration of this possibility through research and clinical practice [55].

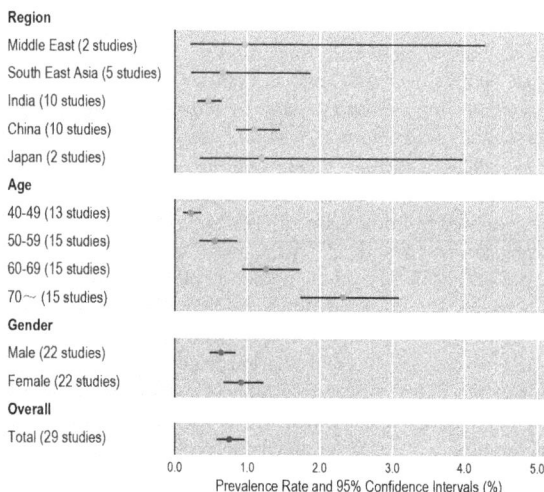

Nevertheless, this systematic review provides a current evidence-based estimate of PACG prevalence in Asian populations. In the past, the number of PACG worldwide probably was misestimated. PACG affects approximately 0.75% adult Asian populations, and the prevalence rates vary greatly by ethnic region. The findings of this present systematic review provide benefit to estimate the burden of PACG in Asia.

## Author Contributions

Conceived and designed the experiments: JWC YZ YYZ RLW. Performed the experiments: JWC YZ YYZ RLW. Analyzed the data: JWC YZ YYZ. Contributed reagents/materials/analysis tools: JWC YZ YYZ. Contributed to the writing of the manuscript: JWC YZ YYZ RLW.

**Figure 3. Ethnicity-, age- and gender-specific pooled prevalence rates of primary angle closure glaucoma.**

# References

1. Quigley HA, Broman AT (2006) The number of people with glaucoma worldwide in 2010 and 2020. Br J Ophthalmol 90: 262–267.

2. Wong TY, Loon SC, Saw SM (2006) The epidemiology of age related eye diseases in Asia. Br J Ophthalmol 90: 506–511.

3. Z Zhou Q, Friedman DS, Lu H, Duan X, Liang Y, et al. (2007) The epidemiology of age-related eye diseases in Mainland China. Ophthalmic Epidemiol 14: 399–407.

4. Foster PJ, Baasanhu J, Alsbirk PH, Munkhbayar D, Uranchimeg D, et al. (1996) Glaucoma in Mongolia. A population-based survey in Hövsgöl province, northern Mongolia. Arch Ophthalmol 114: 1235–1241.

5. Shiose Y, Kitazawa Y, Tsukahara S, Akamatsu T, Mizokami K, et al. (1991) Epidemiology of glaucoma in Japan—a nationwide glaucoma survey. Jpn J Ophthalmol 35: 133–155.

6. Hu CN (1989) An epidemiologic study of glaucoma in Shunyi County, Beijing. Zhonghua Yan Ke Za Zhi 25: 115–119.

7. Dandona L, Dandona R, Mandal P, Srinivas M, John RK, et al. (2000) Angle-closure glaucoma in an urban population in southern India. The Andhra Pradesh eye disease study. Ophthalmology 107: 1710–1716.

8. Foster PJ, Buhrmann R, Quigley HA, Johnson GJ (2002) The definition and classification of glaucoma in prevalence surveys. Br J Ophthalmol 86: 238–242.

9. He M, Foster PJ, Johnson GJ, Khaw PT (2006) Angle-closure glaucoma in East Asian and European people. Different diseases? Eye 20: 3–12.

10. Stroup DF, Berlin JA, Morton SC, Olkin I, Williamson GD, et al. (2000) Meta-analysis of observational studies in epidemiology: a proposal for reporting. Meta-analysis Of Observational Studies in Epidemiology (MOOSE) group. JAMA 283: 2008–2012.

11. Moher D, Liberati A, Tetzlaff J, Altman DG; PRISMA Group (2009) Preferred reporting items for systematic reviews and meta-analyses: the PRISMA statement. BMJ 339: b2535.

12. Rudnicka AR, Mt-Isa S, Owen CG, Cook DG, Ashby D (2006) Variations in primary open-angle glaucoma prevalence by age, gender, and race: a Bayesian meta-analysis. Invest Ophthalmol Vis Sci 47: 4254–4261.

13. Cheng JW, Cheng SW, Ma XY, Cai JP, Li Y, et al. (2013) The prevalence of primary glaucoma in mainland China: a systematic review and meta-analysis. J Glaucoma 22: 301–306.

14. Hoy D, Brooks P, Woolf A, Blyth F, March L, et al. (2012) Assessing risk of bias in prevalence studies: modification of an existing tool and evidence of interrater agreement. J Clin Epidemiol 65: 934–939.

15. Hoy D, Bain C, Williams G, March L, Brooks P, et al. (2012) A systematic review of the global prevalence of low back pain. Arthritis Rheum 64: 2028–2037.

16. von Elm E, Altman DG, Egger M, Pocock SJ, Gøtzsche PC, et al. (2007) The Strengthening the Reporting of Observational Studies in Epidemiology (STROBE) statement: guidelines for reporting observational studies. PLoS Med 4: e296

17. Vandenbroucke JP, von Elm E, Altman DG, Gøtzsche PC, Mulrow CD, et al. (2007) Strengthening the Reporting of Observational Studies in Epidemiology (STROBE): explanation and elaboration. PLoS Med 4: e297.

18. Higgins JPT, Green S (2011) Cochrane Handbook for Systematic Reviews of Interventions Version 5.1.0. The Cochrane Collaboration. Available from www.cochrane-handbook.org. Accessed 11 July 2011.

19. Higgins JP, Thompson SG (2002) Quantifying heterogeneity in a meta-analysis. Stat Med 21: 1539–1558.

20. Higgins JP, Thompson SG, Deeks JJ, Altman DG (2003) Measuring inconsistency in meta-analyses. BMJ 327: 557–560.

21. DerSimonian R, Laird N (1986) Meta-analysis in clinical trials. Control Clin Trials 7: 177–188.

22. Mantel N, Haenszel W (1959) Statistical aspects of the analysis of data from retrospective studies of disease. J Natl Cancer Inst 22: 719–748.

23. Ramakrishnan R, Nirmalan PK, Krishnadas R, Thulasiraj RD, Tielsch JM, et al. (2003) Glaucoma in a rural population of southern India. The Aravind comprehensive eye survey. Ophthalmology 110: 1484–1490.

24. Devereux JG, Foster PJ, Baasanhu J, Uranchimeg D, Lee PS, et al. (2000) Anterior chamber depth measurement as a screening tool for primary angle-closure glaucoma in an East Asian population. Arch Ophthalmol 118: 257–263.

25. Foster PJ, Oen FT, Machin D, Ng TP, Devereux JG, et al. (2000) The prevalence of glaucoma in Chinese residents of Singapore: a cross-sectional population survey of the Tanjong Pagar district. Arch Ophthalmol 118: 1105–1111.

26. Bourne RR, Sukudom P, Foster PJ, Tantisevi V, Jitapunkul S, et al. (2003) Prevalence of glaucoma in Thailand: a population based survey in Rom Klao District, Bangkok. Br J Ophthalmol 87: 1069–1074.

27. Rahman MM, Rahman N, Foster PJ, Haque Z, Zaman AU, et al. (2004) The prevalence of glaucoma in Bangladesh: a population based survey in Dhaka division. Br J Ophthalmol 88: 1493–1497.

28. Yamamoto T, Iwase A, Araie M, Suzuki Y, Abe H, et al. (2005) The Tajimi Study report 2: prevalence of primary angle closure and secondary glaucoma in a Japanese population. Ophthalmology 112: 1661–1669.

29. Bai ZL, Ren BC, Yan JG, He Y, Chen L, et al. (2005) Epidemiology of primary angle-closure glaucoma in a rural population in Shaanxi Province of China. Guo Ji Yan Ke Za Zhi 5: 872–880.

30. Raychaudhuri A, Lahiri SK, Bandyopadhyay M, Foster PJ, Reeves BC, et al. (2005) A population based survey of the prevalence and types of glaucoma in rural West Bengal: the West Bengal Glaucoma Study. Br J Ophthalmol 89: 1559–1564.

31. Vijaya L, George R, Arvind H, Baskaran M, Ve Ramesh S, et al. (2006) Prevalence of primary angle-closure disease in an urban south Indian population and comparison with a rural population. The Chennai Glaucoma Study. Ophthalmology 115: 655–660.e1.

32. He M, Foster PJ, Ge J, Huang W, Zheng Y, et al. (2006) Prevalence and clinical characteristics of glaucoma in adult Chinese: a population-based study in Liwan District, Guangzhou. Invest Ophthalmol Vis Sci 47: 2782–2788.

33. Casson RJ, Newland HS, Muecke J, McGovern S, Abraham L, et al. (2007) Prevalence of glaucoma in rural Myanmar: the Meiktila Eye Study. Br J Ophthalmol 91: 710–714.

34. Khandekar R, Jaffer MA, Al Raisi A, Zutshi R, Mahabaleshwar M, et al. (2008) Oman Eye Study 2005: prevalence and determinants of glaucoma. East Mediterr Health J 14: 1349–1359.

35. Shen SY, Wong TY, Foster PJ, Loo JL, Rosman M, et al. (2008) The prevalence and types of glaucoma in malay people: the Singapore Malay eye study. Invest Ophthalmol Vis Sci 49: 3846–3851.

36. Casson RJ, Baker M, Edussuriya K, Senaratne T, Selva D, et al. (2009) Prevalence and determinants of angle closure in central Sri Lanka: the Kandy Eye Study. Ophthalmology 116: 1444–1449.

37. Sah RP, Badhu BP, Pokharel PK, Thakur SK, Das H, et al. (2007) Prevalence of glaucoma in Sunsari district of eastern Nepal. Kathmandu Univ Med J 5: 343–348.

38. Senthil S, Garudadri C, Khanna RC, Sannapaneni K (2010) Angle closure in the Andhra Pradesh Eye Disease Study. Ophthalmology 117: 1729–1735.

39. Wang YX, Xu L, Yang H, Jonas JB (2010) Prevalence of glaucoma in North China: the Beijing Eye Study. Am J Ophthalmol 150: 917–924.

40. Qu W, Li Y, Song W, Zhou X, Kang Y, et al. (2011) Prevalence and risk factors for angle-closure disease in a rural Northeast China population: a population-based survey in Bin County, Harbin. Acta Ophthalmol 89: e515–520.

41. Liang Y, Friedman DS, Zhou Q, Yang XH, Sun LP, et al. (2011) Prevalence and characteristics of primary angle-closure diseases in a rural adult Chinese population. the Handan Eye Study. Invest Ophthalmol Vis Sci 52: 8672–8679.

42. Song W, Shan L, Cheng F, Fan P, Zhang L, et al. (2011) Prevalence of glaucoma in a rural northern china adult population: a population-based survey in kailu county, inner mongolia. Ophthalmology 118: 1982–1988.

43. Kim JH, Kang SY, Kim NR, Lee ES, Hong S, et al. (2011) Prevalence and characteristics of glaucoma among Korean adults. Korean J Ophthalmol 25: 110–115.

44. Al-Mansouri FA, Kanaan A, Gamra H, Khandekar R, Hashim SP, et al. (2011) Prevalence and determinants of glaucoma in citizens of qatar aged 40 years or older: a community-based survey. Middle East Afr J Ophthalmol 2011;18: 141–9.

45. Kim YY, Lee JH, Ahn MD, Kim CY; Namil Study Group, Korean Glaucoma Society. (2012) Angle closure in the Namil study in central South Korea. Arch Ophthalmol 130: 1177–1183.

46. Thapa SS, Paudyal I, Khanal S, Twyana SN, Paudyal G, et al. (2012) A population-based survey of the prevalence and types of glaucoma in Nepal: the Bhaktapur Glaucoma Study. Ophthalmology 119: 759–764.

47. Sawaguchi S, Sakai H, Iwase A, Yamamoto T, Abe H, et al. (2012) Prevalence of primary angle closure and primary angle-closure glaucoma in a southwestern rural population of Japan: the Kumejima Study. Ophthalmology 119: 1134–1142.

48. Zhong H, Li J, Li C, Wei T, Cha X, et al. (2012) The prevalence of glaucoma in adult rural Chinese populations of the Bai nationality in Dali: the Yunnan Minority Eye Study. Invest Ophthalmol Vis Sci 53: 3221–3225.

49. Nangia V, Jonas JB, Matin A, Bhojwani K, Sinha A, et al. (2013) Prevalence and associated factors of glaucoma in rural central India. The Central India Eye and Medical Study. PLoS One 8: e76434.

50. Narayanaswamy A, Baskaran M, Zheng Y, Lavanya R, Wu R, et al. (2013) The prevalence and types of glaucoma in an urban Indian population: the Singapore Indian Eye Study. Invest Ophthalmol Vis Sci 54: 4621–4627.

51. Pakravan M, Yazdani S, Javadi MA, Amini H, Behroozi Z, et al. (2013) A Population-based Survey of the Prevalence and Types of Glaucoma in Central Iran: The Yazd Eye Study. Ophthalmology 120: 1977–1984.

52. Cassard SD, Quigley HA, Gower EW, Friedman DS, Ramulu PY, et al. (2012) Regional variations and trends in the prevalence of diagnosed glaucoma in the Medicare population. Ophthalmology 119: 1342–1351.

53. Day AC, Baio G, Gazzard G, Bunce C, Azuara-Blanco A, et al. (2012) The prevalence of primary angle closure glaucoma in European derived populations: a systematic review. Br J Ophthalmol 96: 1162–1167.

54. Foster PJ, Aung T, Nolan WP, Machin D, Baasanhu J, et al. (2004) Defining "occludable" angles in population surveys: drainage angle width, peripheral anterior synechiae, and glaucomatous optic neuropathy in east Asian people. Br J Ophthalmol 88: 486–490.

55. Foster P, He M, Liebmann J (2006) Epidemiology, classification and mechanism. In: Weinreb RN, Friedman DS, editors. Angle Closure and Angle-Closure Glaucoma: Reports and Consensus Statements of the 3rd Global AIGS Consensus Meeting on Angle Closure Glaucoma. The Netherlands: Kugler Publications. pp.1–20.

# 20

# Association of a Polymorphism in the *BIRC6* Gene with Pseudoexfoliative Glaucoma

**Humaira Ayub[1], Shazia Micheal[2], Farah Akhtar[3], Muhammad Imran Khan[4], Shaheena Bashir[1], Nadia K. Waheed[5], Mahmood Ali[3], Frederieke E. Schoenmaker-Koller[2], Sobia Shafique[1], Raheel Qamar[1,6], Anneke I. den Hollander[2,4]***

1 Department of Biosciences, COMSATS Institute of Information Technology, Islamabad, Pakistan, 2 Department of Ophthalmology, Radboud University Nijmegen Medical Centre, Nijmegen, The Netherlands, 3 Al-Shifa Trust Eye Hospital, Rawalpindi, Pakistan, 4 Department of Human Genetics, Radboud University Nijmegen Medical Centre, Nijmegen, The Netherlands, 5 Department of Ophthalmology, Tufts University School of Medicine, Boston, Massachusetts, United States of America, 6 Al-Nafees Medical College & Hospital, Isra University, Islamabad, Pakistan

## Abstract

Recently an association was observed between alleles in genes of the unfolded protein response pathway and primary open angle glaucoma (POAG). The goal of the current study is to investigate the role of these two genes, protein disulphide isomerase A member 5 (*PDIA5*) and baculoviral IAP repeat containing 6 (*BIRC6*), in different forms of glaucoma. 278 patients with POAG, 132 patients with primary angle closure glaucoma (PACG) and 135 patients with pseudoexfoliative glaucoma (PEXG) were genotyped for single nucleotide polymorphisms (SNPs) rs11720822 in *PDIA5* and 471 POAG, 184 PACG and 218 PEXG patients were genotyped for rs2754511 in *BIRC6*. Genotyping was done by allelic discrimination PCR, and genotype and allele frequencies were calculated. Logistic regression analyses were performed using R software to determine the association of these SNPs with glaucoma. The allele and genotype frequencies of rs11720822 in *PDIA5* were not associated with POAG, PACG or PEXG. The TT genotype of rs2754511 in *BIRC6* was found to be protective for PEXG (p = 0.05, OR 0.42 [0.22–0.81]) in the Pakistani population, but not for POAG or PACG. This study did not confirm a previously reported association of risk alleles in *PDIA5* and *BIRC6* with POAG, but did demonstrate a protective role of the T allele of rs2754511 in the *BIRC6* gene in PEXG. This supports a role for the unfolded protein response pathway and regulation of apoptotic cell death in the pathogenesis of PEXG.

**Editor:** Robert Lafrenie, Sudbury Regional Hospital, Canada

**Funding:** This work was supported by grant no. PSF/RES/C-COMSATS/MED(280) awarded to R.Q. by the Pakistan Science Foundation and a core grant from the COMSATS Institute of Information Technology. The funders had no role in study design, data collection and analysis, decision to publish, or preparation of the manuscript.

**Competing Interests:** The authors have declared that no competing interests exist.

* Email: anneke.denhollander@radboudumc.nl

## Introduction

Glaucoma is an optic neurodegenerative disorder [1] that leads to gradual loss of vision due to degeneration of the retinal ganglion cells [2]. Two subtypes of primary glaucoma can be distinguished, primary open angle glaucoma (POAG) and primary angle closure glaucoma (PACG), which are associated with different anatomical defects [3]. The most common form of secondary glaucoma is pseudoexfoliative glaucoma (PEXG), which is generally characterized by the appearance of dandruff-like grayish white flakes deposited over the iris, lens, and ciliary epithelium. This material collecting in the anterior angle has been related to raised intra ocular pressure (IOP) and ultimately glaucoma [4–6].

With advancing age, the exposure of the eye to various stress-inducing factors increases, which can damage the integrity of the trabecular meshwork. These majorly include free radicals, reactive oxygen species (ROS) [7,8] and protein aggregation [9], which elevate oxidative stress in the eye. In PEXG and POAG the damage due to oxidative stress [8] can also succumb into mitochondrial damage and neuronal death of retinal ganglion cells eventually leading to vision loss [10–12].

A previous genome-wide analysis in a *Drosophila* ocular hypertension model identified transcripts with altered regulation, and showed induction of the unfolded protein response (UPR) upon overexpression of transgenic human glaucoma-associated myocilin [13,14]. Single nucleotide polymorphisms (SNPs) in two genes involved in reduction of endoplasmic reticulum (ER) stress, protein disulphide isomerase family A member 5 (*PDIA5*) and Baculoviral inhibitor of apoptosis repeat-containing 6 (*BIRC6*), have been recently shown to be significantly associated with POAG [15,16]. Since no other studies have yet attempted to replicate this finding, we investigated both SNPs in a cohort of POAG patients from Pakistan. In addition, we extended the analysis to patients with PACG and PEXG, as recent studies have suggested that common genetic factors might contribute to various forms of glaucoma [17]. The aim of this study was to investigate the role of rs11720822 in *PDIA5* and rs2754511 in *BIRC6* in POAG, PACG and PEXG patients from the Pakistani population.

## Methods

### Ethics statement

This study has been approved by the Department of Biosciences, Ethics Review Committee and conforms to all of the norms of the Helsinki Declaration. Written informed consent was obtained from all participants.

### Patients and control individuals

In the present study 471 POAG, 184 PACG and 218 PEXG patients were recruited from different ophthalmological centers in Pakistan. The diagnosis of POAG and PACG was made as described previously [18]. PEXG was diagnosed on the basis of clinical history, cup-to-disc ratio (CDR) and intraocular pressure (IOP) measurements. In order to detect the exfoliative deposits on the pupillary border and the iris, slit lamp biomicroscopy was initially performed without dilation of the pupil, and subsequently after pupil dilation the patients were re-examined to detect the presence of white deposits on the anterior lens surface. Angles were measured with gonioscopy to discriminate between narrow and open angles. 160 unaffected controls, belonging to the same ethnic background as the patients, were classified on the basis of absence of any exfoliate deposits, normal gonioscopic observations and normal CDR and IOP values. The processing and DNA isolation from whole blood was performed as described previously [18].

### Genotyping

Two intronic SNPs, rs11720822 in *PDIA5* and rs2754511 in *BIRC6*, were genotyped in the POAG, PACG, PEXG patients and control individuals using Taqman allelic discrimination assays performed by Real-time PCR (Applied Biosystems 7900HT Fast System and Sequence Detection Systems Software v2.3, Foster City, CA). The polymerase chain reaction (PCR) amplification was performed according to the protocol of the manufacturer using 10 ng of DNA in a reaction mixture of 4 µl. After an initial denaturation step of 12 minutes at 95°C, 50 cycles of amplification were performed for 15 seconds at 92°C and termination for 90 seconds at 60°C.

### Statistical Analysis

Allele frequencies between the unaffected controls and the three patient groups (POAG, PACG and PEXG) were compared with the Pearson $\chi 2$ test using online free link available (http://statpages.org/ctab2x2.html). The Genotype frequencies were calculated by logistic regression analysis keeping age and gender as covariates. The data was statistically analyzed by using R software (R Core Team (2012). R: A language and environment for statistical computing. R Foundation for Statistical Computing, Vienna, Austria. ISBN 3-900051-07-0, URL http://www.R-project.org/). Moreover Bonferoni correction was applied to the individual p-values generated from logistic regression analysis.

## Results and Discussion

Patients and controls included in the current study were age and gender matched (table 1). The mean age ($\pm$ standard deviation) of the controls was 48.1±13.2 years, of patients with POAG 48.3±16.5 years, PACG 45.5.±16.5 years and PEXG 50.09±14.1 years. In total 321 healthy subjects (52% males and 48% females), 471 patients with POAG (51% males and 49% females), and 184 patients with PACG patients (49.5% males and50.5% females) and 218 PEXG (48% males and 52% females) were enrolled in the study. The majority of the patients was treated

**Table 1.** Demographic and clinical features of the control, POAG, PACG and PEXG cohorts.

| | Controls | POAG | p-value | PACG | p-value | PEXG | p-value |
|---|---|---|---|---|---|---|---|
| Age | 48.1±13.2 | 48.3±16.5 | >0.05 | 45.5.±16.5 | >0.05 | 50.09±14.1 | >0.05 |
| Gender | | | | | | | |
| Males | 52% | 51% | >0.05 | 49.5% | >0.05 | 48% | >0.05 |
| Females | 48% | 49% | | 50.5% | | 52% | |
| IOP | 16.4±2.3 | 30.5±11.6 | <0.05 | 26.4±10.2 | <0.05 | 28.4±10.5 | <0.05 |
| CDR | 0.39±0.18 | 0.85±.63 | <0.05 | 0.67±.27 | <0.05 | 0.76±.23 | <0.05 |

**Table 2.** Results of logistic regression analysis for Genotype and allele frequency of SNPs rs11720822 in *PDIA5* and rs2754511 in *BIRC6* in POAG, PCAG and PEXG patients and control individuals.

| *PDIA5* rs11720822 | POAG Est. | Z value | OR(95%CI) | P-value/p[b] | PACG Est. | Z value | OR(95%CI) | p-value/p[b] | PEXG Est. | Z value | OR(95%CI) | p-value/p[b] |
|---|---|---|---|---|---|---|---|---|---|---|---|---|
| CC | 0.07 | 0.16 | 0.9 (0.37–2.26)[a] | 0.86/1.00[b] | 0.22 | −0.45 | 0.79 (0.29–2.13)[a] | 0.64/1.00[b] | 0.60 | 1.30 | 1.82(0.74–4.48)[a] | 0.18/1.00[b] |
| CT | 17.90 | 0.02 | 5.95(0.00-Inf)[a] | 0.98/1.00[b] | 12.89 | 0.01 | 3.69 (0.00-Inf)[a] | 0.98/1.00[b] | 15.55 | 0.01 | 5.68(0.00-Inf)[a] | 0.98/1.00[b] |
| TT | - | - | | | - | - | | | - | - | | |
| **Allele Frequency** | | | | | | | | | | | | |
| C | - | - | 0.74 (0.41–1.34)[c] | 0.28/1.00[b] | - | - | 1.00 (0.51–1.96)[c] | 0.99/1.00[b] | - | - | 1.15 (0.60–2.19)[c] | 0.66/1.00[b] |
| T | - | - | | | - | - | | | - | - | | |
| ***BIRC6* rs2754511** | | | | | | | | | | | | |
| AA | 0.39 | −2.53 | 0.67 (0.49–0.91)[a] | 0.01/0.06[b] | 0.05 | −0.28 | 0.94 (0.62–1.41)[a] | 0.77/1.00 | 0.35 | −1.87 | 0.70 (0.48–1.01)[a] | 0.06/0.36[b] |
| AT | 0.18 | 0.81 | 0.83 (0.52–1.30)[a] | 0.41/1.00[b] | 0.18 | 0.59 | 1.20 (0.65–2.22)[a] | 0.54/1.00[b] | 0.84 | 2.58 | 0.42 (0.22–0.81)[a] | 0.009/0.05[b] |
| TT | - | - | | | - | - | | | - | - | | |
| **Allele Frequency** | | | | | | | | | | | | |
| A | - | - | 0.85 (0.68–1.06)[c] | 0.15/0.90[b] | - | - | 0.95(0.72–1.26)[c] | 0.28/1.00[b] | - | - | 0.72 (0.55–0.94)[c] | 0.01/0.06[b] |
| T | - | - | | | - | - | | | - | - | | |

[a]Age and gender adjusted OR and (95%CI) from multivariate logistic regression analysis; p[b]Bonferoni corrected p values; [c]OR and (95%CI) from univariate logistic regression analysis; Est., estimates

with medications such as β-blockers, or underwent surgery (trabeculectomy) to lower IOP.

The allele and genotype frequencies of rs11720822 in *PDIA5* were not significantly different between POAG, PACG and PEXG compared to control individuals (Table 2). The T allele of rs2754511 in *BIRC6* was found on 35% of control alleles, while it was found on 32% of POAG alleles, 35% of PACG alleles, and 28% of PEXG alleles. The frequency of the T allele is significantly lower in PEXG patients as compared to controls (p = 0.01; OR 0.72 [95% CI 0.55–0.94]), suggesting it has a protective effect (Table 2), however this association did not remain significant when Bonferoni correction was applied to the data (p = 0.06).

"Logistic regression analysis was conducted to adjust for age and gender which showed that the homozygous TT genotype of the studied *BIRC6* polymorphism is protective for PEXG (p = 0.009), which remained significant even after the Bonferoni correction (p = 0.05)."

Addition of 163 controls, 194 POAG cases, 47 PACG cases and 88 PEXG cases to the previous data improved the statistical power and supported the previous association (p = 0.03) of PEXG with the BIRC6 SNP rs2754511 (p = 0.01). Moreover the application of logistic regression analysis further strengthened the results (p = 0.009).

The two SNPs in *PDIA5* and *BIRC6* were previously associated with POAG in the Salt Lake City and San Diego populations [16]. Since recent studies have suggested that common genetic factors might contribute to various forms of glaucoma, we extended our study to PACG and PEXG. We did not find an association of these SNPs with either POAG or PACG in our population, nor did we find an association of the *PDIA5* gene polymorphism with PEXG. According to the dbSNP database, occurrence of the T allele of rs11720822 in *PDIA5* is very rare in various populations of the world including the Asian and African populations (http://www.ncbi.nlm.nih.gov/projects/SNP/snp_ref.cgi?rs = rs11720822), which supports our finding, as we also do not see high occurrence of the allele in our population. Our study did detect a moderate association of the *BIRC6* rs2754511 polymorphism with PEXG in the Pakistani population (p = 0.05). In agreement with the previous findings in the Salt Lake City and San Diego populations, demonstrating a protective effect of the T allele of rs2754511 on the development of POAG [16], this allele in homozygous form (TT) was also found to be protective for PEXG in our study. In this study, we investigated only the SNPs that were significantly associated with POAG in both the San Diego and Salt Lake City cohorts. We therefore cannot exclude that other SNPs in *BIRC6* or *PDIA5* may be associated with glaucoma in the Pakistani population.

BIRC6 is ubiquitin carrier protein involved in the protection of the cell against apoptosis and reduces cellular stress [16,19]. Increased intraocular pressure, ROS and free radicals create a stressful environment in the eye [8,20]. In the ER, stress can be accompanied by the aggregation of misfolded proteins. The accumulation of misfolded proteins can activate a cytoprotective signal response known as unfolded protein response (UPR), which triggers the activator functions like adaptation, alarm and apoptosis [12]. When stress is prolonged and adaptation and alarm fail to pull the cell back to normal condition, the UPR results in activation of apoptosis [21] and also elicits an inflammatory response in order to restore the normal environment of the cell. This mechanism has been found to be involved in the pathogenesis of many neurodegenerative disorders like Alzhei-

mer's disease, Parkinson's disease and cerebral ischemic insults [22].

In PEXG and POAG the damage due to oxidative stress can succumb into mitochondrial damage [8,10,11]. The extracellular matrix of the trabecular meshwork is disrupted as a consequence of damage to the mitochondria, a characteristic mechanism involved in the pathogenicity of POAG and PEXG [8]. Konstas *et al.* [23] have observed excessive mitochondrial alterations in PEXG. The highest level of mitochondrial damage and mitochondrial loss per cell was seen in PEXG as compared to POAG, which justifies its more aggressive nature.

Zenkel *et al* have reported differential expression of ECM proteins and stress response genes in eyes of PEXG patients compared to eyes of normal healthy controls [24]. The expression of ECM genes is upregulated, resulting in aggregation of ECM proteins. Glutathione S-transferase 1, which is involved in protection from oxidative stress, is downregulated [24]. In addition, clusterin, an efficient extracellular chaperone, is downregulated in PEXG eyes, resulting in aggregation of pathologic ECM proteins [25]. Consequently, abnormal proteins accumulate, resulting in the formation of pseudoexfoliative material [25]. In the anterior chamber this hinders the outflow of aqueous humor by clogging the trabecular meshwork, which results in elevation of the IOP [26,27]. All these stresses succumb in severe degenerative changes in PEXG.

Apoptosis might be one of the various mechanisms that is involved in the degeneration of retinal ganglion cells in PEXG. BIRC6 is an anti-apoptotic protein, which promotes cell survival by inhibiting caspases [28]. Downregulation of BIRC6 by various polymorphisms and mutations leads to upregulation of p53, resulting in mitochondrial-mediated apoptotic cell death [29]. As a consequence of stress, cytochrome C is released from mitochondria, which activates caspases and thus resulting in the degeneration and death of the cells [30].

Recent GWAS studies by Nakano *et al.*, for the Japanese population [31], Gibson *et al.*, for British population [32], Ramdas *et al.*, Dutch population [33] have shown few loci and SNPs to be associated with Glaucoma but these studies did not find any association of the BIRC6 gene polymorphism rs2754511 with the POAG cohort. It was seen that the BIRC6 SNP was not covered in the maps used in those studies therefore that might be the reason of not finding rs275411 association. Contrary to the studies mentioned above we and Carbone et al found significant association of the SNP with PEXG and POAG respectively. As SNPs have individual, ethnicity and population specific role in disease etiology, therefore the association that we found could be due to divergent background of the studied populations [34].

In conclusion, our study demonstrates that the T allele of the rs2754511 in the *BIRC6* gene plays a protective role in PEXG patients of the Pakistani population. This supports a role for the UPR pathway and regulation of apoptotic cell death in the pathogenesis of PEXG.

## Acknowledgments

We thank all the patients for their cooperation in the current study.

## Author Contributions

Conceived and designed the experiments: HA SM RQ AIdH. Performed the experiments: HA SM FESK SS. Analyzed the data: HA SM FESK SB. Contributed reagents/materials/analysis tools: HA SM MIK NKW MA FA. Wrote the paper: HA RQ AIdH.

# References

1. Gupta N, Yucel YH (2007) Glaucoma as a neurodegenerativedisease. Curr Opin Ophthalmol 18:110–4.
2. Chang EE, Goldberg JL (2012) Glaucoma 2.0: neuroprotection, neuroregeneration, neuro enhancement. Ophthalmology 119:979–86.
3. Yousaf S, Khan MI, Micheal S, Akhtar F, Ali SH, et al. (2011) XRCC1 and XPD DNA repair gene polymorphisms: a potential risk factor for glaucoma in the Pakistani population. Mol Vis17:1153–63.
4. Lee RK (2004) The molecular pathophysiology of pseudoexfoliation glaucoma. Curr opin optholmol 19:95–101.
5. Manishi AD, Richard KL (2008) The medical and surgical management of pseudoexfoliation glaucoma. Int Ophthalmol Clin 48: 95–113.
6. Micheal S, Khan MI, Akhtar F, Ali M, Ahmed A, et al (2012) Role of lysyloxidase-like 1 gene polymorphisms in Pakistani patients with pseudoexfoliative glaucoma. Mol Vis 18:1040–1044.
7. Zenkel M, Lewczuk P, Jünemann A, Kruse FE, Naumann GO, et al (2010) Proinflimmatory cytokines are involved in the initiation of the abnormal matrix process in pesudoexfoliation syndrome/glaucoma. Am J Pathol 176:2868–79.
8. Izzotti A, Longobardi M, Cartiglia C, Saccà SC (2011) Mitochondrial damage in the trabecular meshwork occurs only in primary open-angle glaucoma and in pseudoexfoliative glaucoma. PLoSOne 20:14567.
9. Ovodenko B, Rostagno A, Neubert TA, Shetty V, Thomas S (2007) Proteomic analysis of exfoliation deposits. Invest Ophthalmol Vis Sci 48:1447–1457.
10. Niizuma K, Endo H, Chan PH (2009) Oxidative stress and mitochondrial dysfunction as determinants of ischemic neuronal death and survival. J Neurochem 1:133–138.
11. Chen SD, Yang DI, Lin TK, Shaw FZ, Liou CW (2011) Roles of oxidative stress, apoptosis, PGC-1α and mitochondrial biogenesis in cerebral ischemia. Int J Mol Sci12:7199–7215.
12. Xu C, Bailly-Maitre B, Reed JC (2005) Endoplasmic reticulum stress: cell life and death decisions. J Clin Invest 115:2656–2664.
13. Borrás T, Morozova TV, Heinsohn SL, Lyman RF, Mackay TF (2003) Transcription profiling in Drosophila eyes that overexpress the human glaucoma associated trabecular meshwork inducible glucocorticoid response protien/myociline (TIGR/MYOC). Genetics163:637–645.
14. Carbone MA, Ayroles JF, Yamamoto A, Morozova TV, West SA (2009) Overexpression of myocilin in the Drosophila eye activates the unfolded protein response: implications for glaucoma. PLoSOne 4:4216.
15. Liu CH, Goldberg AL, Qiu XB (2007) New insights into the role of the ubiquitin-proteasome pathway in the regulation of apoptosis. Chang Gung Med J 30:469–79.
16. Carbone MA, Chen Y, Hughes GA, Weinreb RN, Zabriskie NA, et al (2011) Genes of the unfolded protein response pathway harbor risk alleles for primary open angle glaucoma. PLoSOne 6:e20649.
17. Patel HY, Richards AJ, De Karolyi B, Best SJ, Danesh-Meyer HV, et al (2012) Screening glaucoma genes in adult glaucoma suggests a multi allelic contribution of CYP1B1 to open-angle glaucoma phenotypes. Clin Experiment Ophthalmol 40:e208–217.
18. Ayub H, Khan MI, Micheal S, Akhtar F, Ajmal M, et al (2010) Association of eNOS and HSP70 gene polymorphisms with glaucoma in Pakistani cohorts. Mol Vis 16:18–25.
19. Lamers F, Schild L, Koster J, Speleman F, Ora I, et al (2012) Identification of BIRC6 as a novel intervention target for neuroblastoma therapy. BMC Cancer 12:285.
20. Sacca SC, Izzoti A, RossiPietro, Traverso C (2007) Glaucomtous outflow pathway and oxidative stress. Exp Eye Res 84:389–99.
21. Kim I, Xu W, Reed JC (2008) Celldeath and endoplasmic reticulum stress: disease relevance and therapeutic opportunities. Nat Rev Drug Discov 7:1013–1030.
22. Wang S, Kaufman RJ (2012) The impact of the unfolded protein response on human diseaseJCellBiol 25:857–67.
23. Kontas AG, Mantziris DA,Stewart WC (1997) Diurnal intraocular pressure in untreated exfoliation and primary open-angle glaucoma. Arch Ophthalmol 115:182–185.
24. Zenkel M, Poschl E, von der Mark K, Hofmann-Rummelt C, Naumann GO, et al (2005) Differential gene expression in pseudoexfoliation syndrome. InvestOphthalmol Vis Sci 46:3742–3752.
25. Zenkel M, Kruse FE, JunemannAG,Naumann GO, Schlötzer-Schrehardt U (2006) Clusterin deficiency in eyes with pseudoexfoliation syndrome may be implicated in the aggregation and deposition of pseudoexfoliative material. Invest Ophthalmol Vis Sci 47:1982–1990.
26. Streeten BW, Li ZY, WallaceRN, Eagle RC,Jr, Keshgegian AA (1992) Pseudoexfoliative fibrillopathy in visceralorgans of a patient with pseudoexfoliation Syndrome. Arch Opthalmol 110:1757–1762.
27. Streeten BW, Dark AJ, WallaceRN, Li ZY, Hoepner JA. (1990) Pseudoexfoliative fibrillopathy in the skin of patients with ocular pseudoexfoliation. Am J Opthalmol 110:490–499.
28. Ishiwata K, Imamiya K, Mizukami T, Abiko Y (2011) Reduction of BIRC6 Gene expression by reactive oxygen stress in osteoblasts. Int J Oral-Med Sci 10:67–71.
29. Ren J, Shi M, Liu R, Yang QH, Johnson T (2005) The BIRC6 (Bruce) gene regulates p53 and the mitochondrial pathway of the apoptosis and is essential for mouse embryonic development. PNAS 102:565–570.
30. Hao Y, Sekine K, Kawabata A, Nakamura H, Ishioka T, et al (2001) Apollon ubiquitinates SMAC and caspase-9, and has an essential cytoprotection function. Nat Cell Biol 6:849–860.
31. Nakano M, Ikeda Y, Taniguchi T, Yagi T, Fuwa M, et al (2009) Three susceptible loci associated with primary open-angle glaucoma identified by genome-wide association study in a Japanese population. Proc Natl Acad Sci 106: 12838–12842.
32. Gibson J, Griffiths H, Salvo D G, Cole M, Jacob A, et al (2012) Genome-wide association study of primary open angle glaucoma risk and quantitative traits. Mol Vis 18: 1083–1092.
33. Ramdas WD, van Koolwijk LM, Lemij HG, Pasutto F, Cree AJ, et al (2011) Common genetic variants associated with open-angle glaucoma. Hum Mol Genet 20: 2464–2471.
34. Qamar R, Ayub Q, Mohyuddin A, Helgason A, Mazhar K, et al (2002) Y-chromosomal DNA variation in Pakistan. Am J Hum Genet. 70: 1107–1124.

# 21

# Binocular Glaucomatous Visual Field Loss and its Impact on Visual Exploration - A Supermarket Study

**Katrin Sippel**[1,9], **Enkelejda Kasneci**[1*,9], **Kathrin Aehling**[2], **Martin Heister**[2], **Wolfgang Rosenstiel**[1], **Ulrich Schiefer**[2,3], **Elena Papageorgiou**[2,4]

1 Computer Engineering Department, University of Tübingen, Tübingen, Germany, 2 Centre for Ophthalmology, Institute for Ophthalmic Research, University of Tübingen, Tübingen, Germany, 3 Competence Centre "Vision Research", Study Course "Ophthalmic Optics/Audiology", University of Applied Sciences Aalen, Aalen, Germany, 4 Department of Ophthalmology, University of Leicester, Leicester Royal Infirmary, Leicester, United Kingdom

## Abstract

Advanced glaucomatous visual field loss may critically interfere with quality of life. The purpose of this study was to (i) assess the impact of binocular glaucomatous visual field loss on a supermarket search task as an example of everyday living activities, (ii) to identify factors influencing the performance, and (iii) to investigate the related compensatory mechanisms. Ten patients with binocular glaucoma (GP), and ten healthy-sighted control subjects (GC) were asked to collect twenty different products chosen randomly in two supermarket racks as quickly as possible. The task performance was rated as "passed" or "failed" with regard to the time per correctly collected item. Based on the performance of control subjects, the threshold value for failing the task was defined as $\mu+3\sigma$ (in seconds per correctly collected item). Eye movements were recorded by means of a mobile eye tracker. Eight out of ten patients with glaucoma and all control subjects passed the task. Patients who failed the task needed significantly longer time (111.47 s $\pm$12.12 s) to complete the task than patients who passed (64.45 s $\pm$13.36 s, t-test, p<0.001). Furthermore, patients who passed the task showed a significantly higher number of glances towards the visual field defect (VFD) area than patients who failed (t-test, p<0.05). According to these results, glaucoma patients with defects in the binocular visual field display on average longer search times in a naturalistic supermarket task. However, a considerable number of patients, who compensate by frequent glancing towards the VFD, showed successful task performance. Therefore, systematic exploration of the VFD area seems to be a "time-effective" compensatory mechanism during the present supermarket task.

**Editor:** Ranji Cui, Jilin University, China

**Funding:** PFIZER Pharma GmbH, Berlin, Germany, and MSD, SHARP & DOHME GmbH, Haar, Germany provided financial support to this study. This funding was used for compensation of the recruited subjects. The funders had no role in study design, data collection and analysis, decision to publish, or preparation of the manuscript.

**Competing Interests:** The authors have the following interests. PFIZER Pharma GmbH, Berlin, Germany, and MSD, SHARP & DOHME GmbH, Haar, Germany provided financial support to this study. There are no patents, products in development or marketed products to declare.

* Email: enkelejda.kasneci@uni-tuebingen.de

9 These authors contributed equally to this work.

## Introduction

Glaucoma is a progressive optic neuropathy leading to characteristic visual field defects, and blindness if left untreated. Glaucoma usually leads to (arcuate) visual field defects that follow the course of the affected retinal nerve fibers. In advanced stages of glaucoma the areas of monocular field defects may spatially coincide and thus result in binocular field loss. The central visual field (VF) and the visual acuity are usually spared even up to end-stage glaucoma.

Patients with binocular glaucomatous visual field loss may experience severe difficulties in activities of daily living such as reading, mobility, or driving [1–8]. Furthermore, due to demographic aging, the number of people suffering from glaucoma is expected to increase. According to Quigley and Broman 2006 [9] the number of people who will be bilaterally blind from open-angle glaucoma is expected to rise to 5.9 million by 2020.

Therefore, the impact of glaucoma on everyday activities and on the quality of life of affected individuals is being investigated intensively during the last years. Many studies have assessed the impairment of patients with glaucoma in everyday activities by means of questionnaires [5,6,10–17], simulators, or under laboratory conditions [18]. Their results suggest that visual search behavior of affected subjects plays a decisive role in coping with everyday activities. The most realistic attempt to assess the functional impairment of patients with glaucoma in everyday activities is by conducting real-world experiments, mostly regarding driving fitness [1,3,19,20–22]. The above previous studies agree on certain aspects: (i) the task performance varies among individuals, (2) binocular visual field defects do not always lead to poorer performance, and (3) binocular visual field defects can be compensated by effective head and eye movement strategies. However, the results of driving studies may not reflect patients' visual behavior in other everyday activities, because compensatory gaze patterns are highly specific and intrinsically related to the specific task [23]. Furthermore, there is variability in patients' compensatory strategies during activities of daily living. Since real-world experiments are expensive, time-consuming, and difficult to standardize, to date only few everyday activities have been investigated.

A common scenario in everyday life involving visual search is shopping, where we permanently search for specific items. Most prior work on visual search during shopping has aimed at understanding the consumer's psychology, e.g., [24–27]. To the best of our knowledge no studies investigating the visual search of patients with binocular glaucomatous visual field defects during shopping tasks have been conducted up to date. Assessment of activities of daily living is necessary for a better understanding of the compensatory strategies of patients with binocular glaucoma. Hence, evaluation of visual exploration during daily activities will be helpful in evaluating global, vision-targeted QOL, in order to improve the correlation between visual function and its perception, design training strategies for improvement of daily functioning, and develop examination tools for usage in the clinical setting.

Therefore, the aim of this pilot study was to assess the visual search performance of patients with binocular glaucomatous visual field loss in a supermarket special offer search task. The patients' performance was compared to that of healthy-sighted control subjects. Furthermore, we investigated the factors affecting task performance and studied features of the visual search strategy. We hypothesize that the performance of patients with binocular glaucoma is not primarily associated to the extent of the visual field defect, but is mainly related to their visual scanning strategy.

## Methods

### Participants

Twenty participants were enrolled in this study: ten patients with glaucoma (we refer to this group as GP, age $60.7 \pm 8.7$ years) and ten healthy-sighted control subjects (GC, age $59.9 \pm 9.1$ years), matched with respect to age and gender (Table S1). All participants were recruited by the Neuro-Ophthalmology service of the University of Tübingen.

To be included in the study all participants were required to be at least 18 years old, have a Minimental Status Examination Score above 24, to have the ability to understand and comply with the requirements of the study, and normal function and morphology of the anterior visual pathways, as evaluated by ophthalmological tests (fundus and slit-lamp examinations, ocular alignment, ocular motility). Color vision should be normal using the Ishihara isochromatic color plates. The age- and gender-matched control subjects should additionally have normal visual fields, normal cup-to-disc ratio (less or equal to 0.5) and no history of brain injury or physical impairment. The best corrected monocular distant visual acuity of control subjects should be >20/20 for those aged-up to 60 years, >20/25 for those aged between 60–70 years and >20/33 for those aged more than 70 years. Patients' best corrected monocular distant visual acuity should be at least 20/40. Glaucoma patients had a confirmed diagnosis of primary open angle glaucoma based on optic nerve damage and visual field loss. Only glaucoma patients with advanced binocular visual field loss were included (stages II-IV according to the Aulhorn classification [28]). Mean time since first glaucoma diagnosis was 12.3 years ($\pm 7.47$ years).

Visual fields were assessed by means of binocular semi-automated $90°$ kinetic perimetry (SKP) obtained with the OCTOPUS 101 Perimeter (background luminance 10 cd/m$^2$, angular velocity $3°$/s, Fa. HAAG-STREIT, Koeniz, Switzerland).

We used the binocular kinetic visual field because it provides more realistic information about the visual field which is needed in daily activities [29].

The research study was approved by the Institutional Review Board of the University of Tübingen (Germany) and was performed according to the Declaration of Helsinki. Following verbal and written explanation of the experimental protocol, all subjects gave their written consent with the option of withdrawing from the study at any time. Clinical Trial Registration http://www.clinicaltrials.gov. Unique identifiers: NCT01372319, NCT01372332.

### Supermarket Search Task

The experiment was performed in a drugstore in the city center of Tübingen. Twenty different special-offer products were chosen randomly among other products in two racks (one right-hand and one left-hand rack) along a corridor of 7.5 m length and 1.3 m width (Figure 1). Furthermore, each of these racks included 6 shelves at different heights as presented in Figure 1. The products of interest varied in color, shape, and size and were marked by orange tags (Figure 1). The products were distributed homogeneously over height and width of both shelves.

The subjects were asked to collect all marked products in both shelves as quickly as possible by walking through the corridor only once. Hence, the main task was to locate the orange tags and collect the above standing product. Eye movements were recorded by means of a Dikablis mobile eye tracker (Ergoneers Inc., Manching, Germany). The eye-tracking device is a light-weighted, head-mounted monocular unit, which does not interfere with glasses.

The supermarket search task was repeated four times by each participant. In order to record the eye movements of subjects during the search task, an eye tracker was worn during the first run. The remaining three runs were performed without eye-tracking equipment due to a very tight time schedule. More specifically, the experiments were conducted in the mornings between 7 and 9 a.m. (i.e., before the supermarket opened). During the last three runs of a subject, the eye-tracking device was calibrated for the next subject. For each trial, the time, the item description, the number of collected items, and the number of wrongly collected items were documented.

### Performance Assessment

The performance of subjects was assessed by means of the following parameters: (i) average number of correctly collected items $N_c$ over all runs, (ii) average performance time $t$ over all runs, and (iii) average time per correctly collected item $T_C = t/N_C$.

**Passing criterion.** The $T_C$ values followed a normal distribution with (mean) $\mu = 3.28$ s and (SD) $\sigma = 0.88$ s in the control group (Shapiro-Wilk test). Based on performance of the control subjects, the threshold value of $T_C$ for failing the task was chosen as $T_C$-failed = $\mu + 3\sigma$. More specifically, $T_C$-failed = 5.92 s, i.e., a subject who needed longer than 5.92 seconds per correctly collected item failed the task.

In order to identify parameters associated with successful task performance, $N_C$, $t$ and $T_C$ were compared across glaucoma control subjects who passed (GCp), glaucoma patients who passed (GPp), and glaucoma patients who failed (GPf) the task by one-way ANOVA. Subsequent post-hoc comparisons were performed using the Tukey's HSD test. As multiple tests were carried out, the significance level was adjusted using a Bonferroni correction to an alpha-level of 0.05 for multiple comparisons. All data sets were tested for normality by the Shapiro-Wilk test; for non-normally distributed data, the Mann-Whitney U test and the Kruskal-Wallis

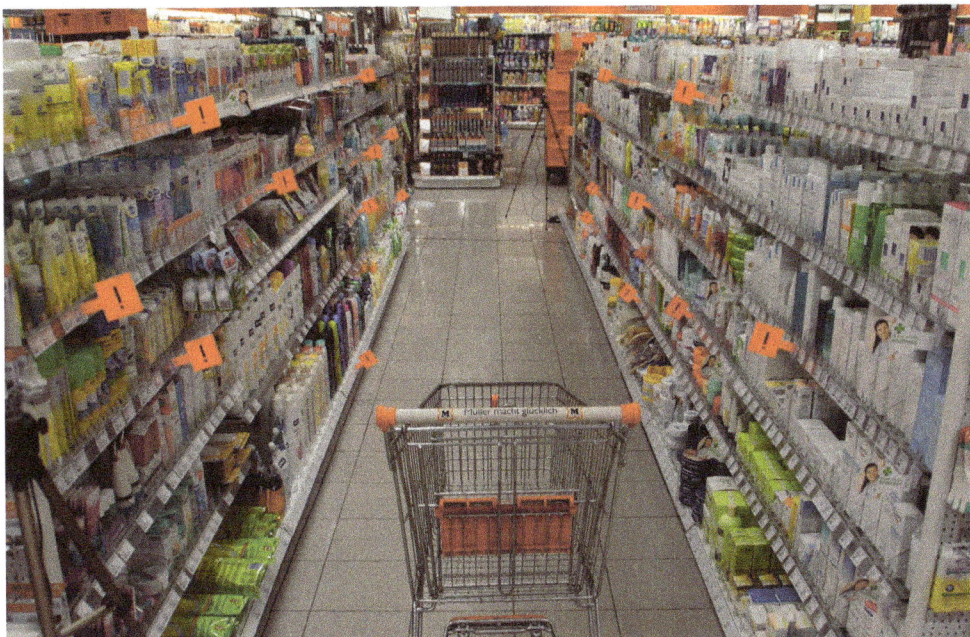

**Figure 1. The drug store corridor with all marked special-offer products (orange signs) on two racks (each containing six shelves).** Two cameras (marked by blue circles) at the beginning and the end of the corridor were used to record navigation of the subjects during the task.

test for multiple comparisons were used. In addition, dependencies between eye-movement-related parameters and performance-related parameters ($N_c$, t, and $T_c$) were also assessed using linear regression (Pearson Correlation Coefficient) in the patient group. Matlab R2013b was used for data analysis.

In order to investigate the effect of the visual field defect on task performance, the size of the binocular visual field defect was calculated from measurements obtained by means of binocular semi-automated 90° kinetic perimetry (SKP) as described above (see Table S1). Only the stimulus III/4e was used, since this is a functionally relevant target that is typically used to define driving fitness and legal blindness in Germany.

## Analysis of Eye Movement Data

Eye movements were recorded using the D-Lab software tool (Ergoneers Inc, Manching, Germany) at a frequency of 25 frames per second. The recorded data was analyzed using both D-Lab and self-developed algorithms. For the detection of fixation clusters and saccades from raw eye-tracking data we applied a Bayesian learning algorithm [30–32]. In order to quantify the frequency and duration of saccades towards the area of visual field defect or towards the peripheral visual field, we superimposed the area of visual field defect as Area Of Interest (AOI) for each participant. These models were transferred into D-Lab to analyze the viewing behavior of participants towards such regions in terms of glance proportion and frequency. We assessed the following gaze-related parameters:

**Horizontal Gaze Activity (HGA).** In order to investigate the horizontal exploration ability of a subject, we assessed the horizontal standard deviation of the pupil, which was expressed as Horizontal Gaze Activity (HGA).

**Glance Proportion in percentage (PGP).** PGP describes the percentage of glance duration in a defined AOI during a given time interval. We computed the PGP for the area of visual field defect (PGP-VFD), for the visual field area beyond 30° (PGP-30c), and for the visual field area beyond 60° (PGP-60c).

Glance Frequency (GF). GF describes the average number of glances towards a defined AOI during the time unit of one second. Similar to PGP, we computed the GF for the area of visual field defect (GF-VFD), the visual field area beyond 30° (GF-30c), and the visual field area beyond 60° (GF-60c).

## Results

### Task performance

For each subject subgroup, Figure 2 presents (a) the average number of correctly collected items $N_C$, (b) the average time t to complete the task, and (c) the average time per correctly collected item $T_C$.

**Number of correctly collected items ($N_C$).** None of the subjects was able to collect all 20 items successfully (Figure 2a). However, contrary to our expectation, the general task performance regarding Nc was good, e.g., the worst performer collected 13 out of 20 items. Furthermore, we found no significant differences in the number of correctly collected items between the glaucoma patients and control subjects. For GPp, we found a strong negative correlation between $N_c$ and the size of the visual field defect (VFDsize) (r = 0.81), indicating that the number of correctly collected objects decreases with increasing size of the visual field defect.

The number of wrongly collected items was very small, there were overall only 7 wrongly collected items for all participants and all runs (three times one error, two times two errors), therefore no further analyses were performed.

**Average performance time (t).** Regarding the overall performance time, we found a highly significant difference between the glaucoma subgroups GCp, GPp, and GPf (p< 0.001, Table 1). GCp needed on average 55.94 s to complete the task, GPp 64.45 s, while GPf needed almost twice as long as GPp to complete the task. In summary, control subjects (GCp) and patients who passed the supermarket search task (GPp) needed

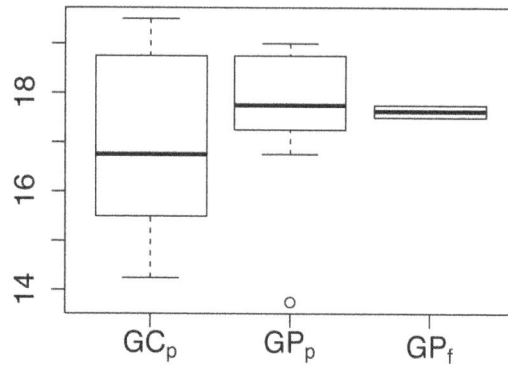

(a) Average number of correctly collected items (*Nc*)

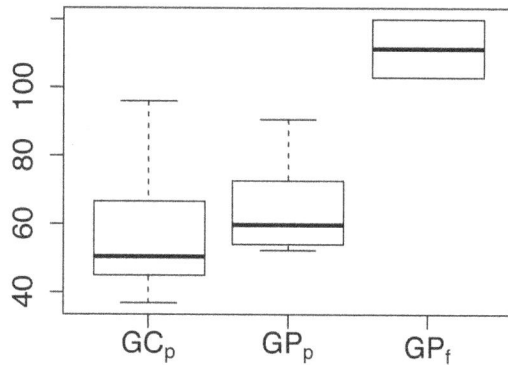

(b) Average time to complete the task (*t*) (sec)

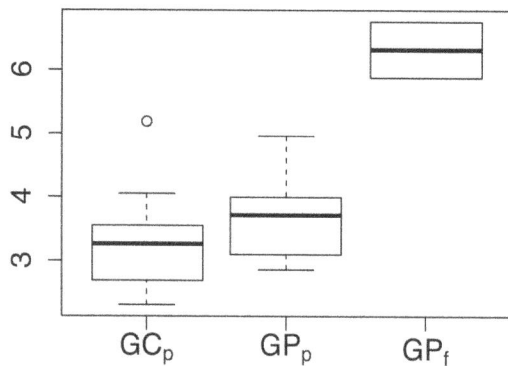

(c) Average time per correctly collected item (*Tc*) (sec)

**Figure 2. Value range for (a) the average number of correctly collected items over all runs, (b) the average time needed to complete the supermarket search task over all runs, and (c) the average time (over all runs) per correctly collected item.** The participant subgroups are marked by GCp/GPp (glaucoma controls/patients who passed), GPf (glaucoma patients who failed).

considerably less time to complete the trial than patients who failed the task (GPf).

**Average time per correctly collected object (T$_C$).** According to the passing threshold of $T_C = 5.92$ sec (see Section Methods) all control subjects completed the supermarket search task successfully and displayed significantly shorter t and Tc values than the patient group. The success rate for glaucoma patients was 80%. Since the parameter $T_c$ depends on $t$, we found

the same significant differences between subject subgroups as for $t$. More specifically, subjects who passed the task (GCp) needed significantly shorter time per collected item than subjects who failed the task (p<0.001, Table 1).

In summary, these results suggest that binocular glaucomatous visual field loss is mainly associated with longer search time. However, a subgroup of patients performed indistinguishably from conytol subjects, possibly by means of efficient gaze compensation.

**Table 1.** Performance and gaze-related parameters for glaucoma control subjects who passed (GCp), glaucoma patients who passed (GPp), and glaucoma patients who failed the task (GPf).

| | $GC_p$ - $GP_p$ - $GP_f$ |
|---|---|
| $N_c$ | n. s. |
| T | *** |
| $T_c$ | *** |
| HGA | n. s. |
| PGP - $60^c$ | n. s. |
| PGP - $30^c$ | n. s. |
| PGP – VFD | n. s. |
| GF - $60^c$ | n. s. |
| GF - $30^c$ | n. s. |
| GF – VFD | * |

Statistical comparisons were made between the groups.
*$p<0.05$; ***$p<0.001$, n.s: indicates non-significant comparisons.

## Gaze-related parameters

**Horizontal Gaze Activity (HGA).** Contrary to our expectations, no difference was found in the horizontal gaze activity between the participant subgroups (see Table 1).

Furthermore, no significant relationship was found between HGA and Nc or the average time per correctly collected object (Tc) in any of the subject subgroups. Thus, it seems that HGA does not influence task performance.

**Proportion of Glances in Percent (PGP).** There was no significant difference between the subject subgroups regarding the proportion of glances beyond the 30° visual field (PGP-30c) and towards the visual field defect (PGP-VFD), see Table 1.

Furthermore, we found a strong positive relationship between Nc and the PGP towards the VFD in GPp ($r = 0.77$), which indicates that patients who passed the task demonstrated more efficient exploration of the VFD area, i.e., the longer duration of glances towards the VFD enables the detection of more target objects.

**Glance Frequency (GF).** There was no significant difference between the subject subgroups in glance frequency (GF) beyond 30° (GF-30c) and beyond 60° (GF-60c).

A significant difference in GF towards the visual field defect area (GF-VFD) was found between GPp and GPf (Table 1). Glaucoma patients who passed (GPp) performed more glances towards their visual defect area than patients who failed (GPf), ($p<0.05$, Table 1).

## Discussion

We investigated the performance of patients with binocular glaucomatous visual field loss in comparison with healthy-sighted control subjects during a special-offer supermarket search task. Our study is novel, because visual search behavior of patients with binocular visual field loss during real-life tasks has not been quantified by means of eye-tracking equipment so far. With a pass rate of 80%, a considerable number of patients with glaucoma managed to pass the test despite their binocular visual field loss. This finding is in accordance with prior studies [3,19] reporting the performance of patients with glaucomatous visual field defects in driving tasks.

With regard to the number of correctly collected items, no significant differences were found between the subject subgroups. Thus, when time is not restricted, patients with glaucomatous visual field loss perform indistinguishably from a control group. However, in many real-life scenarios there is time pressure. Therefore, we defined a time-related passing criterion based on the performance of normal subjects. According to this criterion, the control group needed on average a shorter time per correctly collected item (Tc) than the patient group. Although binocular glaucomatous visual field defects is in general associated with longer search time, a subgroup of patients completed the task within the defined time period (GPp), while patients who failed (GPf) needed considerably longer time to complete the task. On the other hand, glaucoma patients who passed the test (GPp) displayed more efficient exploration of the visual field defect area. Therefore, they managed to locate the target object faster than glaucoma subjects who failed. One might expect that increased scanning activity could be time-demanding and lead to longer task duration. However, our findings suggest that systematic visual search towards the areas, which are considered to be "problematic" in glaucoma patients, namely the areas of the VFD, can be time-effective. In contrast, failure to systematically scan those areas leads to disorganised scan patterns that prove to be time-consuming and ineffective in everyday tasks.

Furthermore, glaucoma patients who passed the task (GPp) showed a gaze bias towards their visual defect area, as indicated by the higher glance frequency (GF) towards the VFD. By directing their gaze towards the area of visual field loss, patients manage to bring more visual elements into their seeing field and thus detect more target objects, which might be obstructed by the VFD. This result is in accordance with our recent on-road study, where we also found increased glances towards the VFD area in patients with binocular visual field loss who passed a driving test [19].

There is limited literature on gaze patterns of patients with glaucomatous visual field loss during real-life tasks. In accordance with our results, Crabb et al. [33] have also reported that patients with bilateral glaucomatous visual field loss made more saccades than a control group when viewing driving scenes during a hazard perception test, in an attempt to compensate for their restricted field of view [33]. These authors also suggested that a glaucomatous visual field defect may cause detection deficits, which could be compensated by gaze movements, since there were revealing cases where patients failed to see a hazard in relation to their binocular visual field defect. Similar detection deficits and longer reaction times in patients with mild to severe glaucoma were also reported in the driving simulator study conducted by Vega et al. [34] in 2013. These authors did not find compensatory visual search patterns for patients [34]. However, gaze compensation was possibly less required in the above study, because the driving simulation did not include other traffic [34]. Despite this, only nine out of 23 participants had binocular field loss.

Vargas-Martin and Peli [35] reported in 2006 that patients with severe VFD due to retinitis pigmentosa (RP) exhibited narrower horizontal eye-position dispersions than normal subjects during walking in real environments, due to the absence of peripheral visual stimulation and the simultaneous use of head movements [35]. In our study, the horizontal extent of exploratory eye movements did not differ between the participant subgroups, as indicated by similar HGA values, which was calculated from the horizontal standard deviation of the pupil. A possible explanation for differences found in [35] is that the above study included RP patients with more severe visual field loss (less than 20° total extent of horizontal and vertical visual field in both eyes). In addition, visual field defects in RP are due to damage of the photoreceptors and the retinal pigment epithelium, while glaucoma is associated with a lesion of the retinal ganglion cells. Hence, the site of lesion in the visual pathway and the different adaptation state (nyctalopia in RP) may lead to distinct exploratory patterns. Furthermore, the above study included a walking route with segments in unfamiliar indoor environments and city streets [35]. In contrast, our participants had to detect and collect specific items, which were placed in expected spatial locations, namely the two supermarket racks. Therefore they could focus on the specific task and their scanning strategy was therefore probably more organized and target-oriented due to possible top-down influences. Compensation was achieved by means of more frequent and longer glances towards the VFD and towards the peripheral visual field. This finding supports the hypothesis presented by Luo et al. [36], who indeed stressed the importance of the top-down mechanism influence on eye-movement control. They also found very frequent beyond-VF saccades in people with tunnel vision, which could not be triggered by instantaneous visual salience [36]. In addition, the nature of the present everyday task would indeed point towards implementation of top-down information based on prior knowledge and intention, in order to provide guidance to eye movements [37]. We therefore agree with the study of Luo et al. [36] that scanning of non-seeing areas may not necessarily lead to instant, accurate detection of the target. However, this approach increases the chances of bringing the desired targets into the seeing field, in order to guide saccades based on bottom-up saliency.

On the other hand, Wiecek et al. 2012 [38] found that patients with peripheral visual field loss (PVFL) due to glaucoma or optic nerve drusen showed a biased directional distribution that was not directly related to the locus of vision loss, challenging feed-forward models of eye movement control. In addition, total search duration, fixation duration, saccade size, and number of saccades showed no difference between PVFL patients and normal subjects. This inconsistency with our results may be attributed to the difference in stimuli (e.g., $26° \times 11°$ images versus natural environment), design of the experiment (use of a chin rest versus free navigation) and monocular versus binocular visual search [38]. Finally, the authors have explained that their visual search task was specifically designed to minimize the role of top-down factors and observers frequently made eye movements into areas of vision loss, although this finding did not reach statistical significance [38].

Task duration in the current experiment was longer in glaucoma patients than in controls, which confirms prior work by Smith et al. [18], suggesting slower performance for glaucoma patients compared to control subjects during visual search tasks. Prior studies by Cornelissen et al. (2005) [39] and Coeckelbergh et al. 2002 [40] on the impact of central and peripheral visual field defects in visual search tasks also reported an increase in search times in patients compared to controls and an additional increase in the number of errors with increasing visual field deficits. Our results are in accordance with these findings, since we also found that the number of correctly collected objects (Nc) decreases with an increase in the glaucomatous visual field defect size.

In summary, gaze pattern analysis revealed that successful task performance of glaucoma patients is associated with longer and frequent glancing towards the VFD.

## Limitations of the study

The above findings should be interpreted in the light of some study limitations. Despite the considerable total number of participants (20 subjects), the number of participants in the subgroups was relatively small. Thus, further studies involving a larger number of subjects have to be conducted. An important issue that will be investigated in our future work concerns the role of head movements during natural visual search tasks. From driving studies there is evidence that patients with binocular VFD compensate by head movements, especially when the task requires exploration of a wide horizontal FOV [19]. In the present task, no differences were found in HGA, which expresses the horizontal standard deviation of the pupil and is an indirect measure of eye movement (saccadic) amplitudes. This points towards the use of head movements in order to reach eccentric locations of the field of view. Therefore, in future studies we will integrate head tracking devices to study the contribution of head movements in natural search tasks. In addition, one should address the motor component of the present task, when trying to interpret trial duration. Subjects were required to identify the item location, then collect the item, and finally move towards the end of the corridor. Although there is no reason to assume any motor differences between groups, the trial duration included the visual search plus the motor response. Finally, some of the participants had some degree of macular sparing, which might affect gaze movement strategies. However, due to the free navigation of participants in a natural environment and the need to locate targets in the far periphery, immediate visual input from the area of macular sparing is unlikely, as also shown by the gaze bias towards the area of the VFD.

## Conclusion

Binocular glaucomatous visual field loss may critically interfere with quality of life. In a special-offer supermarket search task we investigated the performance of ten patients with glaucoma and ten healthy-sighted, age- and gender-related control subjects. 80% of the patients completed the task successfully despite their visual impairment. We found that binocular glaucomatous visual field loss was on average associated with longer search time. However, analysis of eye-tracking data revealed that patients who are able to compensate for their visual field defect employ frequent glancing towards the area of the visual field defect.

## Supporting Information

**Table S1   Demographic data and visual fields of glaucoma patients who participated in the study.** t represents the time since first diagnosis of glaucoma.

## Acknowledgments

The authors would like to thank Müller Ltd. & Co. KG for enabling this study. Clinical Trial Registration http://www.clinicaltrials.gov. Unique identifiers: NCT01372319, NCT01372332.

## Author Contributions

Conceived and designed the experiments: US EP KA MH. Performed the experiments: KS EK KA MH US. Analyzed the data: KS EK. Contributed reagents/materials/analysis tools: KS EK. Contributed to the writing of the manuscript: KS EK WR US EP.

# References

1. Friedman D, Freeman E, Munoz B, Jampel HD, West SK (2007) Glaucoma and Mobility Performance: The Salisbury Eye Evaluation Project. Ophthalmology 114(12): 2232–2237.

2. Haymes SA, LeBlanc RP, Nicolela MT, Chiasson LA, Chauhan BC (2007) Risk of falls and motor vehicle collisions in glaucoma. Investigative Ophthalmology & Visual Science 48(3): 1149–1155.

3. Haymes S, LeBlanc R, Nicolela M, Chiasson L, Chauhan B (2008) Glaucoma and on-road driving performance. Investigative Ophthalmology & Visual Science 49(7): 3035–3041.

4. Johnson CA, Keltner JL (1983) Incidence of visual field loss in 20,000 eyes and its relationship to driving performance. Archives of Ophthalmology 101(3): 371–375.

5. Nelson P, Aspinall P, O'Brien C (1999) Patients' perception of visual impairment in glaucoma: a pilot study. Br J Ophthalmol 83: 546–552.

6. Ramulu PY (2009) Glaucoma and disability: which tasks are affected, and at what stage of disease? Current Opinion in Ophthalmology 20(2): 92–98.

7. Szlyk J, Mahler CL, Seiple W, Edward DP, Wilensky JT (2005). Driving performance of glaucoma patients correlates with peripheral visual field loss. Journal of Glaucoma 14(2): 145–150.

8. Viswanathan AC, McNaught AI, Poinoosawmy D, Fontana L, Crabb DP, et al. (1999). Severity and stability of glaucoma: patient perception compared with objective measurement. Archives of Ophthalmology 117(4): 450–454.

9. Quigley H, Broman A (2006) The number of people with glaucoma worldwide in 2010 and 2020. British Journal of Ophthalmology 90(3): 262–267.

10. Bechetoille A, Arnould B, Bron A, Baudouin C, Renard JP, et al. (2008) Measurement of health-related quality of life with glaucoma: validation of the Glau-QoL© 36-item questionnaire. Acta Ophthalmol 86(1): 71–80.

11. Jampel H, Friedman D, Quigley H, Miller R (2002) Correlation of the binocular visual field with patient assessment of vision. Investigative Ophthalmology & Vision Science 43(4): 1059–1067.

12. McGwin GJ, Mays A, Joiner W, DeCarlo DK, Hall TA, et al. (2005) Visual field defects and the risk of motor vehicle collisons among patients with glaucoma. Investigative Ophthalmology & Visual Science 46(12): 4437–4441.

13. McGwin GJ, Mays A, Joiner W, DeCarlo DK, McNeal S, et al. (2004). Is glaucoma associated with motor vehicle collision involvement and driving avoidance? Investigative Ophthalmology & Visual Science 45(11): 3934–3939.

14. Noe G, Ferraro J, Lamoureux E, Rait J, Keeffe J (2003) Associations between glaucomatous visual field loss and participation in activities of daily living. Clin Experiment Ophthalmol 31(6): 482–486.

15. Owsley C, Ball K, McGwin G, Sloane ME, Roenker DL, et al. (1998) Visual processing impairment and risk of motor vehicle crash among older adults. JAMA: The Journal of the American Medical Association 279(14): 1083–1088.

16. Spaeth G, Walt J, Keener J (2006) Evaluation of quality of life for patients with glaucoma. Am J Ophthalmol 141(1): 3–14.

17. Warrian K, Spaeth GL, Lankaranian D, Lopes J, Steinmann W (2009) The effect of personality on measures of quality of life related to vision in glaucoma patients. Br J Ophthalmol 93(3): 310–315.

18. Smith N, Crabb DP, Garway-Heath DF (2011) An exploratory study of visual search performance in glaucoma. Ophthalmic and Physiological Optics 31(3): 225–232.

19. Kasneci E, Sippel K, Aehling K, Heister M, Rosenstiel W, et al. (2014) Driving with Binocular Visual Field Loss? A Study on a Supervised On-road Parcours with Simultaneous Eye and Head Tracking, PLoS ONE 9(2): e87470. doi:10.1371/journal.pone.0087470.

20. Ramulu P, West S, Munoz B, Jampel H, Friedman D (2009). Driving cessation and driving limitation in glaucoma: the Salisbury Eye Evaluation Project. Ophthalmology 116(10): 1846–1853.

21. Ramulu P, West S, Munoz B, Jampel H, Friedman D (2009) Glaucoma and reading speed: the Salisbury Eye Evaluation Project. Arch Ophthalmol 127(1): 82–87.

22. Wood JM, Black AA, Lacherez P, Mallon K, Thomas R, et al. (2014) On-road Driving Performance in Older Adults with Glaucoma. Abstract Number 3537, ARVO 2014.

23. Schuett S, Kentridge RW, Zihl J, Heywood CA (2009) Adaptation of eye movements to simulated hemianopia in reading and visual exploration: Transfer or specificity? Neuropsychologia 47(7): 1712–1720.

24. Degeratu AM, Rangaswamy A, Wu J (2000) Consumer choice behavior in online and traditional supermarkets: The effects of brand name, price, and other search attributes. International Journal of Research in Marketing 17(1): 55–78.

25. Tonkin C, Duchowski AT, Kahue J, Schiffgens P, Rischner F (2011) Eye tracking over small and large shopping displays. In Proceedings of the 1st International Workshop on Pervasive Eye Tracking & Mobile Eye-Based Interaction. ACM. 49–52.

26. Reutskaja E, Nagel R, Camerer CF, Rangel A (2011) Search dynamics in consumer choice under time pressure: An eye-tracking study. The American Economic Review 101(2): 900–926.

27. Clement J, Kristensen T, Grønhaug K (2013) Understanding consumers' in-store visual perception: The influence of package design features on visual attention. Journal of Retailing and Consumer Services 20(2): 234–239.

28. Aulhorn E, Karmeyer H (1977) Frequency distribution in early glaucomatous visual field defects. Doc Ophtamol Proc Ser. 14: 75–83.

29. Esterman B (1982) Functional scoring of the binocular field. Ophthalmology 89(11): 1226–1234.

30. Tafaj E, Kasneci G, Rosenstiel W, Bogdan M (2012) Bayesian online clustering of eye movement data. In: Proceedings of the Symposium on Eye Tracking Research and Applications. ETRA '12. ACM, New York, NY, USA, 285–288. DOI = 10.1145/2168556.2168617http://doi.acm.org/10.1145/2168556.2168617.

31. Tafaj E, Kübler TC, Kasneci G, Rosenstiel W, Bogdan M (2013) Online Classification of Eye Tracking Data for Automated Analysis of Traffic Hazard Perception, Artificial Neural Networks and Machine Learning – ICANN 2013. Springer Berlin Heidelberg, 2013. 442–450.

32. Kasneci E, Kasneci G, Kübler T, Rosenstiel W (2014) The Applicability of Probabilistic Methods to the Online Recognition of Fixations and Saccades in Dynamic Scenes. In: Proceedings of the Symposium on Eye Tracking Research and Application, ETRA '14. ACM, New York, NY, USA, 323–326.

33. Crabb DP, Smith ND, Rauscher FG, Chisholm CM, Barbur JL, et al. (2010) Exploring Eye Movements in Patients with Glaucoma When Viewing a Driving Scene. PLoS ONE 5(3): e9710. doi:10.1371/journal.pone.0009710.

34. Vega RP, van Leeuwen PM, Vélez ER, Lemij HG, de Winter JC (2013) Obstacle avoidance, visual detection performance, and eye-scanning behavior of glaucoma patients in a driving simulator: A preliminary study. PloS one, 8(10), e77294.

35. Vargas-Martín F, Peli E (2006) Eye movements of patients with tunnel vision while walking. Investigative Ophthalmology & Visual Science 47(12): 5295–5302.

36. Luo A, Parra L, Sajda P (2009) We find before we look: Neural signatures of target detection preceding saccades during visual search. Journal of Vision 9(8): 1207–1207.

37. Rothkopf CA, Ballard DH, Hayhoe MM (2007) Task and context determine where you look. Journal of Vision 7(14): 16. doi:10.1167/7.14.16.

38. Wiecek E, Pasquale LR, Fiser J, Dakin S, Bex PJ (2012) Effects of peripheral visual field loss on eye movements during visual search. Frontiers in Psychology 3: 472. doi: 10.3389/fpsyg.2012.00472.

39. Cornelissen FW, Bruin KJ, Kooijman AC (2005) The influence of artificial scotomas on eye movements during visual search. Optom. Vis. Sci 82(1): 27–35.

40. Coeckelbergh TRM, Cornelissen FW, Brouwer WH, Kooijman AC (2002) The effect of visual field defects on eye movements and practical fitness to drive. Vision Research 42(5): 669–677.

# 22

# Anatomic vs. Acquired Image Frame Discordance in Spectral Domain Optical Coherence Tomography Minimum Rim Measurements

**Lin He**[1][9], **Ruojin Ren**[1][9], **Hongli Yang**[1,2], **Christy Hardin**[1], **Luke Reyes**[1], **Juan Reynaud**[1,2], **Stuart K. Gardiner**[2], **Brad Fortune**[2], **Shaban Demirel**[2], **Claude F. Burgoyne**[1,2]*

**1** Optic Nerve Head Research Laboratory, Legacy Health, Portland, Oregon, United States of America, **2** Discoveries in Sight Research Laboratories of the Devers Eye Institute, Legacy Health, Portland, Oregon, United States of America

## Abstract

***Purpose:*** To quantify the effects of using the fovea to Bruch's membrane opening (FoBMO) axis as the nasal-temporal midline for 30° sectoral (clock-hour) spectral domain optical coherence tomography (SDOCT) optic nerve head (ONH) minimum rim width (MRW) and area (MRA) calculations.

***Methods:*** The internal limiting membrane and BMO were delineated within 24 radial ONH B-scans in 222 eyes of 222 participants with ocular hypertension and glaucoma. For each eye the fovea was marked within the infrared reflectance image, the FoBMO angle ($\theta$) relative to the acquired image frame (AIF) horizontal was calculated, the ONH was divided into 30° sectors using a FoBMO or AIF nasal/temporal axis, and SDOCT MRW and MRA were quantified within each FoBMO vs. AIF sector. For each sector, focal rim loss was calculated as the MRW and MRA gradients (i.e. the difference between the value for that sector and the one clockwise to it divided by 30°). Sectoral FoBMO vs. AIF discordance was calculated as the difference between the FoBMO and AIF values for each sector. Generalized estimating equations were used to predict the eyes and sectors of maximum FoBMO vs. AIF discordance.

***Results:*** The mean FoBMO angle was $-6.6 \pm 4.2°$ (range: $-17°$ to $+7°$). FoBMO vs. AIF discordance in sectoral mean MRW and MRA was significant for 7 of 12 and 6 of 12 sectors, respectively ($p < 0.05$, Wilcoxon test, Bonferroni correction). Eye-specific, FoBMO vs. AIF sectoral discordance was predicted by sectoral rim gradient ($p < 0.001$) and FoBMO angle ($p < 0.001$) and achieved maximum values of 83% for MRW and 101% for MRA.

***Conclusions:*** Using the FoBMO axis as the nasal-temporal axis to regionalize the ONH rather than a line parallel to the AIF horizontal axis significantly influences clock-hour SDOCT rim values. This effect is greatest in eyes with large FoBMO angles and sectors with focal rim loss.

**Editor:** Jost B. Jonas, Medical Faculty Mannheim of the University of Heidelberg, Germany

**Funding:** National Institutes of Health Grants R01-EY021281 (CFB) and R01-EY019674 (SD), Legacy Good Samaritan Foundation, unrestricted research support from Heidelberg Engineering, the Alcon Research Institute and the Sears Medical Trust. The funders had no role in study design, data collection and analysis, decision to publish, or preparation of the manuscript.

**Competing Interests:** The authors have declared that no competing interests exist.

* E-mail: cfburgoyne@deverseye.org

9 These authors contributed equally to this work.

## Introduction

Since the introduction of the concept of the 'cup/disc ratio' by Armaly in the 1960s [1], clinical disc examination has required the identification of the outer and inner borders of the neuroretinal rim, (the optic disc margin and optic disc cup, respectively). The amount of rim tissue is then estimated within the apparent plane of the disc margin as either the rim width (expressed in mm) or as the ratio of the size of the cup to the size of the disc (expressed as a cup/disc ratio using either diameter or area measurements) [1] or as rim area (expressed in mm²) [2,3]. Rim measurements are regionalized relative to a nasal temporal axis that is assumed to be parallel to the horizontal axis of the acquired image frame (AIF), whether the image frame is acquired through fundus imaging or

slit lamp biomicroscopy, without regard to the anatomic relationship between the optic nerve head (ONH) and the fovea.

Recent spectral domain optical coherence tomography (SDOCT) findings call into question the current concepts of the clinical disc margin, rim quantification and its regionalization from both anatomic [4] and geometric [5–8] perspectives. Based on these findings, and previous work by other groups on retinal anatomy and its relationship to structure-function correlation [9–14], we have argued for making minimum rim width (MRW) and area (MRA) measurements relative to SDOCT Bruch's Membrane Opening (BMO) [8,15–17] and linking ONH neuroretinal rim as well as peripapillary and macular retinal nerve fiber layer (RNFL) regionalization to the axis between the centroid of BMO

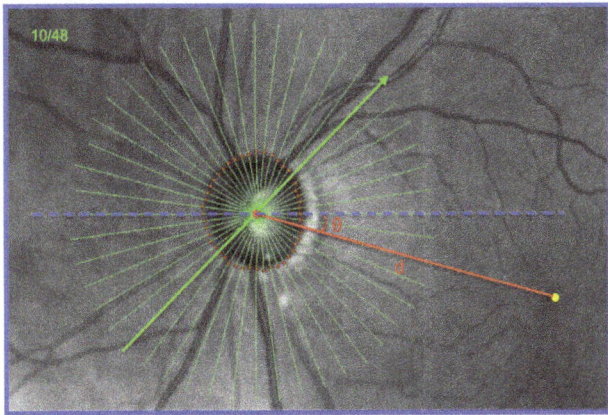

**Figure 1. Identification of the fovea-to-BMO centroid (FoBMO) axis (red) relative to the Acquired Image Frame (AIF- blue outline) horizontal axis (dashed blue line), the FoBMO angle (θ) and the FoBMO distance (d) on the infrared (IR) fundus image of a representative study eye (DIS368).** In each study eye, the FoBMO axis, the FoBMO angle and the FoBMO distance were digitally generated relative to the SDOCT ONH data set through the following steps. 1) The fovea (yellow dot) was digitally identified on the IR image by one clinician (CFB). 2) The delineated BMO points from 24 of the 48 acquired SDOCT B-scans were projected onto the IR image plane allowing the geometric center (BMO centroid - large red dot) to be located relative to the acquired SDOCT data. 3) The FoBMO axis was defined to be the line (red) connecting the fovea and BMO centroid. 4) The FoBMO angle (θ) was defined to be the angle between the FoBMO axis and the AIF horizontal axis (blue dashed line). The FoBMO distance (d) was defined to be the distance between the BMO centroid and the assigned fovea. The FoBMO angle is −16° and the FoBMO distance is 4.3 mm in this eye (see Figure 4).

and the fovea, which we term the foveal-BMO or FoBMO axis (Figure 1) [18].

In clinical fundus images, the fovea is located below the level of the ONH (relative to the horizontal axis of the AIF) in most individuals (Figure 1). In a series of previous studies, the mean angle between the fovea and the center of the ONH was most commonly −6 to −7° (the fovea being 6–7° below, causing the blind spot to be below the horizontal midline during functional testing), with a range between −17° (below) and +7° (above) (reviewed in [18]). The position of these two structures relative to the AIF may may by as much as 6.4±3.8° within images of the same eye obtained on the same imaging day due to cyclotorsion and head tilt [14]. Their position also varies considerably between subjects due to differences in retinal anatomy. However, because the anatomic path of the RNFL axon bundles between the fovea and the ONH is organized relative to the FoBMO axis [9,19,20], it is an anatomically consistent landmark for the regionalization of the ONH and retinal tissues in all human eyes.

Current clinical examination, image acquisition and data analysis algorithms assume that neuroretinal rim width and area in a given sector refer to approximately the same anatomic location in all human eyes. However, this assumption is only true when the ONH of each individual eye is regionalized using the FoBMO axis as the Nasal/Temporal horizontal midline (Figures 1 and 2). Within an individual eye, as the FoBMO angle increases relative to the AIF horizontal axis, the anatomic discordance (the difference in the anatomic location being measured) of an individual sector using AIF vs. FoBMO regionalization may be large (Figure 2). Because AIF sector positions can refer to measurements from different anatomic locations in different eyes,

artificially large inter-individual differences in sectoral neuroretinal rim width and area in normative databases may be introduced by AIF regionalization. As a result, the limits of normal variation in these measurements are likely increased, which may decrease their diagnostic accuracy.

One of the hallmarks of glaucomatous neuroretinal rim loss is that it can be focal or sectoral in character, leading to sectoral rim thickness changes within a damaged eye that are more abrupt than sectoral rim thickness variation within normal ONHs [21]. We propose the term sectoral rim gradient to refer to the magnitude of focal rim loss calculated as the difference in rim anatomy between a sector and its neighboring sectors within an individual eye. To quantify this phenomenon by sector, we introduce the parameters *minimum rim width gradient* and *minimum rim area gradient* which are related to but different from previously described strategies for quantifying retinal nerve fiber layer thickness RNFLT [22,23] and visual field sensitivity gradients [24].

The purpose of the present study was to quantify the eye-specific effects of using FoBMO versus AIF regionalization of SDOCT ONH neuroretinal rim data from 222 eyes of 222 participants with high-risk ocular hypertension and glaucoma enrolled in the Portland Progression Project (P3 study). Our hypothesis was that a combination of FoBMO angle and rim gradient would predict the sectors (and eyes) with greatest FoBMO vs. AIF rim discordance. Our data suggest that the frequency and magnitude of FoBMO vs. AIF sectoral SDOCT MRW and MRA discordance are substantial and greatest within sectors that display elevated rim gradients (i.e. focal rim loss) from eyes with the largest FoBMO axis.

## Methods

All data were obtained from an ongoing longitudinal study, the Portland Progression Project (P3 study) [25]. The P3 study, funded by the National Institutes of Health, is an ongoing longitudinal study of the course and risk factors for glaucomatous progression. Participants with high-risk ocular hypertension and glaucoma (defined below) have been recruited prospectively from the Devers Eye Institute, or other ophthalmic practices in the Portland, OR metropolitan area as previously described [26,27]. At the time of recruitment, all participants were fully informed of the potential risks and benefits of the study and provided their voluntary written consent. All P3 study procedures follow the tenets of the Declaration of Helsinki, are in accordance with the Health Insurance Portability and Accountability Act and were approved by the Institutional Review Board at Legacy Health.

At study entry, participants either had early glaucoma with visual field loss less severe than −6 decibels (dB) for mean deviation (MD) or ocular hypertension (untreated IOP greater than 22 mm Hg) plus one or more risk factors for glaucoma as determined by their clinician. Risk factors for ocular hypertension included: age >70, systemic hypertension, migraine, diet-controlled diabetes, peripheral vasospasm, African ancestry, self-reported family history of glaucoma and suspicious optic nerve head appearance (cup-disc ratio asymmetry >0.2, neuroretinal rim notching or narrowing or disc hemorrhage). All participants also met the following criteria for both eyes: best corrected visual acuity of 20/40 or better and spectacle refraction < ±5.00-D sphere and < ±2.00-D cylinder [26,27]. Potential participants were excluded if they had any other previous or current ocular or neurologic disease likely to affect the visual field and previous ocular surgery (except uncomplicated cataract surgery).

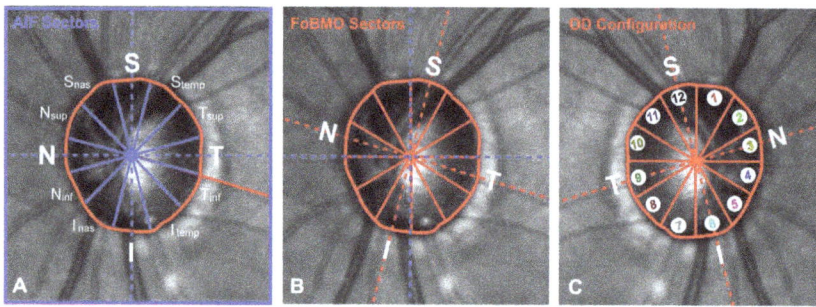

**Figure 2. AIF versus FoBMO 30° ONH regionalization of a representative study eye (DIS368).** This is the same eye (DIS368) as shown in Figure 1. (A) AIF (blue outline) regionalization with the naming convention for the twelve 30° sectors. (B) FoBMO regionalization of the same eye. Note that for this eye the actual anatomy being measured within the Superior (S) sector (as an example) is different within the AIF (A) compared to the FoBMO (B) regions. (C) FoBMO 30° sectors from the left eye shown in panel B, flipped into OD configuration and numbered with separate colors in the manner in which the data for all 222 eyes are presented in Figure 9.

## SDOCT Imaging

Standard Spectralis 870 nm SDOCT (Heidelberg Engineering GmBH, Heidelberg, Germany) was used to image both eyes of all 222 patients. Forty-eight radial B-scans were acquired over a 15° area. Each B-scan consisted of 768 A-scans and was the average of 9 repetitions. All acquired SDOCT datasets had a quality score above 15. If both eyes in each patient met the above inclusion criteria, the eye with the better SDOCT image quality was selected for further quantification.

## SDOCT Delineation and Parameterization

The internal limiting membrane (ILM), RNFL, and BMO were delineated in 24 of the 48 B-scans (every other B-scan) by technicians masked to the clinical status, refractive error and FoBMO angle of the eye. Two SDOCT neuroretinal rim parameters were defined and quantified as previously described [8,16]. BMO Minimum rim width (BMO-MRW) was defined to be the shortest distance from the BMO to the ILM within each B-scan (Figure 3A) [5–8,15,28]. The four sectoral measures within each 30° sector were averaged to give the sector measure for BMO-MRW. This measure occurs at an angle above the BMO plane (blue in Figure 3A and 3B, magnified view in Figure 3C). It should be noted that BMO-MRW is the minimum rim width measured from BMO, which is an anatomically consistent landmark in most SDOCT ONH B-scans. The actual minimum rim width at any location may occur deeper within the neural canal but cannot be consistently visualized[16].

Sectoral minimum rim areas (MRA, yellow areas in Figure 3B, 3C and 3D) [16] were calculated as the area of a trapezium at angle $\varphi$ above the BMO plane (shown for simplicity as $\varphi$ equaling $\theta$, though this may not be the case for a given sector). The height of this trapezium was set equal to the rim width at this angle, $RW_\varphi$. In the event that $\varphi = \theta$, $RW_\varphi = MRW_{sec}$. The long base of the trapezium (bounded by the BMO) equaled the BMO circumference within that sector, $\dfrac{2\pi r}{48}$, where r represents the distance from BMO centroid (red cross in Figure 3B) to the BMO point. The short base of the trapezium (bounded by the ILM) was calculated from these accounting for the inclination angle $\varphi$, giving length $\dfrac{2\pi r}{48} \times (r - RW_\varphi \times \cos\varphi)$. The area of each trapezium is calculated using the formula (Figure 3D):

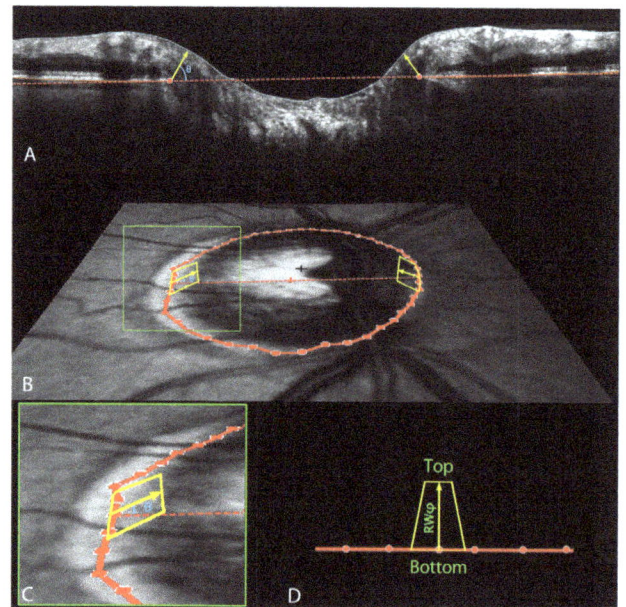

**Figure 3. SDOCT ONH neuroretinal rim parameterization.** A. Within each radial scan, Bruch's Membrane Opening (BMO) was delineated (red circles). The minimum rim width within that sector ($MRW_{sec}$) was calculated, by finding the shortest distance from the BMO to the ILM (yellow arrow in Panel A). Within each section, the measures were averaged across sectors to give the sector measure BMO-MRW. This measure occurs at angle $\theta$ above the BMO plane (blue in Panels A and B, zoomed-in view in Panel C). Sectoral minimum rim areas (yellow areas in panels B, C and D) were calculated as the area of a trapezium at angle $\varphi$ above the BMO plane (shown for simplicity as $\varphi$ equaling $\theta$, though this may not be the case for a given sector). The height of this trapezium was set equal to the rim width at this angle, $RW_\varphi$. In the event that $\varphi = \theta$, $RW_\varphi = MRW_{sec}$. The base of the trapezium (bounded by the BMO) equaled the BMO circumference within that sector, $\dfrac{2\pi r}{48}$, where $r$ represents the distance from BMO centroid (red cross in Panel B) to the BMO point. The top of the trapezium (bounded by the ILM) was calculated from these accounting for the inclination angle $\varphi$, giving length $\dfrac{2\pi r}{48} \times (r - RW_\varphi \times \cos\varphi)$. The area of each trapezium is calculated using the formula: $Area = \dfrac{Base_{ILM} + Base_{BMO}}{2} \times RW_\varphi$ (Panel D).

$$Area = \frac{Base_{ILM} + Base_{BMO}}{2} \times RW_\varphi$$
$$= \frac{2\pi r}{48} \times \frac{r - RW_\varphi \times \cos\varphi + r}{2} \times RW_\varphi$$

Both MRW and MRA were calculated on a 30° degree (12 clock-hours) sector basis.

## SDOCT ONH Regionalization

Separate AIF and FoBMO 30° regionalization of the SDOCT ONH rim data for each eye (Figure 2) were performed as follows.

## FoBMO Axis Identification (Figure 1)

For each eye in the study, one experienced clinician (CFB) identified the position of the fovea within the infrared Scanning Laser Ophthalmoscopy (SLO) reflectance image (IR image) acquired by the Spectralis as part of the SDOCT scan recording. The pixel closest to the point identified was recorded as the position of the fovea for that eye; 2) the delineated BMO points from 24 of the 48 acquired SDOCT B-scans were projected onto the IR image plane allowing the geometric center (BMO centroid) to be located; 3) the FoBMO axis was defined to be the line connecting the fovea and BMO centroid; 4) the FoBMO angle was defined to be the angle between the FoBMO axis and the AIF horizontal axis; and 5) the FoBMO distance was defined to be the distance between the BMO centroid and the assigned fovea.

## Intra- and Inter-delineator Reproducibility of FoBMO Axis Identification

Because the location of the fovea was retrospectively identified within an IR image rather than having been identified at the time of image acquisition on the basis of 3D information available from SDOCT scans (i.e. as the geometric center of the foveal pit [18]), intra- and inter-delineator reproducibility of this post hoc procedure was assessed as follows. Intra-delineator reproducibility was assessed by having the primary foveal delineator (CFB) separately identify the fovea in all 222 study eyes, 2 weeks after and masked to the first foveal delineation. Inter-delineator variability was assessed by having a second clinician (BF) separately delineate the fovea in all 222 study eyes. Intra-delineator variability was defined to be due to the difference between the primary delineator's two sets of foveal marks. Inter-delineator variability was defined to be due to the difference between the primary delineator's initial set of marks and the second delineator's marks.

**FoBMO vs. AIF 30° Sectoral SDOCT Rim Tissue Regionalization (Figure 2).** Using the primary delineator's initial set of foveal marks, the SDOCT ONH rim data (MRW and MRA) for each eye were separately calculated for each 30° sector using either the AIF horizontal or the FoBMO axis as the Nasal-Temporal axis.

## FoBMO vs. AIF 30° Sectoral SDOCT Rim Discordance (Figure 2)

The magnitude of FoBMO vs. AIF discordance in the MRW and MRA measurements for each sector of each eye was calculated as the percent of the average of the two volumes, using the following formulas:

$$MRW : \frac{MRW_{FoBMO} - MRW_{AIF}}{(MRW_{FoBMO} + MRW_{AIF})/2} \times 100\%$$

$$MRA : \frac{MRA_{FoBMO} - MRA_{AIF}}{(MRA_{FoBMO} + MRA_{AIF})/2} \times 100\%$$

## Data Analysis

Intra- and inter-delineator limits-of-agreement were determined by Bland-Altman analysis for both FoBMO axis and distance [29]. Wilcoxon non-parametric t-tests were used to compare the rim values for all 222 eyes aligned to the FoBMO axis against the 222 rim values aligned to AIF for each 30° sector. The significance of each of the 12 t-tests was corrected for multiple comparisons using the Bonferroni method. The mean, 95% CI and range of sectoral, eye-specific discordance between FoBMO and AIF rim data for the 222 eyes were calculated. Percentage of eyes with a minimum of 1, 2 or 3 sectors in which the FoBMO vs. AIF rim data differed by greater than ±20% were identified.

## Quantifying Sectoral Neuroretinal Rim Gradient

To quantify sectoral rim gradient using both MRW and MRA, rim data for all eyes were converted to right eye orientation. A *one-sided* sectoral gradient for MRW and MRA was calculated ($MRW_{FoBMO}'$ and $MRA_{FoBMO}'$) for each sector as the difference in rim width between the value for that sector and the one clockwise to it, then divided by 30° for each sector. Using the superior sector as an example, $MRW_S' = \frac{MRW_{Snas} - MRW_S}{30}$ ($\mu m/°$). All analyses were performed using FoBMO sectoral regionalization of each study eye.

## Predicting FoBMO vs. AIF Discordance

A generalized estimating equation (GEE) model was applied to predict the magnitude of sectoral FoBMO versus AIF discordance, using two hypothesized factors: FoBMO angle ($\theta$) and sectoral rim gradient while accounting for intra-eye inter-sector correlations. Interaction of the two factors was also taken account. The GEE model was implemented in RStudio (RStudio, Inc., Boston, MA) using the package 'geepack'. Models were constructed separately using the FoBMO axis angle ($\theta$), one-sided rim gradient ($MRW_{FoBMO}'$) and the interaction of FoBMO axis angle and one-sided rim gradient ($\theta \times MRW_{FoBMO}'$).

## Results

Table 1 summarizes the demographic information of the study participants. Two hundred and twenty-two eyes, of 222 individuals were included in the study, ranging from 33.7 to 89.8 years old (mean ± SD, 64.3±11.1). Mean IOP (± SD) on the day of imaging was 17.4±3.5 mmHg (range: 5.0 to 29.0 mmHg). Visual field MD (± SD) was −0.7±2.9 dB (range: −16.5 to 3.3 dB) while pattern standard deviation (PSD) (± SD) was 2.8±2.7 dB (range: 0.9 to 14.8 dB).

## Distribution of FoBMO axis angle and distance (Figure 4)

The FoBMO Axis Angle data in this report appeared within a previous publication [18] as part of a written communication.

**Table 1.** Demographic and glaucoma-related characteristics of the cohort.

| Parameter | Count/Mean ± SD |
|---|---|
| Number of eyes/participants | 222/222 |
| Eye: left/right (%) | 51.3/48.7 |
| Gender: M/F | 92/130 |
| Self-identified ethnicity (%): | |
|     Caucasian | 93.2 |
|     African descent | 2.7 |
|     Asian descent | 0.9 |
|     Hispanic descent | 0.9 |
|     Native American | 1.8 |
|     Others | 0.5 |
| Age (yrs) | 64.3±11.1 |
| Intraocular pressure (mmHg) | 17.4±3.5 |
| Mean deviation (dB) | −0.7±3.5 |
| Pattern standard deviation (dB) | 2.8±2.7 |
| Central corneal thickness (μm) | 557±40 |

Histograms of the FoBMO axis angle (A) and distance (B) data for all 222 eyes are presented in Figure 4. FoBMO angle and distance data were normally distributed by Shapiro-Wilk normality test (p = 0.291 and p = 0.294, respectively). The FoBMO angle ranged from −17° to 7° (mean ± SD, −6.6°±4.2°) and the FoBMO distance ranged from 3378 μm to 5269 μm (mean ± SD: 4330±428 μm). Twelve of the 222 eyes (5.4%) demonstrated a positive FoBMO axis angle (fovea above the ONH) and 210 of the 222 eyes (94.6%) demonstrated a negative FoBMO axis angle (fovea below the ONH). Forty nine eyes (22.1%) demonstrated a FoBMO angle more negative than −10°.

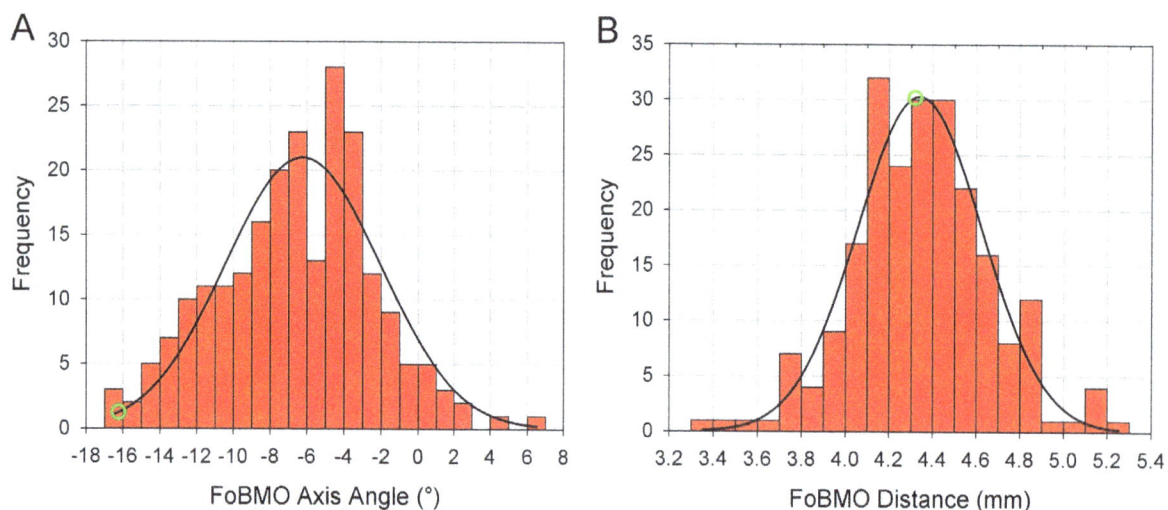

## FoBMO axis angle and distance intra and inter-delineator variability (Figure 5)

Bland-Altman plots of intra- and inter-delineator variability in FoBMO axis and distance are presented in Figure 5. FoBMO axis angle intra-delineator limits-of-agreement were −2.8° to 2.4°. FoBMO axis angle inter-delineator limits of agreement were −2.7° to 4.1° FoBMO distance intra- and inter-delineator limits-of-agreement were −439.2 μm to 467.7 μm and −402.0 μm to 402.7 μm, respectively.

Median interclass correlation coefficients (ICC) for intra-delineator and inter-delineator FoBMO axis angle were 0.949 and 0.899 (Table 2). Median ICC for intra-delineator and inter-delineator FoBMO distance were 0.788 and 0.738.

## Eye-Specific neuroretinal rim gradient by FoBMO sectors (Figure 6)

Within these 222 high-risk ocular hypertensive and glaucoma eyes, median sectoral MRW gradient was largest in the $I_{temp}$ (−2.1 μm/°) and $T_{sup}$ (1.6 μm/°) sectors (Figure 2C). The absolute value of eye-specific, sectoral MRW and MRA gradients ranged from −6.8 to 5.3 μm/° and −2991 to 2811 μm²/° respectively. The inferior and temporal sectors (right half of Figure 6A and 6B) demonstrated larger gradients compared to the nasal and superior sectors (left half of Figures 6A and 6B) for both MRW and MRA.

## FoBMO vs. AIF 30° sectoral rim discordance (Figures 7 and 8)

The difference between the sectoral mean MRW (n = 222 eyes) calculated on the basis of FoBMO vs. AIF regionalization varied by sector (Figure 7, left) but were generally small, ranging from 0 to 13 μm (Supplemental Table S1) but achieved statistical significance in 7 of 12 sectors (Wilcoxon non-parametric test with Bonferroni correction, p<0.05). FoBMO vs. AIF differences in sectoral mean MRA values for each sector (Figure 8, right), were also small ranging from 268 to 7052 μm² (Supplemental Table S1) but achieved statistical significance in 6 of 12 segments (Wilcoxon

**Figure 4. Histograms of FoBMO axis angle (A) and distance (B).** FoBMO axis angle ranges from −17° to 7° (corresponding to "θ" in Figure 2A) while FoBMO distance ranges from 3.4 mm to 5.4 mm (corresponding to "d" in Figure 2B). The black lines are the Gaussian fits for the histograms. Shapiro-Wilk normality test finds p = 0.291 for FoBMO angle and p = 0.294, suggesting both histograms are normally distributed. The green circle represents the eye "DIS368" (Figures 1 and 2). The FoBMO Axis Angle data (panel A) appeared within a previous publication as part of a written communication (*Chauhan BC and Burgoyne CF (2013) From clinical examination of the optic disc to clinical assessment of the optic nerve head: a paradigm change. Am J Ophthalmol 156: 218-227 e212.*).

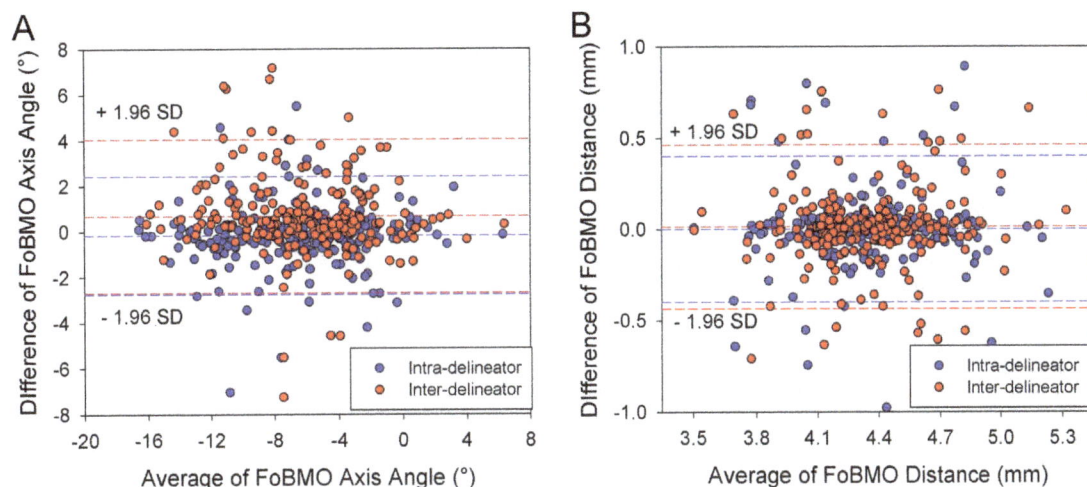

**Figure 5. Bland-Altman plots of intra-observer and inter-observer agreement for FoBMO axis angle (A) and FoBMO distance (B).** For FoBMO axis angle, intra-delineator limits of agreement (LOA) was −2.8° to 2.4° while inter-delineator LOA was −2.7° to 4.1°. For FoBMO distance, intra-delineator LOA was −439.2 μm to 467.7 μm while inter-delineator LOA was −402.0 μm to 402.7 μm.

signed-rank test with Bonferroni correction, p<0.05) (Figure 8B). Five sectors demonstrated significant FoBMO vs. AIF differences for both MRW and MRA sectoral means ($N_{inf}$, $I_{temp}$, $T_{inf}$, $T_{sup}$ and $S_{temp}$ sectors – Supplemental Table S1). FoBMO vs. AIF discordance in the sectoral means of both MRW and MRA occurred in the $I_{temp}$ sector (Figure 7).

While the differences in the overall mean sectoral values were small, eye-specific discordance was more substantial (Figure 8). Eye-specific sectoral discordance between FoBMO-based and AIF-based derivations of MRW exceeded ±20% in at least 1 sector in 24 eyes (10.8%), exceeded ±20% in at least 2 sectors in 11 eyes (4.9%) and exceeded ±20% in at least 3 sectors in 6 eyes (2.7%) (data not shown). Eye-specific discordance for MRA (Figure 8, lower) exceeded ±20% in at least 1 sector in 87 eyes (39.1%), in at least 2 sectors in 38 eyes (17.1%) and in at least 3 sectors in 27 eyes (12.2%) (data not shown). Qualitative inspection of sectoral, eye-specific discordance (Figure 9) suggests that most of the eyes exceeding ±20% difference were in the I, $I_{temp}$ and the $T_{inf}$ sectors, which are the same sectors that demonstrated the largest rim gradients.

### Factors affecting the magnitude of eye-specific FoBMO vs. AIF rim parameter discordance (Figure 9)

The results of GEE modeling to predict eye-specific FoBMO vs. AIF MRW discordance are shown in Table 3, and illustrated in Figure 9. Three models were tested: 1) FoBMO angle (θ) alone; 2) rim gradient ($MRW_{FoBMO}$') alone; and 3) their interaction (θ × $MRW_{FoBMO}$'). Figure 9E shows that the interaction term θ ×

$MRW_{FoBMO}$' best predicted FoBMO vs. AIF MRW discordance and yielded a slope coefficient close to unity, expressed as *0.94 × (θ × $MRW_{FoBMO}$')−1.08*. Using the same definitions, the best fit model for MRA discordance was *1.07 × (θ × $MRA_{FoBMO}$')−731* (Figure 9F). The coefficients and corresponding p-values for MRA discordance are also listed in Table 3. Taken together, these data suggest that sectoral FoBMO vs. AIF MRW and MRA discordance is highest in sectors with high rim gradients from eyes with large FoBMO angles.

After accounting for FoBMO angle and rim gradient (as outlined above) sectoral differences were found to independently contribute to AIF vs. FoBMO MRW and MRA discordance (MRW: $\chi^2 = 742$, p<0.001; MRA: $\chi^2 = 314$, p<0.001).

### Discussion

Ideally, a reference axis for regionalization of ONH and retinal structural measurements should be based on meaningful anatomical features that are also readily detectable by clinical imaging, stable over time and consistent between eyes. The reason to use the FoBMO axis to standardize ONH regionalization in all human eyes is to minimize the intra- and inter-individual variation caused by the combined effects of cyclotorsion and/or anatomic differences in the relationship between the ONH and fovea. When the head tilts, the AIF axis changes its position relative to the tissues of the ONH, RNFL and macula. The FoBMO angle changes, (because the AIF axis has changed), but the relation of the FoBMO axis relative to the fovea, RNFL and ONH remains constant. It is thus reasonable to predict that the confidence

**Table 2.** Intra- and inter-delineator agreement for FoBMO axis angle and distance.

| | | FoBMO Axis Angle | | FoBMO Distance | |
|---|---|---|---|---|---|
| | | Intra-delineator | Inter-delineator | Intra-delineator | Inter-delineator |
| ICC | Median | 0.949 | 0.899 | 0.788 | 0.738 |
| | 95% CI | 0.934–0.961 | 0.871–0.922 | 0.733–0.833 | 0.671–0.792 |
| P-value | Paired t-test | 0.060 | **<0.001** | 0.979 | 0.356 |

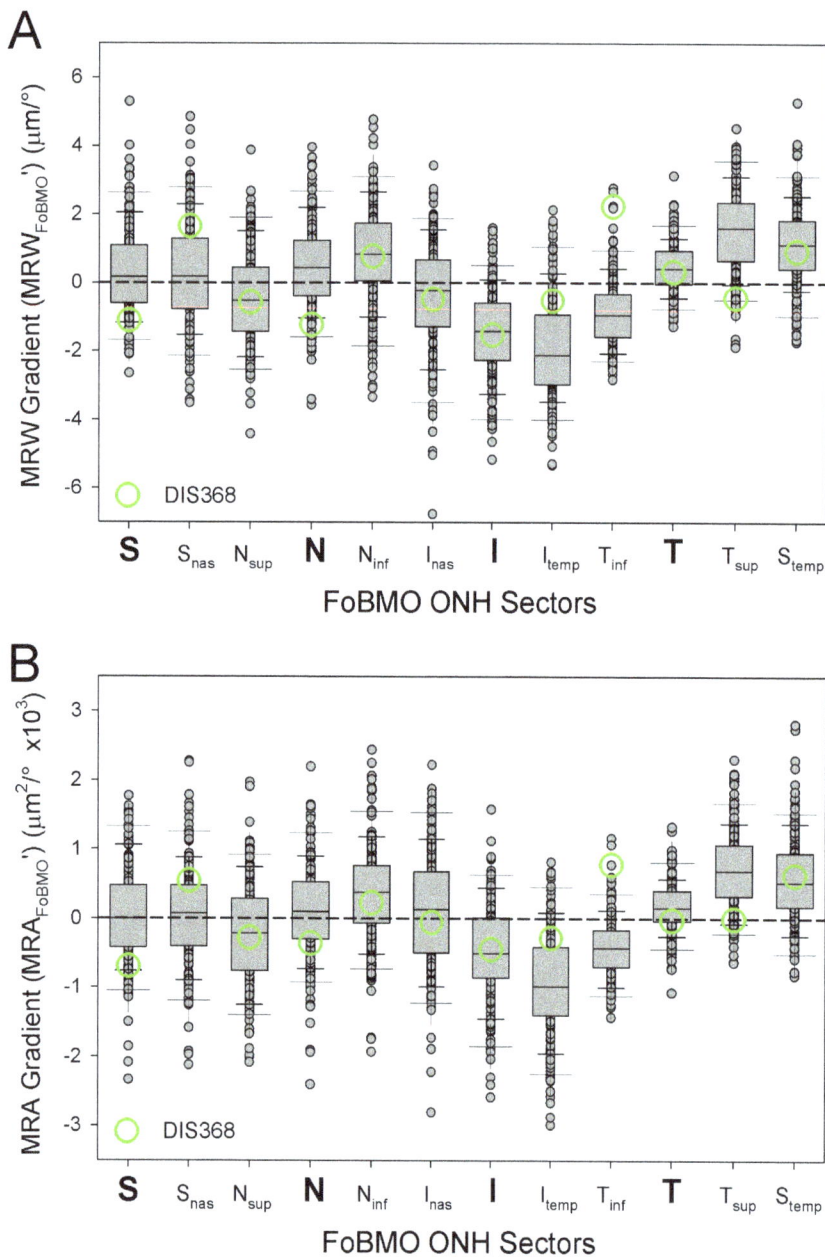

**Figure 6. SDOCT MRW (upper) and MRA (lower) gradient in actual values by FoBMO 30° sector for all 222 eyes.** Median sectoral MRW gradient was largest in the $I_{temp}$ ($-2.1$ $\mu m/°$) and $T_{sup}$ (1.6 $\mu m/°$) sectors. Median sectoral MRA gradient was also largest in the $I_{temp}$ ($-988$ $\mu m^2/°$) and $T_{sup}$ (689 $\mu m^2/°$) sectors.

intervals of reference databases that are regionalized relative to the FoBMO axis should tighten (improving diagnostic performance) and that structure/structure correlations in normal and glaucomatous eyes should be enhanced.

This study expands upon previous descriptions of the importance of the anatomic relationship between the position of the optic disc and fovea and the axis connecting the two [9,11,13,14,19]. Herein we report descriptive statistics of the FoBMO axis angle and distance within SDOCT images from a population of 222 eyes of 222 participants with high-risk ocular hypertension and glaucoma. To do so we retrospectively identified the fovea within the infrared image associated with SDOCT ONH datasets in which BMO had been hand-delineated. We then

characterized eye-specific ONH neuroretinal rim gradient within each eye. Finally, we quantified the magnitude of 30° sectoral discordance in FoBMO versus AIF regionalization of SDOCT MRW and MRA data, and sought predictive factors influencing their magnitude and location. The principal findings of these studies are as follows.

First, while the median FoBMO angle in these eyes was $-6.6°$, the range encompassed 24° (from $-17°$ to $+7°$) which is almost equivalent to one full 30° sector (i.e. one clock-hour). Second, the gradient of rim width (and subsequent derivation to rim area) varied by sector, being greatest in the inferior-temporal and temporal-superior sectors. Third, though the differences between FoBMO and AIF-based measurements of ONH rim tissue were

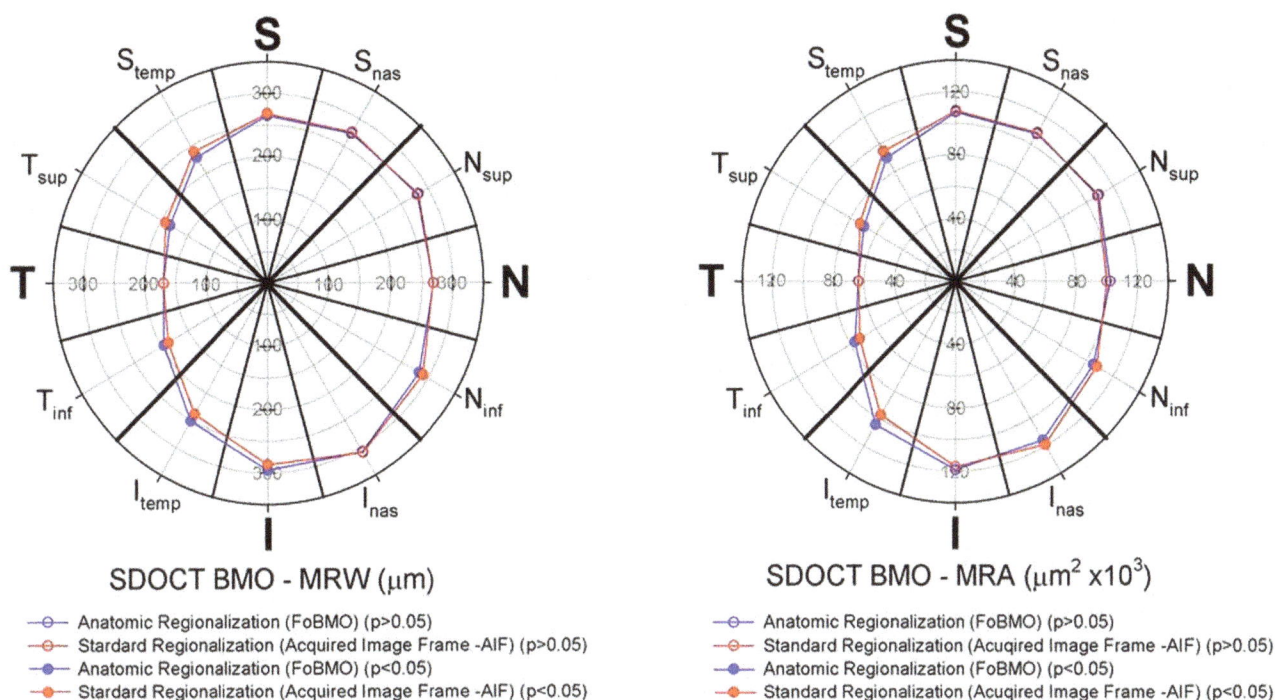

**Figure 7. Mean sectoral MRW (left) and MRA (right) for FoBMO regionalization (red) and AIF regionalization (blue) for all 222 study eyes.** Wilcoxon signed rank test with Bonferroni correction was applied to compare the two means in the twelve sectors. Sectors of which differences were statistically significant (p<0.05) were shown in solid symbols while sectors of which differences were not statistically significant (p>0.05) were shown in open symbols. These data suggest that when reported as the means of all 222 eyes, the sectoral discordance between AIF and FoBMO regionalization is statistically significant but small. (See Supplemental Table S1 for the sectoral mean values and p values).

generally small for the population averages in each of the 30° sectors, the variation in the magnitude of eye specific discordance among the 222 eyes was substantial with 10.8% of the eyes demonstrating a 20% difference in FoBMO vs. AIF MRW in at least one sector and 39.2% demonstrating a similar difference in MRA. Fourth, in general sectors from the inferior and superior quadrants demonstrated the highest FoBMO vs. AIF discordance. Fifth, a combination of FoBMO angle and rim gradient best predicted the sectors (and eyes) in which FoBMO vs. AIF rim discordance exceeded 20%.

The median value and range of FoBMO axis and distance that we report are similar to a series of previous studies which made a measurement of the ONH-foveal axis using techniques that were different than ours [9,11,13,14,19]. Initial studies of the angle and distance between the fovea and the center of the ONH have been based on the clinical disc margin within a clinical photograph [19,30,31], or SLO reflectance image [5,9,32]. Patel et al[14] used the SDOCT-determined neural canal opening [33–35] (previous terminology that is equivalent to BMO) and fovea to co-localize RNFLT measurements from two different SDOCT instruments. However in this study, the range of the FoBMO angle relative to the AIF was not a primary outcome and was not reported.

The FoBMO axis angle in the current study was retrospectively determined using BMO as delineated within SDOCT ONH radial B-scans and by clinical (2D) identification of the fovea within the corresponding IR CSLO image. Despite these methodological differences, the range of the FoBMO angle observed here among 222 eyes is similar to the range of the fovea-to-disc angle (relative to the AIF) within the current Heidelberg Spectralis RNFL normative database (mean −6°, range −15° to +3°) [36] as well as the range of an anatomically determined FoBMO angle (−17° to

+2°) within a new Heidelberg Spectralis ONH normative database that is based on 246 eyes of 246 normal Caucasian participants (personal communication from Dr. Gerhard Zinser, President of Heidelberg Engineering GmBH, Heidelberg, Germany).

Though the concept and clinical importance of focal and/or regional rim loss in glaucoma has been well known for many years, to our knowledge, eye-specific, sectoral SDOCT rim gradient has not previously been quantitatively characterized. In this study we defined 30°sectoral rim gradient to be the difference in rim width or rim area relative to its neighboring sectors. The purpose of eye-specific rim gradient quantification in this report was to assess its contribution to AIF vs. FoBMO rim discordance. The one-sided approach was chosen because it gave the best prediction of FoBMO vs. AIF discordance. While other strategies for rim gradient quantification such as a two-sided or absolute percent approach demonstrated prediction slopes that were far from unity, they may better discriminate early glaucoma. In the future, we will quantify the same parameter in a series of normative databases so as to assess its potential contribution to the detection of glaucomatous damage in eyes that either have early glaucomatous visual field loss or are clinically determined to be at risk for its development.

The fact that the discordance between sectoral ONH rim parameters derived using the FoBMO reference frame versus the AIF was substantial for individual eyes but not for the population average value has clinical importance. Prior studies have found that study population average values for ONH rim measurements made within stereophotos [32] or confocal scanning laser tomography (CSLT) [37] compare favorably with those made by SDOCT. However, eye-specific discordance revealed a substantial number of eyes in which differences were large, though the

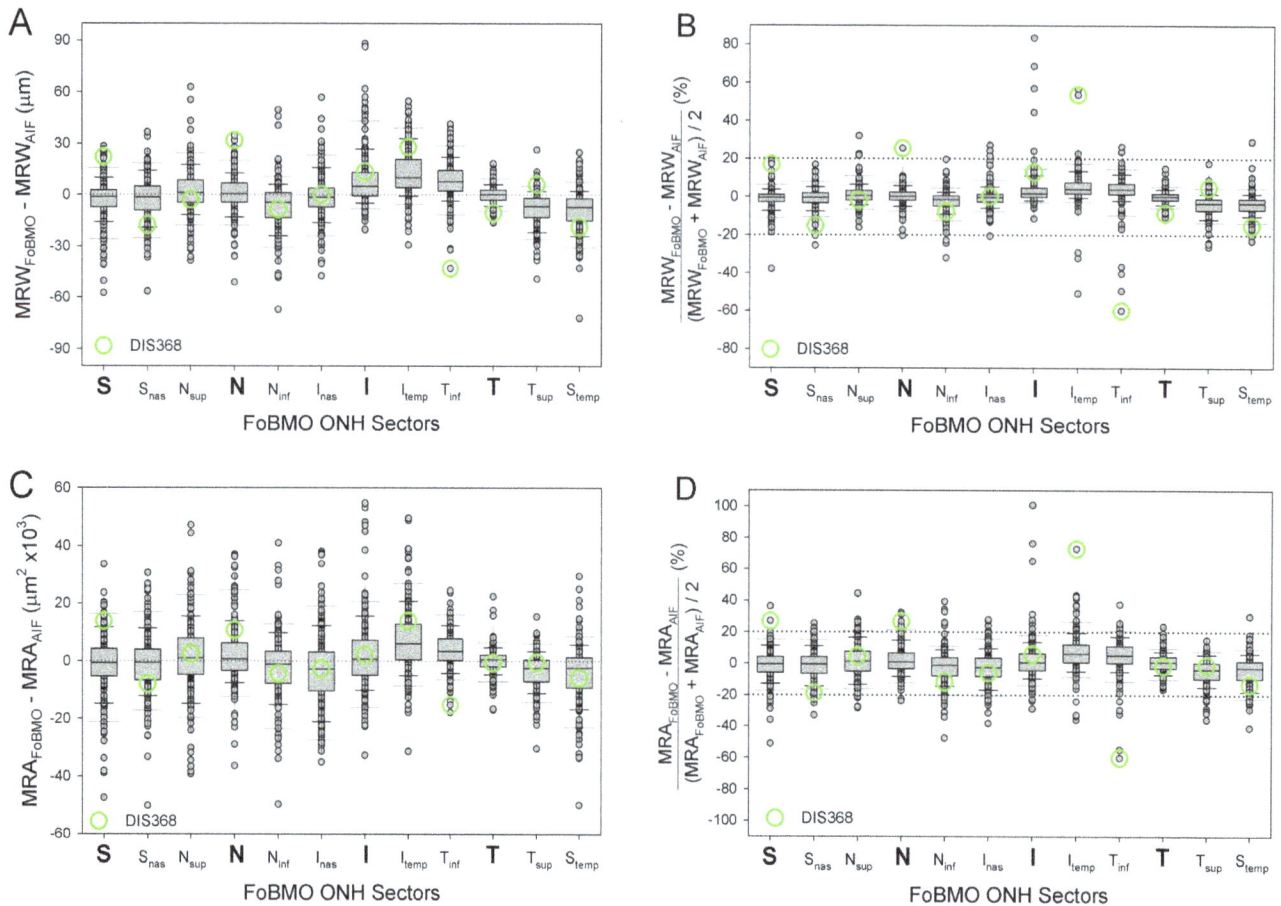

**Figure 8. Distribution of Eye-specific, AIF vs. FoBMO discordance for MRW (above) and MRA (below) by 30° sector in actual values (left) and percentage (right).** At each sector, the long whiskers correspond to the lowest 5% and upper 95% of the distribution while the short whiskers correspond to the lowest 10% and upper 90%, respectively. The bars with the separator in the middle correspond to lower quartiles (25%), upper quartiles (75%) and medians (50%). The percentage difference in most eyes for both MRW and MRA are within ±20% (horizontal dotted lines). However, in some eyes, the difference can be up to 80%. Eye DIS368, (green circles – and also seen in Figures 1 and 2), has three sectors with a difference of more than 20% for MRW and four for MRA. These data suggest that while the overall mean differences reported in Figure 7 can be small, eye-specific discordance within sectors for a subset of eyes is substantial.

magnitude and opposing polarity of these differences averaged close to zero. In our study, the small FoBMO vs. AIF differences for population average values similarly mask the important clinical finding that eye-specific differences can be substantial.

The fact that sectors from the inferior and superior quadrants demonstrated the highest FoBMO vs. AIF discordance (Figure 9) is important because numerous studies have shown that onset and progression of glaucomatous ONH damage most commonly occurs within these sectors [38]. Our study eyes represent a spectrum of glaucomatous damage that ranges from suspicious discs to moderate visual field loss. They also demonstrate the greatest rim gradients within these regions. Our rim gradient data may therefore be a reflection of the location of early to moderate glaucomatous rim change in these eyes. Future studies comparing these eyes to age and population matched normal databases will be necessary to understand the importance of this result.

Our study has the following limitations. SDOCT ONH datasets were not acquired relative to the FoBMO axis, nor was the location of the fovea anatomically determined using SDOCT. The logic for acquiring SDOCT datasets relative to the FoBMO axis has been the subject of a previous report [18]. While that capability has recently been accomplished as part of a separate,

SDOCT ONH, peripapillary retinal and macular normative database collection, (a collaborative manuscript is in preparation), it was not available in 2009 and 2010 when this study's SDOCT datasets were acquired. The importance of FoBMO acquisition of SDOCT ONH data remains to be determined and will be the subject of future reports.

We could not perform complete corrections for the transverse magnification of each individual eye in this study because axial length was not measured; only corneal curvatures were entered into the instrument's calculation of transverse magnification. While the FoBMO distance data reported here are thus not completely corrected for eye-specific transverse magnification, the FoBMO axis angle data should not be affected by differences in transverse magnification.

While BMO anatomy was manually delineated within the SDOCT ONH datasets, we did not have macular SDOCT datasets in these eyes from which to identify the fovea geometrically in 3D. Therefore, the fovea was retrospectively identified within the IR CSLO image acquired simultaneously with the SDOCT ONH B-scans. This was done first by a single clinician and the FoBMO axis for each eye was determined using this foveal location and the centroid of the 48 delineated BMO

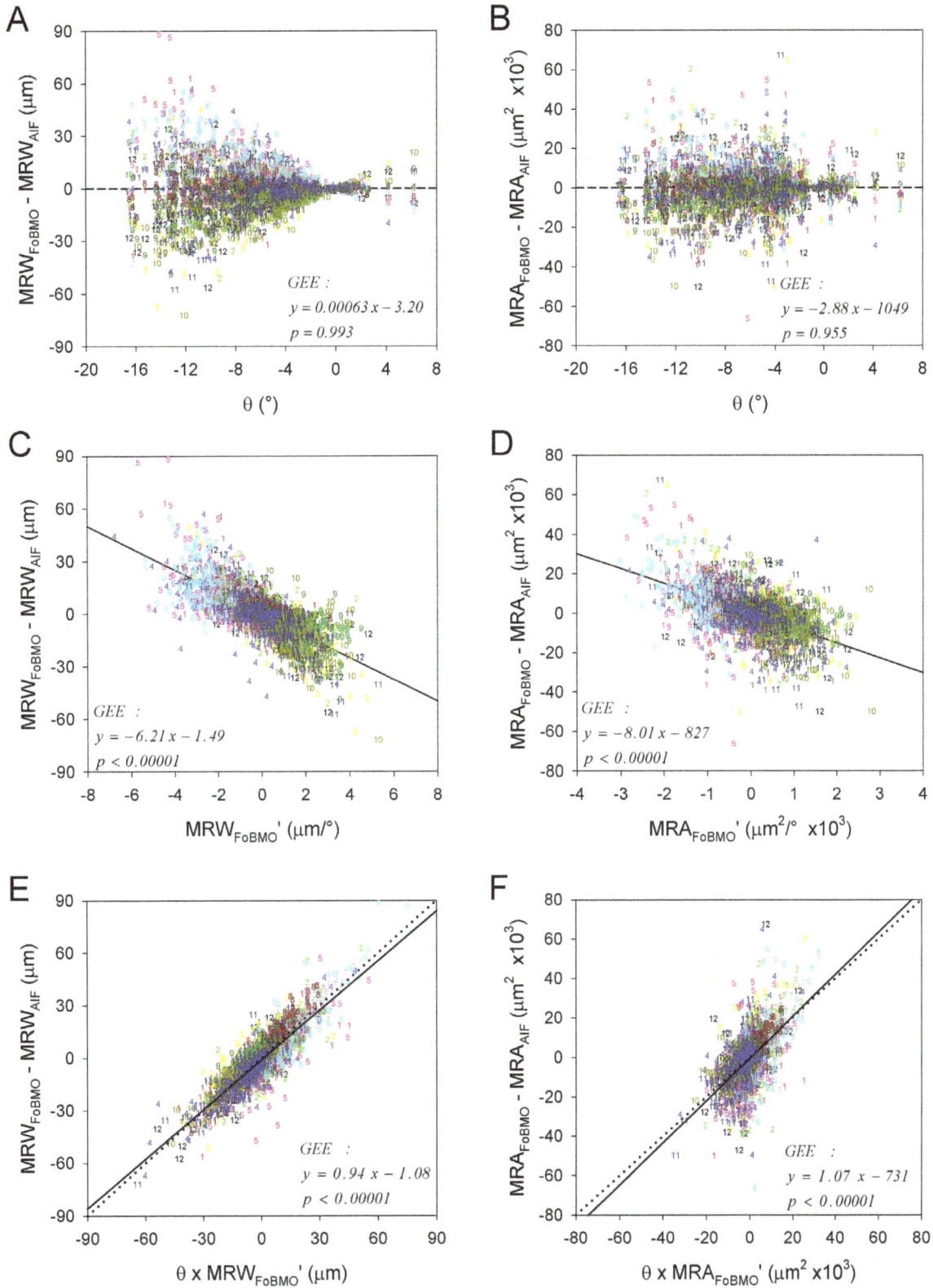

**Figure 9. Sectoral FoBMO vs. AIF discordance for MRW (left) and MRA (right) predicted by a univariate generalized estimating equation (GEE) model using FoBMO angle (A & B), one-sided rim gradient (C & D) (see methods) and the interaction of both (E & F).** The color coded numbers (1–12) correspond to the FoBMO 30° sectors of each study eye in right eye configuration (Figure 8A and B) expressed as clock-hours (12 - superior, 3 - nasal, 6 - inferior and 9 – temporal, see Figure 2). Eye-specific sectoral AIF vs. FoBMO discordance for both MRW and MRA is better predicted by a combination of FoBMO angle (θ) and one-sided sectoral rim gradient (E & F) than by either, alone. Qualitative inspection of these data suggests that sectors from the inferior and superior quadrants commonly demonstrate the highest sectoral AIF versus FoBMO discordance for both MRW and MRA.

**Table 3.** Generalized estimating equation (GEE) slope coefficients (b₁) and p-values for the prediction of sectoral AIF vs. FoBMO sectoral discordance using FoBMO angle and a one-sided definition of rim gradient (Figure 7).

| | $MRW_{FoBMO}$ - $MRW_{AIF}$ | | $MRA_{FoBMO}$ - $MRA_{AIF}$ | |
|---|---|---|---|---|
| | $b_1$ | $p$ | $b_1$ | $p$ |
| FoBMO angle ($\theta$) | −0.00063 | 0.993 | −2.88 | 0.955 |
| Rim Gradient ($MR_{FoBMO}'$) | −6.21 | <0.00001 | −8.01 | <0.00001 |
| $\theta \times MR_{FoBMO}'$ | 0.94 | <0.00001 | 1.07 | <0.00001 |

points. This foveal delineation was then repeated by the primary delineator 2 weeks later and by a secondary delineator to characterize the intra and inter-delineator reproducibility. While inter-delineator variation was significantly larger than intra-delineator variation, both the intra-delineator and inter-delineator ICCs were 0.899 or above suggesting that our retrospective approach to identifying the FoBMO axis was reliable.

Given the fact that the 95% CI of the FoBMO axis angle among the 222 eyes spanned nearly 17° and the FoBMO axis angle inter-delineator limits of agreement were −2.7° to 4.1°, FoBMO angle variation caused by foveal delineation may be up to one-third of that caused by actual variation in foveal-ONH anatomy. However, anatomic assignment of the BMO centroid, fovea and FoBMO axis, at the time of SDOCT image acquisition [6], will reduce this component of FoBMO variability in future studies.

AIF vs. FoBMO rim discordance will likely be less important using Garway-Heath ONH sectors [30] because they are larger, ranging from 40 to 110 degrees, and therefore less strongly influenced by focal rim gradient. We believe that FoBMO-based, Garway-Heath regional analysis will continue to be important. However, we also believe that by combining anatomic consistency (the use of the FoBMO axis as the Nasal-Temporal Axis) and eye tracking [39], 30° anatomic precision in regional rim characterization both within and between eyes is now technologically feasible. In correlating to the 12 clock-hours, 30° sectors are clinically intuitive and easy to visualize [18]. Their size allows for a "focal" rather than a "regional" rim gradient characterization. While reproducibility studies are necessary and underway, future studies to assess the performance of 30° and sub-30° FoBMO

regionalization in the discrimination of glaucoma, its progression and the enhancement of structure/structure and structure/function relations are also warranted.

In summary, we quantitatively characterized both the FoBMO axis and eye-specific ONH sectoral rim gradient in high risk ocular hypertensive and glaucomatous human eyes so as to characterize their effect on FoBMO versus AIF discordance in SDOCT rim assessment. We found that 10.8% (using SDOCT MRW) and 39.2% (using SDOCT MRA) of the 222 studied eyes demonstrated a 20% difference in AIF vs. FoBMO values in at least one 30° sector. We also found that this occurred most commonly in sectors from the inferior and superior quadrants and specifically within sectors with the greatest sectoral rim gradient and/or eyes with the greatest FoBMO angle. Studies to assess the effects of using FoBMO vs. AIF regionalization and sectoral rim gradient in the discrimination of glaucoma suspect, glaucoma and normal eyes are underway.

## Supporting Information

**Table S1   Mean and SD of sectoral MRW and MRA using FoBMO axis and AIF horizontal axis and their differences.** Wilcoxon signed-rank test with Bonferroni correction was applied to compare the means and sectoral calculated p-values are listed.

## Acknowledgments

The authors wish to thank Joanne Couchman for her assistance in preparing the manuscript. The authors also wish to thank Cindy Blachly and Michael Whitworth for collecting the Portland Progression Project SDOCT data.

Aspects of this paper were presented at the 2013 Annual Meeting of the Association for Research in Vision and Ophthalmology (ARVO) in Seattle, Washington. The FoBMO axis angle data in Figure 4 previously appeared in an invited editorial: *Chauhan BC, Burgoyne CF. From Clinical Examination of the Optic Disc to Clinical Assessment of the Optic Nerve Head: A Paradigm Change. Am J Ophthalmol 2013;156:218–227.*

## Author Contributions

Conceived and designed the experiments: LH RR HY SKG BF SD CFB. Performed the experiments: RR LR BF CH JR CFB. Analyzed the data: LH HY SKG BF SD CFB. Contributed reagents/materials/analysis tools: JR LH. Wrote the paper: LH RR HY CFB.

## References

1. Armaly MF (1967) Genetic determination of cup/disc ratio of the optic nerve. Arch Ophthalmol 78: 35–43.
2. Balazsi AG, Drance SM, Schulzer M, Douglas GR (1984) Neuroretinal rim area in suspected glaucoma and early chronic open- angle glaucoma. Correlation with parameters of visual function. Arch Ophthalmol 102: 1011–1014.
3. Caprioli J, Miller JM (1988) Correlation of structure and function in glaucoma. Quantitative measurements of disc and field. Ophthalmology 95: 723–727.
4. Reis AS, Sharpe GP, Yang H, Nicolela MT, Burgoyne CF, et al. (2012) Optic disc margin anatomy in patients with glaucoma and normal controls with spectral domain optical coherence tomography. Ophthalmology 119: 738–747.
5. Chen TC (2009) Spectral domain optical coherence tomography in glaucoma: qualitative and quantitative analysis of the optic nerve head and retinal nerve fiber layer (an AOS thesis). Trans Am Ophthalmol Soc 107: 254–281.
6. Povazay B, Hofer B, Hermann B, Unterhuber A, Morgan JE, et al. (2007) Minimum distance mapping using three-dimensional optical coherence tomography for glaucoma diagnosis. J Biomed Opt 12: 041204.
7. Strouthidis NG, Fortune B, Yang H, Sigal IA, Burgoyne CF (2011) Longitudinal change detected by spectral domain optical coherence tomography in the optic nerve head and peripapillary retina in experimental glaucoma. Invest Ophthalmol Vis Sci 52: 1206–1219.
8. Reis AS, O'Leary N, Yang H, Sharpe GP, Nicolela MT, et al. (2012) Influence of clinically invisible, but optical coherence tomography detected, optic disc

margin anatomy on neuroretinal rim evaluation. Invest Ophthalmol Vis Sci 53: 1852–1860.
9. Jansonius NM, Nevalainen J, Selig B, Zangwill LM, Sample PA, et al. (2009) A mathematical description of nerve fiber bundle trajectories and their variability in the human retina. Vision Res 49: 2157–2163.
10. Hood DC, Kardon RH (2007) A framework for comparing structural and functional measures of glaucomatous damage. Prog Retin Eye Res 26: 688–710.
11. Turpin A, Sampson GP, McKendrick AM (2009) Combining ganglion cell topology and data of patients with glaucoma to determine a structure-function map. Invest Ophthalmol Vis Sci 50: 3249–3256.
12. Harwerth RS, Wheat JL, Fredette MJ, Anderson DR (2010) Linking structure and function in glaucoma. Prog Retin Eye Res 29: 249–271.
13. Jonas JB, Nguyen NX, Naumann GO (1989) The retinal nerve fiber layer in normal eyes. Ophthalmology 96: 627–632.
14. Patel NB, Wheat JL, Rodriguez A, Tran V, Harwerth RS (2012) Agreement between retinal nerve fiber layer measures from Spectralis and Cirrus spectral domain OCT. Optom Vis Sci 89: E652–666.
15. Chauhan BC, O'Leary N, Almobarak FA, Reis AS, Yang H, et al. (2013) Enhanced detection of open-angle glaucoma with an anatomically accurate optical coherence tomography-derived neuroretinal rim parameter. Ophthalmology 120: 535–543.

16. Gardiner SK, Ren R, Yang H, Fortune B, Burgoyne CF, et al. (2013) A Method to Estimate the Amount of Neuroretinal Rim Tissue in Glaucoma: Comparison With Current Methods for Measuring Rim Area. Am J Ophthalmol Accepted for Publication.

17. He L, Yang H, Gardiner SK, Williams G, Hardin C, et al. (2014) Longitudinal detection of optic nerve head changes by spectral domain optical coherence tomography in early experimental glaucoma. Invest Ophthalmol Vis Sci 55: 574–586.

18. Chauhan BC, Burgoyne CF (2013) From clinical examination of the optic disc to clinical assessment of the optic nerve head: a paradigm change. Am J Ophthalmol 156: 218–227 e212.

19. Hood DC, Raza AS, de Moraes CG, Liebmann JM, Ritch R (2013) Glaucomatous damage of the macula. Prog Retin Eye Res 32: 1–21.

20. Airaksinen PJ, Tuulonen A, Werner EB (1996) Clinical evaluation of the optic disc and retinal nerve fiber layer. In: R. . Ritch, M. B. . Shields and T. . krupin, editors. The Glaucomas. St. Louis: Mosby. pp. 617–657.

21. Harizman N, Oliveira C, Chiang A, Tello C, Marmor M, et al. (2006) The ISNT rule and differentiation of normal from glaucomatous eyes. Arch Ophthalmol 124: 1579–1583.

22. Essock EA, Sinai MJ, Bowd C, Zangwill LM, Weinreb RN (2003) Fourier analysis of optical coherence tomography and scanning laser polarimetry retinal nerve fiber layer measurements in the diagnosis of glaucoma. Arch Ophthalmol 121: 1238–1245.

23. Medeiros FA, Susanna R Jr (2003) Comparison of algorithms for detection of localised nerve fibre layer defects using scanning laser polarimetry. Br J Ophthalmol 87: 413–419.

24. Wyatt HJ, Dul MW, Swanson WH (2007) Variability of visual field measurements is correlated with the gradient of visual sensitivity. Vision Res 47: 925–936.

25. Gardiner SK, Johnson CA, Demirel S (2012) Factors Predicting the Rate of Functional Progression in Early and Suspected Glaucoma. Invest Ophthalmol Vis Sci 53: 3598–3604.

26. Gardiner SK, Johnson CA, Cioffi GA (2005) Evaluation of the structure-function relationship in glaucoma. Invest Ophthalmol Vis Sci 46: 3712–3717.

27. Spry PG, Johnson CA, Mansberger SL, Cioffi GA (2005) Psychophysical investigation of ganglion cell loss in early glaucoma. J Glaucoma 14: 11–19.

28. Yang H, Qi J, Hardin C, Gardiner SK, Strouthidis NG, et al. (2012) Spectral-domain optical coherence tomography enhanced depth imaging of the normal and glaucomatous nonhuman primate optic nerve head. Invest Ophthalmol Vis Sci 53: 394–405.

29. Bland JM, Altman DG (1986) Statistical methods for assessing agreement between two methods of clinical measurement. Lancet 1: 307–310.

30. Garway-Heath DF, Poinoosawmy D, Fitzke FW, Hitchings RA (2000) Mapping the visual field to the optic disc in normal tension glaucoma eyes. Ophthalmology 107: 1809–1815.

31. Schiefer U, Flad M, Stumpp F, Malsam A, Paetzold J, et al. (2003) Increased detection rate of glaucomatous visual field damage with locally condensed grids: a comparison between fundus-oriented perimetry and conventional visual field examination. Arch Ophthalmol 121: 458–465.

32. Sharma A, Oakley JD, Schiffman JC, Budenz DL, Anderson DR (2011) Comparison of Automated Analysis of Cirrus HD OCT Spectral-Domain Optical Coherence Tomography with Stereo Photographs of the Optic Disc. Ophthalmology 118: 1348–1357.

33. Strouthidis NG, Grimm J, Williams GA, Cull GA, Wilson DJ, et al. (2010) A comparison of optic nerve head morphology viewed by spectral domain optical coherence tomography and by serial histology. Invest Ophthalmol Vis Sci 51: 1464–1474.

34. Hu Z, Abramoff MD, Kwon YH, Lee K, Garvin MK (2010) Automated segmentation of neural canal opening and optic cup in 3D spectral optical coherence tomography volumes of the optic nerve head. Invest Ophthalmol Vis Sci 51: 5708–5717.

35. Downs JC, Yang H, Girkin C, Sakata L, Bellezza A, et al. (2007) Three-dimensional histomorphometry of the normal and early glaucomatous monkey optic nerve head: neural canal and subarachnoid space architecture. Invest Ophthalmol Vis Sci 48: 3195–3208.

36. Valverde-Megias A, Martinez-de-la-Casa JM, Serrador-Garcia M, Larrosa JM, Garcia-Feijoo J (2013) Clinical Relevance of Foveal Location on Retinal Nerve Fiber Layer Thickness Using the New FoDi Software in Spectralis Optical Coherence Tomography. Invest Ophthalmol Vis Sci 54: 5771–5776.

37. Moghimi S, Hosseini H, Riddle J, Lee GY, Bitrian E, et al. (2012) Measurement of Optic Disc Size and Rim Area with Spectral-Domain OCT and Scanning Laser Ophthalmoscopy. Invest Ophthalmol Vis Sci.

38. Hood DC, Wang DL, Raza AS, de Moraes CG, Liebmann JM, et al. (2013) The Locations of Circumpapillary Glaucomatous Defects Seen on Frequency-Domain OCT Scans. Invest Ophthalmol Vis Sci 54: 7338–7343.

39. Helb HM, Charbel Issa P, Fleckenstein M, Schmitz-Valckenberg S, Scholl HP, et al. (2010) Clinical evaluation of simultaneous confocal scanning laser ophthalmoscopy imaging combined with high-resolution, spectral-domain optical coherence tomography. Acta Ophthalmol 88: 842–849.

# Permissions

# List of Contributors

**Keiko Fujikawa**
Department of Pathology and Immunology, Hokkaido University Graduate School of Medicine, Sapporo, Japan
Faculty of Health Science, Hokkaido University, Sapporo, Japan
Department of Ophthalmology and Visual Sciences, Washington University School of Medicine, St. Louis, Missouri, United States of America

**Hanako Kadotani**
Department of Pathology and Immunology, Hokkaido University Graduate School of Medicine, Sapporo, Japan

**Takeshi Iwata and Masakazu Akahori**
National Institute of Sensory Organs, National Hospital Organization Tokyo Medical Center, Tokyo, Japan

**Kaoru Inoue**
Faculty of Health Science, Hokkaido University, Sapporo, Japan

**Masahiro Fukaya and Masahiko Watanabe**
Department of Anatomy, Hokkaido University Graduate School of Medicine, Sapporo, Japan

**Qing Chang and Edward M. Barnett**
Department of Ophthalmology and Visual Sciences, Washington University School of Medicine, St. Louis, Missouri, United States of America

**Wojciech Swat**
Department of Pathology and Immunology, Washington University School of Medicine, St. Louis, Missouri, United States of America

**Yibo Yu and Ke Yao**
Eye Center of the 2nd Affiliated Hospital, Zhejiang University School of Medicine, Hangzhou, China

**Yu Weng**
Department of Clinical Laboratory, Sir Run Run Shaw Hospital, Zhejiang University School of Medicine, Hangzhou, China

**Jing Guo and Guangdi Chen**
Department of Public Health, Zhejiang University School of Medicine, Hangzhou, China

**Alexandre Denoyer, José A. Sahel and Christophe Baudouin**
UPMC University Paris 6, Institut de la Vision, UMRS968, Paris, France
INSERM, U968, Paris, France
CNRS, U7210, Paris, France
Quinze-Vingts National Ophthalmology Hospital, Paris, France

**David Godefroy, Julie Frugier, Julie Degardin, Serge Picaud and William Rostène**
UPMC University Paris 6, Institut de la Vision, UMRS968, Paris, France
INSERM, U968, Paris, France
CNRS, U7210, Paris, France
Isabelle Célérier Team 1, Centre de Recherche des Cordeliers, INSERM, U872, Paris, France

**Jeffrey K. Harrison**
Department of Pharmacology & Therapeutics, College of Medicine, University of Florida, Gainesville, Florida, United States of America

**Francoise Brignole-Baudouin**
UPMC University Paris 6, Institut de la Vision, UMRS968, Paris, France
INSERM, U968, Paris, France
CNRS, U7210, Paris, France
Department of Toxicology, Faculty of Biological and Pharmacological Sciences, University René Descartes Paris 05, Paris, France

**Francoise Baleux**
Unité de chimie des biomolécules, Institut Pasteur, CNRS 2128, Paris, France

**Suddhasil Mookherjee, Moulinath Acharya, Deblina Banerjee, Ashima Bhattacharjee and Kunal Ray**
Molecular & Human Genetics Division, CSIR-Indian Institute of Chemical Biology, Kolkata, India

**Verena Prokosch and Maurice Schallenberg**
Institute of Experimental Ophthalmology, School of Medicine, University of Münster, Albert-Schweitzer-Campus 1, Münster, Germany

**Solon Thanos**
Institute of Experimental Ophthalmology, School of Medicine, University of Münster, Albert-Schweitzer-Campus 1, Münster, Germany
Interdisciplinary Center for Clinical Research, Albert-Schweitzer-Campus 1, Münster, Germany

**Alberto Izzotti, Mariagrazia Longobardi and Cristina Cartiglia**
Department of Health Sciences, Faculty of Medicine, University of Genoa, Genoa, Italy

**Federico Rathschuler and Sergio Claudio Saccà**
Ophthalmology Unit, Department of Head/Neck Pathologies, St. Martino Hospital, Genoa, Italy

**Ellen E. Freeman and Mark R. Lesk**
Maisonneuve-Rosemont Hospital Research Center, Montreal, Quebec, Canada
Department of Ophthalmology, University of Montreal, Montreal, Quebec, Canada

**Marie-Hélène Roy-Gagnon**
CHU Sainte-Justine Research Center, University of Montreal, Montreal, Quebec, Canada
Department of Social and Preventive Medicine, University of Montreal, Montreal, Quebec, Canada

**Denise Descovich**
Maisonneuve-Rosemont Hospital Research Center, Montreal, Quebec, Canada
Hugues Massé CHU Sainte-Justine Research Center, University of Montreal, Montreal, Quebec, Canada

**Janey L. Wiggs, Bao Jian Fan, Dan Yi Wang, Dayse R. Figueiredo Sena and Louis R. Pasquale**
Department of Ophthalmology, Harvard Medical School, Massachusetts Eye and Ear Infirmary, Boston, Massachusetts, United States of America

**Alex W. Hewitt**
Centre for Eye Research Australia, University of Melbourne, Royal Victorian Eye and Ear Hospital, Melbourne, Australia

**Colm O'Brien**
School of Medicine and Medical Science, University College of Dublin, Dublin, Ireland

**Anthony Realini**
Department of Ophthalmology, West Virginia University School of Medicine, Morgantown, West Virginia, United States of America

**Jamie E. Craig and David P. Dimasi**
Department of Ophthalmology, Flinders University, Flinders Medical Centre, Adelaide, Australia

**David A. Mackey**
Centre for Ophthalmology and Visual Science, University of Western Australia, Lions Eye Institute, Perth, Australia

**Jonathan L. Haines**
Center for Human Genetics Research, Vanderbilt University School of Medicine, Nashville, Tennessee, United States of America

**Hiroshi Murata, Hiroyo Hirasawa, Yuka Aoyama, Chihiro Mayama and Ryo Asaoka**
Department of Ophthalmology, University of Tokyo Graduate School of Medicine, Tokyo, Japan

**Kenji Sugisaki**
Department of Ophthalmology, University of Tokyo Graduate School of Medicine, Tokyo, Japan
Tokyo Koseinenkin Hospital, Tokyo, Japan

**Makoto Araie**
Department of Ophthalmology, University of Tokyo Graduate School of Medicine, Tokyo, Japan
Kanto Central Hospital, The Mutual Aid Association of Public School Teachers, Tokyo, Japan

**Makoto Aihara**
Department of Ophthalmology, University of Tokyo Graduate School of Medicine, Tokyo, Japan
Shirato Eye Clinic, Tokyo, Japan

**Francisco G. Junoy Montolio and Christiaan Wesselink**
Dept. of Ophthalmology, University Medical Center Groningen, University of Groningen, Groningen, The Netherlands

**Nomdo M. Jansonius**
Dept. of Ophthalmology, University Medical Center Groningen, University of Groningen, Groningen, The Netherlands
Dept. of Epidemiology, Erasmus Medical Center, Rotterdam, The Netherlands

**Meredith S. Gregory, Caroline G. Hackett, Emma F. Abernathy, Alexander Jones, Paraskevi Kolovou, Dong Feng Chen and Bruce R. Ksander**
The Schepens Eye Research Institute, Department of Ophthalmology, Harvard Medical School, Boston, Massachusetts, United States of America

**Karen S. Lee and Andreas M. Hohlbaum**
Department of Microbiology, Boston University School of Medicine, Boston, Massachusetts, United States of America

**Maura W. Hobson**
The Schepens Eye Research Institute, Department of Ophthalmology, Harvard Medical School, Boston, Massachusetts, United States of America
Department of Microbiology, Boston University School of Medicine, Boston, Massachusetts, United States of America

**Rebecca R. Saff**
Department of Medicine, Harvard Medical School, Boston, Massachusetts, United States of America

**Ann Marshak-Rothstein**
Department of Medicine, University of Massachusetts Medical School, Worcester, Massachusetts, United States of America

**Krishna-sulayman L. Moody**
Department of Microbiology, Boston University School of Medicine, Boston, Massachusetts, United States of America
Department of Medicine, University of Massachusetts Medical School, Worcester, Massachusetts, United States of America

**Saoussen Karray**
Institut National de la Sante et de la Recherche Medicale (INSERM) Unite 580, Hopital Necker, Paris, France

**Andrea Giani**
Massachusetts Eye and Ear Infirmary, Department of Ophthalmology, Harvard Medical School, Boston, Massachusetts, United States of America

**Simon W. M. John**
Howard Hughes Medical Institute, Jackson Laboratory, Bar Harbor, Maine, United States of America

**Christopher Bowd, Robert N. Weinreb, Madhusudhanan Balasubramanian, Intae Lee, Siamak Yousefi, Linda M. Zangwill, Felipe A. Medeiros and Michael H. Goldbaum**
Hamilton Glaucoma Center, Department of Ophthalmology, University of California, San Diego, La Jolla, California, United States of America

**Giljin Jang**
Hamilton Glaucoma Center, Department of Ophthalmology, University of California, San Diego, La Jolla, California, United States of America
School of Electrical and Computer Engineering, Ulsan National Institute of Science and Technology, Ulsan, South Korea

**Christopher A. Girkin**
Department of Ophthalmology, University of Alabama at Birmingham, Birmingham, Alabama, United States of America

**Jeffrey M. Liebmann**
Department of Ophthalmology, New York University School of Medicine, New York, New York, United States of America
New York Eye and Ear Infirmary, New York, New York, United States of America

**Alena Z. Minton, Nitasha R. Phatak, Dorota L. Stankowska, Shaoqing He, Colby Brownlee and Raghu R. Krishnamoorthy**
Department of Cell Biology and Anatomy, University of North Texas Health Science Center, Fort Worth, Texas, United States of America

**Hai-Ying Ma, Brett H. Mueller, Ming Jiang, Robert Luedtke and Shaohua Yang**
Department of Pharmacology and Neuroscience, University of North Texas Health Science Center, Fort Worth, Texas, United States of America

**K. David Kennedy, S. A. Anitha Christy, LaKisha K. Buie and Teresa Borrás**
Department of Ophthalmology, University of North Carolina School of Medicine, Chapel Hill, North Carolina, United States of America

**Françoise Brignole-Baudouin**
INSERM, U968, Paris, France
UPMC Univ Paris 06, UMR_S 968, Institut de la Vision, Paris, France
CNRS, UMR_7210, Paris, France
Centre Hospitalier National d'Ophtalmologie des Quinze-Vingts, INSERM-DHOS CIC 503, Paris, France
Chimie Toxicologie Analytique et Cellulaire, EA 4463, Faculté des Sciences Pharmaceutiques et Biologiques, Université Paris Descartes, Paris, France

**Nicolas Desbenoit**
INSERM, U968, Paris, France
UPMC Univ Paris 06, UMR_S 968, Institut de la Vision, Paris, France
CNRS, UMR_7210, Paris, France
Centre de recherche de Gif, Institut de Chimie des Substances Naturelles, CNRS, Gif-sur-Yvette, France

**Hong Liang**
INSERM, U968, Paris, France
UPMC Univ Paris 06, UMR_S 968, Institut de la Vision, Paris, France
CNRS, UMR_7210, Paris, France
Centre Hospitalier National d'Ophtalmologie des Quinze-Vingts, INSERM-DHOS CIC 503, Paris, France

**Alain Brunelle, Vincent Guerineau and David Touboul**
Centre de recherche de Gif, Institut de Chimie des Substances Naturelles, CNRS, Gif-sur-Yvette, France

**Jean-Pierre Both**
Laboratoire d'Intégration des Systèmes et des Technologies, CEA-LIST, Gif-sur-Yvette, France

**Isabelle Fournier, Maxence Wisztorski and Michel Salzet**
Laboratoire de Spectromé trie de Masse Biologique, Fondamentale et Appliquée, EA 4550, Universite´ Lille Nord de France – Université Lille 1, Villeneuve d'Ascq, France

**Gregory Hamm, Raphael Legouffe and Jonathan Stauber**
Imabiotech Campus Cité Scientifique, Villeneuve d'Ascq, France

**Olivier Laprevote**
Chimie Toxicologie Analytique et Cellulaire, EA 4463, Faculté des Sciences Pharmaceutiques et Biologiques, Université Paris Descartes, Paris, France

**Christophe Baudouin**
INSERM, U968, Paris, France
UPMC Univ Paris 06, UMR_S 968, Institut de la Vision, Paris, France
CNRS, UMR_7210, Paris, France
Centre Hospitalier National d'Ophtalmologie des Quinze-Vingts, INSERM-DHOS CIC 503, Paris, France
Université Versailles Saint-Quentin-en-Yvelines, Versailles, France
Assistance Publique - Hôpitaux de Paris Hôpital Ambroise Paré, Service d'Ophtalmologie, Boulogne-Billancourt, France

**Jen-Hao Cheng**
Department of Ophthalmology, Tri-Service General Hospital, National Defense Medical Center, Taipei, Taiwan

**Ming-Cheng Tai, Yi-Hao Chen, Chang-Min Liang, Jiann-Torng Chen, Ching-Long Chen and Da-Wen Lu**
Department of Ophthalmology, Tri-Service General Hospital, National Defense Medical Center, Taipei, Taiwan
Graduate Institute of Medical Science, National Defense Medical Center, Taipei, Taiwan

**Yinwei Song, Junming Wang, Zhiqi Chen, Xiaoqin Yan and Hong Zhang**
Department of Ophthalmology, Tongji Hospital, Tongji Medical College, Huazhong University of Science and Technology, Wuhan, China

**Ketao Mu, Yonghong Hao and Wenzhen Zhu**
Department of Radiology, Tongji Hospital, Tongji Medical College, Huazhong University of Science and Technology, Wuhan, China

**Fuchun Lin**
Wuhan Center for Magnetic Resonance, State Key Laboratory of Magnetic Resonance and Atomic and Molecular Physics, Wuhan Institute of Physics and Mathematics, Chinese Academy of Sciences, Wuhan, China

**Ya Xing Wang, Liang Xu, Lei Shao, Ya Qin Zhang, Hua Yang and Jin Da Wang**
Beijing Institute of Ophthalmology, Beijing Tongren Hospital, Capital Medical University, Beijing, China

**Jost B. Jonas**
Beijing Institute of Ophthalmology, Beijing Tongren Hospital, Capital Medical University, Beijing, China
Department of Ophthalmology, Medical Faculty Mannheim of the Ruprecht-Karls-University, Heidelberg, Germany

**Wen Bin Wei**
Beijing Tongren Eye Center, Beijing Tongren Hospital, Capital Medical University, Beijing, China

**Jin-Wei Cheng and Rui-Li Wei**
Department of Ophthalmology, Shanghai Changzheng Hospital, Second Military Medical University, Shanghai, China

**Ying Zong**
Department of Health Toxicology, Second Military Medical University, Shanghai, China

**You-Yan Zeng**
School of Nursing, Second Military Medical University, Shanghai, China

**Humaira Ayub, Shaheena Bashir and Sobia Shafique**
Department of Biosciences, COMSATS Institute of Information Technology, Islamabad, Pakistan

**Shazia Micheal and Frederieke E. Schoenmaker-Koller**
Department of Ophthalmology, Radboud University Nijmegen Medical Centre, Nijmegen, The Netherlands

**Farah Akhtar Mahmood Ali and Muhammad Imran Khan**
Al-Shifa Trust Eye Hospital, Rawalpindi, Pakistan

**Nadia K. Waheed**
Department of Ophthalmology, Tufts University School of Medicine, Boston, Massachusetts, United States of America

**Raheel Qamar**
Department of Biosciences, COMSATS Institute of Information Technology, Islamabad, Pakistan
Al-Nafees Medical College & Hospital, Isra University, Islamabad, Pakistan

**Anneke I. den Hollander**
Department of Ophthalmology, Radboud University Nijmegen Medical Centre, Nijmegen, The Netherlands
Department of Human Genetics, Radboud University Nijmegen Medical Centre Nijmegen, The Netherlands

**Katrin Sippel, Enkelejda Kasneci and Wolfgang Rosenstiel**
Computer Engineering Department, University of Tübingen, Tübingen, Germany

**Kathrin Aehling and Martin Heister**
Centre for Ophthalmology, Institute for Ophthalmic Research, University of Tübingen, Tübingen, Germany

**Ulrich Schiefer**
Centre for Ophthalmology, Institute for Ophthalmic Research, University of Tübingen, Tübingen, Germany
Competence Centre "Vision Research", Study Course "Ophthalmic Optics/Audiology", University of Applied Sciences Aalen, Aalen, Germany

**Elena Papageorgiou**
Centre for Ophthalmology, Institute for Ophthalmic Research, University of Tübingen, Tübingen, Germany
Department of Ophthalmology, University of Leicester, Leicester Royal Infirmary, Leicester, United Kingdom

**Lin He, Ruojin Ren, Christy Hardin and Luke Reyes**
Optic Nerve Head Research Laboratory, Legacy Health, Portland, Oregon, United States of America

**Stuart K. Gardiner, Brad Fortune and Shaban Demirel**
Discoveries in Sight Research Laboratories of the Devers Eye Institute, Legacy Health, Portland, Oregon, United States of America

**Hongli Yang, Juan Reynaud and Claude F. Burgoyne**
Optic Nerve Head Research Laboratory, Legacy Health, Portland, Oregon, United States of America
Discoveries in Sight Research Laboratories of the Devers Eye Institute, Legacy Health, Portland, Oregon, United States of America

# Index

www.ingramcontent.com/pod-product-compliance
Lightning Source LLC
Chambersburg PA
CBHW080626200326
41458CB00013B/4525